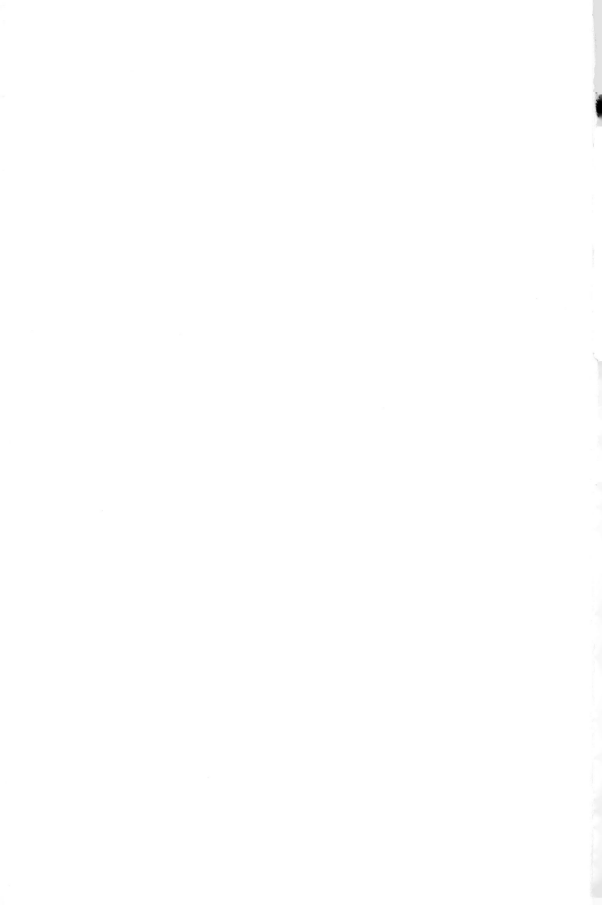

Hans Flaatten | Rui P. Moreno
Christian Putensen | Andrew Rhodes
(Eds.)

Organisation and Management
of Intensive Care

Medizinisch Wissenschaftliche Verlagsgesellschaft

Hans Flaatten | Rui P. Moreno
Christian Putensen | Andrew Rhodes
(Eds.)

Organisation and Management of Intensive Care

with contributions from:

MG Abate | S Afonso de Carvalho | A Aneman | DC Angus | A Artigas | DJ Baker | J Ball
O Barbosa da Silva | DM Baron | P Bauer | A Beishuizen | P Biban | SI Blot | G Brattebø
M Cecconi | J Chen | MD Christian | G Citerio | K Colpaert | J Creteur | WE Dager | J Decruyenaere
D Dewald | JR Dichter | AC Diogo | Y Donchin | S Dray | R Endacott | P Ferdinande | R Ferrer
H Flaatten | ARJ Girbes | CD Gomersall | U Guenther | B Guidet | AP Gurses | M Haisjackl
M Hamilton | C de Haro | GT Henriques-Filho | M Hiesmayr | K Hillman | J Jacobi | M Jonas
GM Joynt | L-P Kamolz | L Keating | MM Kennedy | K Klöcker | E Knobel | M Knobel | SO Labeau
B Lawless | M Makdisse | ML Martinez | PGH Metnitz | RP Moreno | CW Mutz | A Navas
Y-L Nguyen | M Palomar Martínez | R Pearse | PJ Pronovost | C Putensen | IJ Rechner | J Rello
A Rhodes | JL da Rocha Paranhos | HU Rothen | S Rubertsson | J Scholes | R Shulman
B Singer | A Soury-Lavergne | L Spagnesi | S Streat | N Theuerkauf | J Trpkovski | DA Vagts
A Valentin | J-L Vincent | C Waldmann | J Wernerman | M Wittmann | H Wunsch | JG Zijlstra

Medizinisch Wissenschaftliche Verlagsgesellschaft

Editors

Hans Flaatten, MD, PhD
Department of Anaesthesia and Intensive Care
Haukeland University Hospital
Jonas Liesvei 65
5021 Bergen, Norway

Rui P. Moreno, MD, PhD
Unidade de Cuidados Intensivos Polivalente
Hospital de Santo António dos Capuchos
Centro Hospitalar de Lisboa Central E.P.E.
Alameda de Santo António dos Capuchos
1169-050 Lisboa, Portugal

Christian Putensen, Prof., MD
Universitätsklinikum Bonn
Klinik und Poliklinik für Anästhesiologie und Operative
Intensivmedizin
Sigmund-Freud-Str. 35
53105 Bonn, Germany

Andrew Rhodes, FRCA FRCP
Department of Intensive Care Medicine
St George's Hospital
Blackshaw Road
London SW17 0QT, UK

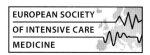

European Society of Intensive Care Medicine
19, rue Belliard
1040 Brussels, Belgium
Tel: 0032 2 559 03 50 – Fax: 0032 2 559 03 79
E-mail: public@esicm.org
www.esicm.org

MWV Medizinisch Wissenschaftliche Verlagsgesellschaft mbH & Co. KG
Zimmerstraße 11
D- 10969 Berlin
www.mwv-berlin.de

ISBN 978-3-941468-27-6

These publications are listed in: Deutsche Nationalbibliothek
Detailed bibliographical information is available via internet http://dnb.d-nb.de.

Any necessary errata are published at the publisher's website www.mwv-berlin.de.

Project management: Claudia Leonhardt, Berlin
Editorial office: Frauke Budig, Monika Laut-Zimmermann, Berlin
Copy editing: Dr. Michael Kastner, acaman.de, Berlin | Jan K. Schwing, readytoread.de, Hamburg
Layout and typesetting: eScriptum GmbH & Co KG – Publishing Services, Berlin
Printing: druckhaus köthen GmbH, Köthen

Reply and complaints to:
MWV Medizinisch Wissenschaftliche Verlagsgesellschaft mbH & Co. KG, Zimmerstraße 11, D- 10969 Berlin, lektorat@mwv-berlin.de

Contents

Introduction _____ 1
Hans Flaatten, Rui P. Moreno and Andrew Rhodes

A. Concepts   5

What is an ICU? _____ 7
Rui P. Moreno, Ben Singer and Andrew Rhodes

Concepts: intensive care units (ICUs) and intermediate care units _____ 15
Jean-Louis Vincent and Jacques Creteur

The role of the intensive care unit in the modern hospital _____ 21
Jan Wernerman

Interfacing the intensive care unit and evaluating it – admission and discharge policies _____ 27
Rui P. Moreno and Andrew Rhodes

Interfacing the ICU with the next of kin_____ 35
Albertus Beishuizen and Armand R.J. Girbes

The rapid response system (management, organisation)_____ 41
Anders Aneman

Integrating elective workloads into an emergency setting in the intensive care unit_____ 53
Gavin M. Joynt and Charles D. Gomersall

Special admission paths: sepsis _____ 65
Ricard Ferrer, Ana Navas, Maria Luisa Martinez, Candelaria de Haro and Antonio Artigas

Special admission paths: trauma _____ 73
Jonathan Ball, Rupert Pearse, Andrew Rhodes and Rui P. Moreno

Special admission paths: acute brain injury _____ 79
Maria Giulia Abate and Giuseppe Citerio

The ICU without walls _____ 87
Ken Hillman, Jack Chen and Anders Aneman

B. Structures, monitoring, and personnel   97

How to design a new ICU _____ 99
Michael Hiesmayr, Philipp G.H. Metnitz and Markus Haisjackl

Minimal structural requirements for ICUs and HDUs _____ 107
Patrick Ferdinande

Contents

Minimal training requirements for ICU physicians _____ 117
Armand R.J. Girbes, Albertus Beishuizen and Jan G. Zijlstra

Minimal training requirements for ICU nurses _____ 123
Ruth Endacott and Julie Scholes

Preparation and training of critical care pharmacists_____ 133
William E. Dager, Rob Shulman and Judith Jacobi

Requirements and standards for treating children in intensive care units (ICUs) _____ 143
Paolo Biban

Do we need specific cardiac (non-operative) ICUs?_____ 155
Elias Knobel, Marcia Makdisse and Marcos Knobel

Do we need specific neurocritical ICUs? _____ 167
Jorge Luiz da Rocha Paranhos, Gustavo Trindade Henriques-Filho and Odin Barbosa da Silva

Designing burn ICUs _____ 175
David M. Baron, Lars-Peter Kamolz and Philipp G.H. Metnitz

Design features of the ICU from the patient and family perspective_____ 181
Nils Theuerkauf, Ulf Guenther and Christian Putensen

Minimal standards for physiological monitoring in the intensive care unit_____ 191
Maurizio Cecconi, Lorenzo Spagnesi, Mark Hamilton, Rui P. Moreno and Andrew Rhodes

Medical work patterns: The impact on quality and burnout _____ 197
Dierk A. Vagts, Kristina Klöcker and Christian W. Mutz

Nursing work patterns_____ 205
Yên-Lan Nguyen, Sandrine Dray, Aude Soury-Lavergne and Bertrand Guidet

Physician extenders _____ 213
Maria Wittmann, Daniela Dewald and Christian Putensen

Organising the workflow in an ICU_____ 225
Hans U. Rothen

Evaluating staff performance in the ICU _____ 241
Armand R.J. Girbes and Jan G. Zijlstra

C. Processes   249

The role of ergonomics in modern medicine _____ 251
Yoel Donchin

Creating the ideal ward round _____ 259
Martha M. Kennedy, Deborah J. Baker, Ayse P. Gurses and Peter J. Pronovost

Smoothing the way: Improving admission to and discharge from the ICU_____ 269
Hannah Wunsch, Yên-Lan Nguyen and Derek C. Angus

Contents

Surge management for critical care leaders _____ 277
Michael D. Christian, Bernard Lawless, Julie Trpkovski and Jeffrey R. Dichter

Evaluating and improving the effectiveness of our practices _____ 295
Stephen Streat

The contribution of technology assessment _____ 307
Carl Waldmann, Max Jonas, Liza Keating and Ian J. Rechner

Evaluating and improving organizational outcome _____ 317
Hans Flaatten

Education and training teamwork using simulation _____ 323
Guttorm Brattebø

Electronic prescribing: minimal requirements _____ 335
Kirsten Colpaert and Johan Decruyenaere

Should research be together with clinical practice? _____ 345
Sten Rubertsson

D. Outcomes   349

Patient safety – An essential paradigm in intensive care medicine _____ 351
Andreas Valentin

Evaluating and reporting nosocomial infections _____ 359
Stijn I. Blot, Sonia O. Labeau and Jordi Rello

Self-reporting of errors and adverse events in the intensive care unit (ICU) ___ 369
Hans Flaatten

Benchmarking the intensive care unit _____ 375
Rui P. Moreno, Ana Cristina Diogo, Susana Afonso de Carvalho and Andrew Rhodes

Nosocomial infection: outcome indicator? _____ 383
Mercedes Palomar Martínez

The role of risk profile management in the evaluation of the intensive care units ___ 391
Rui P. Moreno, Philipp G.H. Metnitz, Andrew Rhodes and Peter Bauer

E. Future approaches   397

The intensive care unit of the future _____ 399
Rui P. Moreno and Andrew Rhodes

Hans Flaatten, Rui P. Moreno and Andrew Rhodes

Introduction

Medicine used to be simple, ineffective and relatively safe. It is now complex, effective and potentially dangerous.

(Professor Sir Cyril Chantler)

Since its beginnings not more than half a century ago, intensive care medicine has undergone remarkable changes. It is now considered to be a "standard of care", and most hospitals worldwide have one or more intensive care units (ICUs) within their structure.

The citation above is more than anything else an excellent summary of the developments in our field of medicine. In addition, one is tempted to add that medicine once used to be inexpensive, and now it has become quite expensive. Many countries use around 10% of their gross domestic product (GDP) for medical care in general, and up to 25% of a hospital's budget has been reported to be used on intensive care and intermediate care, due to the very labour-intensive characteristics of these units. It is no wonder that funding agencies, governmental bodies and others have begun to ask the question as to whether we get "value for money" from medicine in general, and in particular from intensive care medicine.

Notwithstanding these high costs, it is important to understand the dynamics of the current population changes and to anticipate an increase in the number of patients requiring intensive care. A closer look at the probable demographic changes for the coming 15–20 years shows that the most striking change will be the increase in the cohorts above 70 years of age. Since the aged population at present is the largest consumer of intensive care resources, this demand can easily exhaust the current capacity in most countries. This is a particular challenge, because research shows that the elderly population also benefit from intensive care, although their ICU and hospital mortality rates are higher, and their hospital stay remains longer in comparison with their younger counterparts. This can easily generate a large ethical dilemma concerning how much of these ICU resources can we afford to use in regard to the very old patients above 80 years of age.

Although intensive care is in fact very similar from hospital to hospital, there are several important differences. Organisation varies considerably, and this is often a consequence of the type of medical speciality or specialities from which it is anchored. In some countries nearly all ICUs "belong" to one speciality, as is the case in the Scandinavian countries, while in others there exist both "medical" and "surgical" ICUs with different bonds within the same hospital. A further consequence is that education of intensive care physicians and nurses differs; and not necessarily to the same standard even within one region.

Intensive care produces a high number of survivors, usually with an acceptable quality of life. The cost for an additional surviving year is not very high, and is often less than prescribing a number of drugs e.g. for any cardiovascular disease. These facts are in particular important to highlight in the future. In addition, a formidable challenge is to produce intensive care in a more cost-efficient way; probably, the best way will involve the capacity to afford the increase in services needed on a budget that is close to the limit. In this context, the use of resources like personnel is probably one of the most important factors. Another important factor is to use new technologies, devices, and drugs in a more cost effective manner.

A major difference between different regions is the availability of ICU beds. Even between countries on the same economic level, the availability differs 5 to 10-fold from the "bottom" to the "top". This is of importance since the availability of ICU beds seems to impact the quality of the outcome. One of the biggest costs to the ICU budget, is the one related to staffing, which often attributes as much as 75% of the overall running expenses. It is interesting, therefore how much staffing of the ICU varies within a reported range of nurse to patient ratios from > 1:1 up to 1:3. Some units are only staffed with specially trained ICU nurses, while others also employ respiratory technicians, physiotherapists, pharmacists and other health personnel.

The availability of enough personnel to work in our ICUs will probably become a major problem in the future. The demographic changes in most western European nations will not only lead to an increase in the numbers of elderly people, but it will simultaneously decrease the number of young people available to dedicate their life to careers for the health service.

The competition for health care workers such as nurses will be very hard, and in particular our labour-intensive ICUs will be quite vulnerable to this phenomenon. Even the well-situated countries will be confronted with a probable lack of qualified personnel. As the prime minister of Norway recently commented: "It is not doctors and nurses we pump up from our oilfields". Other countries do not even have any oil to pump and will not be able to cope with this increase in costs.

All of the above will be important issues for the delivery of intensive care in the future. It is also of great importance to make intensive care more visible within the structure of European health care. As of today, there are no references at all to intensive care or critical care within the medical content of the European directive on the recognition of professional qualifications (EU Directive 2005/36). It has been suggested to make intensive care a medical field of "particular qualification" within this directory, but this is still not in operation.

Like to all fields of medicine, the coming 15–20 years will bring additional challenges to our "speciality". First, there is a growing acceptance that the part of a country's GDP used on health care has reached its limits. It is not self-evident that spending more money on health care will necessarily improve public health; it is possible that investment in other areas of the society will pay off more. This will obviously hit intensive care medicine, since this involves an expensive treatment, reported to range from below 1000 € to more than 3000 € per day in the ICU.

To this end, understanding the organizational challenges of intensive care medicine is a key issue in providing more cost-effective intensive care. We hope that this book may provide the reader with in-depth knowledge of important aspects related to how the ICU functions and how it should be managed. We also hope the information here may be of help to shape ICUs for the future, by discussing further important and highly relevant themes which are related as well to the structure, work-flow and outcome after intensive care.

The authors

Hans Flaatten, MD, PhD[1]
Rui P. Moreno, MD, PhD[2]
Andrew Rhodes, FRCP FRCA[3]
[1]Department of Anaesthesia and
Intensive Care | Haukeland University
Hospital | Bergen, Norway
[2]Unidade de Cuidados Intensivos
Polivalente | Hospital de Santo António
dos Capuchos | Centro Hospitalar de Lisboa
Central, E.P.E. | Lisbon, Portugal
[3]General Intensive Care | St George's
Hospital | London, UK

Address for correspondence
Hans Flaatten
Haukeland University Hospital
Department of Anaesthesia and
Intensive Care
Jonas Liesvei 65
5021 Bergen, Norway
E-mail: hans.flaatten@kir.uib.no

A. Concepts

What is an ICU? _____ 7
Rui P. Moreno, Ben Singer and Andrew Rhodes

Concepts: intensive care units (ICUs) and intermediate care units _____ 15
Jean-Louis Vincent and Jacques Creteur

The role of the intensive care unit in the modern hospital_____ 21
Jan Wernerman

Interfacing the intensive care unit and evaluating it – admission and discharge policies _____ 27
Rui P. Moreno and Andrew Rhodes

Interfacing the ICU with the next of kin_____ 35
Albertus Beishuizen and Armand R.J. Girbes

The rapid response system (management, organisation)_____ 41
Anders Aneman

Integrating elective workloads into an emergency setting in the intensive care unit_____ 53
Gavin M. Joynt and Charles D. Gomersall

Special admission paths: sepsis _____ 65
Ricard Ferrer, Ana Navas, Maria Luisa Martinez, Candelaria de Haro and Antonio Artigas

Special admission paths: trauma _____ 73
Jonathan Ball, Rupert Pearse, Andrew Rhodes and Rui P. Moreno

Special admission paths: acute brain injury _____ 79
Maria Giulia Abate and Giuseppe Citerio

The ICU without walls _____ 87
Ken Hillman, Jack Chen and Anders Aneman

Rui P. Moreno, Ben Singer and Andrew Rhodes

What is an ICU?

Introduction

Intensive care medicine (ICM) is the science and the art of detecting and managing critically ill patients while preventing further deterioration, in order to achieve the best possible outcomes. Delivering high-level quality care to these patients demands the perfect match of two factors:

- An open and holistic approach from the intensivist, looking to detect, evaluate, integrate and develop a set of priorities and objectives of care for the patient, both in the short, medium and long term;
- A dedicated area, in which all monitoring and therapeutic devices required are immediately available, together with a large, multidisciplinary, highly specialised team of professionals, with a high nurse-to-patient and physician-to-patient ratio: the intensive care unit (ICU).

Even today, at a time in which critical care knowledge and skills are increasingly required and used outside the ICU, from pre-hospital care to long-term follow-up clinics (a process that Ken Hillman immortalised with the words "critical care without walls" [1]), the ICU is still needed as an independent unit inside the hospital.

From the concept of high-vigilance bed to the first intensive care units

The nurse Florence Nightingale was best known as 'the lady with the lamp' for her habit of making rounds at night to tend to injured soldiers during the Crimean war (Oct. 1853–Feb. 1856). Perhaps her most important contribution towards the development of intensive care medicine was her recognition of the fact that some patients needed more frequent and careful monitoring than others. As a consequence she started to place these patients closer to the nursing station [2]. This insight also appeared in the late 19th century in other places of the world [3]. Subsequently, as a consequence of the treatment of respiratory failure associated with the 1952 Copenhagen poliomyelitis epidemic [4, 5], hospitals started to create the first spaces specifically designed and adapted to provide this kind of organ support. The introduction of this new branch of medical science (both physiological and technological) quickly required the development of a new setting for these skills and the subsequent creation of a designated area in the hospital, known today as the ICU.

This area of the hospital was conceived to provide continuous monitoring and high-intensity therapy, as required, for instance, in the case of those patients with poliomyelitis needing artificial ventilation, the replacement of a physiological function (in this case respiration). This represented an organisational revolution for hospitals, as we argue in another chapter of this book (see chapter A "Interfacing the intensive care unit and evaluating it – admission and discharge policies"). What followed in the development of intensive care medicine is well known: Vladimir Negovsky [6], Peter Safar, Max Harry Weil, amongst others, created the science of re-animatology [7] in the late 1950s and early 1960s, of which we are the heirs. These pioneers together with subsequent generations of clinicians and nurses have continued to develop new knowledge and skills as well as the technology required to transform this diverse series of competencies into an integrated package of care, now known as the art and science of intensive care medicine.

The ICU of today

Given the objectives and scope of intensive care, the ICU is critically involved with many areas and specialties within the hospital. The location chosen for the ICU, however, commonly reflects the need for proximity to the more acute areas such as the emergency department and operating theatres, as well as required diagnostic facilities such as the radiology department, minimising the distances that critically ill patients have to be transferred. In addition, the availability of biological tests 24 hours a day, 7 days a week, and easy access to blood transfusion facilities are mandatory. Most ICUs today have facilities and equipment located within the unit to perform immediate analysis of arterial blood gas samples and some basic biochemistry and haematology.

Since most situations in intensive care medicine are critically time-dependent, the successful provision of care is reliant on good relationships and communications between the ICU and the other services and departments of the hospital; this is required both for optimising the timing of referrals and admissions of the patients to the ICU and for the safe and effective discharge of patients to a less intensive area of the hospital, a process in which the monitoring of resolving organ dysfunction/failure is very important [8]. A higher level of vigilance with respect to these recently discharged patients by both ward doctors and nurses is necessary to identify and prevent any deterioration early; failure to do so can compromise all the benefits of the ICU stay [9, 10]. Another risk to the recovering intensive care patient is inappropriate early discharge to the ward, due to lack of beds or time constraints [11], and although this is controversial [12, 13], it has been demonstrated that there is room for improvement [14]. This need for an effective interface between the ICU and the other departments of the hospital not only has physical and architectural implications, it also has a crucial impact on human resource factors, both outside and inside the ICU, on stress management, professionalism in facing and coping with rotating working patterns [15], and fatigue [16, 17]. All these issues are now being addressed and disclosed, an attitude that was virtually unthinkable a couple of decades ago and that will have a major impact on the organisation of our work.

The fact that the last European recommendations on minimal requirements for intensive care departments [18] were published in 1977 (and are just being revised this year), in a field that changes so quickly, indicates how low this has been on the scientific agenda of intensive care professionals as well as the political agenda of regulatory agencies and healthcare managers. Fortunately, in most European countries some recommendations are in place, although usually limited and locally designed, not integrated, and developed using less than optimal consensus techniques.

The concept of levels of care

The concept of levels of care (LOC) was initially proposed by Lockward in 1960 [19] and defined for the first time by a National Institute of Health (NIH) consensus conference on critical care medicine, the Bethesda Conference in 1983 [20]. Based on differences in staffing, available technology and professional organisational structures of the ICUs, the Bethesda Conference proposed the division of intensive care facilities into four groups: intensive care, high care, medium care, and low care (usually no longer considered an ICU).

Two main criteria were used in this classification: the availability of technological resources (type and intensity of use of specific monitoring and therapeutic interventions) and the availability of human resources (training and coverage by medical leadership and nurse-to-patient ratio). Underlying this classification was the concept of complexity of care: patients were moved around the system according to the complexity of the care they needed at a given point in their hospital stay.

On the European side, also during the 1980s, a task force of the European Society of Intensive Care Medicine chaired by Dinis Miranda considered this classification insufficient for purposes of organisational and policy-making decisions [21]. Arguing that it did not provide sufficient information for comparing ICUs and was inadequate for purposes of effective regionalisation of intensive care, this task force proposed a new classification based entirely on the amount of nursing manpower required by the patients: three LOC were proposed, level I with a patient/nurse (P/N) ratio of 4:1, level II, with a P/N ratio of 2.5:1 and level III with a P/N ratio of 1:1. The rationale behind the choice of this criterion was that the nurses represent the largest part of the fixed resources allocated to ICUs and consequently was the most comparable element of the permanent staff of an ICU. Also, despite the fact that the use of nursing staff is dependent on the various activities provided to each patient in each ICU, these activities depend to a large extent on the number and typology of the admitted patients and on the standing practices and policies of care in each ICU. Consequently, nursing workload can be seen as the most important and quantifiable limiting factor in the provision of care inside the ICU. Several years later, this concept developed to integrate the fact that inside the same ICU co-existed patients requiring different P/N ratios. Thus, ICUs should be classified by the mean level of care they provide and not by the maximum amount of care that can be provided (as is the case if the type and amount of available technology is used to classify ICUs) [22].

This methodology was subsequently tested by Dinis Miranda et al. in a large national study in the Netherlands at the beginning of the 1990s [23]. In this study, three LOCs were identified after determining the P/N ratios for the participating ICUs. These LOCs correlated with the size and type of hospital in which the respective ICUs were operating and discriminated significantly for the different medical activities developed in each LOC. Another interesting finding was that when comparing units under the classical definition of intensive, high and medium care that ICUs classified as 'medium care' could have a larger organisation and provide a greater frequency and intensity of care than other ICUs identified as 'intensive care'. One important implication of this was the inappropriate allocation of staff to some units and the resulting mismatch between available and required resources.

A further development of these concepts was derived from the analysis of the database of the Foundation for Research on Intensive Care in Europe (FRICE) concerning data collected during a Concerted Action of the Biomed 1 Program of the Commission of the European Communities, called EURICUS-I (BMH1-CT93-1340), addressing the effects of organisation and management on the effectiveness and efficiency of ICUs in Europe [24]. This database included data from 89 ICUs in 12 European countries. In this study the evaluation of the use of nursing manpower was done using the Nine Equivalents of Nursing Manpower use Score (NEMS), developed and validated for this specific purpose [25]. Since the Therapeutic Intervention Scoring System (TISS) had been demonstrated to be accurately related to the amount of nursing workload used [26] and NEMS previously shown to be highly related to TISS [25], they share the same limitation: they measure the amount of nursing workload used and not the amount of nursing workload required or the appropriateness of their use. This could be seen as a limitation of all methods of ICU classification and evaluation based on nursing workload use. Based on the available number of nurses, on the amount of work one nurse can perform in each shift (the equivalent of 46 NEMS points in 24 hours) and on the amount of NEMS points used during the study period, the efficiency of nursing manpower use was evaluated by the work utilisation ratio (WUR) [27]. This measure can be defined as the ratio between the produced workload and the available workload in the ICU, and is computed as:

$$\text{Work utilisation ratio} = \frac{\Sigma \text{ NEMS points used during one year}}{\text{Number of nurses} \times 200 \times \frac{46}{3}}$$

in which 200 is the annual number of working days for each nurse, 46 is the maximum number of NEMS points a nurse can perform in a day and 3 is the usual number of nursing shifts (8 hours) per 24 hours.

During the same study, the planned level of care of the ICUs was computed based on the appointed number of nurses in relation to the number of beds. Briefly, the planned number of beds to be assisted by one nurse (planned patient/nurse ratio) was computed for each ICU according to the formula:

$$\text{Number of beds assisted by one nurse} = \frac{A \times B \times C \times D \times E}{F \times G}$$

Therein:
A: Number of shifts per day (set to 3)
B: Number of beds in the unit
C: Number of days the unit is operating per week (set to 7)
D: Occupancy rate (set to 85 %)
E: Extra manpower for holidays, illness, etc. (set to 25 %, i.e. E = 1.25)
F: Number of nurses in the ICU
G: Number of days that each professional is working per week

Based on these data, the three LOC proposed by the Bethesda Consensus Conference meeting [20] were computed and compared with the operative level of care of the ICUs, computed for each ICU by dividing the number of NEMS points equivalent to the nursing activities of one nurse per shift (46 daily points) by the mean value of daily NEMS in the ICU during the study period.

This work has the advantage of replacing a subjective classification with a more objective system (to distinguish what is "limited invasive monitoring" from "all necessary invasive and non-invasive monitoring" [20] as proposed by the Bethesda classification?). Moreover, the classification of ICUs according to the complexity of care defines each LOC as an area of "medical competence of care". Accordingly, with this criterion some ICUs should have the competence for the implementation of all techniques and therapies, others only for a limited set of them. This distinction is against the rationale behind the concept of good practice of intensive care regardless of the level of care. The development of intensive care medicine in Europe is based on the concept that intensive care should be practised where and when necessary, by professionals with the right amount of knowledge and skills. In 1998 it was proposed that the limiting factor on the practice of intensive care at ICU level is the amount and not the complexity of the work that can be performed. This concept implies that two ICUs with the same amount of nursing manpower available may treat groups of patients with different severity of illness (requiring care of distinct complexity) if other variables such as occupancy rate and/ or length of stay are also taken into account. This is nothing different than what happens in daily practice, when the degree of physiologic derangement and the complexity of the patients usually decrease over time during the ICU stay. Therefore, one ICU operating at a low LOC may be able to treat a newly admitted patient requiring much more nursing care than the average patient on that ICU. It is the overall daily amount of work (which depends on the total number and the relative proportion of patients in each category) that limits the provision of more differentiated (and more nursing workload-consuming) care [22]. The application of this concept also helps managers to address the goal of the classification of ICUs into LOCs: in order to match demand and provision of resources. Finally, being easily quantifiable, it allows for evaluation and comparison of the planned versus the operative levels of the ICUs, which is nothing more than the effectiveness of the use of nursing workload resources in each ICU. In any case, the most adequate patient-to-nurse ratio for each patient and each clinical condition should be found, or we may otherwise end up with unacceptably high rates of nosocomial infections, mortality, postoperative complications, and unplanned extubations [28]. As in all domains of life, the right balance, the optimal match between what is needed and what must be provided is the key, not always identifiable but crucial to the system, defined by Donabedian as the point of optimal balance between cost and effectiveness. It is also important to conceptually separate two important concepts that are unduly mixed in the current classification of ICUs: operative capability and medical competence. Operative capability is a continuous measurement that can be lower or higher than the average for any given ICU. Medical competence is a rather dichotomous question (yes/no), that must be evaluated by the standing professional regulatory mechanisms. To create intermediate degrees of competence implies conceptually that some patients may not get enough. So where do we set the cut-off point? Should a patient be treated with at least 70% (or 60 or 80%) of medical competence? M. Fisher raised the question [29], "do intensivists matter?" The answer is: Yes they do, if they are allowed to apply their knowledge in the place they work.

Since the method proposed by Moreno and Miranda was regarded as complex, Iapichino et al. tried and achieved a classification of patients into just two groups (also based on the amount of nursing workload used): high-dependency and low-dependency patients [30, 31]. This brings the number of LOC from three to two, as previously proposed by other authors (based on different arguments) [23, 24, 32, 33].

Once the problem of medical (and nursing) competency is solved, then the system must address the issue of regionalisation versus centralisation: We need to have the expertise available anywhere it is needed in order to recognise and quickly stabilise the patient with a critical illness. This early recognition and early stabilisation should then be followed, given the relationship between volume and outcome [34–38], by adequate and timely transfer to a reference centre, a problem that may overload the system [39–45].

Of course, ultimately this has the side effect of an unavoidable fusion (or closure) of small ICUs [37, 46–49] and re-arrangement of existing ICUs and services into large networks, regularly assessed for organisational performance and not just for clinical performance [50]. Good examples of this can be seen in the effects of extra-corporeal membrane oxygenation on survival in patients with severe lung injury as demonstrated recently by the results of the CESAR trial [51].

Why we need intensive care units

It is the concentration of the skills, expertise and resources (human and technical) together in one designated area that makes an intensive care unit. This concentration allows optimal care and management of patients to occur. There is reasonable evidence now showing that the care of critically ill patients by both intensivists and/or critical care trained nurses can improve many patient-related outcomes, as well as achieving a more efficient use of the available resources. These improved outcomes include a reduced rate of infections, decreased complications, reduced length of stay and decreased mortality. If these resources are not concentrated, but rather spread evenly throughout the hospital, with a few beds on each ward, then this 'improvement by quantity' is reduced, with a less efficient use of resources and a decreased level of care being delivered to the patients.

Obviously, we do not want to take the risk of working with our backs turned on the rest of the professionals and services of the hospital, so dialogue and cooperation should be mandatory. The four walls around the ICU are there simply to allow a more cost-effective use of the resources, and not to block communication and interaction.

Conclusion

At the end of the day, managing an ICU is like driving a world rally championship car: Hardware, technical issues and teamwork certainly are important, but above all, results come from the state of mind that produces champions; an ability to fight for victory, with the constant awareness that the work of many hours could be lost in a few moments of distraction.

The authors

Rui P. Moreno, MD, PhD[1]
Ben Singer, MD[2]
Andrew Rhodes, FRCA FRCP[2]
   [1]Unidade de Cuidados Intensivos
   Polivalente | Hospital de Santo António
   dos Capuchos | Centro Hospitalar de Lisboa
   Central, E.P.E. | Lisbon, Portugal
   [2]General Intensive Care | St George's
   Hospital | London, UK

Address for correspondence
   Rui P. Moreno
   Unidade de Cuidados Intensivos Polivalente
   Hospital de Santo António dos Capuchos
   Centro Hospitalar de Lisboa Central, E.P.E.
   Alameda de Santo António dos Capuchos
   1169-050 Lisbon, Portugal
   E-mail: r.moreno@mail.telepac.pt

References

1. Hillman K. Critical care without walls. Curr Opin Crit Care 2002;8:594–9.
2. Nightingale F. Notes on hospitals. 3rd ed. London: Longman, Green, Longman, Roberts, and Green, 1863:89.
3. Takala J. Organisation of intensive care. In: Kuhlen R, Moreno R, Ranieri M, Rhodes A, eds. 25 Years of Progress and Innovation in Intensive Care Medicine. Berlin: Medizinisch Wissenschaftliche Verlagsgesells-chaft, 2007:343–50.
4. Lassen HCA. A preliminary report on the 1952 epidemic of poliomyelitis in Copenhagen with special reference to the treatment of acute respiratory insufficiency. Lancet 1953;1:37–41.
5. Ibsen B. The anaesthetist's viewpoint on the treatment of respiratory complications in poliomyelitis during the epidemic in Copenhagen, 1952. Proc R Soc Med 1954;47:72–4.
6. Negovsky VA. Some Physiopathologic Regularities in the Process of Dying and Resuscitation. Circ Metab Cerveau 1961;23:452–7.
7. Negovsky VA. Essays on Reanimatology. Moscow: MIR Publishers, 1986
8. Moreno R, Miranda DR, Matos R, Fevereiro T. Mortality after discharge from intensive care: the impact of organ system failure and nursing workload use at discharge. Intensive Care Med 2001;27:999–1004.
9. Moreno R, Agthé D. ICU discharge decision-making: are we able to decrease post-ICU mortality? Intensive Care Medicine 1999;25:1035–6.
10. Iapichino G, Morabito A, Mistraletti G, Ferla L, Radrizzani D, Miranda RR. Determinants of post-inten-sive care mortality in high-level treated critically ill patients. Intensive Care Med 2003;29:1751–6.
11. Goldfrad C, Rowan K. Consequences of discharges from intensive care at night. Lancet 2000;355:1138–42.
12. Bell CM, Redelmaier DA. Mortality among patients admitted to hospitals on weekends as compared with weekdays. N Engl J Med 2001;345:663–8.
13. Arabi Y, Alshimemeri A, Taher S. Weekend and weeknight admissions have the same outcome of weekday admissions to an intensive care unit with onsite intensivist coverage. Crit Care Med 2006;34:605–11.
14. Perren A, Conte P, De Bitonti N, Limoni C, Merlani P. From the ICU to the ward: cross-checking of the physician's transfer report by intensive care nurses. Intensive Care Med 2008;34:2054–61.
15. Harrocks N, Pounder R. Working the night shift: preparation, survival and recovery – a guide for junior doctors. Clin Med 2006;6:61–7.
16. West CP, Tan AD, Habermann TM, Sloan JA, Shanafelt TD. Association of Resident Fatigue and Distress With Perceived Medical Errors. JAMA 2009;302:1294–300.
17. Gaba DM, Howard SK. Fatigue among clinicians and the safety of patients. N Engl J Med 2002;347:1249–55.
18. Ferdinande P, Members of the Task Force of the European Society of Intensive Care Medicine. Recommendations on minimal requirements for Intensive Care Departments. Intensive Care Med 1997;23:226–32.
19. Lockward HJ, Giddings L, Thoms EJ. Progressive patient care: a preliminary report. JAMA 1960;172:132–7.
20. NIH Consensus Development Conference on Critical Care Medicine. Crit Care Med 1983;11:466–9.
21. Reis Miranda D, Williams A, Loirat P, eds. Management of Intensive Care. Guidelines for better use of resources. Dordrecht/Boston/London: Kluwer Academish Publishers, 1990.
22. Moreno R, Reis Miranda D. Nursing staff in intensive care in Europe. The mismatch between planning and practice. Chest 1998;113:752–8.
23. Reis Miranda D, Gimbrere J. Quality, efficiency, and organization of intensive care units in The Netherlands: an interdisciplinary study on medical and business aspects (Dutch language). In: Reis Miranda D, Spangenberg JFA, eds. Groningen: Van Denderen, 1992.
24. Reis Miranda D, Ryan DW, Schaufeli WB, Fidler V, eds. Organization and management of Intensive Care: a prospective study in 12 European countries. Berlin Heidelberg: Springer-Verlag, 1997 (vol 29).
25. Reis Miranda D, Iapichino G, Moreno R. Nine Equivalents of Nursing Manpower use Score (NEMS). Validation on the EURICUS-I database [abstract]. Intensive Care Med 1996;22:S296.
26. Reis Miranda D, de Rijk A, Schaufeli W. Simplified Therapeutic Intervention Scoring System: The TISS 28 items – Results from a multicenter study. Crit Care Med 1996;24:64–73.
27. Reis Miranda D, Gimbrere J. The Netherlands. New Horiz 1994;2:357–63.
28. Aragon Penoyer D. Nurse staffing and patient outcomes in critical care: A concise review. Crit Care Med 2010;38:1521–8.
29. Fisher M. Intensive care: do intensivists matter? Intensive Care World 1995;12:71–2.
30. Iapichino G, Radrizzani D, Ferla L, Pezzi A, Porta F, Zanforlin G, Miranda DR. Description of trends in the course of illness of critically ill patients. Markers of intensive care organization and performance. Intensive Care Med 2002;28:985–9.
31. Guccione A, Morena A, Pezzi A, G I. I carichi di lavoro infermieristico [The assessment of nursing workload]. Minerva Anestesiol 2004;70:411–6.
32. Haupt MT, Bekes CE, Bayly RW, Brilli RJ, Carl LC, Diringer MN, Greenbaum DN, Jacobi J, Jastremski MS, Nasraway SA, Nikas DL, Scott WS, Spevetz A, Stone JR, Warren J, Wedel SK. Critical care services and personnel. Recommendations based on a system of categorization

into two levels of care. American College of Critical Care Medicine of the Society of Critical Care Medicine. Crit Care Med 1999;27:422–6.

33. Haupt MT, Bekes CE, Brilli RJ, Carl LC, Gray AW, Jastremski MS, Naylor DF, Rudis M, Spevetz A, Wedel SK, Horst M. Guidelines on critical care services and personnel: Recommendations based on a system of categorization of three levels of care. Crit Care Med 2003;31:2677–83.

34. Jones J, Rowan K. Is there a relationship between the volume of work carried out in intensive care and its outcome? Int J Technol Assess Health Care 1995;11:762–9.

35. The UK Neonatal Staffing Study Group. Patient volume, staffing, and workload in relation to risk adjusted outcomes in a random stratified sample of UK neonatal intensive care units: a prospective evaluation. Lancet 2002;359:99–107.

36. Kahn JM, Goss CH, Heagerty PJ, Kramer AA, O'Brien CR, Rubenfeld GD. Hospital volume and the outcomes of mechanical ventilation. N Engl J Med 2006;355:41–50.

37. Lindenauer PK, Behal R, Murray CK, Nsa W, Houck PM, Bratzler DW. Volume, Quality of Care, and Outcome in Pneumonia. Ann Intern Med 2006;144:262–9.

38. Bagshaw SM, Bellomo R. The influence of volume management on outcome. Curr Opin Crit Care 2007;13:541–8.

39. Besserman E, Teres D, Logan A, Brennan M, Cleaves S, Bayly R, Brochis D, Nemeth B, Grare J, Ngo D. Use of flexible intermediate and intensive care to reduce multiple transfers of patients. Am J Crit Care 1999;8:170–9.

40. Surgenor SD, Corwin HL, Clerico T. Survival of patients transferred to tertiary intensive care from rural community hospitals. Crit Care 2000;5:100–4.

41. Uusaro A, Parviainen I, Takala J, Ruokonen E. Safe long-distance interhospital ground transfer of critically ill patients with acute severe unstable respiratory and circulatory failure. Intensive Care Med 2002;28:1122–5.

42. Bekes C. Transfer surcharge. Crit Care Med 2007;35:1612–3.

43. Calgary Health Region. ICU Interfacility Transfer Checklist, Calgary Health Region. 2007.

44. Chalfin DB, Trzeciak S, Likourezos A, Baumann BM, Dellinger RP, for the DELAY-ED study group. Impact of delayed transfer of critically ill patients from the emergency department to the intensive care unit. Crit Care Med 2007;35:1477–83.

45. Golestanian E, Scruggs JE, Gangnon RE, Mak RP, Wood KE. Effect of interhospital transfer on resource utilization and outcomes at a tertiary care referral center. Crit Care Med 2007;35:1470–6.

46. Aujesky D, Mor MK, Geng M, Fine MJ, Renaud B, Ibrahim SA. Hospital volume and patient outcomes in pulmonary embolism. Can Med Assoc J 2008;178:27–33.

47. Glance LG, Dick AW, Osler TM, Mukamel DB. The relation between surgeon volume and outcome following off-pump vs on-pump coronary artery bypass graft surgery. Chest 2005;128:829–37.

48. Kahn JM. Volume and outcome in intensive care. In: Chice J-D, Moreno R, Putensen C, Rhodes A, eds. Patient Safety and Quality of Care In Intensive Care Medicine. Berlin: Medizinisch Wissenschaftiche Verlagsgesells-chaft, 2009:161–70.

49. Matti R, Sari K, Tero V, Ilkka P, Esko R, Marjut V, Tero A-K, Ville P. Are small hospitals with small intensive care units able to treat patients with severe sepsis? Intensive Care Med 2009;36:673–9.

50. Minvielle E, Aegerter P, Dervaux B, Boumendil A, Retbif A, Jars-Guincestre MC, Guidet B, for the CUB-REA network. Assessing organizational performance in intensive care units: A French experience. J Crit Care 2008;23:236–44.

51. Peek GJ, Mugford M, Tiruvoipati R, Wilson A, Allen E, Thalanany MM, Hibbert CL, Truesdale A, Clemens F, Cooper N, Firmin RK, Elbourne D, for the CESAR trial collaboration. Efficacy and economic assessment of conventional ventilatory support versus extracorporeal membrane oxygenation for severe adult respiratory failure (CESAR): a multicentre randomised controlled trial. Lancet 2009.

Jean-Louis Vincent and Jacques Creteur

Concepts: intensive care units (ICUs) and intermediate care units

Introduction

The concept of intensive care was developed only just over 50 years ago. Initially, it was often just one or two beds in the corner of a general ward, but the value of being able to combine the necessary technology and trained staff together in one dedicated area of the hospital soon resulted in the creation of separate areas of the hospital for critically ill patients, and the intensive care unit (ICU) came into being. Since those early days, intensive care medicine has developed into a specialty in its own right and the ICU is now a key feature in almost every hospital, looking after patients who need "intensive" care in terms of equipment and high staff-to-patient ratios. With advances in medicine and improved life-support systems, patients are now surviving diseases and trauma from which in the past they would have succumbed, and the need for and use of intensive care has never been greater. The aging population and increased numbers of patients receiving immunosuppressive drugs have also increased the demand for ICU beds. Hence, the number of ICU beds is still increasing worldwide, whereas the total number of hospital beds is decreasing.

However, intensive care is expensive with new drugs, expensive technologies, and specialized clinical care all contributing to ever-increasing health care expenditures [1]. Any strategies that could reduce or retain costs are therefore worthy of consideration. One such approach has been the development of so-called "intermediate care units", often synonymous with "high-dependency" or "step-down" units, although some hospitals may have both a high-dependency unit as an immediate step down from intensive care and then an intermediate care unit. Such units are used for patients who need more care than a general ward can provide, but not full intensive care. However, the question arises as to whether the intermediate care unit is really a valid solution to ICU bed shortages and does it really benefit patient care and patient costs? In this chapter we will consider some of the pros and cons of intermediate care units (see box below).

Box: pros and cons of intermediate care units

Pros
- They can facilitate earlier ICU discharge of patients no longer needing full ICU care but who are not yet ready for the general floor
- They may decrease the need for ICU admission of patients who only need extra monitoring or nursing such as that available on the general floor
- They may be associated with improved patient comfort
- They may reduce costs

Cons

- They may precipitate premature discharge of patients
- They result in fragmentation of ICU equipment and staff skills
- They may be associated with increased patient anxiety
- They require additional patient transfer
- They may be associated with decreased staff morale and job satisfaction
- They may reduce the role of the intensivist
- They may actually increase costs

Intermediate care units: pros

Intermediate care units generally have higher staff-to-patient ratios and more specialized equipment, notably for monitoring, than the general ward does but less than the ICU theoretically making it a more cost-effective option for patients not needing full ICU facilities. Perhaps one of the first documented intermediate care units was the non-invasive respiratory care unit established by Bone and Balk primarily for the monitoring of patients with respiratory disorders as they were weaned from ventilatory support, using a nurse-to-patient ratio of 1:3 or 4 [2]. Intermediate care units have now been adopted by many hospitals, particularly for specific patient groups, such as cardiac, neurosurgical, or respiratory patients. The use of such units may enable earlier discharge of some ICU patients who no longer need full ICU facilities but are not ready to be discharged to the general ward (step-*down* unit). They could also be used for the often considerable numbers of patients who are admitted to the ICU just for intensive monitoring and are unlikely to need active therapy [3]. Another use is for the early admission of patients requiring more intensive management than is available on the general floor but not yet needing full intensive care (step-*up* unit). The presence of an intermediate care unit could, therefore, help to free up ICU beds for those patients who need them most.

Many authors have supported the use of intermediate care units as a means of reducing pressure on overloaded ICUs at a cost-saving because of the reduced staff and equipment needed without negative effect on patient care. However, there appear to be relatively few published stud-ies that have directly assessed the value of intermediate care units, and even fewer which have compared intermediate with intensive care. In an early study, Franklin et al. [4] reported that the opening of an intermediate care unit was associated with an overall decrease in the case fatality rate in the medical service, largely because of a decrease in the mortality rate in general medical wards. The authors suggested that this was because unstable ICU patients who would normally have been discharged to the general ward were being more appropriately managed on the intermediate care unit. Byrick et al. [5] reported an increase in the number of ICU admissions with low severity of illness after closure of an intermediate care unit for budgetary reasons. The perceived increase in inefficient use of staff and resources led to the intermediate care unit being reopened. Fox et al. [6] reported that the opening of a high dependency unit reduced the number of ICU readmissions, again supporting the suggestion that without the intermediate unit, intensive care patients were being discharged too early to the general floor. Beck et al. [7] found that patients with high severity scores who were discharged to hospital wards had a higher risk (1.31; CI: $1.02-1.83$) of in-hospital death compared with patients discharged to a high dependency unit. More recently, Eachempati et al. [8] noted that in their surgical ICU, the opening of a step-down unit was associated with an increase in emergency admissions and in the overall severity of illness of the patients admitted to the ICU, without increased mortality. These authors suggested that the increase in total critical care beds with the opening of the step-down unit enabled patients to be admitted who would otherwise have been transferred to other units, hence the increased severity of illness. Ranhoff and colleagues [9] reported that creation of a "sub intensive care unit" within their care for the elderly department was associated with improved patient outcomes and suggested that this could help reduce ICU overcrowding.

The increased efficiency of use of ICU beds associated with availability of an intermediate care unit has often been promoted as a means of reducing costs. In a prospective study, Bertolini et al. reported that, for patients with exacerbation of chronic obstructive pulmonary disease (COPD), the total cost per patient was lower in a respiratory intermediate care unit than in an ICU

[10]. Such units may also be potentially associated with increased patient comfort in terms of less technology, less ambient noise, more privacy, and more open visiting hours [11], although the sudden decrease in nurse-to-patient ratios and monitoring equipment can lead to feelings of insecurity among patients and their families [12].

Intermediate care units: cons

Despite the arguments that intermediate care units may help reduce costs and improve use of ICU resources, creation of intermediate care units to limit ICU overflow could be seen simply as a means of diverting the problem rather than solving it. In an early systematic review of the literature, Keenan et al. concluded that there were insufficient data to demonstrate a definite improvement in cost-effectiveness with the use of intermediate care units compared to traditional ICUs and general ward beds [13]. More recently, in a before-after study, introduction of an intermediate care unit was actually associated with increased total hospital costs per patient [14]. The authors suggested that this was likely due to an increase in severity of illness of patients admitted in the period after introduction of the intermediate unit and longer lengths of ICU stays, and not related to the introduction of the intermediate care unit per se [14]. However, as the intermediate care unit consumes a relatively low proportion of total ICU costs, total intensive care costs are unlikely to be altered much by introduction of an intermediate care unit [14, 15]; the majority of ICU resources is consumed by the most severely ill patients, and reducing the number of less sick patients will therefore have relatively little impact on overall ICU spending. Similarly, hospital costs are unlikely to decrease and may, in fact, increase a little because many of the intermediate care patients would otherwise have been treated in the general ward using fewer resources, especially in terms of staffing [16], at a considerably lower cost. Moreover, larger units, combining "intensive" with "intermediate" beds, may be associated with reduced costs when compared to smaller units [17].

There are several other reasons why separate intermediate care units may not be the best solution to ICU overload problems. First, a larger unit caring for a mix of intensive care patients is more able to adapt to changes in workload than a smaller unit can, thus allowing more efficient use of available resources. Moreover, mortality rates in larger ICUs with high annual patient volumes have been reported to be lower than in smaller units with lower annual patient volumes [18–21]. Secondly, the presence of an intermediate care unit may provide a (false) sense of security and encourage early discharge of patients from the ICU who would never have qualified for ward transfer. In their audit of 4,736 patients discharged alive from the ICU, Campbell and colleagues [22] reported that discharge to a high-dependency unit was an independent risk factor for early ICU readmission, suggesting that these patients had been discharged prematurely. Importantly, ICU readmission is associated with increased mortality [23]. Thirdly, although the ICU environment, with its high impact technology and invasive procedures, can be stressful for patients and their families, this same setting can, in fact, be reassuring as patients receive constant monitoring and staff attention and care [12]. Leaving this secure environment can be associated with increased anxiety. Moreover, transfer to an intermediate unit necessitates an extra break in the continuity of care for the patient and their family, who will have to adapt again to new surroundings and staff when they are then transferred to the general ward. Fourthly, intensive care trained nursing staff may feel that working on the intermediate care unit is less "important" than having a position in the ICU, and working on a mixed unit with more heterogeneous patient populations may be associated with greater job satisfaction. One of the most important psychological aspects for all health staff is of course to see that patients recover; transferring patients to an intermediate unit can remove this positive continuity of care. Intermediate care unit patients may also potentially be seen as less 'urgent' than their ICU counterparts with the risk that medical rounds will be rushed to allow more time on the ICU. Alternatively, if the intermediate care unit falls outside the remit of the intensivist, patients may lose the advantages on outcomes that have been associated with full-time intensivist-led care [24]. Combining intermediate with intensive care beds will ensure that patient management remains optimal.

Conclusion

The organisation of intensive care unit (ICU) facilities varies hugely within and among various countries, and the optimal approach will vary according to local demand and available facilities. Intermediate care units have been introduced into many hospitals, largely to ease the pressure on ICUs and to provide a cost-effective means of treating patients who need more care than a general ward can provide, but who do not require full ICU facilities. Such units can be developed as freestanding in a hospital area distant from the ICU, adjacent to the ICU, or integrated within a department of intensive care [25]. We believe that this latter approach offers a more efficient and effective model for the reasons outlined above. By combining intensive and intermediate care beds in one mixed unit, equipment and staff skills are focused into one clear area rather than being fragmented into separate units.

Whatever the systems' approach to ICU facilities, development and implementation of strict admission and discharge criteria is essential to ensure efficient utilization of resources and optimal outcomes for all patients [26, 27]. Ultimately, each patient should be able to receive exactly the amount of care they require at all times during their hospital stay [28]. However, many patients with no reasonable chance of survival are still admitted to ICUs, and yet will not benefit from intensive care [29]; reducing these and other unnecessary admissions must be a priority to improve the cost-effectiveness and efficiency of our ICUs, and to ensure adequate provision of ICU beds for those who will indeed benefit.

The authors

Jean-Louis Vincent, Prof.
Jacques Creteur, MD
    Department of Intensive Care | Erasme Hospital | Université libre de Bruxelles, Belgium

Address for correspondence
    Jean-Louis Vincent
    Department of Intensive Care
    Erasme Hospital
    Route de Lennik 808
    B-1070, Brussels, Belgium
    E-mail: jlvincen@ulb.ac.be

References

1. Kahn JM, Angus DC. Reducing the cost of critical care: new challenges, new solutions. Am J Respir Crit Care Med 2006;174:1167–1168.
2. Bone RC, Balk RA. Noninvasive respiratory care unit. A cost effective solution for the future. Chest 1988;93:390–394.
3. Zimmerman JE, Kramer AA. A model for identifying patients who may not need intensive care unit admission. J Crit Care 2010;25:205–213.
4. Franklin CM, Rackow EC, Mamdani B, Nightingale S, Burke G, Weil MH. Decreases in mortality on a large urban medical service by facilitating access to critical care. An alternative to rationing. Arch Intern Med 1988;148:1403–1405.
5. Byrick RJ, Mazer CD, Caskennette GM. Closure of an intermediate care unit. Impact on critical care utilization. Chest 1993;104:876–881.
6. Fox AJ, Owen-Smith O, Spiers P. The immediate impact of opening an adult high dependency unit on intensive care unit occupancy. Anaesthesia 1999;54:280–283.
7. Beck DH, McQuillan P, Smith GB. Waiting for the break of dawn? The effects of discharge time, discharge TISS scores and discharge facility on hospital mortality after intensive care. Intensive Care Med 2002;28:1287–1293.
8. Eachempati SR, Hydo LJ, Barie PS. The effect of an intermediate care unit on the demographics and outcomes of a surgical intensive care unit population. Arch Surg 2004;139:315–319.
9. Ranhoff AH, Rozzini R, Sabatini T, et al. Subintensive care unit for the elderly: a new model of care for critically ill frail elderly medical patients. Intern Emerg Med 2006;1:197–203.
10. Bertolini G, Confalonieri M, Rossi C, et al. Costs of the COPD. Differences between intensive care unit and respiratory intermediate care unit. Respir Med 2005;99:894–900.
11. Rudy EB, Daly BJ, Douglas S, Montenegro HD, Song R, Dyer MA. Patient outcomes for the chronically critically ill: special care unit versus intensive care unit. Nurs Res 1995;44:324–331.
12. Chaboyer W, James H, Kendall M. Transitional care after the intensive care unit: current trends and future directions. Crit Care Nurse 2005;25:16–2, 24.
13. Keenan SP, Massel D, Inman KJ, Sibbald WJ. A systematic review of the cost-effectiveness of noncardiac transitional care units. Chest 1998;113:172–177.
14. Solberg BC, Dirksen CD, Nieman FH, van Merode G, Poeze M, Ramsay G. Changes in hospital costs after introducing an intermediate care unit: a comparative observational study. Crit Care 2008;12:R68.
15. Zimmerman JE, Wagner DP, Knaus WA, Williams JF, Kolakowski D, Draper EA. The use of risk predictions to identify candidates for intermediate care units.

Implications for intensive care utilization and cost. Chest 1995;108:490–499.

16. Zimmerman JE, Wagner DP, Sun X, Knaus WA, Draper EA. Planning patient services for intermediate care units: insights based on care for intensive care unit low-risk monitor admissions. Crit Care Med 1996;24:1626–1632.

17. Jacobs P, Rapoport J, Edbrooke D. Economies of scale in British intensive care units and combined intensive care/high dependency units. Intensive Care Med 2004;30:660–664.

18. Jones J, Rowan K. Is there a relationship between the volume of work carried out in intensive care and its outcome? Int J Technol Assess Health Care 1995;11:762–769.

19. Peelen L, de Keizer NF, Peek N, Scheffer GJ, van der Voort PH, de Jonge E. The influence of volume and intensive care unit organization on hospital mortality in patients admitted with severe sepsis: a retrospective multicentre cohort study. Crit Care 2007;11:R40.

20. Reinikainen M, Karlsson S, Varpula T, et al. Are small hospitals with small intensive care units able to treat patients with severe sepsis? Intensive Care Med 2010;36:673–679.

21. Wunsch H, Angus DC, Harrison DA, et al. Variation in critical care services across North America and Western Europe. Crit Care Med 2008;36:2787–2789.

22. Campbell AJ, Cook JA, Adey G, Cuthbertson BH. Predicting death and readmission after intensive care discharge. Br J Anaesth 2008;100:656–662.

23. Rosenberg AL, Hofer TP, Hayward RA, Strachan C, Watts CM. Who bounces back? Physiologic and other predictors of intensive care unit readmission. Crit Care Med 2001;29:511–518.

24. Pronovost PJ, Angus DC, Dorman T, Robinson KA, Dremsizov TT, Young TL. Physician staffing patterns and clinical outcomes in critically ill patients: a systematic review. JAMA 2002;288:2151–2162.

25. Haupt MT, Bekes CE, Brilli RJ, et al. Guidelines on critical care services and personnel: Recommendations based on a system of categorization of three levels of care. Crit Care Med 2003;31:2677–2683.

26. American Thoracic Society Fair allocation of intensive care unit resources. Am J Respir Crit Care Med 1997;156:1282–1301.

27. Task Force of the American College of Critical Care Medicine SoCCM. Guidelines for intensive care unit admission, discharge, and triage. Crit Care Med 1999;27:633–638.

28. Moreno R, Agthe D. ICU discharge decision-making: are we able to decrease post-ICU mortality? Intensive Care Med 1999;25:1035–1036.

29. Vincent JL. Forgoing life support in western European intensive care units: the results of an ethical questionnaire. Crit Care Med 1999;27:1626–1633.

Jan Wernerman

The role of the intensive care unit in the modern hospital

Introduction

This volume covers a number of different aspects of organization and management of intensive care. It is inevitable that overlaps occur. In this chapter focusing upon the role of the ICU in the modern hospital it has been necessary to elaborate over what the modern hospital will be or develop into in different health care systems. That is perhaps the unique task of this chapter, but besides that the distinction between the ICU and the high dependency unit, or perhaps the grey zone between the two as well as the relation between the ICU and different outreach activities will also be covered with the risk of overlap of other entries in this volume.

Relation between ICU, hospital and health care system

Starting up with the role of the individual hospital within different health care systems it is easy to see differences. Any hospital with an emergency unit would need an intensive care facility. Related to the size of the emergency unit and/or the availability of alternative emergency units in the same area, the intensive care facility will be different. There is a strong tendency towards increasing the size of emergency units in the western world in order to reach a critical mass for handling complicated emergency cases [1]. This is best illustrated by the level one trauma units which may or may not at the same time handle non trauma emergencies. In other parts of the world the need of intensive care facilities may be different. Sometimes intensive care facilities are totally out of the economic possibilities. Here the type of health care system in use will be a strong determinant of the intensive care facility. In most hospitals dealing with emergency cases or major surgery within a health care system where patients (families) pay directly or via private insurance there will be an intensive care facility as a part of the business plan also in countries with a low BNP per capita on the average.

In countries with a general health care system, public or private, but accessible to all inhabitants, the situation is different and decision making is different [2]. Again the roles of the ICU in the hospital are related to whether there is a uniform public insurance system or of insurances are individualized on different levels. Expensive parts of hospital care, as in this case a stay in the ICU, may differ in availability in an individualized insurance system. This may then also be a part of the local business plan. It may be attractive for some individuals to sign up for a health insurance that covers for ICU care on broad indications. The cost for such insurance may not be feasible and/or attractive for everybody.

ICU and high dependency care

It seems important to differentiate between the role of an intensive care unit which serves its purpose from strictly medical indications and when the purpose is a combination of medical indication and a business plan. In any public health care system, whether financed by the tax bill or by public insurance systems, where admissions to the ICU rest solidly on medical grounds this will be a limiting resource. The role of the ICU and the ICU physician will be to make use of the resource as efficiently as possible. The patients that have the best need of these resources at any time point will ideally be the ones in the ICU. The size of the ICU resource parallel to outpatient activities, ordinary wards and high dependency unit must be properly analysed. Again, depending upon the size and profile of the hospital, the optimal solution may be very different [3].

The ICU registry as a tool

Other chapters in this volume will try to define what intensive care medicine is and what the ICU is. Still, as a reflection of the hospital profile, the optimal solution may be a combined intensive care and high dependency unit. This is particularly true in sparsely populated areas where transport logistics will favour comparatively small hospitals with comparatively broad medical responsibility. The same situation may occur in hospitals confined to elective admittance or major surgery only, where the optimal solution may be a combined recovery room high dependency and ICU.

A major achievement during the last ten years is the use of computerized information systems and the development of databases reflecting ICU care. Characterization of patients, activities and outcome can be studied with an epidemiological perspective [4]. For the first time, systematic information from clinical practice becomes available for decision making. As with any data-

base, a lot of flaws and pitfalls are unavoidable in databases, and these may disguise important information. Inevitable comparisons between the use of resource and the performance within given resources come up to discussion in economical as well as in political perspectives. Although these epidemiological data are still far from perfect, they add new dimensions into the discussion of the role of the ICU in the modern hospital. As ICU physicians and nurses, we should embrace this possibility and engage ourselves and make the registration and follow up as accurately and detailed as we can.

Beside obvious limitations in databases, such as low quality input in terms of imperfect registrations, there are system-related limitations. These limitations may be that a certain ICU facility is not accessible to everybody or that the decision of admittance is made only partly on medical grounds, or there may be other selection criteria that limit the generalizability of data.

Furthermore, when discussing performance, ICU outcome is far from being one-dimensional [5]. In addition to mortality and morbidity, quality of life must be considered. As a part of the epidemiology, the long term outcome after intensive care is an important part of the basis for decision making concerning the role of the ICU in the modern hospital. The long term outcome is an important perspective when admittance criteria are discussed. It is covered by other chapters in this volume: which patients should be admitted to the ICU, particularly when there are restraining levels of care and treatments.

Transporting ICU patients

Another issue to consider is how and when to transport or transfer patients in need of intensive care facilities [6]. Knowledge about the safety of transport of critical ill patients is rapidly increasing, but still the risks involved are not sufficiently characterized. It is possible to transport patients on ECMO with a higher level of safety as compared to a transport of the same patients on artificial ventilation with 100 % oxygen and a borderline oxygenation. There are reports that any transport carries the risk of adding to morbidity and to prolonging the ICU stay. Here it is often difficult to separate the transport itself from the indication for the transport [7]. In some areas, transports between hospitals are carried out for no other reason than shortage of ICU beds. The triage behind the choice for such a patient transport has, to our knowledge, not yet been sufficiently studied. This is in particular the case when such bedside decisions must often be made under the pressure of time and where only limited information is available. These are often decisions of triage which are dependent on several levels.

There are also situations when decisions are merely about the availability of competence and resources on one hand and the risk of transport on the other hand. Techniques involved and competence during transport have increased rapidly. Transport between units and hospitals will probably be more common in the future. This involves a number of problems, where safety is just one. The acceptance inside the ICU, inside the hospital, as well as among patient relatives and people in general represented by politicians must all be considered in this process. The need for these transports comes out of an urge to optimize the use of medical resources as well as that of economical resources. From a patient and relative perspective any transport that is not motivated by access to a higher level of resources and competences, is questioned and poorly accepted. In this regard, an ICU organization that involves an increased need of transports must constantly seek support from taxpayers and politicians.

Flexibility as a success factor

When the role of the ICU in the hospital in the future is discussed it is important to remember that flexibility historically has been a success factor. There is no reason to believe that the future will be any different. Hospitals with an ICU organization and an ICU resource that can adapt to new situations are usually successful [8]. Rigid systems in terms of organization, staffing, localities and use of technique have usually been less successful. General statements like this may be interpreted very differently and therefore such a statement must be developed a little bit further. For a successful ICU management, medical competence is essential. Management and leadership in general may be organized in multiple ways but it is the involvement and medical com-

petence in the decision making which remains most essential.

The flexibility may be dependent on the level of number of patients and on the level of care. Today, scoring systems to differentiate between categories of patients are operational to allow ICUs to optimize the number of patients in relation to resources. The obvious problem is the non-linearity of the scoring and the fact that nurse-to-patient ratios can only involve whole number such as 1:1, 1:2, 1:3 etc. [9]. Flexibility may also be in terms of single-patient rooms and multiple-patient rooms and the different need for staffing related to that.

Flexibility on another level may be how to handle a change in demand. How can we find the optimal critical mass in a new situation? Here, the ability to analyse ICU need on the hospital level is a critical success factor. The number of holy grails and hidden agendas in a given hospital will increase the painfulness-delay rational solutions. Very often no effective solution will achieved at all. Strong professional organizations of doctors as well as nurses are necessary to guaranty quality. Besides that, the structure how to use the resource in an optimal way is the key to success.

Health economy

In a health care system where > 70 % of the total costs refers to payment for nurses and doctors, optimal staffing competes over any other factor in calculations of cost-effectiveness [10]. The role of ICU in the hospital will then be to care for the patients in need of its full resources and to always have a high occupancy of its beds. However this equation is not complete without introduction of a proper time axis. The term optimal care refers to a level of care, but in addition also to a length of care. ICUs that are understaffed with doctors and nurses tend to have a longer length of stay (LOS). Optimal care also refers to a correct level of care in terms of restrains meaning withholding and sometimes even withdrawing treatment.

It is obvious that defining the correct level of care will be a critical success factor in the future. To make this process meaningful in economical terms, the corresponding levels of care must be available. A proper analysis of the demand for ICU beds, high dependency beds and perhaps also units for ventilated single organ failure patients. With good planning, such units may provide care for patients with need of mechanical ventilation, but with no other organ failure demanding approximately the same staffing as a high dependency unit. These patients often have neuro-muscular diseases and they may be candidates for home ventilator treatment.

Optimal level of care as soon as possible

If priority and effort are directed to optimizing the level of treatment for each individual patient, we now come to the problem of how this decision is to be reached. It is highly likely that patients and relatives will demand the highest possible level of care, at least initially. This is also reasonable until a thorough evaluation of each individual patient has been performed and a subsequent decision of the optimal level of care is made. It will then not be possible to immediately house every patient inside the ICU at every time point. For the availability of various outreach services, or an ICU so to say without walls you can and must offer the solution yourself. Patients should not be admitted to high dependency care unless having been fully evaluated in a setting with full ICU resources available, not necessarily utilizing all technical resources in all cases. Sometimes such an evaluation process may be facilitated if the patient is well known to the hospital or to the referring doctor.

It will come naturally that a system as described above will need full medical competence around the clock. Senior intensivist competence will be needed for doing the correct priorities. A competence on a similar level will also be needed to evaluate the underlying pathology, in particular the chronic health evaluation is critical. Again the type of health care system will favour different solutions of this problem. The cost and availability for senior doctors will make the difference.

Conclusions

The modern hospital will serve a defined purpose and that will also define the intensive care facility needed. Economy will necessitate that patients are transferred to the optimal level of care as soon as possible. Initial ob-

servation, diagnosis and treatment should be offered with access to full resources, but thereafter a different level of care may be optimal for the individual patient. Various kinds of out-reach facilities may be needed to fulfil the task of initial handling with access to full resources. Consequently, median ICU stay will be short, which calls for a high medical competence around the clock and a highly flexible organization of care. As early intensive treatment has the potential to shorten the need for ICU stay, this will be a priority. Related to the mission of the hospital the ICU may be organized as a specialized unit or a combined intensive care and high dependency unit. The size of the unit is probably not critical as long as it fits the defined purpose of the hospital.

The author

Jan Wernerman, MD, PhD
    Professor of Intensive Care Medicine
    Department of Anaesthesiology and
    Intensive Care Medicine
    Karolinska University Hospital Huddinge
    Stockholm, Sweden
    E-mail: Jan.wernerman@karolinska.se

References

1. Ala-Kokko TI, et al. Improved outcome after trauma care in university-level intensive care units. Acta Anaesthesiol Scand, 2009;53(10):1251–6.
2. Angus DC, et al. International comparisons of critical care outcome and resource consumption. Crit Care Clin, 1997;13(2):389–407.
3. Wunsch H, et al. Variation in critical care services across North America and Western Europe. Crit Care Med, 2008;36(10):2787–93, e1–9.
4. Fakhry SM. Kercher KW, and Rutledge R. Survival, quality of life, and charges in critically Ill surgical patients requiring prolonged ICU stays. J Trauma, 1996;41(6):999–1007.
5. Carson SS. Outcomes research: methods and implications. Semin Respir Crit Care Med, 2010;31(1):3–12.
6. Beckmann U, et al. Incidents relating to the intra-hospital transfer of critically ill patients. An analysis of the reports submitted to the Australian Incident Monitoring Study in Intensive Care. Intensive Care Med, 2004;30(8):1579–85.
7. Belway D, et al. The role of transport intervals in outcomes for critically ill patients who are transferred to referral centers. J Crit Care, 2008;23(3):287–94.
8. Sprung CL, et al. Recommendations for intensive care

unit and hospital preparations for an influenza epidemic or mass disaster: summary report of the European Society of Intensive Care Medicine's Task Force for intensive care unit triage during an influenza epidemic or mass disaster. Intensive Care Med, 2010;36(3):428–43.

9. Pirret AM. Utilizing TISS to differentiate between intensive care and high-dependency patients and to identify nursing skill requirements. Intensive Crit Care Nurs, 2002;18(1):19–26.

10. Kahn JM. Understanding economic outcomes in critical care. Curr Opin Crit Care, 2006;12(5):399–404.

Rui P. Moreno and Andrew Rhodes

Interfacing the intensive care unit and evaluating it – admission and discharge policies

Introduction

The practice of intensive care medicine began in Europe in the late 1950s, as a consequence of the treatment of respiratory complications of poliomyelitis during the 1952 Copenhagen epidemic [1, 2]. One of the first consequences of the introduction of this new resource rich branch of medical science (both human and material), requiring a new set of knowledge and skills, was the creation of a separate area in the hospital, the intensive care unit (ICU). In this area, patients needing artificial replacement of a physiological function (in this case respiration) were placed together. This represented for hospitals a significant organizational revolution (much more than a scientific revolution). Although it had previously been recognized by Florence Nightingale in 1863 [3], amongst others [4], that at risk, patients were better placed near to the nursing station to enable more frequent and intense observation, that was the first time that this increased monitoring was combined with a systematic method of providing support to modify the delivery of care. The subsequent development of methods for providing cardiovascular support and resuscitation by Vladimir Negovsky [5], Peter Safar, Max Harry Weil and many other pioneers of our discipline resulted in the creation in the late 1950s and early 1960s of the science of reanimatology [6] from which we are the

heirs. These pioneers and subsequent generations of clinicians have further increased this need for the concentration of skill sets, and transformed this diverse series of competencies into an integrated package of care that is now known as the art and science of critical care medicine (CCM).

The closed ICU

Until the 20th century, hospitals were places which offered a specialised space, where a doctor (or a team of doctors lead by a well known figure) admitted patients and visited them occasionally (rarely more that once every few days). Over time, the possibility to perform more complex and aggressive interventions to an increasingly older and sicker population, often with several co-morbidities, created the concept of team working: instead of isolated professionals working as individuals, teams were created, with a very clear leadership that soon evolved to yield multi-disciplinary and even multi-professional teams. The ICU, and the ICU professionals in particular, were pioneers in this movement, especially in Europe, where the concept of the closed ICU was created and flourished from the 1960s to the

1980s. During this period, the speciality grew inside the four walls of the ICU, developing and applying a significant body of knowledge, based primarily on a group of physiological principles that were applied at the bed-side, that progressed to allow specific therapies and – more important-ly – the development and definition of a unique group of knowledge and skills. It is very impor-tant to note that, since the early days, the need for accurate accounting and audit, became very clear. Thus, it soon became obvious that as im-portant as tracking the effects and outcomes of the diverse practices performed in the ICU, there was a need for rigorous criteria for admission and discharge from the ICU and for an accurate evaluation of the case-mix.

Today, a significant number of ICUs in Europe (and also in Australia and New Zealand) are directed by a full-time, fully trained intensiv-ist, leading a multi-professional team of experts in the field, able to provide 24 hours a day, 7 days a week all interventions potentially required by the patient. These professionals are also more and more involved in the management of unsta-ble patients outside the ICU [7–10] in a move-ment called by Ken Hillman "critical care with-out walls" [10]. In the United States the situation is slightly different, with a significant number of ICUs still using the so-called open model [11]. In this system, the care and therapy is often su-pervised by nurses and younger physicians (only sometimes with a mandatory or optional consul-tation with an intensive care professional), but under the direction and orientation of a primary physician, not member of the ICU permanent staff; it is paradoxically a system that the litera-ture suggests as providing less effective care [12].

The closed ICU and the need for objective admission criteria

Intensive care is an expensive and often-scarce resource, therefore ensuring that capacity is re-served for those most likely to benefit from it is very important. There is therefore a significant responsibility on the intensivist to triage patients appropriately so that those most likely to benefit are admitted, and those less likely to, are not. Of-ten, however, the situation is more complex. ICU is but one part of the patient journey that takes

in many differing parts of the hospital together with multiple professional consultations and in-terventions. ICU admission criteria must there-fore be able to cope with not just the sick emer-gency patient but often also the elective patient who has been planned even before hospital ad-mission.

The first scientific society to develop and publish guidelines for ICU admission and dis-charge was the Society of Critical Care Medicine (SCCM, in USA) in 1988 [13]. These guidelines were subsequently revised in 1999 [14] together with guidance on admission to adult intermedi-ate care units [15], and to guidelines for devel-oping admission and discharge policies for the paediatric intensive care unit [16]. Other socie-ties, such as the Canadian Critical Care Society, have also developed their own set of guidelines [17]. In Europe, despite the development of some national guidelines [18], no common European Guidelines have yet been published, a task that should be possibly undertaken by the European Society of Intensive Care Medicine.

The development of admission (and dis-charge) criteria is a very complex issue, full of ethical implications, both to the patient and to society. Being a potentially life-saving asset, an ICU bed is also a scarce and costly resource that should be used in the most cost-effective way. Consequently, all possible expertise should be used when deciding as to whether a certain pa-tient should, or should not, be admitted to an ICU, a decision that is notoriously difficult to get right with any precision [19]. Usually, several ob-jective and subjective factors – both ICU-related and patient-related – have an impact on this de-cision, such as the number of beds available, the admission diagnosis, the severity of illness, age and operative status [20].

In a recent multicentre study in France, Maité Garrouste-Orgeas demonstrated that the decision to deny ICU admission to a certain patient was common (23.8%), explained both by the patient being too well to benefit (55.4%), too sick to ben-efit (37.2%), the unit is too busy (6.5%), and/or there is refusal by the family (0.7%). The same authors demonstrated in a multivariate analysis that the two patient-related factors more strong-ly associated with ICU refusal were dependency and metastatic cancer and that the most impor-tant organizational factors were the unit's fullness, the specific centre, phone rather than face-to-face referral, and daytime admission (OR, 0.52; 95% CI, 0.32–0.84) [21]. The organization of the health care system inside a certain region plays an important role, since when a hospital is lacking a bed to admit a patient that may eventually meet criteria for ICU admission, a system should be in place to find an ICU bed for that patient, as it is very clear that the survival of a patient with critical illness is completely different inside or outside an ICU [22, 23]. Despite these facts, in the SAPS 3 study almost two thirds of the admissions were classified as unplanned [24]. What is clear is that general outcome prediction models, given their probabilistic nature, should not be used exclusively to make this decision [25–27].

Usually, intensivists, still based mainly on the 1999 SCCM recommendations [14], use a combination of the following prioritizing criteria:

- **Priority 1** is assigned to patients who are critically ill, unstable, in need of intensive treatment and monitoring that cannot be provided outside of the ICU. No limits are generally placed on the extent of the therapy that these patients can receive. This category should also include patients where brain death is diagnosed, or expected, in order to optimise the quality of the organs retrieved [28];
- **Priority 2** is assigned to patients who are requiring intensive monitoring, and may potentially need immediate intervention. This category includes, for instance, patients who are at risk concerning intubation and invasive mechanical ventilation. No therapeutic limits are generally placed for these patients;
- **Priority 3** is assigned to patients with underlying disease and/or acute illness with a reduced likelihood of recovery. Due to their long-term outcome, they may receive intensive treatment to relieve acute illness, but limits on therapeutic efforts may be set;
- **Priority 4** is assigned to those who are generally not appropriate for ICU admission, either because they are "too well to benefit" or "too sick to benefit". This level also includes those patients who have the capacity to make decisions and who decide to refuse aggressive interventions, although they still require 'comfort' care at a level not deliverable on a normal ward setting.

Given the uncertainty of all these decisions, several authors have proposed in recent years to patients with very severe disease, especially to those with cancer, that the so called "ICU trial" be used; in other words, patients are admitted and fully treated for a limited period of time and then reassessed for the continuation of life-sustaining therapy [29, 30]. If the patient is not benefiting from the ICU care, then appropriate decisions with regards end-of-life-care should be made, according to the state of the art, the law, and religious preferences, a process quite heterogeneous in different cultures [31–34].

Other prioritizing models have been proposed but are used less often, such as the diagnosis model (which uses specific conditions or diseases to determine appropriateness of ICU admission) and the objective parameters model (which uses a long list of arbitrary criteria) [14]. Also, for situations where the demand of intensive care could largely exceed the supply of intensive care services in a short period of time, as happened during SARS in Hong-Kong [35] and in Toronto [36], or in certain places of the world during the recent pandemic influenza A (H1N1)v [37, 38], contingency plans should exist in anticipation for both the need to increase the capacity of intensive care services and also for triage of patients that could benefit more from ICU admission, ideally based on objective and pre-defined criteria [39, 40].

The closed ICU and the need for objective discharge criteria

During the ICU stay, all the patients must be continuously evaluated for the need to remain in the ICU. According to consensus definitions, a discharge decision should be taken *"when a patient's physiologic status has stabilized and the need for ICU monitoring and care is no longer necessary"* [14]. However, this issue is more complex than it seems at first glance. Since the 1980s, many published outcome studies have presented data both on vital status at intensive care unit (ICU) discharge and also at hospital discharge. Consequently, it has become clear that a significant number of patients either deteriorated or died following ICU discharge but before leaving the hospital (the so-called post-ICU discharge mortality or occult mortality). Several published studies have raised attention to the magnitude of this phenomenon that can be as high as 36.7% of all deaths [24]. Some patients deteriorate and then need to be re-admitted to the ICU often soon after ICU discharge [41–44], again a common phenomenon, and one which carries with it a large associated mortality [45].

Until the early 2000s, little research was published about the main determinants of post-ICU mortality. The fact that these deaths occurred after discharge from the ICU leads many authors to look for factors out of the ICU sphere [46]. In the beginning of this decade, Smith et al. [47] refocused the problem raising the hypothesis that the problem lies in the ICU, or more precisely in an inappropriate discharge of some patients from the ICU to the ward. Based on a small cohort of patients from one centre, the authors concluded that a high demand for nursing activities, such as that measured by the therapeutic intervention scoring system (TISS) at ICU discharge was associated with an increased risk of in-hospital mortality and that this group of patients should eventually be transferred to a high dependency unit (HDU), since the amount of nursing workload required by them at discharge from the ICU could not be provided in the general ward [48]. However, when Moreno studied the issue based on data from the EURICUS-II study, he was able to demonstrate in a multivariate analysis that the need for high nursing-workload use was just a (non-significant) proxy for the amount of residual organ dysfunction/failure presented by the patient at ICU discharge [49]. Similar results have also been found by others [45]. Even today, organizational factors remain important, with a high percentage of patients still being discharged in an unplanned way (8.15%), i.e., without at least a 12-hour planning window [24], or at night and weekends, a fact that seems to be also associated with a higher post-ICU discharge mortality [50, 51], a phenomenon also described for in-hospital cardiac arrests [52]. However there is still controversy here, and the issue is not yet closed [53, 54].

A pragmatic rule would be to decide to discharge a patient when the amount of residual organ dysfunction is low and can thus be met by the facility that will receive the patient after discharge [55, 56]. An alternative view is that discharge can be allowed after a consensus has been reached that further intensive care is unlikely to lead to further benefit and the patient should be allowed to die [29]. In this process, the clinician responsible for the decision to transfer a patient from the ICU, especially when under pressure due to the need to admit another patient waiting for an intensive care bed – that can result in a premature discharge of the patient – should balance and weigh the contract he has made with the patient that is already been cared in the ICU with the rights of a patient, still outside the ICU. In this issue, at the cutting edge of medical ethics, the value of the individual and the need for distributive justice could eventually clash, forcing the physician to take complex decisions [57]. In any case, more and better dialogue around the discharge process is needed, since errors in this process happen in almost one third of all cases [58]. There is an important role for developing systems that enable care to be provided by intensive care trained clinicians in the ward following ICU discharge, such as critical care outreach teams, to allow earlier identification of the patients that are deteriorating [59]. There is also a role for improving our understanding with regards patient processes and flows [60] in order to make early discharge safer [61].

Conclusions

The decisions to admit patients to and discharge them from ICU are extremely complex and depend on multiple variables, some regarding the patient, some the health care professional and some the organization and the health care system. There is an urgent need to improve these processes, by defining European guidelines for ICU admission and discharge and by optimizing the processes involved in the interface of the ICU and the ward, both before and after ICU discharge. These rules should balance the duties and rights of the patients already in the ICU, while keeping the balance with the increasing number of patients that, due to eventual present and future shortages of ICU resources, have an equal right to share the benefits of ICU admission and discharge at the right moment in their disease process, in what John McMillan and Tony Hope called recently the "Justice-based obligations in intensive care" [57].

The authors

Rui P. Moreno, MD, PhD[1]
Andrew Rhodes, FRCP FRCA[2]
[1] Unidade de Cuidados Intensivos
Polivalente | Hospital de Santo António
dos Capuchos | Centro Hospitalar de Lisboa
Central, E.P.E. | Lisbon, Portugal
[2] General Intensive Care | St George's
Hospital | London, UK

Address for correspondence
Rui P. Moreno
Unidade de Cuidados Intensivos Polivalente
Hospital de Santo António dos Capuchos
Centro Hospitalar de Lisboa Central, E.P.E.
Alameda de Santo António dos Capuchos
1169-050 Lisbon, Portugal
E-mail: r.moreno@mail.telepac.pt

References

1. Lassen HCA. A preliminary report on the 1952 epidemic of poliomyelitis in Copenhagen with special reference to the treatment of acute respiratory insufficiency. Lancet 1953;1:37–41.
2. Ibsen B. The anaesthetist's viewpoint on the treatment of respiratory complications in poliomyelitis during the epidemic in Copenhagen, 1952. Proc R Soc Med 1954;47:72–4.
3. Nightingale F. Notes on hospitals. 3rd ed. London: Longman, Green, Longman, Roberts, and Green, 1863:89.
4. Takala J. Organisation of intensive care. In: Kuhlen R, Moreno R, Ranieri M, Rhodes A, eds. 25 Years of Progress and Innovation in Intensive Care Medicine. Berlin: Medizinisch Wissenschaftliche Verlagsgesell-schaft, 2007:343–50.
5. Negovsky VA. Some Physiopathologic Regularities in the Process of Dying and Resuscitation. Circ Metab Cerveau 1961;23:452–7.
6. Negovsky VA. Essays on Reanimatology. Moscow: MIR Publishers, 1986
7. Hourihan F, Bishop GF, Hillman KM, Daffurn K, Lee AJ. The medical emergency team: a new strategy to identify and intervene in high-risk patients. Clin Intensive Care 1995;6:269–72.
8. Lee AJ, Bishop GF, Hillman KM, Daffurn K. The Medical Emergency Team. Anaesthesia and Intensive Care Medicine 1995;23:183–6.
9. Hillman K, Parr M, Flabouris A, Bishop G, Stewart A. Redefining in-hospital resuscitation: the concept of the medical emergency team. Resuscitation 2001;48:105–10.
10. Hillman K. Critical care without walls. Curr Opin Crit Care 2002;8:594–9.
11. Capuzzo M, Valentin A, Alvisi R. Open versus closed units. In: Chice J-D, Moreno R, Putensen C, Rhodes A, eds. Patient Safety and Quality of Care In Intensive Care Medicine. Berlin: Medizinisch Wissenschaftiche Verlagsgesellschaft, 2009:177–88.
12. Pronovost P, Angus DC, Dorman T, Robinson KA, Dremsizov TT, Young TL. Physician Staffing Patterns and Clinical Outcomes in Critically Ill Patients. A Systematic Review. JAMA 2002;288:2151–62.
13. Task Force on Guidelines. Society of Critical Care Medicine. Recommendations for intensive care unit admission and discharge criteria. Crit Care Med 1988;16:807–8.
14. Task Force on Guidelines. Society of Critical Care Medicine. Recommendations for intensive care unit admission and discharge criteria. Crit Care Med 1999;27:633–8.
15. Nasraway SA, Cohen IL, Dennis RC, Howenstein MA, Nikas D, Warren J, Wedel S, American College of Critical Care Medicine of the Society of Critical Care Medicine. Guidelines on admission and discharge for adult intermediate care units. Crit Care Med 1998;26:607–10.
16. American Academy of Pediatrics Committee on Hospital Care and Section on Critical Care, Society of Critical Care Medicine Pediatric Section Admission Criteria Task Force. Guidelines for Developing Admission and Discharge Policies for the Pediatric Intensive Care Unit. Pediatrics 1999;193:840–2.
17. Canadian Critical Care Society. Critical care Unit/ Program/Dept. Statement of Service and admission and discharge policy. 2000.
18. Gruppo di studio ad hoc della Commissione di Bioetica della Società Italiana di Anestesia Analgesia Rianimazione e Terapia Intensiva. SIAARTI guidelines for admission to and discharge from Intensive Care Units and for the limitation of treatment in intensive care. Minerva Anestesiol 2003;69:101–18.
19. Joynt GM, Gomersall CD, Tan PSK, Lee A, Cheng CAY, Wong ELY. Prospective evaluation of patients refused admission to an intensive care unit: triage, futility and outcome. Intensive Care Med 2001;27:1459–65.
20. Sprung CL, Geber D, Eidelman LA, Baras M, Pizov R, Nimrod A, Oppenheim A, Epstein L, Cotev S. Evaluation of triage decisions for intensive care admission. Crit Care Med 1999;27.
21. Garrouste-Orgeas M, Montuclard L, Timsit J-F, Reignier J, Desmettre T, Karoubi P, Moreau D, Montesino L, Duguet A, Boussat S, Ede C, Monseau Y, Paule T, Misset B, Carlet J, for the French ADMISSIONREA Study Group. Predictors of intensive care unit refusal in French intensive care units: A multiple-center study. Crit Care

Med 2005;33:750–5 10.1097/01. CCM.0000157752.26180.F1.

22. Simchen E, Sprung CL, Galai N, Zitser-Gurevich Y, Bar-Lavi Y, Gurman G, Klein M, Lev A, Levi L, Zveibil F, Mandel M, Mnatzaganian G. Survival of critically ill patients hospitalized in and out of intensive care units under paucity of intensive care unit beds. Crit Care Med 2004;32:1654–61.

23. Simchen E, Sprung CL, Galai N, Zitser-Gurevich Y, Bar-Lavi Y, Levi L, Zveibil F, Mandel M, Mnatzaganian G, Goldschmidt N, Ekka-Zohar A, Weiss-Salz I. Survival of critically ill patients hospitalized in and out of intensive care. Crit Care Med 2007;35:449

24. Metnitz PG, Moreno RP, Almeida E, Jordan B, Bauer P, Campos RA, Iapichino G, Edbrooke D, Capuzzo M, Le Gall JR, SAPS 3 Investigators. SAPS 3. From evaluation of the patient to evaluation of the intensive care unit. Part 1: Objectives, methods and cohort description. Intensive Care Med 2005;31:1336–44.

25. Suter P, Armagandis A, Beaufils F, Bonfill X, Burchardi H, Cook D, Fagot-Lereault A, Thijs L, Vesconi S, William A. Predicting outcome in ICU patients: consensus conference organized by the ESICM and the SRLF. Intensive Care Med 1994;20:390–7.

26. Vincent J-L, Moreno R. Clinical review: Scoring systems in the critically ill. Crit Care 2010;14.

27. Moreno R, Metnitz P. Severity Scoring Systems: Tools for the Evaluation of Patients and Intensive Care Units. In: Parrillo JE, Dellinger RP, eds. Principles of Diagnosis and Management in the Adult, 3rd Edition. Philadelphia: Mosby, Elsevier, 2008:1547–65.

28. Najafizadeh K, Shadmehr MB, Daneshvar A, Malekmohammad M, Arab M, Ahmadi ZH, Shafaghi SH, Ghorbani F, Assari S, Moghani-Lankarani M. Lung donation and causes behind its failure: a single-center experience. Tranplant Proc 2009;41:2726–8.

29. Lecuyer L, Chevret S, Thiery G, Darmon M, Schlemmer B, Azoulay E. The ICU Trial: A new admission policy for cancer patients requiring mechanical ventilation. Crit Care Med 2007;35:808–14.

30. Azoulay E, Bele N, Thiery G, Schlemmer B. An alternative to refusing ICU admission of cancer patients. In: Kuhlen R, Moreno R, Ranieri M, Rhodes A, eds. 25 Years of Progress and Innovation in Intensive Care Medicine. Berlin: Medizinisch Wissenschaftliche Verlagsgesellschaft, 2007:449–58.

31. Azoulay E, Metnitz B, Sprung C-L, Timsit J-F, Lemaire F, Bauer P, Schlemmer B, Moreno R, Metnitz P. End-of-life practices in 282 intensive care units: data from the SAPS 3 database. Intensive Care Med 2009;35:623–30.

32. Sprung CL, Woodcock T, Sjokvist P, Ricou B, Bulow H-H, Lippert A, Maia P, Cohen S, Baras M, Hovilehto S, Ledoux D, Phelan D, Wennberg E, Schobersberger W. Reasons, considerations, difficulties and documentation of end-of-life decisions in European intensive care units: the ETHICUS Study. Intensive Care Med 2008;34:271–7.

33. Bülow H-H, Sprung C-L, Reinhart K, Prayag S, Du B, Armaganidis A, Abrouq F, Levy MM. The world's major religions' points of view on end-of-life decisions in the intensive care unit. Intensive Care Med 2008;34:423–30.

34. Randall Curtis J. End-of-life care for patients in the Intensive Care Unit. In: Kuhlen R, Moreno R, Ranieri M, Rhodes A, eds. 25 Years of Progress and Innovation in Intensive Care Medicine. Berlin: Medizinisch Wissenschaftliche Verlagsgesellschaft, 2007:469–79.

35. Tsang KW, Ho PL, Ooi GC, Yee WKS, Wang T, Chan-Yeung M, Lam WK, Seto WH, Yam LY, Cheung TM, Wong PC, Lam B, Ip MS, Chan J, Yuen KY, Lai KN. A Cluster of Cases of Severe Acute Respiratory Syndrome in Hong Kong. N Engl J Med 2003;348:1977–85.

36. Skowronski DM, Petric M, Daly P, Parker RA, Bryce E, Doyle PW, Noble MA, Roscoe DL, Tomblin J, Yang TC, Krajden M, Patrick DM, Pourbohloul B, Goh SH, Bowie WR, Booth TF, Tweed SA, Perry TL, McGeer A, Brunham RC. Coordinated response to SARS, Vancouver, Canada. Emerging Infectious Diseases 2006;12:55–8.

37. Rello J, Rodriguez A, Ibanez P, Socias L, Cebrian J, Marques A, Guerrero J, Ruiz-Santana S, Marquez E, del Nogal-Saez F, Alvarez-Lerma F, Martinez S, Ferrer M, Avellanas M, Granada R, Maravi-Poma E, Albert P, Sierra R, Vidaur L, Ortiz P, Prieto del Portillo I, Galvan B, Leon-Gil C, The H1N1 SEMICYUC working group. Intensive care adult patients with severe respiratory failure caused by Influenza A (H1N1) in Spain. Crit Care 2009;13.

38. Webb SAR, Seppelt IM, for the ANZIC Influenza Investigators. Pandemic (H1N1) 2009 influenza ("swine flu") in Australian and New Zealand intensive care. Crit Care Resusc. 2009;11:170–2.

39. Eastman N, Philips B, Rhodes A. Triaging for adult critical care in the event of overwhelming need. Intensive Care Med 2010;36.

40. Sprung CL, Zimmerman JL, Christian MD, Joynt GM, Hick JL, Taylor B, G. A. R, Sandrock C, Cohen R, Adini B. Recommendations for intensive care unit and hospital preparations for an influenza epidemic or mass disaster: summary report of the European Society of Intensive Care Medicine's Task Force for intensive care unit triage during an influenza epidemic or mass disaster. Intensive Care Med 2010;36.

41. Rosenberg AL, Hofer TP, Hayward RA, Strachan C, Watts CM. Who bounces back? Physiologic and other predictors of intensive care readmission. Crit Care Med 2001;29:511–8.

42. Hasan M. Readmission of patients to hospital: still ill defined and poorly understood. Int J Qual Health Care 2001;13:177–9.

43. Rubins HB, Moskowitz MA. Discharge decision-making in a medical intensive care unit. Identifying patients at high risk of unexpected death or unit readmission. Am J Med 1988;84:863–9.

44. Bhatia N, Gombar S, Gombar KK, Thapa D. Why Patients are Readmitted to ICU. Journal of Anaesthesiology Clinical Pharmacology 2010;26:91–3.

45. Metnitz PG, Fieux F, Jordan B, Lang T, Moreno R, Le Gall JR. Critically ill patients readmitted to intensive care units – lessons to learn? Intensive Care Med 2003;29:241–8.

46. Lawrence A, Havill JH. An audit of deaths occurring in hospital after discharge from the intensive care unit. Anaesth Intensive Care 1999;27:185–9.

47. Smith L, Orts CM, O'Neil I, Batchelor AM, Gascoigne AD, Baudouin SV. TISS and mortality after discharge from intensive care. Intensive Care Med 1999;25:1061–5.

48. Moreno R, Agthé D. ICU discharge decision-making: are we able to decrease post-ICU mortality? Intensive Care Medicine 1999;25:1035–6.

49. Moreno R, Miranda DR, Matos R, Fevereiro T. Mortality after discharge from intensive care: the impact of organ system failure and nursing workload use at discharge. Intensive Care Med 2001;27:999–1004.

50. Goldfrad C, Rowan K. Consequences of discharges from intensive care at night. Lancet 2000;355:1138–42.

51. Pilcher DV, Duke GJ, George C, Bailey MJ, Hart G. After-hours discharge from intensive care increases the risk of readmission and death. Anaesthesia and Intensive Care Medicine 2007;35:477–85.

52. Peberdy MA, Ornato JP, Larkin GL, Braithwaite RS, Kashner TM, Carey SM, Meaney PA, Cen L, Nadkarni VM, Praestgaard AH, Berg RA, for the National Registry of Cardiopulmonary Resuscitation Investigators. Survival From In-Hospital Cardiac Arrest During Nights and Weekends. JAMA 2008;299:785–92.

53. Arabi Y, Alshimemeri A, Taher S. Weekend and weeknight admissions have the same outcome of weekday admissions to an intensive care unit with onsite intensivist coverage. Crit Care Med 2006;34:605–11.

54. Morales IJ, Afessa B. Hospital mortality rate and length of stay in patients admitted at night to the intensive care unit. Crit Care Med 2003;31:858–63.

55. Iapichino G, Morabito A, Mistraletti G, Ferla L, Radrizzani D, Miranda RR. Determinants of post-intensive care mortality in high-level treated critically ill patients. Intensive Care Med 2003;29:1751–6.

56. Iapichino G, Attanasio A, Avalli L, Bassi E, Biffi C, Calappi E, Casiraghi ML, Ferrario P, Guarino A, Langer M, Marcora B, Panozzo M, Reschini G, Rotelli S, Sicignano A, Trivellato A, Vesconi S, Miranda DR. Rilevazione giornaliera di procedure come tracciante dell'utilizzo di risorse [Daily survey of procedures as markers of resources utilization]. Minerva Anestesiol 1996;62:289–96.

57. McMillan J, Hope T. The art of medicine. Justice-based obligations in intensive care. Lancet 2010;375.

58. Perren A, Conte P, De Bitonti N, Limoni C, Merlani P. From the ICU to the ward: cross-checking of the physician's transfer report by intensive care nurses. Intensive Care Med 2008;34:2054–61.

59. Ball C, Kirkby M, Williams S. Effect of the critical care outreach team on patient survival to discharge from hospital and readmission to critical care: non-randomised population based study. Br Med J 2003;327:1014-.

60. Rothen HU. Optimisation of patient process and workflow. In: Kuhlen R, Moreno R, Ranieri M, Rhodes A, eds. Controversies in Intensive Care Medicine. Berlin: Medizinisch Wissenschaftiche Verlagsgesellschaft, 2008:323–36.

61. Hiesmayr M, Schmidlin D. Early discharge from the ICU is safe. In: Kuhlen R, Moreno R, Ranieri M, Rhodes A, eds. Controversies in Intensive Care Medicine. Berlin: Medizinisch Wissenschaftiche Verlagsgesellschaft, 2008:343–51.

Albertus Beishuizen and Armand R.J. Girbes

Interfacing the ICU with the next of kin

Introduction

Although the interest of the patient is the primary focus of ICU physicians, interfacing with family is an important part of the job for intensivists and ICU nurses. Admission of a patient in the ICU means by definition that vital functions are in peril and thus, the patient's life is seriously at risk. This is obviously an enormous and threatening event for all those who have a close relationship with the patient. Additionally, the ICU is an awe-inspiring environment for laypersons, and even for doctors not used to working in an ICU. Another important feature is the absolute loss of control of the patient and their relatives over the patient's life. The patients seem totally dependent on the ICU healthcare workers, machines and monitors. The ICU also generally is a noisy environment, with beeps all the time and everywhere, visible alarms on the monitor and nurses and doctors walking on and off, having mysterious conversations using a strange jargon.

It is evident that the patient is the most important person in the ICU, being the 'suffering person' to be cared for. Next of kin are a very important, probably even vital, source of emotional and psychological support, as they can motivate the patient to struggle for survival.

The life situation of the next of kin may change abruptly when their family member is admitted to an ICU, into what is often referred to as a disrupted emotional state characterised by feelings of uncertainty and anxiety, which makes them vulnerable to reduced mental and physical functioning during the ICU period [1].

Family satisfaction in the intensive care unit

The critical care community has shown an increasing interest in the needs of families, recognising that satisfaction with ICU care may be variable [2–5]. The most common and recurrent complaint is poor communication with clinicians [2, 4, 6]. Other factors related to family satisfaction are quality of care, proper meeting rooms, liberal visiting hours, adequate pain management, compassion, courtesy and respect, provision of information and effective communication and the ability to identify and meet the clinicians [2–4, 7]. In several studies the families of patients dying in the ICU reported higher satisfaction with their ICU experience than the families of survivors and the greatest differences were noted for care aspects directly affecting family members. Significant differences were also found for inclusion in decision-making, communication, emotional support, respect and compassion shown toward family, and consideration of family needs [8]. Therefore, efforts to improve support for next of kin in the ICU should focus not only on the families of dying patients but also on the families of patients who survive their ICU stay.

In a prospective cohort study in 6 ICUs across Canada most family members appeared to be highly satisfied with general ICU care and with overall decision-making [4]. Families were least satisfied with waiting room atmosphere and frequency of clinician communication. The main determinants of overall satisfaction were the completeness of information received, respect and compassion shown to patients and families and the amount of healthcare provided. Therefore, factors related to communication and decision-making are most strongly related to satisfaction. Education and training of clinicians' communication skills is one aspect to target in order to improve satisfaction; however, sufficient time to talk to families should be available and most often repeated family-clinician meetings are mandatory [9].

Assessing family needs and satisfaction with ICU care must be part of quality assessments in the ICU [10].

ICU family conferences

Clinician-family communication is central in medical decision-making in the ICU and may have a profound impact on the experience and long-term mental health of the next of kin. To improve this, clinician-family communication and structured ICU family conferences are essential [11]. Conducting these conferences within 72 hours of ICU admission is associated with reduced days in the ICU for patients who die and improved family experience or better assessment of the quality of communication [12, 13]. Other communication factors during these multidisciplinary meetings are: a private place for communication (family rooms), consistency in communication, empathy, time to listen, acknowledgment of family emotions, exploration and focus on patient values and treatment preferences, clear explanation of surrogate decision making, assurance to family members that the patient will not suffer. Five features to enhance clinician-fam-

ily communication have been combined into a mnemonic: VALUE (Value family statements, Acknowledge family emotions, Listen to the family, Understand the patient as a person, and Elicit family questions), which has been applied to improve clinician-family communication and was associated with a reduction of family symptoms of depression, anxiety and post-traumatic stress disorder after a patient died in the ICU [14].

During family conferences, physicians are more likely to effectively discuss issues regarding prognosis (for both quality of life and for survival) with next of kin [15].

Another key element in family conferences is multidisciplinary involvement, such as nurse-physician communication. Improved interdisciplinary communication is associated with less symptoms of depression and anxiety among next of kin, and even with better clinical patient outcomes [16]. Interdisciplinary communication is a key element of end-of-life care in the ICU, which could even be improved when an interdisciplinary intervention was included [13, 17].

Care of families in the intensive care unit: Spiritual care and empowerment

Spiritual care is increasingly recognised as a quality domain for critically ill patients and, in particular, their families. Next of kin were more satisfied with spiritual care if a pastor or spiritual advisor was involved in the last 24 hours of the patient's life [8]. Also, there appeared to be a marked association between satisfaction with spiritual care and satisfaction with the total ICU experience. Spiritual needs of families of patients who are dying in the ICU should be part of an integrative approach. Family satisfaction with ICU care is much higher if these spiritual needs are properly addressed and if spiritual care is provided, such as by hospital pastors [18]. In this respect, cultural competence in communication should be enhanced by exploring cultural beliefs, addressing language barriers, explicit discussion of religion and spirituality and sometimes involvement of religious or family leaders [19]. Use of interpreters in specific cases may be of value, however, even then miscommunication may occur. Pre-conference preparation to inform the interpreter and debriefing in such a cross-cultural setting may help to limit errors in communication [20].

ICU admissions influence entire family structures and the family influences the way severe illness is experienced. Next of kin play important roles in regard to ICU patients' illnesses and they should be considered in direct patient care as their presence may improve feelings of security (inner calmness), protection and well-being. Well-informed next of kin are a valuable resource for both patients and the ICU team as they can transfer knowledge about the patient, calm down the patient and create a link between the patient and reality [21]. Considering the high level of stress the next of kin is exposed to it may be difficult for them to support the patient. Next of kin empowerment, defined as a process to develop a sense of inner strength through connection with others or a model through which strengths and strategies may be developed, was found to be associated with a caring atmosphere providing human warmth and sensitivity [22].

Next of kin experienced the ability to be close to their severely ill family member to be of utmost importance and they were empowered when they felt welcome all the time. Other factors related to the perception of empowerment by next of kin were the quality of information (straightforward, honest), possibility to feel hope, support from other family members, being involved in the care for the patient, and reliance on medical care.

A healing and caring environment should be built, consisting of respectful norms among patients, next of kin and the ICU staff, in addition to a focus on the physical aspects such as light, colour, planning, sound and pictures [23]

Family tutor

Relatives of ICU patients often experience a sudden change in their situation which may be described as a disrupted emotional state (shock and chaos), in particular when they are confronted with a life-threatening situation. They experience feelings of uncertainty, anxiety and often feel powerless at being unable to help the patient and being forced to rely on healthcare professionals. Little is known about what is supportive in these situations from the perspective of the relatives;

however, empowerment through both internal and external resources is essential. Relatives should cope with the situation in their own way, but external support may also be of great value, although data on the experiences of next of kin and optimisation of family care in the ICU are scarce. In general, a warm and positive atmosphere with good relations and sensitivity are essential, as well as closeness to the patient, nursing staff availability at the bedside, and support from the ICU team. Family tutors are primarily focused on the family and they can also take care, apart from emotional issues, of practical and logistical issues with advice and appropriate actions. Family tutors might therefore fill the gap between the medical ICU team and the next of kin, primarily focusing on family support, creating the right atmosphere, caring, taking time to talk and listen to them, offering kindness, providing practical information and guidance (where to sit, about touching the patient and talking to the patient, where to rest, where to eat, etc.) [5]. Family tutors will be present during family visiting hours and take care of the next of kin of new admissions who are often in great distress. They will not replace nursing and medical staff, who often lack the time to give maximum family support, but are adjunctive, approaching the families with compassion, respect and human warmth. Family tutors, who often lack a medical background, will not provide information on medical care and details, but can be present during family conferences if desired by the next of kin.

Psychiatric illnesses in the next of kin of intensive care patients

Symptoms of anxiety and depression are very common in the relatives of critically ill patients [16, 24]. Contributing factors include worry about the patient and the pressure of being involved in decisions about withholding or withdrawing life support [25]. In addition, inadequate communication, unprofessional or disrespectful behaviour by healthcare professionals, frequent rotations, inadequate meeting facilities, and restrictive visiting policies may add to the development of symptoms of anxiety, depression, and post-traumatic stress, which may persist even after discharge from the ICU [2, 6, 26, 27]. Beyond relatively mild symptoms, the prevalence of fully developed psychiatric illness in next of kin appears to be high during and after the ICU stay. The next of kin would be at particular risk for diagnosable psychiatric illness following a loved one's death. Using structured clinical interviews in a cohort of next of kin, 3–12 months after a relative's death in a medical ICU, over 30 % suffered from at least one psychiatric illness (mainly depression, anxiety disorder or complicated grief disorder) and one-forth had major depression [18, 28]. Specific features of the ICU experience are likely to predispose bereaved next of kin to psychiatric illness. Death is often sudden and unexpected, leaving next of kin psychologically unprepared. Dying ICU patients often experience troubling symptoms, such as pain and dyspnoea [7], which can upset relatives and contribute to psychiatric morbidity. Conflicts with the medical staff, often related to poor communication or unprofessional behaviour, can also upset family members. During family meetings, ICU physicians often fail to listen and respond to the needs of next of kin [29]. Because most patients lack decision-making capacity, next of kin, in many countries, often play a major role in end-of-life decision-making. It has been acknowledged that this may contribute to the risk of psychiatric morbidity [7, 29]. In some studies psychiatric symptoms are more prevalent when patients die after end-of-life decisions [25], whilst in others no relation with withdrawal of treatment was found when family participation in end-of-life decisions was standard [28]. Psychiatric symptoms may not be related to the decision process itself but rather to how family meetings are conducted [2, 11, 13, 29]. Risk factors associated with the development of psychiatric illness include: being the patient's spouse, experiencing other major stress events after the loss, illness lasting less than five years, and failure to consider the clinician a source of comfort. Empathic care, in combination with optimal communication and listening skills may limit the psychiatric burden [14, 30].

Next of kin and end-of-life care

End-of-life care in the ICU comprises a high level of expertise, knowledge and competence, and several recommendations have been developed to improve care of ICU patients during the transition from cure to comfort and through the dying process [31]. Increasingly, the ICU has become the place to die. In the USA 22 % of all deaths occur in the ICU [32]. Family-centred care is pivotal in managing end-of-life care acknowledging the social structure within which ICU patients are embedded. Most patients in the ICU are not able to make decisions for themselves and most decisions are made by surrogates on their behalf using the 'substituted judgment standard' or the 'best interest standard'. Legal guidelines regarding end-of-life decisions vary strongly between the various countries; however, in the majority the next of kin are involved in shared decision-making. In Europe end-of-life decisions are primarily based on opinions and expertise of physicians rather than on the wishes of patients and their families, which is considered by some as paternalism. In the USA, a sharp focus prevails on patient autonomy, or self-determination. In any case, families should be offered sufficient time to reach decisions based on optimal information and recommendations by the physicians. End-of-life consensus decisions are for the most part reached when proper communication between clinicians and surrogates/next of kin has taken place. However, conflicts between clinicians and next of kin may arise, such as when families insist on interventions or life-sustaining treatment while the physician considers this inadvisable. In dealing with these conflicts, clarity about the goals of care should be obtained and clearly defined. Consequently, in such a situation the next of kin should express what they hope to achieve: extending life, pain relief or restoring health. Then clinicians can and should provide clear information on prognostication [33]. Regarding family conferences it was noted that in one third of those meetings prognosis for survival was not discussed [15]. In addition, less educated families received less prognostic information. Family members of ICU patients want and should receive clear information about the prognosis of their loved ones, in order to allow them to plan for the future and to participate in treatment decisions in agreement with the patient's values.

Conclusions

Critical care is complex and lacks certainty about outcome in individual patients. The approach to ICU patients and their next of kin has shifted from paternalism to provision of clear, consistent and straightforward information, and their inclusion in the decision-making process. It is important to acknowledge that the family is part of the total team that takes care of the patient, thus offering a way to cope with the situation where dependence on others seems to prevail. Communication with family is of utmost importance and requires extensive training and interdisciplinary teamwork. The quality of communication with the next of kin is determined by effective discussion of prognostication, the setting of multidisciplinary family conferences and the assessment of spiritual needs and cross-cultural barriers. Factors related to communication and decision-making have the strongest impact on family satisfaction. A warm and positive atmosphere appears to be of greatest importance to next of kin. Empowerment of the next of kin is successful when the ICU staff displays a genuine interest and care for the next of kin as well as the patient. Major psychiatric illness, particularly major depressive disorder, is common after the death of a loved one in the ICU. Early recognition and appropriate action and anticipation is therefore desirable.

The authors

Albertus Beishuizen, MD, PhD[1]
Armand R.J. Girbes, MD, PhD[2]
   [1]Consultant in Intensive Care | Department of Intensive Care | University Hospital VU Medical Center | Amsterdam, The Netherlands
   [2]Professor in Intensive Care Medicine | Department of Intensive Care | University Hospital VU Medical Center | Amsterdam, The Netherlands

Address for correspondence
   Armand R.J. Girbes
   Department of Intensive Care
   University Hospital VU Medical Center
   P.O. Box 7057
   1007 MB Amsterdam, The Netherlands
   E-mail: arj.girbes@vumc.nl

References

1. Johansson I, Fridlund B, Hildingh C. What is supportive when an adult next-of-kin is in critical care? Nurs Crit Car 2005;10:289–298.

2. Abbott KH, Sago JG, Breen CM, et al: Families looking back: One year after discussion of withdrawal or withholding of life-sustaining support. Crit Care Med 2001;29:197–201.

3. Nelson JE, Angus DC, Weissfeld LA, et al. End-of-life care for the critically ill: A national intensive care unit survey. Crit Care Med 2006;34:2547–2553.

4. Heyland DK, Rocker GM, Dodek PM, et al. Family satisfaction with care in the intensive care unit: results of a multiple center study. Crit Care Med 2002;30:1413-1418.

5. Davidson JE, Powers K, Hedayat KM, et al. Clinical practice guidelines for support of the family in the patient-centered intensive care unit: American College of Critical Care Task Force 2004–2005. Crit Care Med 2007; 35:605-622.

6. Azoulay E, Chevret S, Leleu G, et al: Half the families of intensive care unit patients experience inadequate communication with physicians. Crit Care Med 2000;28:3044–3049.

7. Levy CR, Ely EW, Payne K, et al. Quality of dying and death in two medical ICUs — Perceptions of family and clinicians. Chest 2005;127:1775–1783.

8. Wall RJ, Engelberg RA, Gries CJ, et al. Spiritual care of families in the intensive care unit. Crit Care Med 2007;35:1084–1090.

9. Quill TE, Townsend P. Bad news: delivery, dialogue and dilemmas. Arch Int Med 1991;151:463–468.

10. Burck R. Family satisfaction surveys to improve the fit between the ICU and its concept. Crit Care Med 2002;30:1650–1651.

11. Curtis JR, White DB. Practical guidance for evidence-based ICU family conferences. Chest 2008;134:835–843.

12. Glavan BJ, Engelberg RA, Downey L, et al. Using the medical record to evaluate the quality of end-of-life care in the intensive care unit. Crit Care Med 2008; 36:1138-1146.

13. Lilly CM, De Meo DL, Sonna LA, et al. An intensive communication intervention for the critically ill. Am J Med 2000;109:469–475.

14. Lautrette A, Darmon M, Megarbane B, et al. A communication strategy and brochure for relatives of patients dying in the ICU. N Engl J Med 2007; 356:469-478.

15. White DB, Engelberg RA, Wenrich MD, et al. Prognostication during physician-family discussions about limiting life support in intensive care units. Crit Care Med 2007;35:442–448.

16. Pochard F, Azoulay E, Chevret S, et al. Symptoms of anxiety and depression in family members of intensive care unit patients: Ethical hypothesis regarding decision-making capacity. Crit Care Med 2001;29:1893–1897.

17. Campbell ML, Guzman JA. Impact of a proactive approach to improve end-of-life care in a medical ICU. Chest 2003;123:266–271.

18. Gries CJ, Curtis JR, Wall RJ, Engelberg RA. Family member satisfaction with end-of-life decision making in the ICU. Chest 2008;133:704–712.

19. Kagawa-Singer M, Blackhall LJ. Negotiating cross-cultural issues at the end of life: "You got to go where he lives". JAMA 2001;286:2993–3001.

20. Pham K, Thornton JD, Engelberg RA, et al. Alterations during medical interpretation of ICU family conferences that interfere with or enhance communication. Chest 2008;134:109–116.

21. Williams C. The identification of family members' contribution to patients' care in the ICU: a naturalistic inquiry. Nurs Crit Care 2005;10:6–14.

22. Wahlin I, Ek A-C, Idvall E. Empowerment from the perspective of next of kin in intensive care. J Clin Nurs 2009;19:2580–2587.

23. Rushton CH. Respect in critical care. A foundational ethical principle. AACN Adv Crit Care 2007;18:149–156.

24. Pochard F, Darmon M, Fassier T, et al. Symptoms of anxiety and depression in family members of intensive care unit patients before discharge or death: A prospective multicenter study. J Crit Care 2005;20:90–96.

25. Azoulay E, Pochard F, Kentish-Barnes N, et al, Risk of post-traumatic stress symptoms in family members of intensive care unit patients. Am J Respir Crit Care Med 2005;171:987–994.

26. Young E, Eddleston J, Ingleby S, et al. Returning home after intensive care: A comparison of symptoms of anxiety and depression in ICU and elective cardiac surgery patients and their relatives. Intensive Care Med 2005;31:86–91.

27. Jones C, Skirrow P, Griffiths RD, et al. Post-traumatic stress disorder-related symptoms in relatives of patients following intensive care. Intensive Care Med 2004;30:456–460.

28. Siegel MD, Hayes E, Vanderwerker LC, et al. Psychiatric illness in the next of kin who die in the intensive care unit. Crit Care Med 2008;36:1722–1728.

29. Curtis JR, Engelberg RA, Wenrich MD, et al. Missed opportunities during family conferences about end-of-life care in the intensive care unit. Am J Respir Crit Care Med 2005; 171:844–849.

30. Lilly CM, Daly BJ. The healing power of listening in the ICU. N Eng J Med 2007;356:513–515.

31. Truog RD, Campbell ML, Curtis JR, et al. Recommendations for end-of-life care in the intensive care unit: a consensus statement by the American College of Critical Care Medicine. Crit Care Med 2008:36:953–963.

32. Angus DC, Barnato AE, Linde-Zwirble WT, et al. Use of Intensive Care at the end of life in the United States: an epidemiologic study. Crit Care Med 2004;32:638–643.

33. Back AL, Arnold RM, Quill TE. Hope for the best, and prepare for the worst. Ann Int Med 2003;138:439–443.

Anders Aneman

The rapid response system (management, organisation)

Clinically effective care?

Both patients treated in-hospital and their medical management are becoming increasingly complex. Furthermore, the demographic profile of patients indicates that age-induced limitation of physiological reserve is likely to be present in a majority of cases. Resource constraints along with demands for a high number of patients passing through hospitals result in patients being in advanced care areas, including the intensive care unit (ICU), for shorter periods of time. Discharge from ICU and high-dependency units to wards out of office hours has been demonstrated to increase the risk for adverse outcomes [1].

Studies in the UK, Australia, Canada and the USA estimate that adverse events, defined as poor outcomes caused by medical error and not progression of disease, occur in approximately 10% of hospitalised patients with a mortality of 5–10%. Up to half of these deaths are judged preventable [2–5]. A similar incidence and severity for adverse events have been reported in Europe [6–8]. The awareness of the rates for adverse events and the desire to participate in measures to reduce their incidence and consequences are the quintessential requirements to initiate changes to improve clinically effective care. All medical staff must share this conviction for a change of healthcare delivery to be successful.

The delivery of clinically effective care involves doing the right thing(s), in the right way, at the right time to the right patient. Very tangible results of failure to deliver such care comprise unplanned admissions to the ICU, cardiac arrests, unexpected deaths and omission of palliative care. The lack of organisation, knowledge and supervision, as well as failure to appreciate clinical urgency, result in less than optimal care in the time preceding ICU admission, which is a major contributor to ICU mortality [9, 10]. The level of care required rather than the location of care provided should prompt management as underlined in the notion "the ICU without walls" [11]. In addition to obvious matters such as nurse-to-patient ratios, access to specialist medical competence and level of patient monitoring, less apparent issues impeding clinically effective care might include hierarchic and undefined routes of communication as well as emotional, cultural or political obstacles.

Rapid response systems

A proposed solution to overcome some of the problems in delivering clinically effective care as outlined above has been the implementation of a rapid response system (RRS). A generic plan of the RRS is illustrated in Figure 1 [12]. All components of the RRS require thoughtful consideration from a management and organisational point of view. The afferent arm recognises the patient at risk for an in-hospital emergency using a set of criteria or triggers based on a monitoring strategy and provides a mechanism to alert a response. The efferent arm delivers the staff and equipment necessary to resolve the problem. Finally, components to ensure audit, governance and feedback mechanisms are important to promote education, manage resources and ensure sustainability of the RRS. All four components of the RRS may have variable designs and none have demonstrated unequivocal advantages. Furthermore, it remains unproven whether the effectiveness of an RRS, if indeed factual, relates to the whole system or any of the individual components. In the latter case, the design of single components may have different potential and cost-effectiveness to change clinical outcomes.

Several major stakeholders involved in hospital organisation and patient safety have adopted the generic RRS structure. In Australia, the "Safer Systems-Saving Lives" [13] and "Between the Flags" [14] initiatives are endorsed by the Victorian and New South Wales governments. In the UK, the Department of Health formally promoted an RRS with the publication of Comprehensive Critical Care [15] and the outreach service is supported by the national outreach forum [16]. In the USA, the Institute for Healthcare Improvement through its 100 k and 5 M lives campaigns recommended an RRS as an integral part of the improvement process [17]. In Canada, the government of Ontario has implemented an RRS throughout state hospitals [18]. In Denmark, an RRS was part of the "Operation Life" endorsed by the Danish Society for Patient Safety [19]. The European Resuscitation Council in their 2005 guidelines recommended that the introduction of an RRS should be considered in the adult in-hospital setting [20]. This recommendation may become less compelling following publication of the ongoing 2010 revisions (Dr. Michael Parr, *personal communication*). Most published studies on rapid response systems emanate from Anglo-American healthcare, with fewer publications originating from mainland Europe [21–23].

The afferent arm

A number of studies have demonstrated that premonitory signs of physiological instability are present for several hours preceding ultimate

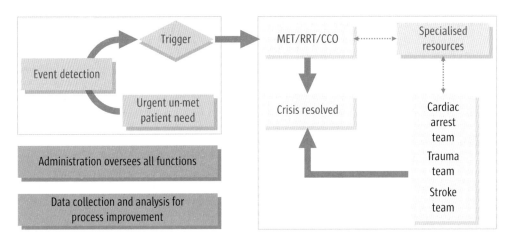

Fig. 1 A generic Rapid Response System (RRS) structure. Urgent un-met patient need(s) are detected by the afferent arm and triggers a systematic response. The efferent arm delivers the staff and equipment necessary to resolve the problem. Components to ensure audit, governance and feedback mechanisms are important to promote education, manage resources and sustainability of the RRS. [From Devita MA, Bellomo R, Hillman K et al. Findings of the first consensus conference on medical emergency teams. Crit Care Med 2006;34:2464 with kind permission.]

deterioration such as cardiac or respiratory arrest [24–26]. This provides a window of opportunity to intervene given greater potential for reversibility of disease when detected early rather than late. The organisation of the afferent arm needs to take into account monitoring strategy and which criteria should be used to determine when and how to alert a response. Ideally, any system to detect the patient at risk should be simple and quick, integrated in daily ward routines, and with a sensitivity and specificity sufficient to identify a condition while still amendable to therapeutic interventions and yet avoiding over-triage.

Documentation of vital signs is often incomplete and infrequent [27, 28]. This appears surprising since most medical staff would agree that such documentation is an integral part of standard care and does help identify patients at risk for adverse events [10, 29]. The introduction of an RRS has been demonstrated to improve assessment and documentation of vital signs, in particular for respiratory rate [30, 31]. An important aspect in organising the afferent arm is to consider which variables should and could be monitored, particularly for a hospital-wide RRS. The nurse-to-patient ratio and the technology available are likely to vary between ward areas. In addition, the appropriate clinical triggers may vary between medical and surgical patients [32, 33].

Documentation of heart rate, blood pressure, respiratory rate, and level of consciousness are common to most RRSs. In addition, pulse oximetry, urine output and occurrence of seizures are frequently incorporated. A subjective "worry" criterion is often used in addition to the objective vital signs in order to empower the staff to alert the RRS for a patient that causes significant concern although the objective criteria are not fulfilled. The "worried" criterion has been reported to represent close to one-third of the total number of RRS alerts, typically related to signs of respiratory distress. Most patients meeting the "worried" criterion still remained in a general ward area following review by the RRS team and significantly fewer patients meeting the "worried" criterion compared to any objective criteria ultimately progressed to cardiac arrest [34]. A high proportion of "worried" calls should also encourage RRS managers to survey training and education on trigger criteria. In a post-hoc analysis of the MERIT study (see

below, [72]), the "worried" criterion was found to trigger close to 40 % of RRS activations [35]. Such a high proportion of "worried" calls may reflect successful empowerment and vigilance of all staff to call the RRS, and to do this early in the disease before progression to overt physiological aberrations has occurred.

The trigger criteria for alerting a response should ideally be evaluated in terms of prevalence to estimate the impact on workload before the RRS is implemented. In one single-centre study using standard RRS calling criteria, the presence of deviating vitals signs in a cohort of 1,097 patients was associated with a 10-fold increase in mortality one month later [36]. A major increase in the potential workload for an RRS was demonstrated using extended criteria encompassing a wider physiological range, while the sensitivity to detect deaths within one month was actually decreased. A similar decrease in sensitivity was also observed using restricted criteria. This study, while not being able to assess the "worried" criterion, illustrates a useful prevalence study approach to tune physiological calling criteria before launching an RRS. Another study, using a nested matched case (n = 450) versus control (n = 520) design, demonstrated that the combination of heart rate (> 140), respiratory rate (> 36), systolic blood pressure (< 90 mm Hg) and a greater than two point reduction in GCS identified cardiac arrest, unplanned ICU admission or unexpected death with a specificity > 90 % but with a less than 50 % sensitivity and a less than 10 % positive predictive value. The best positive predictive value achievable by modifying cut-off values or by adding threatened airway and seizures to the criteria was still below 16 % [37]. In addition to single-parameter systems with defined threshold values, physiological track and trigger systems may also rely on multiple parameters, which are aggregated to give a weighted score, or combinations of such designs. There is no clear evidence to indicate which system is best and the extent to which existing systems are valid, and reliable tools for detecting patients at risk for deterioration remain largely undetermined. Significant variation in reproducibility, particularly for aggregate scores, has been reported [38]. A systematic review of track and trigger systems identified 25 distinct designs and highlighted limited adherence to methodological quality standards in 36 publications [39].

A consensus document on the afferent arm of the RRS has recently been published recommending a core set of physiological data to be monitored as outlined above. Assessments should be made at least every 12 hours and be easily available to clinical staff. The monitoring strategy should furthermore allow for modifications in terms of variables, frequency and response to meet individual patients' needs [40].

The Clinical Excellence Commission recently launched the Between the Flags programme as a safety net in all public hospitals in New South Wales to detect deteriorating patients on wards [14]. This initiative represents a second tier to the RRS with similar but lower thresholds to trigger a clinical review by the patient's parent ward team. The RRS team is not involved unless it is considered needed following initial assessment. The consequences of introducing a two-tiered RRS model remain to be evaluated.

The effectiveness of any RRS relies heavily on the performance of the afferent arm. This component deserves further research and needs careful consideration and continuous evaluation when organising and managing an RRS.

The efferent arm

Once the afferent arm of an RRS has detected a medical in-hospital emergency, the efferent arm operates to deliver adequate resources to meet the needs of the patient. Such resources may include staff with special training, experience and skills to support vital functions as well as equipment and means to escalate therapy if indicated. Similar to the case of the afferent arm, no universal design exists for the composition of the efferent limb.

In most RRSs, a team linked to the ICU represents the efferent arm. An intensivist-led team enables airway management, central venous access, and advanced therapy on a par with basic intensive care to be initiated bedside. The medical emergency team (MET) is typically based on such designs as reported from Australia/New Zealand, Canada and Denmark [13, 18, 19]. In the UK, critical care outreach teams are mainly nurse-based [41]. In the US, the team is usually nurse-led but may also include emergency or respiratory physicians or a hospitalist [17]. The organisation of the efferent limb needs to take into account that the team must be immediately available and its members can thus not have competing responsibilities. The level of care to be made available bedside must also be decided as well as what authority the team is empowered with to change plans for the management of the patient. This is particularly important if the team is to have admitting rights to the ICU or to authorise not-for-resuscitation (NFR) orders [42, 43]. The efferent arm may provide anything from advice on further medical management to the ward staff looking after the patient to decisive action on therapy including admission to the ICU or limitation of ongoing care. Furthermore, the hospital areas and the working hours the team should cover will also dictate resource allocation. The organisation of an RRS deploying a team to respond to medical emergencies in specified clinical areas out of office hours will obviously be very different from an RRS with hospital-wide cover 24 hours a day, seven days a week. In most institutions where an RRS has been introduced, the efferent arm is identical to or even replaces the cardiac arrest team.

A pivotal key to success of the efferent arm is effective, succinct and assertive communication. Breakdown of communication has been identified as a major problem within deterioration incidents [44]. Several structured ways to train and establish effective communication have been recommended, including the RSVP (Reason-Story-Vital Signs-Plan system) [45] and the SBAR (Situation-Background-Assessment-Recommendation) model [46]. The management of an RRS should include recommendations for and training in medical communication. This facet of the RRS is not clarified in many reports of the efferent arm. In general, the best model for training of the team representing the efferent arm has been sparsely investigated. The ALERT (Acute Life-Threatening Events Recognition and Treatment) [47–49] and CCrISP (Care of the Critically Ill Surgical Patient) [50] courses as well as high-fidelity computer simulations [51] represent various initiatives to standardise team competencies and attitudes. Sufficient knowledge and abilities in the areas pertinent to operating an RRS are pivotal for successful implementation.

Audit and governance

The fact that no detailed generic model for an RRS exists means that most hospitals will have to adopt RRS solutions that are tailored to meet local needs and resources. It is vital that appropriate systems for audit and governance are organised to document effectiveness, ensure sustainability and support further development of the RRS. The management of the RRS should thus include identified responsibilities to collate and present clinical data that represent valuable feedback to the members of the RRS as well as the users on clinical wards.

A minimum dataset for documentation has been recommended to assist further interpretations, comparisons, reviews and changes to various forms of rapid response systems [52, 53]. It has been argued that similar data need to be collected for all in-hospital patients, notably patients at risk who do not trigger the RRS and do not experience an adverse event, in order to further outline the effects of the RRS [54]. Such stringency would make a significantly more complex system for hospital-wide patient monitoring necessary.

The importance of consistent and continuous collection of RRS data is further highlighted by several studies demonstrating that the rates for cardiac arrest and unexpected deaths continue to change over several years following the introduction of an RRS. In a single-centre study, the cardiac arrest rate decreased within two years while unexpected hospital deaths decreased within a four-year time period [55]. Another single-centre study documented progressive and significant reductions in cardiac arrest rates compared to historical controls during and up to four years after RRS implementation, with improved survival up to 1,500 days [33, 56].

The systematic review of RRS data may also enable identification of common problems or "syndromes" [57] that can be used to develop algorithms for managing the ward patient with tachycardia, hypotension, hypoxia and dyspnoea [58], low urinary output and altered level of consciousness [59]. Furthermore, targeted efforts for education and training can be directed to specific clinical areas.

Do rapid response systems reduce in-hospital adverse events?

The literature on rapid response systems is rapidly expanding. A PubMed search using the terms "Rapid Response Team" or "Medical Emergency Team" yielded 239 hits including 26 reviews as per February 2010. In contrast, a search of clinical trials (www.clinicaltrials.gov) only identified one trial on the effects of introducing an RRS (medical emergency team) for patients undergoing major surgery and two trials on wireless patient monitoring systems.

The vast majority of studies on the effects of introducing rapid response systems are single-centre, non-randomised, based on a historical control population (before-and-after design), and usually report outcomes in terms of rates for cardiac arrests, unexpected deaths, and unplanned ICU admissions. The single-centre before-and-after design renders the results susceptible to the Hawthorne effect. The outcomes may not reflect total in-hospital mortality and omit the impact on morbidity. Systematic reviews and meta-analyses of RRSs often point out the paucity of level 1 evidence (randomised controlled trials) supporting the RRS. Although a systematic review found rapid response systems to be associated with reduced mortality and cardiac arrests [60], the heterogeneity of the studies assessed as well as the wide confidence intervals precluded a firm conclusion to recommend an RRS as an effective intervention. Notwithstanding, RRSs have been widely adopted not only in general wards but also in paediatric [61, 62], obstetric [63] and emergency wards [64] and specific areas such as an otolaryngology service [65]. Furthermore, the generic principle of an RRS has recently been suggested as an additional "bundle" to improve outcomes for septic patients [66]. Several extensive reviews on RRSs have been published [67–71].

The largest study to date on rapid response systems is the Medical Early Response Intervention Therapy (MERIT) study [72]. This cluster-randomised trial of 23 hospitals in Australia included 56,756 patients admitted to control hospitals (not using RRS but cardiac arrest teams) and 68,376 patients admitted to hospitals running a medical emergency team (MET). No differences were found between MET and control hospitals for the composite of cardiac arrest, unexpected death or unplanned ICU admission as the primary outcome, nor for the individual events of the composite as secondary outcomes. For the hospital contemplating introducing an RRS, the MERIT study results may provide an argument for absence of evidence of benefit. However, this should not be misconstrued as evidence of absence of benefit. The lack of effect of RRSs in the MERIT trial has been attributed to insufficient power to detect a difference, particularly since the incidence of the outcome variables decreased in all hospitals during the study period, rendering the estimates used in the power calculations invalid. In addition, the periods for baseline assessment (2 months), education (4 months) and evaluation (6 months) might have been too short for such a complex healthcare intervention. A low rate of MET calls preceding unplanned ICU admissions and unexpected deaths, despite MET calling criteria being fulfilled and documented, suggests a lack of compliance to the protocol.

The MERIT study is the largest of its kind targeting a hospital-wide population evaluated for outcomes very relevant to the operations of an ICU. Eight studies have to date been published on data from the MERIT study population including analyses of the triggers [35], timing and interventions [73], impact for the documentation of vital signs [30] and not-for-resuscitation orders [42]. In the context of organisation and management, the MERIT study and subsequent follow-up studies thus highlight several issues that should be considered when planning, designing, implementing and evaluating an RRS.

The critical care outreach service initiative launched in the UK has been extensively reviewed [41]. The comprehensive report concluded that presence of an outreach service was associated with a significant decrease in cardiopulmonary resuscitation episodes in the 24 hours prior to ICU admission, the number of out-of-hours admissions and a reduced severity of illness on admission. These effects did not translate into mortality benefits nor reduced re-admissions for patients discharged alive from the ICU. Visits by the outreach service for patients discharged from the ICU were associated with decreased hospital mortality and hospital length of stay. These effects were considered cost-effective. The published observational study did not find any clear evidence that outreach services had a significant impact on clinical outcomes and no characteristics of an optimal service could be discerned [74]. It should be noted that RRS team composition was variable and less often physician-led compared to RRS medical emergency team models.

The medical and organisational complexity of the RRS might compromise the applicability of traditional randomised controlled trial (RCT) designs to determine efficacy. The Cochrane review on RRSs [75] identified 35 potentially relevant studies but only included two for further evaluation, based on RCT inclusion criteria. In addition to the MERIT trial, another ward-clustered randomised trial [76] was analysed. It was concluded that most studies investigating RRSs suffered from methodological diversity and poor quality. Based on the two trials analysed, no support for rapid response systems reducing overall mortality was found. A recent systematic review and meta-analysis including 18 studies in adult and paediatric populations, involving close to 1.3 million hospital admissions, reported a significant effect of RRSs in reducing cardiac arrests outside the ICU. The fact that hospital mortality was not consistently lowered in a similar fashion suggests that the RRS may have resulted in increased NFR orders or that while initial cases of cardiac arrest could be prevented, the overall survival of severely ill patients was not altered, albeit no longer labelled as unexpected or cardiac arrest deaths [77].

Complex interventions such as an RRS are notoriously difficult to research [78]. The combined quantitative and qualitative research methodologies of health services research, rather than multi-centre RCTs, might be more suitable for further assessments of RRSs [79, 80]. Such expertise should ideally be part of the organisation to maintain and develop an RRS.

Although the RCT design may be fallible in evaluating the effectiveness of rapid response systems, a conventional dose-response relationship has still been reported between RRS activity and clinical outcome [81]. The number of RRS activations per 1,000 hospital admissions inversely correlated to the number of cardiac arrests and unexpected deaths [82]. No such relationship was found for unplanned ICU admissions or for the composite of all three outcomes. Hospitals using a mature RRS typically report a "RRS dose" between 25.8 and 56.4 activations per 1,000 hospital admissions [81] for physician-led teams. In comparison, the RRS dose in the MERIT study was only 8.3 activations per 1,000 admissions during the study period. It seems clinically intuitive that the effectiveness of the RRS would be dose-dependent, similar to many other medical interventions. If the dose is inadequate, no response should be expected, and as a general rule of thumb, the RRS dose needs to be equal to or exceed the number of adverse events in the patient population targeted.

Other effects of implementing rapid response systems

A systems intervention like the RRS may have several implications for the delivery of healthcare in addition to the potential to manage medical emergencies on the wards. Tools for detecting and characterising adverse events are typically based on retrospective chart reviews that may be limited by missing information. Such quality assurance initiatives require considerable investments in time and money. The RRS was recently reported as a tool to capture real-time data on adverse events at the time of consultation [83]. The contemporaneous evaluation of adverse events in conjunction with an RRS response can identify important opportunities for improvement of the delivery of healthcare at the ward level with a much higher rate and precision than is achieved by routine incident-reporting systems. In the reported model, a standardised form was filled out during the RRS call during a five-minute debriefing. Weekly one-hour audits were used to identify room for improvement in antecedent clinical care.

Improved safety awareness as well as workplace satisfaction among nurses have been demonstrated following the implementation of an RRS. The benefits reported by nurses surveyed included immediate attention to patients' needs and easy access to medical expertise that was believed to improve outcome and reduce adverse events [84, 85]. Additional education on the management of medical crises was identified as an area for improvement. This is important as evidence suggests that nurses are more likely to activate an RRS response if they have attended dedicated educational sessions [86]. Routes and competencies for effective communication are

emphasised in several reports, as is maintaining a blameless culture when the RRS is activated to build rapprochement between all team members involved [87]. Reassurance to ward staff was among the most quoted impacts in the outreach service report [41]. A sense of empowerment on the part of ward staff through enhanced educational activities was also reported, as well as improved mutual understanding of activities both in the ICU and on wards. Hence, the aspiration towards "critical care without walls" had a definitive organisational and social meaning for which there was considerable evidence of achievement.

Concern has been raised that an RRS may lead to reduced autonomy and education for registrars, which could result in insufficient opportunities to gain and maintain clinical skills to manage medical emergencies. Medical registrars are more likely to be involved with the RRS than their surgical colleagues and tend to have a more favourable view of it. Neither medical nor surgical registrars perceived that an RRS negatively affected their skills or education in critical care and resuscitation [88]. Registrars in intensive care have also reported that RRS involvement favourably influenced their training, although shortcomings such as lack of supervision and senior engagement was pointed out. Notably, serious concern was expressed that RRS duties during on call, when ICU staffing levels are at their lowest, had a negative impact on the ability of registrars to attend ICU patients' needs and placed additional stress on medical staff [89].

The outreach services report demonstrated that timely identification of patients with impending critical illness to potentially avoid or at least facilitate ICU admission was ranked as the two most important priorities for the RRS by more than 80 % of clinical staff [41]. In contrast, the sharing of critical care skills, bedside and formal teaching received top ranking by only 40 % down to 20 % of participants. These findings emphasise the need to further explore educational issues in RRS-related healthcare services research.

Conclusion

Rapid response systems (RRS) are gaining increased worldwide acceptance despite variable, or arguably

Tab. 1   These questions illustrate some key management and organisational issues that need to be clarified in consideration
of implementing a rapid response system (RRS)

What is the problem?

What is the adverse event rate?

What types of patients are at risk? (e. g. medical, surgical, recently discharged from ICU)

What clinical outcomes are targeted? (e. g. cardiac arrest rate, unexpected death, unplanned ICU admission,
death in hospital, length of stay in hospital, inappropriate decisions for end-of-life care)

How to detect the problem?

How are vital signs monitored? (e. g. which signs, frequency, adjustments for individual patients, wireless technologies)

How are vital signs documented?

What triggers should be used and how? (e. g. threshold triggers, aggregate scores, clinical signs, laboratory values)

One- or two-tiered review? (e. g. mandatory clinical review by parent team before RRS)

How are advanced care directives decided and documented?

How to get further assistance?

Who can call the team? (e. g. clinical staff or any hospital staff/relatives/visitors)

How should clinical communication be performed? (e. g. structure for call and handover)

What should be done while waiting for further help?

How to solve the problem?

Who should be member of the team?

Who is leading the team? (e. g. physician – "ramp down", nurse – "ramp up")

What level of care/resources should be made available bedside (e. g. airway management, vascular access)

What clinical authority is given to the team? (e. g. ICU admission rights, limitation/withdrawal of care)

How is the parent ward team involved? (e. g. define clinical responsibilities including follow-up)

Will the team be available 24/7?

What other commitments will the team have? (e. g. can appropriate ICU cover be maintained?)

How to document?

What clinical documentation is made? (e. g. notes in medical records, use of separate forms, use of templates)

Will any cause analysis be performed simultaneously?

How are team activities collated? (e. g. database construction)

How to educate and train?

What teaching will be provided? (e. g. bedside, formal lectures, short courses, simulation)

What skills are targeted? (e. g. initial clinical management, communication, crew resource management)

What feedback is provided to parent teams? (e. g. weekly rounds, clinical case reviews, e-mails)

How to reinforce and sustain?

What statistics for which clinical outcomes will be distributed?

How to ensure sustainability while clinical outcomes change? (e. g. RSS may evolve during several years)

How to engage clinical champions? (e. g. clinical key opinion makers, stakeholders) even insufficient, level of evidence to support their effectiveness. The heterogeneous organisational nature of hospitals as well as significant differences in patient case mix, trigger criteria, team composition, educational support, supervision, audit and governance make research into rapid response systems challenging. However, this should not discourage much needed initiatives to delineate optimal RRS models, including specific attention to design, consumption of resources and cost-benefit analyses. One RRS model is very unlikely to fit all hospitals and careful consideration by management and organisation leaders/champions is needed before implementing an RRS to ensure optimal benefits in individual hospitals.

The author

Anders Aneman, MD, PhD, EDIC, FCICM
Staff specialist in Intensive Care | Liverpool Hospital | Sydney South West Area Health Service | Liverpool, Australia
Conjoint associate professor | Faculty of Medicine | SWS Clinical School | University of New South Wales | Sydney, Australia

Address for correspondence
Anders Aneman
Liverpool Hospital
Sydney South West Area Health Service
Locked Bag 7103
Liverpool BC, NSW 1871, Australia
E-mail: anders.aneman@sswahs.nsw.gov.au

References

1. Goldfrad C, Rowan K. Consequences of discharges from intensive care at night. Lancet 2000;355:1138–42.
2. Vincent C, Neale G, Woloshynowych M. Adverse events in British hospitals: preliminary retrospective record review. BMJ 2001;322:517–9.
3. Wilson RM, Runciman WB, Gibberd RW et al. The Quality in Australian Health Care Study. Med J Aust 1995;163:458–71.
4. Baker GR, Norton PG, Flintoft V et al. The Canadian Adverse Events Study: the incidence of adverse events among hospital patients in Canada. CMAJ 2004;170:1678–86.
5. Kohn L, Corrigan J, Donaldson M, eds. To Err is Human: Building a Safer Health System. Washington DC: National Academy Press 2000.
6. Zegers M, de Bruijne MC, Wagner C et al. Adverse events and potentially preventable deaths in Dutch hospitals: results of a retrospective patient record review study. Qual Saf Health Care 2009;18:297–302.
7. Aranaz-Andres JM, Aibar-Remon C, Vitaller-Murillo J et al. Incidence of adverse events related to health care in Spain: results of the Spanish National Study of Adverse Events. J Epidemiol Community Health 2008;62:1022–9.
8. Soop M, Fryksmark U, Koster M, Haglund B. The incidence of adverse events in Swedish hospitals: a retrospective medical record review study. Int J Qual Health Care 2009;21:285–91.
9. McQuillan P, Pilkington S, Allan A et al. Confidential inquiry into quality of care before admission to intensive care. BMJ 1998;316:1853–8.
10. Goldhill DR, White SA, Sumner A. Physiological values and procedures in the 24 h before ICU admission from the ward. Anaesthesia 1999;54:529–34.
11. Hillman K. Critical care without walls. Curr Opin Crit Care 2002;8:594–9.
12. Devita MA, Bellomo R, Hillman K et al. Findings of the first consensus conference on medical emergency teams. Crit Care Med 2006;34:2463–78.
13. Safer Systems – Saving Lives, State Government of Victoria, Department of Health. http://www.health.vic. gov.au/sssl. Accessed 9 March, 2010.
14. Clinical Excellence Commission, New South Wales, Department of Health. http://www.cec.health.nsw.gov.au/ programs/between-the-flags.html. Accessed 9 March, 2010.
15. Comprehensive Critical Care: a review of adult critical care services. Department of Health, London, UK. http:// www.dh.gov.uk/en/Publicationsandstatistics/ Publications/PublicationsPolicyAndGuidance/ DH_4006585. Accessed 9 March, 2010.
16. The National Outreach Forum. http://www.norf.org.uk. Accessed 9 March, 2010.

17. Institute for Healthcare Improvement. http://www.ihi. org/IHI/Topics/CriticalCare/IntensiveCare. Accessed 9 March, 2010.

18. Ministry of Health and Long-Term Care, Government of Ontario. Canada. http://www.health.gov.on.ca/english/ providers/program/critical_care/cct_response.html. Accessed 9 March, 2010.

19. Danish Society for Patient Safety. Operation Life. http:// www.operationlife.dk/English.aspx. Accessed 9 March, 2010.

20. Nolan JP, Deakin CD, Soar J, Böttiger BW, Smith G. European Resuscitation Guidelines for Resuscitation 2005. Section 4. Adult Advanced Life Support. Resuscitation 2005;67S1:S39-S86.

21. Konrad D, Jaderling G, Bell M et al. Reducing in-hospital cardiac arrests and hospital mortality by introducing a medical emergency team. Intensive Care Med 2010;36:100-6.

22. Campello G, Granja C, Carvalho F et al. Immediate and long-term impact of medical emergency teams on cardiac arrest prevalence and mortality: a plea for periodic basic life-support training programs. Crit Care Med 2009;37:3054-61.

23. Nurmi J, Harjola VP, Nolan J, Castren M. Observations and warning signs prior to cardiac arrest. Should a medical emergency team intervene earlier? Acta Anaesthesiol Scand 2005;49:702-6.

24. Hillman KM, Bristow PJ, Chey T et al. Antecedents to hospital deaths. Intern Med J 2001;31:343-8.

25. Kause J, Smith G, Prytherch D et al. A comparison of antecedents to cardiac arrests, deaths and emergency intensive care admissions in Australia and New Zealand, and the United Kingdom - the ACADEMIA study. Resuscitation 2004;62:275-82.

26. Harrison GA, Jacques T, McLaws ML, Kilborn G. Combinations of early signs of critical illness predict in-hospital death-the SOCCER study (signs of critical conditions and emergency responses). Resuscitation 2006;71:327-34.

27. Harrison GA, Jacques TC, Kilborn G, McLaws ML. The prevalence of recordings of the signs of critical conditions and emergency responses in hospital wards - the SOCCER study. Resuscitation 2005;65:149-57.

28. McGain F, Cretikos MA, Jones D et al. Documentation of clinical review and vital signs after major surgery. Med J Aust 2008;189:380-3.

29. Hillman KM, Bristow PJ, Chey T et al. Duration of life-threatening antecedents prior to intensive care admission. Intensive Care Med 2002;28:1629-34.

30. Chen J, Hillman K, Bellomo R et al. The impact of introducing medical emergency team system on the documentations of vital signs. Resuscitation 2009;80:35-43.

31. McBride J, Knight D, Piper J, Smith GB. Long-term effect of introducing an early warning score on respiratory rate charting on general wards. Resuscitation 2005;65:41-4.

32. Schmid-Mazzoccoli A, Hoffman LA, Wolf GA et al. The use of medical emergency teams in medical and surgical patients: impact of patient, nurse and organisational characteristics. Qual Saf Health Care 2008;17:377-81.

33. Jones D, Opdam H, Egi M et al. Long-term effect of a Medical Emergency Team on mortality in a teaching hospital. Resuscitation 2007;74:235-41.

34. Santiano N, Young L, Hillman K et al. Analysis of medical emergency team calls comparing subjective to "objective" call criteria. Resuscitation 2009;80:44-9.

35. Chen J, Bellomo R, Hillman K et al. Triggers for emergency team activation: A multicenter assessment. J Crit Care 2010, in press.

36. Bell MB, Konrad D, Granath F et al. Prevalence and sensitivity of MET-criteria in a Scandinavian University Hospital. Resuscitation 2006;70:66-73.

37. Cretikos M, Chen J, Hillman K et al. The objective medical emergency team activation criteria: a case-control study. Resuscitation 2007;73:62-72.

38. Subbe CP, Gao H, Harrison DA. Reproducibility of physiological track-and-trigger warning systems for identifying at-risk patients on the ward. Intensive Care Med 2007;33:619-24.

39. Gao H, McDonnell A, Harrison DA et al. Systematic review and evaluation of physiological track and trigger warning systems for identifying at-risk patients on the ward. Intensive Care Med 2007;33:667-79.

40. Devita MA, Smith GB, Adam SK et al. "Identifying the hospitalised patient in crisis" - A consensus conference on the afferent limb of Rapid Response Systems. Resuscitation 2010;81:375-82.

41. Evaluation of outreach services in critical care. Project SDO/74/2004. http://www.sdo.nihr.ac.uk/files/ project/74-final-report.pdf. Accessed 9 March, 2010.

42. Chen J, Flabouris A, Bellomo R et al. The Medical Emergency Team System and not-for-resuscitation orders: results from the MERIT study. Resuscitation 2008;79:391-7.

43. Jones DA, McIntyre T, Baldwin I et al. The medical emergency team and end-of-life care: a pilot study. Crit Care Resusc 2007;9:151-6.

44. Safer care for the acutely ill patient: learning from serious incidents. The fifth report from the Patient Safety Observatory. http://www.nrls.npsa.nhs.uk/ EasySiteWeb/getresource.axd?AssetID=60140&type=full &servicetype=Attachment. Accseesed 9 March, 2010.

45. Featherstone P, Chalmers T, Smith GB. RSVP: a system for communication of deterioration in hospital patients. Br J Nurs 2008;17:860-4.

46. Dunsford J. Structured communication: improving patient safety with SBAR. Nurs Womens Health 2009;13:384-90.

47. Featherstone P, Smith GB, Linnell M et al. Impact of a one-day inter-professional course (ALERT) on attitudes and confidence in managing critically ill adult patients. Resuscitation 2005;65:329–36.

48. Smith GB, Osgood VM, Crane S. ALERT – a multiprofessional training course in the care of the acutely ill adult patient. Resuscitation 2002;52:281–6.

49. Smith GB, Poplett N. Impact of attending a 1-day multi-professional course (ALERT) on the knowledge of acute care in trainee doctors. Resuscitation 2004;61:117–22.

50. Zotti MG, Waxman BP. A qualitative evaluation of the Care of the Critically Ill Surgical Patient course. ANZ J Surg 2009;79:693–6.

51. DeVita MA, Schaefer J, Lutz J et al. Improving medical emergency team (MET) performance using a novel curriculum and a computerized human patient simulator. Qual Saf Health Care 2005;14:326–31.

52. Cretikos M, Parr M, Hillman K et al. Guidelines for the uniform reporting of data for Medical Emergency Teams. Resuscitation 2006;68:11–25.

53. Peberdy MA, Cretikos M, Abella BS et al. Recommended guidelines for monitoring, reporting, and conducting research on medical emergency team, outreach, and rapid response systems: an Utstein-style scientific statement: a scientific statement from the International Liaison Committee on Resuscitation (American Heart Association, Australian Resuscitation Council, European Resuscitation Council, Heart and Stroke Foundation of Canada, InterAmerican Heart Foundation, Resuscitation Council of Southern Africa, and the New Zealand Resuscitation Council); the American Heart Association Emergency Cardiovascular Care Committee; the Council on Cardiopulmonary, Perioperative, and Critical Care; and the Interdisciplinary Working Group on Quality of Care and Outcomes Research. Circulation 2007;116:2481–500.

54. Peet H, Smith GB, Pryterch D, Featherstone PI, Schmidt P. Proposed guidelines for uniform reporting of Medical Emergency Team data are inadequate. Resuscitation 2006; 70: 291–2.

55. Santamaria J, Tobin A, Holmes J. Changing cardiac arrest and hospital mortality rates through a medical emergency team takes time and constant review. Crit Care Med 2010;38:445–50.

56. Jones D, Egi M, Bellomo R, Goldsmith D. Effect of the medical emergency team on long-term mortality following major surgery. Crit Care 2007;11:R12.

57. Jones D, Duke G, Green J et al. Medical emergency team syndromes and an approach to their management. Crit Care 2006;10:R30.

58. Quach JL, Downey AW, Haase M et al. Characteristics and outcomes of patients receiving a medical emergency team review for respiratory distress or hypotension. J Crit Care 2008;23:325–31.

59. Downey AW, Quach JL, Haase M et al. Characteristics and outcomes of patients receiving a medical emergency team review for acute change in conscious state or arrhythmias. Crit Care Med 2008;36:477–81.

60. Winters BD, Pham JC, Hunt EA et al. Rapid response systems: a systematic review. Crit Care Med 2007;35:1238–43.

61. Tibballs J, Kinney S. Reduction of hospital mortality and of preventable cardiac arrest and death on introduction of a pediatric medical emergency team. Pediatr Crit Care Med 2009;10:306–12.

62. Hunt EA, Zimmer KP, Rinke ML et al. Transition from a traditional code team to a medical emergency team and categorization of cardiopulmonary arrests in a children's center. Arch Pediatr Adolesc Med 2008;162:117–22.

63. Gosman GG, Baldisseri MR, Stein KL et al. Introduction of an obstetric-specific medical emergency team for obstetric crises: implementation and experience. Am J Obstet Gynecol 2008;198:367.e1–367.e7.

64. Subbe CP, Slater A, Menon D, Gemmell L. Validation of physiological scoring systems in the accident and emergency department. Emerg Med J 2006;23:841–5.

65. Oliver CL, Devita MA, Dunwoody CJ et al. Patient safety on the otolaryngology service: the role of an established rapid response system. Qual Saf Health Care 2009;18:496–9.

66. Funk D, Sebat F, Kumar A. A systems approach to the early recognition and rapid administration of best practice therapy in sepsis and septic shock. Curr Opin Crit Care 2009;15:301–7.

67. Aneman A, Parr M. Medical emergency teams: a role for expanding intensive care? Acta Anaesthesiol Scand 2006;50:1255–65.

68. Cretikos MA, Parr MJ. The Medical Emergency Team: 21st century critical care. Minerva Anestesiol 2005;71:259–63.

69. Hillman K, Parr M, Flabouris A et al. Redefining in-hospital resuscitation: the concept of the medical emergency team. Resuscitation 2001;48:105–10.

70. Sakai T, Devita MA. Rapid response system. J Anesth 2009;23:403–8.

71. Ranji SR, Auerbach AD, Hurd CJ et al. Effects of rapid response systems on clinical outcomes: systematic review and meta-analysis. J Hosp Med 2007;2:422–32.

72. Hillman K, Chen J, Cretikos M et al. Introduction of the medical emergency team (MET) system: a cluster-randomised controlled trial. Lancet 2005;365:2091–7.

73. Flabouris A, Chen J, Hillman K et al. Timing and interventions of emergency teams during the MERIT study. Resuscitation 2010;81:25–30.

74. Gao H, Harrison DA, Parry GJ et al. The impact of the introduction of critical care outreach services in England: a multicentre interrupted time-series analysis. Crit Care 2007;11:R113.

75. McGaughey J, Alderdice F, Fowler R et al. Outreach and

Early Warning Systems (EWS) for the prevention of intensive care admission and death of critically ill adult patients on general hospital wards. Cochrane Database Syst Rev 2007:CD005529.

76. Priestley G, Watson W, Rashidian A et al. Introducing Critical Care Outreach: a ward-randomised trial of phased introduction in a general hospital. Intensive Care Med 2004;30:1398–404.

77. Chan PS, Jain R, Nallmothu BK et al. Rapid Response Teams: A Systematic Review and Meta-analysis. Arch Intern Med 2010;170:18–26.

78. DeVita MA, Bellomo R. The case of rapid response systems: are randomized clinical trials the right methodology to evaluate systems of care? Crit Care Med 2007;35:1413–4.

79. Hillman K, Chen J, Brown D. A clinical model for Health Services Research-the Medical Emergency Team. J Crit Care 2003;18:195–9.

80. Hillman K, Chen J, May E. Complex intensive care unit interventions. Crit Care Med 2009;37:S102–6.

81. Jones D, Bellomo R, DeVita MA. Effectiveness of the Medical Emergency Team: the importance of dose. Crit Care 2009;13:313.

82. Chen J, Bellomo R, Flabouris A et al. The relationship between early emergency team calls and serious adverse events. Crit Care Med 2009;37:148–53.

83. Iyengar A, Baxter A, Forster AJ. Using Medical Emergency Teams to detect preventable adverse events. Crit Care 2009;13:R126.

84. Salamonson Y, van Heere B, Everett B, Davidson P. Voices from the floor: Nurses' perceptions of the medical emergency team. Intensive Crit Care Nurs 2006;22:138–43.

85. Jones D, Baldwin I, McIntyre T et al. Nurses' attitudes to a medical emergency team service in a teaching hospital. Qual Saf Health Care 2006;15:427–32.

86. Cretikos MA, Chen J, Hillman KM et al. The effectiveness of implementation of the medical emergency team (MET) system and factors associated with use during the MERIT study. Crit Care Resusc 2007;9:206–12.

87. Bagshaw SM, Mondor EE, Scouten C et al. A survey of nurses' beliefs about the medical emergency team system in a canadian tertiary hospital. Am J Crit Care 2010;19:74–83.

88. Sarani B, Sonnad S, Bergey MR et al. Resident and RN perceptions of the impact of a medical emergency team on education and patient safety in an academic medical center. Crit Care Med 2009;37:3091–6.

89. Jacques T, Harrison GA, McLaws ML. Attitudes towards and evaluation of medical emergency teams: a survey of trainees in intensive care medicine. Anaesth Intensive Care 2008;36:90–5.

Gavin M. Joynt and Charles D. Gomersall

Integrating elective workloads into an emergency setting in the intensive care unit

Introduction

In an emergency setting, such as a major epidemic, natural disaster or other mass casualty event (MCE), there is a natural focus on the immediate victims of the MCE. Nevertheless it is important that the medical needs of other patients that would normally require emergency admission are not neglected. This includes patients who require intensive care after elective admission. An unavoidable consequence of any significant MCE is that ICU resources will be placed under pressure. If resources are overwhelmed, some sort of just distribution of resources is required [1, 2]. We will attempt to provide a framework from which a consistent approach to integrating emergency and elective workloads can be developed in such an emergency setting.

Although it is acknowledged that macro-allocation of healthcare resources within healthcare systems is important, in the emergency setting, it is front-line healthcare professionals who are tasked with the use and allocation of scarce medical resources, and it is from this perspective that the following opinions are presented. Intensive care workload is proportional to the number of patients admitted, and the intensive care resources consumed per patient. Therefore the contribution of each of these requires consideration, particularly in relation to the magnitude of the medical benefits derived from the ICU resources invested.

The potential effects of cancellation or delay of elective admissions

Many elective surgical patients require intensive care unit (ICU) support post-operatively. In the absence of an available ICU bed, it is usually necessary to cancel or delay elective surgery. The assessment of many factors is required to quantify the resulting potential detrimental effects. It requires an assessment of the net potential benefit of admission for each individual case. This in turn involves a quantitative assessment of the potential outcome of a patient admitted without delay, and the potential outcome of the same patient if refused admission.

When refusal of a post-operative bed results in a delay of the elective surgical procedure, the magnitude or length of this delay is important. Delay of one or two days is likely to have negligible consequences for most patients; however, should the delay be weeks or months, many categories of surgical patients run the risk of suffering substantial additional morbidity and mortality [3]. In particular patients undergoing cardiac, neurological or oncological surgery might be reasonably expected to suffer detrimental effects as a result of progression of the surgical condition [4, 5]. It is important to be aware that this effect may be subtly hidden when a waiting list of a large number of patients is affected by multiple short delays because cumulative delay that results for patients at the end of the queue may be substantial.

Thus, while the length of delay is an important consideration, even long delays must be assessed in the context of their potential effect on the individual patient's surgical outcome. The requirement for ICU admission and elective surgical outcome is likely to be influenced by two main factors, pre-existing disease status and the nature of the operative disease. The contribution of pre-existing disease status and its influence on long-term outcome should be readily comparable with non-elective patients. Assessing the medium- and long-term outcome of the surgical condition itself is more difficult, and often the intensivist relies on the professional judgment of a surgical specialist to assist in the prediction of short- and long-term surgical outcomes. There are some surgical scoring systems applicable in the ICU that may assist in determining outcome in selected high-risk elective surgical patients [6, 7], but they are few and their application to individual patients is difficult. Nevertheless, with consultation, and careful assessment of the pre-morbid and surgical condition, a comprehensive assessment of likely outcome after appropriate post-operative ICU admission should be determined.

Ultimately anticipated length of the delay to surgery, coupled with its likely detrimental effect on outcome has to be interpreted to assess the likely loss of benefit. Thus by way of a simple example the large potential benefit of curative carcinoma surgery in an otherwise well, middle-aged patient may be lost if as a result of repeated ICU refusals, the delay in the operation led to the surgery being non-curative. On the other hand, a patient with severe, end-stage cardio-respiratory morbidity, presenting for a discomfort relieving vascular procedure, may suffer only moderate discomfort despite repeated delays resulting in relatively less loss of benefit.

The last factor to consider is the resource utilisation imposed by the elective admission workload. In general, it might be expected to be relatively small. Most such cases require short-term organ support, very often of the respiratory system, without the need for complicated therapeutic interventions. Thus, while the net benefit derived from intensive care may often be relatively small, resource consumption may be modest and the appropriate designation of low-intensity ICU resources for elective surgery in this setting may be justified. The resource consumption cost of delayed post-operative complications is difficult to assess, but may have to be considered in some cases. For example, the ICU re-admission rate of patients who have undergone elective oesophagectomy is likely to be in the region of 12 % [8].

The nature of the MCE and its likely effect on elective surgery

As only substantial delays are likely to have important effects on the loss of outcome benefit of elective admissions, the predicted duration of the MCE in question has major implications for the need to create alternative strategies for integrating elective workloads. For example, after an explosion or earthquake, victim recovery time may be relatively fast, and ICU length of stay for most victims is expected to be relatively short, perhaps only one to two weeks for the majority. Thus the effect on elective workloads is likely to be minimal as the vast majority of elective surgical cases can be safely deferred. However, epidemics may last several weeks to several months, and possibly have multiple peak periods, depending on the nature of the infectious agent and may therefore have significant detrimental effects if they cause long elective surgical delays.

Certain types of injury such as severe burn injury (mean ICU stays as long as 6–10 weeks), or infectious disease such as SARS (mean ICU stay 14 days) may require a prolonged length of stay in ICU and hospital to achieve successful outcomes [9, 10]. Such heavy ICU resource utilisation, even if by fewer patients, may also result in ICU bed shortages and possible elective surgical delays.

A careful analysis of the potential impact and likely duration of each MCE is therefore necessary in the initial stages to establish possible effects on the elective surgical workload.

The ethical principles of triage

In a number of countries the routine demand for intensive care unit resources exceeds supply [11–

13], and epidemiological evidence suggests that even in well-resourced countries future demands may soon outstrip resources [14]. Therefore during any major epidemic or other MCE available resources may be readily overwhelmed. This section addresses the fair distribution of ICU resources when they become insufficient to meet demands.

In the emergency setting of a MCE there appears to be no pressing moral argument why the interests of other individuals also requiring ICU admission should be compromised. We therefore propose that both MCE victims and elective admissions be prioritised on the same basis.

Prioritisation or triage systems should attempt to develop a process of decision-making that is ethically and morally justifiable [15, 16]. As a result of the complexity of decision-making in ICU triage, a number of different ethically and morally justifiable processes have been proposed [17, 18], without resolution as to which is superior. It is also appealing to try to develop concrete, objective, practical triage protocols that can simply be applied by front-line doctors responsible for triage to determine admission in an emergency setting. Recently an attempt to create such a detailed protocol, based on a clinical outcome scoring system and application of an admission rule has been proposed [19]. Unfortunately, independent assessments of its implementation, when applied in a retrospective manner to representative populations, have demonstrated that it is impractical in its current form [21, 22]. Given the complexity of diseases and the heterogeneous nature of ICU patients, as well as the relative paucity of good quality outcome data, it is not surprising that current protocols are unable to define specific clinical conditions under which individual patient triage decisions should be made. Therefore we propose a method whereby individual doctors adhering to a defined triage framework constructed from broad ethical and moral principles make clinical triage decisions. We believe that when explicitly and transparently applied, the chance of achieving justice and consistency in decision-making is maximised.

Principles of justice

When ICU resources are overwhelmed, there is an inevitable and unavoidable need to triage the use of ICU beds. This means that while some patients who will potentially benefit from ICU care will be able to receive it, other deserving patients will be denied life-saving ICU care. Not treating each individual patient to the very best of our ability is justified by the principle of impossibility or "all other things being equal, one cannot have a duty to do what is impossible under the circumstances that obtain" [23]. Once this principle is fulfilled in emergency setting, the following section sets out the terminology, possible reasons for admission and refusal, and an approach to triage in principle with the primary objective of satisfying recognised norms of justice.

The moral justifications for decision-making in the discussion that follows will rely heavily on the moral principles and ethical reasoning proposed by Beauchamp and Childress [24]. Briefly, four *prima facie* moral principles – beneficence, non-maleficence, autonomy and justice – were used as a framework to assist the interpretation of the ethical problem being considered. While a large body of bioethicists and doctors have adopted this model of ethical justification both for policy-making and individual clinical decisions, it has not been universally accepted [25]. The key principle defining rationing is justice. We have chosen to justify the proposed triage procedural process by using both utilitarian and egalitarian principles of justice, each where their use is most appropriately justified. In the main, we adhere to medical utility (achieving the best possible medical outcome for the greatest number of patients) and social egalitarianism (providing equal treatment on the basis of an individual's socially defining factors) [24]. A possible, justified use of social utility to determine decisions in specific emergency settings is suggested separately. Accepting the difficulties associated with using only broad ethical principles to guide ethical decision making, after we applied and specified relevant principles in the context of triage to develop the initial version of the process described briefly below, we have embarked on a process of 'accountability for reasonableness' [26, 27], to confirm its acceptability and legitimacy, and allow challenges and revision by stakeholders.

Terminology and possible reasons for admission and refusal

It is important to realise that not all cases refused ICU admission are refused as a consequence of resource limitation. Based on relatively simple ethical reasoning three distinct morally justifiable pathways may exist for refusal of ICU admission (see Fig. 1).

The first pathway involves refusal of intensive care admission based on futility – that admission to ICU would not increase the probability of achieving the desired goal and result in provision of pointless treatment. It is not generally considered obligatory for doctors to provide pointless treatment and therefore ICU admission could be justifiably refused. Patients meeting this criterion could be medically well patients, in whom ICU care will provide little or no extra benefit over ward care. At the other end of the spectrum of disease, terminally ill patients who may also

not reasonably be expected to derive any additional medical benefit from ICU care could also be refused admission. While the moral definition and meaning of futility is clear, the difficulty with futility is one of practical implementation [28, 29]. It appears difficult to say with certainty that an intensive care admission will not lead to any benefit being derived by an individual patient, either in survival or quality of life; however, it has been suggested that futility should be seen in a similar way to all other medical decisions that are also based on probability [28]. More specifically, it has been suggested that when doctors conclude that in the last 100 similar cases, a medical treatment has been useless, it could be regarded as futile [30]. This approach to dealing with futility is controversial, and therefore futility is not frequently used for the justification of refusal of intensive care admission.

The second pathway is one where the patient, or their surrogate, makes an autonomous, in-

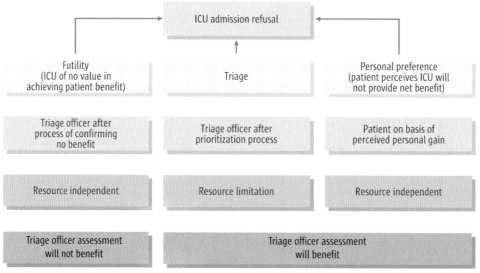

Fig. 1   An explanatory schematic of reasons for ICU admission refusal. The triage officer should be an experienced ICU doctor. Left column: At the time of referral the triage officer makes and initial decision regarding potential medical benefit to the patient if admitted. If the decision is no, once confirmed, the patient is refused admission on the basis that ICU treatment is futile. This is a resource-independent process. Middle column: If the patient will potentially benefit, but does not meet criteria for sufficient benefit to achieve priority for admission, the patient is refused. This is a response directly to resource limitation and constitutes triage. Right column: If the patient will potentially benefit and does meet criteria for sufficient benefit to achieve priority for admission, but after communication of the risks and benefits of ICU admission, declines admission, the patient is refused on the basis of their personal preference. This is a resource-independent process.

formed decision to decline ICU admission. Intensive care and the provision of life support are associated with potential discomfort, pain and suffering, and potential benefits may be small for some patients. After an explanation of the expected burden and benefits of admission to intensive care, some patients or their surrogates may express a wish not to be admitted. This patient preference not to be admitted is an expression of autonomy and should be respected. This discussion should normally take place in situations when the gatekeeper has already decided to accept the patient for intensive care admission and has sufficient resources to provide ICU care, if it is the patient's or surrogate's wish.

The third morally justifiable reason that results in refusal is the process of triage, or prioritisation of patients for admission in the presence of inadequate resources [15]. Random allocation of resources would achieve an egalitarian or "equally fair" chance of ICU admission for all. Prioritisation or triage can utilise a naturally occurring, acceptably random process such as "first come, first served" to determine admission, provided that the patient meets the minimum threshold for benefit from admission. The American Thoracic Society, for example, recommended this approach on the basis that defining degrees of benefit without ambiguity, bias or subjectivity is difficult and therefore morally problematic [18].

The desire to achieve maximum benefit from available ICU resources, however, leads some to preferentially admit patients based on the predicted magnitude of benefit that the individual would derive from ICU care. This approach is based on the utilitarian principle of 'achieving the greatest good for the greatest number' of patients. The Society of Critical Care Medicine proposes that the likely benefit derived by an individual patient from the use of ICU resources should be considered as a primary criterion for prioritisation or triage [17]. Using this model, a patient who will clearly derive more medical benefit from ICU resources should be given priority over one who will derive less benefit (e.g. lower increment in chances of survival). In the emergency setting of severely restricted resources it can be argued on the basis of medical utility that those who consume excess resources to the detriment of others in order to achieve sufficient

worthwhile benefit, could justifiably be denied such excess resources. Thus patients who may ultimately derive meaningful benefit could be prioritised lower than those in whom the same benefit could be achieved at a substantially lower cost of resources (see Fig. 2).

It is important to note that this proposed triage model retains egalitarian principles in the sense that no distinction is made based on socially defining factors such as ethnic origin, race, religion, sex, and social utility. Finally, in circumstances where competing patients would derive similar benefit from the use of similar resources, we would propose a 'first come, first served', egalitarian approach.

As noted above, one argument against using a medical utilitarian approach for triage is that benefit is difficult to assess and that this lack of accuracy introduces unfairness [18]. We accept that triage decisions, as with all clinical decisions made on an individual basis, are subject to arbitrary variations. However, we believe that broad, ethically based guidelines that make the decision process explicit and ensure that it is made with due care reduces the variability of triage decisions, and that medical benefit differences can be acceptably determined in most cases. Nevertheless, any form of prioritisation will result in the interests (and rights to autonomy, beneficence and non-maleficence) of refused patients being overridden. For these reasons, the justification for triage (severe resource limitation) must be strong, and each decision fully documented (see Tab. 1).

The additional use of the process of 'accountability for reasonableness' is recommended to improve the quality of guidelines in response to feedback, assist resolution of conflicts of principle related to the triage process, and promote consistency of decision-making in specific subgroups of patients. It is intended to allow most, and if possible all of the stakeholders to agree on what is fair or just, and consists of four key procedural elements [27]. The need for transparency (all relevant parties, including the public, should have complete access to the decisions and the reasons for the decisions); the use of rationales that all parties can accept are relevant to the fair use of the health resources in question; ensuring that a formal and accessible mechanism exists for appeals or challenges; and lastly, that some sort of

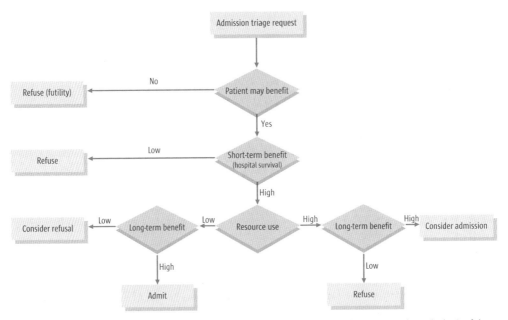

Fig. 2   Algorithm outlining the process of making an individual triage decision. Each decision is made on the basis of the agreed triage threshold for the particular emergency setting (see text). Long-term benefit may include an assessment of expected quality of life, if considered appropriate. When overwhelmed, elective and emergency admissions should be assessed by the same criteria. Before any final decision to admit to ICU, patient preference regarding desire for admission should be explored.

oversight mechanism, preferably external, exists to monitor the first three conditions.

Finally, as doctors we should be aware and resist all inappropriate influences, such as political and economic pressures, that have no place in determining rationing decisions [31].

A practical approach to integrating elective workloads in the emergency setting

Maximisation of ICU resources

The first step to ensure the integration of the elective workload into any emergency setting is to identify and mobilise sufficient resources to accommodate it. This is done by ensuring that all ICU resources are maximally utilised. Not only should all available ICU and other high care beds within the hospital be identified and used, they should also be used in the most efficient way [32]. Attempts should be made to identify, and exclude from the ICU, patients with low illness severity

who may not benefit from ICU care [33]. Specifically, not all post-operative elective admissions for whom admission is routinely requested will benefit from HDU or ICU admission [34], and workloads can be reduced by appropriate exclusion. Vigorous attempts should be made to maximise efficiency with the utilisation of fast-track post-operative approaches, good weaning protocols and rapid recognition of patients fit for transfer to lower levels of care.

The use of a designated facility with limited capability for complicated organ support, such as an intermediate care or high dependency unit (HDU) with mechanical ventilatory capacity may be adequate for the initial support of the majority of elective patients in the first instance. This would allow all ICU beds to be freed for potentially more complex cases associated with the MCE. The physical location of such a unit may be important, especially in the setting of an infectious disease crisis. In the setting of an infectious disease outbreak, identifying and designating units within hospitals with no or minimal infectious disease burdens

Tab. 1   Individual decisions to refuse ICU admission must be clearly documented in the patient's records

An assessment of the diagnosis, prognosis, and outcome

A statement of the degree of benefit expected for the patient if admitted, and supporting evidence for this assessment

A statement clearly making the decision and identifying it as a triage decision

The physician/s responsible for the decision (usually the ICU director or designated senior ICU doctor), after consultation with relevant stakeholders*

A statement confirming that clear communication of relevant factors with the patient/family/other caregivers has taken place – including amongst others inquiry into the patient's current and expected quality of life

A statement that the decision and reason for that decision has been communicated to the family and relevant caregivers should conclude the documentation

*   The minimisation of bias when decisions are made is important and it has been suggested that the ICU director or designate be charged with ultimate responsibility for triage decisions as physicians seeking admission for individual patients are likely to have a bias toward securing resources for their own patients.

specifically to deal with elective workloads may also be appropriate, as this would reduce the risk of cross-infection of uninfected elective patients.

Increasing the number of ICU beds by reallocation of other hospital resources is usually possible to some degree, depending on the type of MCE and complexity of management required for MCE cases [35, 36]. Ability to expand is often overestimated, however, and in the setting of an infectious disease outbreak, it has been estimated that by maximum expansion of fully functional ICU beds after internal hospital reallocation, it is unlikely to be more than about 50 % of initial capacity [36]. At an organisational level, a system of efficient intra-hospital communication and coordination is required to achieve this goal efficiently, and standard operating procedures to guide the development of an intra-hospital coordination structure have recently been published [37]. These structures and systems should be in place, and tested for functionality by simulation exercises, before the emergency occurs [38].

Regional cooperation and coordination

Regional cooperation and coordination, between individual hospitals or clusters of hospitals realistically joined by an inter-hospital transport system, may allow sufficient resources to be mobilised to deal with moderate size MCEs [37, 38]. To determine the best allocation of resources and

ensure efficient use of all resources, a regional emergency incident group in conjunction with advice or instruction from a regional ICU resource group should be activated to gather relevant information and provide regional solutions to resource problems such as facilitation of inter-hospital patient transfer (see Tab. 2). The designation of a single regional facility to accommodate elective admissions may have advantages as it is generally easier to relocate surgical teams and pre-operative patients than critically ill patients, and hospitals with lower infectious disease burdens may have operating rooms and ICUs/HDUs capable of supporting elective workloads, avoiding high cross-infection risks.

Considerations when overwhelmed

If triage is not already a routine practice, broad institutional guidelines based on the framework discussed above that govern front-line triage decisions should be developed. Development should occur prior to the emergency event to allow adequate time for consultation, feedback, adjustment and stakeholder acceptance. The guidelines are best developed by a designated group that should include experienced ICU doctors, if possible with experience of implementing triage, and ethical expertise.

The system we have proposed implies that the front-line ICU doctor (when acting as the triage

Tab. 2   A summary of the essential resource allocation responsibilities of regional and hospital coordinating centres

Quantify the actual and expected MCE workload
- Systems for adequate reporting, data collation, and analysis from within the hospital system
- Interface with community/civil disaster authorities
- Prediction of magnitude and duration of MCE

Quantify actual and expected elective workload
- Records of historical ICU utilisation
- Systems for adequate reporting of current status, data collation, and analysis – including systems to evaluate the urgency and likely outcome of routine and elective patients

Identify all resources that can be mobilised within the region by ICU expansion and reallocation of resources from non-ICU areas
- Based on pre-crisis contingency plans
- Review of current status

Identify all accessible ICU/HDU resources
- Including all ICU resources that can be reasonably reached by patient transfer – regional, national, or rarely international

Identify special requirements or constraints specific to the type of MCE
- In infectious disease outbreaks, it may be advantageous to designate certain hospitals and ICUs for outbreak victims, and others for routine elective workloads

Recommend and implement an appropriate distribution of resources based on the above information
- Expand number of ICU beds if indicated and possible
- Monitor regional ICU bed availability, and facilitate inter-hospital transfers if necessary

Coordinate communication with and approve triage by front-line ICU doctors (designated triage officers) when conditions for triage are met

officer) carries a heavy decision-making burden; however, we believe this is currently unavoidable. While the guidelines clearly identify the key factors required for decision-making, as with any medical decision, it is the clinical judgment of the individual doctor that intuitively establishes the presence of likely benefit, the magnitude of likely benefit, the resource cost of admission, and the patient's desire for admission. The final decision is reached after systematic consideration of these factors, which are explicitly outlined in the guideline (see Fig. 2).

In the emergency setting it becomes necessary to set a 'triage threshold' of acceptable benefit and cost to guide individual triage officers when following the decision-making process outlined in Figure 2. The assessment of mortality benefit is usually the priority in an emergency setting, but outcome in terms of quality of life ben-

efit may also be considered when appropriate. It is usually at the regional and hospital triage committee level that the resource availability in an emergency is best assessed, and a designated hospital or regional triage committee should bear the responsibility for setting appropriate triage thresholds. Some important factors that should be addressed as part of this process are shown in Table 3.

There appears to be no obvious or pressing reason why either one of emergency or elective admissions should receive priority over the other. It appears reasonable and just to integrate and triage elective workloads on the same basis, which is with reference to medical benefit and resource consumption. Thus it is necessary to establish a prediction of the prognosis of elective surgical admission as discussed earlier – estimate the effect of potential refusal of ICU care,

Tab. 3 Major factors to be considered when deciding triage 'threshold levels' for acceptable benefit and resource use

Predicted number of victims

Resources required for successful treatment (estimated length of stay in the ICU)

Resources available

Likely duration of emergency/MCE

Likelihood of benefit (short-term, e.g. hospital survival)

Duration of benefit (e.g. long-term survival, consider incorporating quality of life where appropriate)

Social worth* (e.g. direct multiplier effect of treating emergency caregivers, contribution to social stability of chief of police, military, prime minister, etc.)

* In the emergency setting, the usual egalitarian approach to excluding social worth from influencing triage decisions may require reassessment. If an individual's expected future contribution is indispensable to achieving a major social good, priority on this basis could be considered.

make an assessment of likely resource consumption and arrive at an intuitive assessment of likely net benefit. It is again necessary to compare this with the expected net benefit of an emergency MCE admission and make a priority judgment. This is an enormously complex comparison that we believe currently can only be achieved intuitively by an experienced ICU doctor, with assistance in formulating surgical prognosis from a specialist surgeon. This process should take place on a daily basis in all ICUs independently. Alternatively, an overall assessment of justified elective load for a hospital or region can be made, and all surgical cases allocated to a specific elective facility (of justified size and resources) within a hospital or region. As discussed above, this may have certain advantages.

It must be remembered that triage decisions carry a heavy burden and ICU refusal on the basis of triage is associated with an excess mortality, even after being adjusted for severity of illness [12, 13]. Therefore an appropriate group such as the local or regional triage committee should formally monitor the consequences of triage decisions, and appropriate feedback clearly communicated to the front-line ICU doctors of affected hospitals as well as regional authorities. The number of refused and admitted cases, details of the refusal process, and outcomes (e.g. length of ICU and hospital stay and mortality) should be recorded. Levels of acceptable benefit and cost may require adjustment as the emergency progresses, and a mechanism for appeal or challenge of the process should be available.

Future challenges

Choosing patients on the basis of medical benefit requires careful clinical assessment and estimation of prognosis, and then an intuitive prediction of the magnitude of the beneficial effect of ICU admission. Clinical factors known to be associated with such triage decisions include acute severity of illness, diagnosis, chronic illness status, age, and the likely success or failure of current medical therapy [12, 13, 39]. Although all clinical decisions, including triage, are subject to variability and inconsistency, basing judgements on as much objective data as possible is likely to improve accuracy. Therefore encouraging the accumulation of objective databases to record prognosis and outcome of all significant subgroups of patients after ICU admission, both in terms of mortality and quality of life, is an urgent priority. While some such data is available [40–45], it is currently insufficient to consistently guide individual decisions. Measuring and recording the outcome of comparable subgroups of patients who do not receive ICU care is more difficult, but is also necessary to allow the accurate assessment of the relative magnitude of benefit of ICU admission. Models to predict ICU length of stay would also be beneficial in allowing a more accurate assessment of likely ICU resource utilisation.

If sufficiently large, comprehensive and informative databases are developed, not only would intuitive decision-making be better informed, but comprehensive predictive models capable of being developed into clinical triage tools may become a realistic prospect.

Conclusion

Integrating elective workloads, first at a local and then regional level is best achieved by maximising the use of existing resources. If overwhelmed, it is necessary to prioritise patient admission and therefore, workload, through a justifiable triage process. As a group, neither elective nor emergency admissions intrinsically deserve priority over the other. We believe at this time it is necessary for experienced front-line ICU doctors (designated as triage officers) to make individual clinical triage decisions, guided by prevailing conditions and based on broad guidelines similar to those presented above. Explicit triage protocols that guide triage according to specific clinical rules are potentially desirable, but currently there are none available that function adequately.

The authors

Gavin M. Joynt, MBBCh, CICM, FHKCA(IC)
Charles D. Gomersall, MBBS, CICM, EDIC
    Department of Anaesthesia and Intensive
    Care | The Chinese University of Hong Kong |
    Shatin, Hong Kong

Address for correspondence
    Gavin M. Joynt
    Department of Anaesthesia and Intensive Care
    The Chinese University of Hong Kong
    Shatin, Hong Kong
    E-mail: gavinmjoynt@cuhk.edu.hk

References

1. Devereaux AV, Dichter JR, Christian MD, Dubler NN, Sandrock CE, Hick JL, et al. Definitive care for the critically ill during a disaster: a framework for allocation of scarce resources in mass critical care: from a Task Force for Mass Critical Care summit meeting, January 26–27, 2007, Chicago, IL. Chest 2008;133(5 Suppl):51S–66S.

2. Christian MD, Joynt GM, Hick JL, Colvin J, Danis M, Sprung CL; European Society of Intensive Care Medicine's Task Force for intensive care unit triage during an influenza epidemic or mass disaster. Chapter 7. Critical care triage. Recommendations and standard operating procedures for intensive care unit and hospital preparations for an influenza epidemic or mass disaster. Intensive Care Med 2010;36 Suppl 1:S55–64.

3. Valente R, Testi A, Tanfani E, Fato M, Porro I, Santo M, et al. A model to prioritize access to elective surgery on the basis of clinical urgency and waiting time. BMC Health Serv Res 2009;9:1, doi:10.1186/1472-6963-9-1.

4. MacCormick AD, Collecutt WG, Parry BR. Prioritizing patients for elective surgery: a systematic review. ANZ J Surg 2003;73:633–42.

5. Shelton BK. Admission criteria and prognostication in patients with cancer admitted to the intensive care unit. Crit Care Clin 2010;26:1–20.

6. Copeland GP, Jones D, Walters M. POSSUM: a scoring system for surgical audit. Br J Surg 1991;78:355–60.

7. Roques F, Nashef SA, Michel P, Gauducheau E, de Vincentiis C, Baudet E, et al. Risk factors and outcome in European cardiac surgery: analysis of the EuroSCORE multinational database of 19030 patients. Eur J Cardiothorac Surg 1999;15:816–22.

8. Park DP, Welch CA, Harrison DA, Palser TR, Cromwell DA, Gao F, et al. Outcomes following oesophagectomy in patients with oesophageal cancer: a secondary analysis of the ICNARC Case Mix Programme Database. Crit Care 2009;13 Suppl 2:S1, doi:10.1186/cc7868.

9. Ryan CM, Schoenfeld DA, Thorpe WP, Sheridan RL, Cassem EH, Tompkins RG. Objective estimates of the probability of death from burn injuries. N Engl J Med 1998;338:362–6.

10. Hui DS, Joynt GM, Wong KT, Gomersall CD, Li TS, Antonio G, et al. Impact of severe acute respiratory syndrome (SARS) on pulmonary function, functional capacity and quality of life in a cohort of survivors. Thorax 2005;60:401–9.

11. Metcalfe MA, Sloggett A, McPherson K. Mortality among appropriately referred patients refused admission to intensive care units. Lancet 1997; 50:7–12.

12. Sprung CL, Geber D, Eidelman LA, Baras M, Pizov R, Nimrod A, et al. Evaluation of triage decisions for intensive care admission. Crit Care Med 1999;27:1073–9.

13. Joynt GM, Gomersall CD, Tan P, Lee A, Cheng CA, Wong EL. Prospective evaluation of patients refused admission to an intensive care unit: triage, futility, and outcome. Intensive Care Med 2001;27:1459–65.

14. Angus DC, Kelley MA, Schmitz RJ, White A, Popovich J Jr; Committee on Manpower for Pulmonary and Critical Care Societies (COMPACCS). Caring for the critically ill patient. Current and projected workforce requirements for care of the critically ill and patients with pulmonary disease: can we meet the requirements of an aging population? JAMA 2000;284:2762–70.

15. Iserson KV, Moskop JC. Triage in medicine, part I: Concept, history, and types. Ann Emerg Med 2007;49:275–81.

16. Moskop JC, Iserson KV. Triage in medicine, part II: Underlying values and principles. Ann Emerg Med 2007;49:282–7.

17. Society of Critical Care Medicine Ethics Committee. Consensus statement on the triage of critically ill patients. JAMA 1994;271:1200–3.

18. American Thoracic Society Statement. Fair allocation of intensive care unit resources. Am J Respir Crit Care Med 1997;156:1282–301.

19. Christian MD, Hawryluck L, Wax RS, Cook T, Lazar NM, Herridge MS, et al. Development of a triage protocol for critical care during an influenza pandemic. CMAJ 2006;175:1377-1381.

20. Guest T, Tantam G, Donlin N, Tantam K, McMillan H, Tillyard A. An observational cohort study of triage for critical care provision during pandemic influenza: 'clipboard physicians' or 'evidenced based medicine'? Anaesthesia 2009;64:1199-206.

21. Khan Z, Hulme J, Sherwood N. An assessment of the validity of SOFA score based triage in H1N1 critically ill patients during an influenza pandemic. Anaesthesia 2009;64:1283-8.

22. Kluge EH. Social values, socioeconomic resources, and effectiveness coefficients. An ethical model for statistically based resource allocation. Ann N Y Acad Sci 2000;913:23-31.

23. Beauchamp TL, Childress JF. Principles of biomedical ethics. 5th Ed, 2001. Oxford University press, Oxford.

24. Pellegrino ED. The metamorphosis of medical ethics: a 30 year retrospective. JAMA 1993;269:1158-62.

25. Daniels N, Sabin J. Limits to health care: fair procedures, democratic deliberation, and the legitimacy problem for insurers. Philos Publ Affairs 1997;26:303-50.

26. Daniels N. Accountability for reasonableness, establish-ing a fair process for priority setting is easier than agreeing on principles. BMJ 2000:321:1300-1.

27. Schneiderman LJ, Jecker NS, Jonsen AR. Medical futility: response to critiques.Ann Intern Med 1996;125:669-74.

28. Fine RL, Mayo TW. Resolution of futility by due process: early experience with the Texas Advance Directives Act. Ann Intern Med 2003;138:743-6.

29. Schneiderman U, Jecker NS, Jonsen AR. Medical futility: its meaning and ethical implications. Ann Intern Med 1990;112:949-54.

30. Marshall MF, Schwenzer KJ, Orsina M, Fletcher JC, Durbin CG Jr. Influence of political power, medical provincialism, and economic incentives on the rationing of surgical intensive care unit beds. Crit Care Med 1992;20:387-94.

31. Hick JL, Christian MD, Sprung CL; European Society of Intensive Care Medicine's Task Force for intensive care unit triage during an influenza epidemic or mass disaster. Chapter 2. Surge capacity and infrastructure considerations for mass critical care. Recommendations and standard operating procedures for intensive care unit and hospital preparations for an influenza epidemic or mass disaster. Intensive Care Med 2010;36 Suppl 1:S11-20.

32. Zimmerman JE, Kramer AA. A model for identifying patients who may not need intensive care unit admission. J Crit Care 2009 doi:10.1016/j.jcrc.2009.06.010.

33. Joynt GM, Gomersall CD. Is 'more' always 'better'? Moving towards optimal utilization of high dependency and intensive care beds by selecting the right patients for admission. Anaesth Intensive Care 2006;34:423-5.

34. Rubinson L, Nuzzo JB, Talmor DS, O'Toole T, Kramer BR, Inglesby TV.

35. Augmentation of hospital critical care capacity after bioterrorist attacks or epidemics: recommendations of the Working Group on Emergency Mass Critical Care. Crit Care Med 2005;33:2393-403.

36. Gomersall CD, Tai DY, Loo S, Derrick JL, Goh MS, Buckley TA, et al. Expanding ICU facilities in an epidemic: recommendations based on experience from the SARS epidemic in Hong Kong and Singapore. Intensive Care Med. 2006;32:1004-13.

37. Joynt GM, Loo S, Taylor BL, Margalit G, Christian MD, Sandrock C, et al; European Society of Intensive Care Medicine's Task Force for intensive care unit triage during an influenza epidemic or mass disaster. Chapter 3. Coordination and collaboration with interface units. Recommendations and standard operating procedures for intensive care unit and hospital preparations for an influenza epidemic or mass disaster. Intensive Care Med 2010;36 Suppl 1:S21-31.

38. Sprung CL, Zimmerman JL, Christian MD, Joynt GM, Hick JL, Taylor B, et al. Recommendations for intensive care unit and hospital preparations for an influenza epidemic or mass disaster: summary report of the European Society of Intensive Care Medicine's Task Force for intensive care unit triage during an influenza epidemic or mass disaster. Intensive Care Med 2010;36:428-43.

39. Garrouste-Orgeas M, Montuclard L, Timsit JF, Misset B, Christias M, Carlet J. Triaging patients to the ICU: a pilot study of factors influencing admission decisions and patient outcomes. Intensive Care Med 2003; 29: 774-81.

40. Lemeshow S, Teres D, Klar J, Avrunin JS, Gehlbach SH, Rapoport J. Mortality Probability Models (MPM II) based on an international cohort of intensive care unit patients. JAMA 1993;270:2478-86.

41. Flaatten H, Kvåle R. Survival and quality of life 12 years after ICU. A comparison with the general Norwegian population. Intensive Care Med 2001;27:1005-11.

42. Cuthbertson BH, Scott J, Strachan M, Kilonzo M, Vale L. Quality of life before and after intensive care. Anaesthesia 2005; 60: 332-9.

43. Graf J, Mühlhoff C, Doig GS, Reinartz S, Bode K, Dujardin R, Koch KC, Roeb E, Janssens U. Health care costs, long-term survival, and quality of life following intensive care unit admission after cardiac arrest. Crit Care 2008;12:R92.

44. Cuthbertson BH, Roughton S, Jenkinson D, Maclennan G, Vale L. Quality of life in the five years after intensive care: a cohort study. Crit Care 2010;14:R6.

45. Muller MP, McGeer AJ, Hassan K, Marshall J, Christian M; Toronto Invasive Bacterial Disease Network. Evaluation of pneumonia severity and acute physiology scores to predict ICU admission and mortality in patients hospitalized for influenza. PLoS One. 2010 Mar 5;5(3):e9563.

Ricard Ferrer, Ana Navas, Maria Luisa Martinez,
Candelaria de Haro and Antonio Artigas

Special admission paths: sepsis

Introduction

The successful treatment of acutely ill patients with a high risk of death is predicated on early recognition and treatment. The key role of early intervention has been recognized in the creation of the term "the golden hour" as it relates to therapy of life-threatening conditions. Analogous to the "golden-hour" concept for trauma [1], acute myocardial infarction [2] and stroke [3], a "golden-hour" concept involving early diagnosis and intervention has been proposed to reduce mortality due to septic shock. Over the past 20 years, systems have evolved in order to better recognize patients with these acute illnesses and to accelerate appropriate treatment.

Sepsis is one of the most prevalent conditions among hospitalized patients and one of the main causes of hospital mortality [4]. Severe sepsis accounts for one in five admissions to intensive care units (ICUs) and is a leading cause of death in non-cardiac ICUs [5, 6]. In Spain, the incidence of severe sepsis is 104 cases per 100,000 adult residents per year with a hospital mortality of 20.7%, and the incidence of septic shock is 31 cases per 100,000 adult residents per year with a mortality of 45.7% [7]; these figures are similar to those reported in other European countries [8]. In the United States, both the incidence of severe sepsis (300 cases per 100,000 persons per year) and the mortality rate (28.6% = 215,000 deaths annually) are higher [4]. Sepsis places a signifi-

cant burden on healthcare resources, accounting for 40% of total ICU expenditures; the total cost of treating sepsis in the year 2000 was estimated to be $ 7.6 billion in Europe and $ 16.7 billion in the United States. Surprisingly, a recent survey done in the general population of Europe and United States showed that 88% of the interviewees had never heard of the term "sepsis" and that 58% of those who indeed recognized the term still did not know that sepsis is a leading cause of death [9].

In recent years there have been unprecedented advances in the understanding of the epidemiology, pathophysiology, and treatment of the sepsis syndrome [10, 11]. Several recently published studies have demonstrated that different interventions and treatments can decrease mortality among patients with sepsis. These data from rigorously performed randomized controlled trials, combined with previous data for beneficial interventions not specific to sepsis management, such as prophylaxis against deep vein thrombosis and stress ulcer, show that it is possible to significantly reduce mortality in patients with severe sepsis and septic shock. Early appropriate antibiotic therapy [12, 13], early goal-directed therapy (EGDT) [14], corticosteroids [15], recombinant human activated protein C or drotrecogin alfa (activated) [16], tight glucose control [17], and lung protective ventilation strategies [18] have all been associated with survival benefits.

These and other therapeutic advances led to the development of the Surviving Sepsis Campaign (SSC) Guidelines [19] as part of a plan to reduce severe sepsis mortality by 25% up to the year 2009. To improve the care for patients with sepsis, the SSC and the Institute for Healthcare Improvement recommend implementing two sepsis bundles. A bundle is a group of interventions that produce better outcomes when executed together than when implemented individually. The individual bundle elements are built on evidence-based practices, and the evidence for each element is strong enough for it to be considered a generally accepted practice. Care bundles ensure that strongly evidence-based clinical practice is consistently applied in a sustained pattern to all patients on all occasions. The key target in bundle implementation is to change clinical practice since it recognizes that on the majority of occasions, core clinical interventions are not uniformly applied to all patients. Bundles enable clinicians to more reliably deliver the best possible care against a background where every intervention carries inherent risk through its commission or omission. They are simply means which improve care in a structured way.

The recommended SSC sepsis bundles were elaborated in partnership with the Institute for Healthcare Improvement and are available from its website: http:// www.ihi.org/IHI/Topics/CriticalCare/Sepsis/. There are two bundles: the resuscitation bundle and the management bundle.

- The resuscitation bundle includes lactate determination, early cultures and antibiotics, and EGDT. This bundle describes seven tasks that should begin immediately and must be accomplished within the first 6 hours of presentation of severe sepsis or septic shock. Some items may not be completed if the clinical conditions described in the bundle do not prevail in a particular case, but it is clinicians themselves who must assess these elements.
- The management bundle includes optimization of glycaemic control and respiratory inspiratory plateau pressure, and determination of the need for corticosteroids or drotrecogin alfa (activated). Efforts to accomplish these goals should begin immediately, and these items must be completed within 24 hours of presentation of severe sepsis or septic shock.

Bundled care of sepsis

The first evidence of an effect of sepsis bundles on patient care came from Birmingham, England.

Gao and colleagues [20] conducted a prospective observational study on 101 consecutive adult patients who presented severe sepsis or septic shock on medical or surgical wards, or during emergency care at two acute National Health Service Trust teaching hospitals in England. The main outcome measures were the rate of compliance with the sepsis resuscitation and management bundles and the difference in hospital mortality between patients in whom care was compliant and those in whom it was not. Overall compliance with the sepsis bundles was 52%; compliance was associated with lower hospital mortality when compared with noncompliance (29% vs. 55%, $p = 0.045$). Micek et al. [21] demonstrated that the implementation of a protocol for the management of septic shock in the emergency department was significantly associated with more rigorous fluid resuscitation, greater administration of appropriate initial antibiotic treatment (71.7% vs. 86.76, $p = 0.043$), less need for vasopressors at the time of transfer to the ICU (100% vs. 71.7%, $p < 0.001$), lower 28-day mortality (48.3% vs. 30%, $p = 0.040$), and shorter hospital stay (12.1 + 9.2 days vs. 8.9 + 7.2 days, $p = 0.038$). Kortgen et al. [22] assessed in Germany the impact of a resuscitation algorithm (standard operating procedure) for organ dysfunction and septic shock. These investigators concluded that an approach combining EGDT, intensive insulin therapy, hydrocortisone administration, and rhAPC administration in selected cases improved outcome. Mortality was lower after implementation of the standard operating procedure in comparison with the historical control group (27% vs. 53%, $p < 0.05$). Shapiro and colleagues [23] enrolled 116 septic patients, 79 of whom had septic shock, in a study to evaluate a sepsis treatment protocol that incorporated empirical antibiotics, EGDT, rhAPC, steroids, intensive insulin therapy, and lung protective ventilation (MUST: multiple urgent sepsis therapies). Compared with 51 historical controls, protocol patients received more fluids, earlier antibiotics, more appropriate empiric antibiotic coverage, more vasopressors in the first 6 hours, and tighter glucose control. Although mortality in the protocol group was only 18%, the study was not able to demonstrate a reduction in mortality because it was not adequately powered and the historical control group introduced a potential selection bias. This limitation underlines the need for multicentre trials to establish the collective effect of combining available evidenced-based sepsis therapies. Nguyen and colleagues [24] enrolled 330 patients who met the criteria for severe sepsis or septic shock in a two-year prospective observational cohort study that examined the effect of implementing a severe sepsis bundle in the emergency department. The bundle comprised the following five elements:

1. Initiation of central venous pressure (CVP)/ central venous oxygen saturation (ScvO$_2$) monitoring within 2 hours.
2. Delivery of broad-spectrum antibiotics within 4 hours.
3. Completion of an EGDT trial at 6 hours.
4. Delivery of corticosteroids to vasopressor-dependent patients and to those with suspected adrenal insufficiency.
5. Ongoing monitoring for lactate clearance.

The bundle was introduced as a quality indicator, and regular feedback was routinely provided to modify physicians' behaviour in the early management of severe sepsis and septic shock. Compliance with the bundle increased from zero at the start of the study to 51.2 % at the end of the study period. During the emergency department stay, patients in whom the bundle was completed received more CVP/ScvO$_2$ monitoring, more antibiotics, and more corticosteroids than patients with in whom the bundle was not completed. In a multivariate regression analysis including the five elements of the bundle, completion of EGDT was significantly associated with decreased mortality (odds ratio, 0.36; 95 % CI, 0.17 to 0.79; p = 0.01). In-hospital mortality was lower in patients in whom the bundle was completed than in patients in whom the bundle was not completed (20.8 % vs. 39.5 %, p < 0.01). Also in 2007, Jones et al. [25] published the results of a two-year prospective interventional trial that sought to determine the clinical effectiveness of implementing EGDT as a routine protocol in the emergency department. The authors prospectively recorded pre-intervention clinical and mortality data on consecutive eligible patients for 12 months. Next, they introduced an EGDT protocol and recorded clinical and mortality data for an additional 12 months. Before starting the study, the investigators defined the clinical

effectiveness of the intervention as a 33 % relative reduction in mortality (the reduction in relative mortality found in the original EGDT trial by Rivers et al. [14]). A total of 156 patients were enrolled in the study:

- 79 in the 12 months immediately before the intervention and
- 77 in the 12 months immediately after the intervention.

Patients in the post-intervention period received a significantly greater crystalloid volume and frequency of vasopressor infusion during initial resuscitation than patients in the pre-intervention period. In-hospital mortality was 27 % before the intervention, compared with 18 % after the intervention but this difference did not reach statistical significance.

A recent meta-analysis [26], including all of these studies, done by the group of the National Institutes of Health in the United States, examined the effect of bundle institution on survival. Sepsis care bundles were associated with a consistent and significant increase in survival (odds ratio, 1.91; CI, 1.49–2.45; p < 0.0001). Additionally, the investigators analysed which components of the bundles were responsible for the mortality increase. Antibiotic use was also consistently and significantly improved across the studies. In contrast, this group of investigators found significant heterogeneity in the effect of bundle care on the use of the remaining bundle components analysed. Haemodynamic support with fluids and vasopressors is probably as important as antibiotics in reducing mortality from septic shock [27]. However, resuscitation fluid volumes and the percentage of patients receiving vasopressors were not consistently altered by bundled care. Although bundles in each of these studies targeted a CVP of 8 mmHg to 12 mmHg for fluid administration and a mean arterial pressure ≥ 65 mmHg for vasopressors, levels outside this range were likely employed clinically in some patients and may have contributed to heterogeneity. Importantly, the effectiveness of these targets is being re-evaluated in large, multicentre randomized controlled trials [28]. Likewise, bundled care did not uniformly change low-dose corticosteroid or activated protein C use among trials, and this may also be related to variations in practice. The risk and benefits of these treatments administered alone or together, are being assessed in randomized controlled trials [29]. Besides antibiotic treatment, other unmeasured effects, like earlier recognition of patients requiring surgical intervention or more readily available non-bundled therapies, such as respiratory support, may have changed the outcome.

Multifaceted strategies to deliver bundled care for sepsis

Two studies have analysed the impact of multifaceted strategies in delivering bundled care for severe sepsis on a national or international scale.

A large multicentre sepsis trial (Edusepsis study) in Spain tested the effect of a multifaceted educational program on bundle treatment goals and outcome [30]. Edusepsis-assessed compliance with the SSC guidelines before and after an educational program in 77 medical-surgical ICUs homogeneously distributed around the country. Compliance with the recommendations of the SSC guidelines was measured in a cohort of patients before the educational program, in a cohort after the program, and in a third cohort from a subset of the ICUs one year later. The educational program was a multifaceted intervention that consisted of training physicians and nursing staff from the emergency department, medical and surgical wards, and ICU in the definitions of severe sepsis and sepsis shock, early recognition of severe sepsis and septic shock, and the treatment bundles included in the guidelines. A total of 2,319 patients fulfilled the criteria for severe sepsis or septic shock during the pre-intervention and post-intervention periods. Compliance with process-of-care variables improved after the educational program: Resuscitation bundle (5.3% vs. 10.0%; p < 0.001) and Management bundle (10.9% vs. 15.7%; p = 0.001). In-hospital mortality was also lower after the educational program (44% vs. 39.7%, p = 0.036); however, as in other studies, the decrease in mortality observed in this study might derive from better identification of patients with severe sepsis or from improved compliance with the guidelines or both.

A sub-study of the Edusepsis database analysed the effectiveness of the treatments included in the bundles [31]. Using propensity scores to assess the effectiveness of the treatments, the investigators identified the administration of broad-spectrum antibiotics in all patients and activated protein C in patients with multi-organ failure as the treatments responsible for the reduction in mortality.

The patients from the Spanish database were added to an international registry for the SSC international multifaceted performance improving program, which also showed improved bundle care and survival (hospital mortality decreased from 37.0% to 30.8% in two years) [32]. This huge effort to improve performance in hospitals across Europe, South America and the United States recruited the largest prospective series of severe sepsis patients yet studied. After adjustment for baseline characteristics, administrating broad-spectrum antibiotics, obtaining blood cultures before their initiation, and maintaining blood glucose control were all associated with lower mortality. The administration of activated protein C in the first 24 hours was associated with improved survival in patients in shock, and achieving plateau pressure control was associated with improved outcome in those on mechanical ventilation.

The results of the meta-analysis of single-centre studies [26], the results of the Spanish Edusepsis study [30] and the results of the international SSC study [32] are very consistent in showing that sepsis bundles improve survival by improving the way sepsis treatments are delivered. Early sepsis recognition and administration of broad-spectrum antibiotics in all patients and specific treatments for patients in shock or on mechanical ventilation play a role in improving sepsis outcome (see Tab. 1). Hospitals should recognize this new evidence and design strategies to guarantee bundled care for severe sepsis.

How can delivery of bundle care for severe sepsis be improved? Possible strategies

Despite the above-mentioned initiatives, an augmentation of bundle implementation still remains low. The data support an important role for sepsis care bundles in future management of infection, but the measures included in the bundles must be applied in the context of wider programs rather than isolated solutions. Setting up these multifaceted programs requires a capital

Tab. 1 Treatments associated with lower mortality in studies analysing bundled care for severe sepsis. NIH: National Institutes of Health. SSC: Surviving Sepsis Campaign

Study	Population	Treatment
NIH meta-analysis [26]	All septic patients	Broad-spectrum antibiotic
Edusepsis [31]	All septic patients	Broad-spectrum antibiotic in the first hour
	Multi-organ failure	Activated protein C
International SSC [32]	All septic patients	Broad-spectrum antibiotic
	All septic patients	Tight glucose control
	Septic shock	Activated protein C
	Mechanical ventilation	Low plateau pressure

outlay; however, these expenditures represent an investment that will be outweighed by the resultant benefits. For these programs to succeed, clinical practice must change, and changes in clinical practice depend upon the clinicians' willingness to adopt new ways of working. Health-care organizations traditionally favour investing in new technology and drugs, but are reluctant to invest in organizational development. For sepsis care bundles to succeed, this must change.

Our proposals for improving sepsis survival are:
- To improve the general population's knowledge of sepsis. Prompt consultation in the emergency department about potentially severe septic conditions could help septic patients receive treatment earlier.
- Emergency department staff might be insufficient to deliver bundled care of sepsis [33]. This point should be evaluated and corrected where necessary.
- Earlier recognition and treatment of sepsis. Research in biomarkers: Future trials should include the measurement of biomarkers that could aid in future decisions regarding the use of the agent being tested in the clinical arena; this approach can also help improve our understanding of the natural history of sepsis and of the effects of specific interventions on its biological evolution. As pointed out recently by Marshall and Reinhart [34], a reliable biomarker in sepsis will make it possible to establish a diagnosis to inform a treatment decision and to do so more reliably, more rapidly, or more inexpensively than that achieved

by available methods. Other potential benefits of a sepsis biomarker are: identifying subgroups of patients who may experience greater benefit or harm from therapeutic intervention, measuring the response to an intervention to permit the titration of dose or duration of treatment, and providing a more sensitive measure of the consequences of treatment that can substitute for a direct measure of a patient-cantered outcome.
- Locally driven organizational interventions are urgently needed, along with a wide educational campaign to change behaviours among nurses and doctors working in the emergency department, ICUs, and general and surgical wards. The key to success involves the implementation of a hospital-wide system that recognizes septic patients early, and at the same time rapidly administers effective therapy. This is best accomplished by identifying those physicians and nurses who can turn out to be champions of a sepsis rapid response team [35]. This system should emphasize education, as well as policies and procedures that empower frontline providers to recognize sepsis early, and independently institute basic resuscitation. Creation of a sepsis-rapid response team requires not only various champions to drive it, but also needs an effective structure for its development, education of staff, implementation and continuous process improvement.
- Use of adequate teaching and quality improvement strategies: reminders and interactive dissemination of educational materials, to-

gether with auditing and feedback, produce modest to moderate improvements in care [36]. The sepsis team should design specific multifaceted quality improvement strategies based on cycles of the Plan-Design-Study-Act as proposed by Shewhart [37]. Cycles should be focused on those treatments yielding the greatest impact on survival, such as antibiotics or activated protein C.

■ Computerized clinical decision support: computer technology can provide information to guide specific care at the bedside in real time. This technology has been useful in other scenarios in critical care [38]. Clinical information systems, prescription support systems, or ICU bed monitors could be adequate platforms to assist physicians in delivering bundled care for severe sepsis.

Summary

Bundled care for severe sepsis is associated with better survival. Multifaceted strategies are useful to increase bundled care at the national or international level. However, bundle implementation remains unacceptably low and many lives could be saved each year by improving the way in which we deliver sepsis care.

The challenge that hospitals must now face is how to best implement systems to facilitate this goal.

The authors

Ricard Ferrer, MD, PhD
Ana Navas, MD
Maria Luisa Martinez, MD
Candelaria de Haro, MD
Antonio Artigas, MD, PhD
    Critical Care Center | Hospital de Sabadell |
    CIBER Enfermedades Respiratorias |
    Instituto Universitario Parc Tauli |
    Universidad Autónoma de Barcelona, Spain

Address for correspondence
    Ricard Ferrer
    Critical Care Center
    Hospital de Sabadell
    Parc Tauli s/n
    08208 Sabadell, Spain
    E-mail: rferrer@tauli.cat

References

1. Blow O, Magliore L, Claridge JA, Butler K, Young JS. The golden hour and the silver day: detection and correction of occult hypoperfusion within 24 hours improves outcome from major trauma. J Trauma 1999 Nov;47(5):964–9.
2. Boersma E, Maas AC, Deckers JW, Simoons ML. Early thrombolytic treatment in acute myocardial infarction: reappraisal of the golden hour. Lancet 1996 Sep 21;348(9030):771–5.
3. Meschia JF, Miller DA, Brott TG. Thrombolytic treatment of acute ischemic stroke. Mayo Clin Proc 2002 Jun;77(6):542–51.
4. Angus DC, Linde-Zwirble WT, Lidicker J, Clermont G, Carcillo J, Pinsky MR. Epidemiology of severe sepsis in the United States: analysis of incidence, outcome, and associated costs of care. Crit Care Med 2001 Jul;29(7):1303–10.
5. Brun-Buisson C, Doyon F, Carlet J, Dellamonica P, Gouin F, Lepoutre A, et al. Incidence, risk factors, and outcome of severe sepsis and septic shock in adults. A multicenter prospective study in intensive care units. French ICU Group for Severe Sepsis. JAMA 1995 Sep 27;274(12):968–74.
6. Guidet B, Aegerter P, Gauzit R, Meshaka P, Dreyfuss D. Incidence and impact of organ dysfunctions associated with sepsis. Chest 2005 Mar;127(3):942–51.
7. Esteban A, Frutos-Vivar F, Ferguson ND, Penuelas O, Lorente JA, Gordo F, et al. Sepsis incidence and outcome: contrasting the intensive care unit with the hospital ward. Crit Care Med 2007 May;35(5):1284–9.
8. Alberti C, Brun-Buisson C, Burchardi H, Martin C, Goodman S, Artigas A, et al. Epidemiology of sepsis and infection in ICU patients from an international multicentre cohort study. Intensive Care Med 2002 Feb;28(2):108–21.
9. Rubulotta FM, Ramsay G, Parker MM, Dellinger RP, Levy MM, Poeze M. An international survey: Public awareness and perception of sepsis. Crit Care Med 2009 Jan;37(1):167–70.
10. Abraham E, Singer M. Mechanisms of sepsis-induced organ dysfunction. Crit Care Med 2007 Oct;35(10):2408–16.
11. Wheeler AP. Recent developments in the diagnosis and management of severe sepsis. Chest 2007 Dec;132(6):1967–76.
12. Garnacho-Montero J, Garcia-Garmendia JL, Barrero-Almodovar A, Jimenez-Jimenez FJ, Perez-Paredes C, Ortiz-Leyba C. Impact of adequate empirical antibiotic therapy on the outcome of patients admitted to the intensive care unit with sepsis. Crit Care Med 2003 Dec;31(12):2742–51.
13. Kumar A, Roberts D, Wood KE, Light B, Parrillo JE, Sharma S, et al. Duration of hypotension before initiation of effective antimicrobial therapy is the

critical determinant of survival in human septic shock. Crit Care Med 2006 Jun;34(6):1589–96.

14. Rivers E, Nguyen B, Havstad S, Ressler J, Muzzin A, Knoblich B, et al. Early goal-directed therapy in the treatment of severe sepsis and septic shock. N Engl J Med 2001 Nov 8;345(19):1368–77.

15. Annane D, Sebille V, Charpentier C, Bollaert PE, Francois B, Korach JM, et al. Effect of treatment with low doses of hydrocortisone and fludrocortisone on mortality in patients with septic shock. JAMA 2002 Aug 21;288(7):862–71.

16. Bernard GR, Vincent JL, Laterre PF, LaRosa SP, Dhainaut JF, Lopez-Rodriguez A, et al. Efficacy and safety of recombinant human activated protein C for severe sepsis. N Engl J Med 2001 Mar 8;344(10):699–709.

17. van den Berghe G., Wouters P, Weekers F, Verwaest C, Bruyninckx F, Schetz M, et al. Intensive insulin therapy in the critically ill patients. N Engl J Med 2001 Nov 8;345(19):1359–67.

18. Ventilation with lower tidal volumes as compared with traditional tidal volumes for acute lung injury and the acute respiratory distress syndrome. The Acute Respiratory Distress Syndrome Network. N Engl J Med 2000 May 4;342(18):1301–8.

19. Dellinger RP, Carlet JM, Masur H, Gerlach H, Calandra T, Cohen J, et al. Surviving Sepsis Campaign guidelines for management of severe sepsis and septic shock. Intensive Care Med 2004 Apr;30(4):536–55.

20. Gao F, Melody T, Daniels DF, Giles S, Fox S. The impact of compliance with 6-hour and 24-hour sepsis bundles on hospital mortality in patients with severe sepsis: a prospective observational study. Crit Care 2005;9(6):R764-R770.

21. Micek ST, Roubinian N, Heuring T, Bode M, Williams J, Harrison C, et al. Before-after study of a standardized hospital order set for the management of septic shock. Crit Care Med 2006 Nov;34(11):2707–13.

22. Kortgen A, Niederprum P, Bauer M. Implementation of an evidence-based "standard operating procedure" and outcome in septic shock. Crit Care Med 2006 Apr;34(4):943–9.

23. Shapiro NI, Howell MD, Talmor D, Lahey D, Ngo L, Buras J, et al. Implementation and outcomes of the Multiple Urgent Sepsis Therapies (MUST) protocol. Crit Care Med 2006 Apr;34(4):1025–32.

24. Nguyen HB, Corbett SW, Steele R, Banta J, Clark RT, Hayes SR, et al. Implementation of a bundle of quality indicators for the early management of severe sepsis and septic shock is associated with decreased mortality. Crit Care Med 2007 Apr;35(4):1105–12.

25. Jones AE, Focht A, Horton JM, Kline JA. Prospective external validation of the clinical effectiveness of an emergency department-based early goal-directed therapy protocol for severe sepsis and septic shock. Chest 2007 Aug;132(2):425–32.

26. Barochia AV, Cui X, Vitberg D, Suffredini AF, O'grady NP, Banks SM, et al. Bundled care for septic shock: an analysis of clinical trials. Crit Care Med 2010 Feb;38(2):668–78.

27. Natanson C, Danner RL, Reilly JM, Doerfler ML, Hoffman WD, Akin GL, et al. Antibiotics versus cardiovascular support in a canine model of human septic shock. Am J Physiol 1990 Nov;259(5 Pt 2):H1440-H1447.

28. Delaney A, Angus DC, Bellomo R, Cameron P, Cooper DJ, Finfer S, et al. Bench-to-bedside review: the evaluation of complex interventions in critical care. Crit Care 2008;12(2):210.

29. Finfer S, Ranieri VM, Thompson BT, Barie PS, Dhainaut JF, Douglas IS, et al. Design, conduct, analysis and reporting of a multi-national placebo-controlled trial of activated protein C for persistent septic shock. Intensive Care Med 2008 Nov;34(11):1935–47.

30. Ferrer R, Artigas A, Levy MM, Blanco J, Gonzalez-Diaz G, Garnacho-Montero J, et al. Improvement in process of care and outcome after a multicenter severe sepsis educational program in Spain. JAMA 2008 May 21;299(19):2294–303.

31. Ferrer R, Artigas A, Suarez D, Palencia E, Levy MM, Arenzana A, et al. Effectiveness of treatments for severe sepsis: a prospective, multicenter, observational study. Am J Respir Crit Care Med 2009 Nov 1;180(9):861–6.

32. Levy MM, Dellinger RP, Townsend SR, Linde-Zwirble WT, Marshall JC, Bion J, et al. The Surviving Sepsis Campaign: results of an international guideline-based performance improvement program targeting severe sepsis. Intensive Care Med 2010 Feb;36(2):222–31.

33. McNeill G, Dixon M, Jenkins P. Can acute medicine units in the UK comply with the Surviving Sepsis Campaign's six-hour care bundle? Clin Med 2008 Apr;8(2):163–5.

34. Marshall JC, Reinhart K. Biomarkers of sepsis. Crit Care Med 2009 Jul;37(7):2290–8.

35. Funk D, Sebat F, Kumar A. A systems approach to the early recognition and rapid administration of best practice therapy in sepsis and septic shock. Curr Opin Crit Care 2009 Aug;15(4):301–7.

36. Grimshaw JM, Thomas RE, MacLennan G, Fraser C, Ramsay CR, Vale L, et al. Effectiveness and efficiency of guideline dissemination and implementation strategies. Health Technol Assess 2004 Feb;8(6):iii-72.

37. Best M, Neuhauser D. Walter A Shewhart, 1924, and the Hawthorne factory. Qual Saf Health Care 2006 Apr;15(2):142–3.

38. Sucher JF, Moore FA, Todd SR, Sailors RM, McKinley BA. Computerized clinical decision support: a technology to implement and validate evidence based guidelines. J Trauma 2008 Feb;64(2):520–37.

Jonathan Ball, Rupert Pearse, Andrew Rhodes and Rui P. Moreno

Special admission paths: trauma

Trauma is a leading cause of death and disability worldwide and its prevalence is increasing. In 2007, the UK National Confidential Enquiry into Patient Outcome and Death [1] reported trauma to be the fourth leading cause of death within the first four decades of life with an average of 39 years lost per trauma death. Although trauma is perceived to be a disease of the young, paradoxically, especially for the specialty of critical care, the elderly have a major impact on the overall epidemiology. Unsurprisingly, an older patient with the same severity of injury has a worse outcome [2].

Arguably of even greater importance, trauma is also the most common cause of debilitating long-term injuries, with two patients left permanently disabled for each fatality. The impact, both on health care systems and societies is immense. For the affected individuals and their families, the consequences are frequently life-changing especially following traumatic brain injury. Worldwide, the majority of poly-trauma patients are victims of motor vehicle accidents and the majority suffer some degree of brain injury [3].

The optimal care of a polytrauma patient must involve early and coordinated input from multiple specialties. Trauma deaths have a trimodal distribution. Most immediate and some early deaths are inevitable due to the severity of injury and/or the frailty of the patient and are the province of preventative strategies.

Of the remainder of early deaths, the majority result from uncontrolled haemorrhage. Intermediate deaths result from either catastrophic brain injury and/or multiple organ failure. Late deaths result from secondary complications such as infection and thromboemobolism. Critical care plays a major role not only in minimising death at all these stages, but also and arguably more importantly, in maximising functional outcome in survivors.

For obvious reasons, major advances in both the clinical and organisational management of trauma patients have emerged from military conflicts over the last 100 years. Indeed, these advances have demonstrated dramatic reductions in mortality and long term disability. The most recent military conflicts in Iraq and Afghanistan are no exception. It is a sobering fact that despite the precision and lethality of modern weapons, mortality rates in immediate survivors of conflict injuries have been reduced to 10 % [3]. In civilian medicine however, many of these advances, especially those relating to organisation, have been relatively neglected, and best practice has been only slowly and patchily adopted [1, 4]. Although many of these advances do translate seamlessly into civilian practice, there are also significant differences, and an extrapolation requires thoughtful caution and ongoing clinical trials.

Preventable poor outcomes

Multiple reports from a wide variety of august institutions over the last 10–20 years have all highlighted the same failings in the organisation of trauma care and the unacceptably high rates of preventable death and disability. There is dramatic outcome variability, both within and between countries, with 100–200 % differences in mortality rates for patients with similar injuries. The causes of these excess deaths are complex but do include at least poor organization of services, inappropriate division and distribution of responsibility, poor use of resources and a lack of both education and training into definitive trauma management [5–6].

Sadly, it remains commonplace for severely injured trauma patients to be taken to hospitals which are inadequately equipped to manage them. This results in either suboptimal care or a detrimental/fatal delay in the delivery of such care. Even within multi-specialty hospitals, care is all too often fragmented with a series of single organ doctors merely looking after their own part of the body and nobody taking the overall holistic view that the patient requires. Appropriate management of multiply injured trauma patients requires much more than just a hospital of all the specialties, it requires a specialist hospital.

A systems approach with centralized care

Unequivocal evidence has established that a coordinated, inclusive systems approach, which encompasses every aspect of the trauma patient journey from prevention to pre-hospital care, hospital reception, through to intensive care and onto rehabilitation, optimises patient outcome [7–8]. This is a public health model and involves regions rather than just individual hospitals. The model should provide care for all trauma patients that are injured in a defined population, rather than just those being presented to an individual hospital. It is important to recognize that a trauma system is not just the designation of a "Level I"/Major Trauma Centre (MTC) with the most severely injured patients bypassing local hospitals. It is a coordinated approach that includes local hospitals ("Levels II–IV"/"Trauma Units") who manage less severely injured patients, together with transfer/transport mechanisms and education. If less severely injured patients all end up in the "Level I"/MTC, there is a risk of inferior treatment, due to them being deprioritized within an overloaded hyper-acute setting. Such a geographical system must therefore include all hospitals within a region and ensure that the caseload of each is appropriate for its resources.

Is has been estimated that for an individual hospital to provide optimal "Level I" trauma care for seriously injured polytrauma patients, it should see a throughput of approximately 240 or more such cases per year. This is one of the fields of medicine where the relationship between volume and outcome has been more clearly demonstrated [9–10].

There is evidence suggesting that the institution of regional models of trauma care improves outcomes with mortality reductions of up to 40 % and preventable deaths of less than 1 % of the total [11]. This can be achieved by redeployment of available resources in a more equitable and rational fashion and can even produce a reduction in costs [12]. Incorporating MTCs into an inclusive trauma system consistently achieves an additional 20 % reduction in mortality. It is notable that these benefits are for the entire region rather than just for those patients managed in the MTC.

Trauma registries

National trauma registries are essential to provide standardised quality performance indicators to each institution within a trauma system, and to monitor the performance of the system as a whole and the interfaces between the critical parts of the system. Such registries provide vital data to inform governance structures and facilitate hypothesis generating research. As with other areas of critical care, injury severity scoring is a useful population tool for comparison, generating mortality prediction models and potentially benchmarking [13].

The process of trauma care

The process of trauma care is well established and involves a series of repeated surveys. The primary survey is aimed at detecting and treating immediate life-threatening injuries. The secondary survey aims at cataloguing all other injuries, and the tertiary survey revises this list in light of imaging and expert review including intensivists, surgeons and radiologists [14]

For the severely injured patient, critical care involvement ideally starts in the pre-hospital phase, with rapid assessment, advanced airway management and packaging for transfer to a centre capable of delivering definitive care, thereby avoiding the need for a secondary transfer. Packaging for safe transfer includes a much lower threshold than normal for endotracheal intubation and thoracostomies/pleural drainage, as performing these procedures in transit may be difficult or impossible, especially if helicopter transfer is undertaken. A further major benefit to experienced on-scene critical care is early detailed communication to the receiving hospital to allow a team of appropriate specialists to be assembled to receive the patient and pre-alert imaging, blood transfusion, theatres and critical care to allow them to start preparing for the

patient(s). When only a paramedic response is available, a simple triage decision tree is essential to minimise both under and over triage [14]. The newly established London trauma system uses the following scheme (see Fig. 1) and has a permanently manned coordination desk both to advise on scene crew and direct a patient's destination. This again provides a vital pre-alert to receiving hospitals.

Critical care during the hospital reception phase should provide optimal physiological management during the assessment, imaging and transfer of the patient to either an operative environment or a critical care area. This should employ a "damage control" resuscitation approach [15]. Such an approach may include permissive hypotension during the initial resuscitation (prior to haemorrhage control). However, the evidence base for this approach, especially in the polytrauma patient with brain injury, is controversial. The choice of resuscitation fluid and the optimal ratio of packed red blood cells to fresh frozen plasma and platelets, remains uncertain. However,

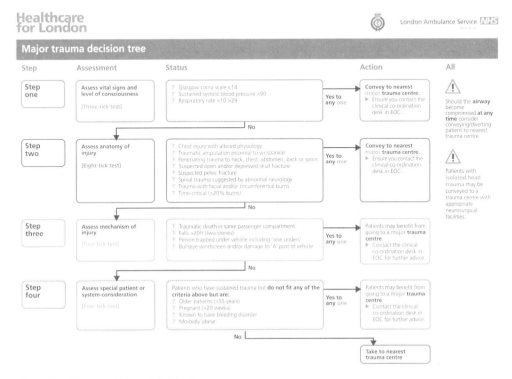

Fig. 1   HfL/LAS trauma triage and decision tree

minimising dilutional coagulopathy (by avoiding crystalloids and colloids) and instead using blood products in physiological (1:1) ratios during the resuscitation phase, is advocated more and more [16–17]. Aggressive measures are often required to maintain normothermia and avoid/minimise metabolic acidosis whilst standardisation of anaesthesia/sedation and vascular access practices are probably beneficial [18–19]. Ideally, the reception area, CT/interventional radiology, theatres and the ICU should be co-located and share equipment, such as monitors, pumps and ventilators. All of these areas should be available within a few minutes of an emergency need. Inevitably, creating such capacity is problematic but it must be sufficiently flexible to permit reasonably predictable fluxes in demand, including a sustainable response to simultaneous/multiple casualties. All of these areas need rapid access to blood transfusion laboratories and a limited unmatched supply of packed red blood cells and fresh frozen plasma. Similarly, the availability of near patient testing for blood gas analysis, co-oximetry and thromboelastography is valuable and regarded by some as essential. A robust and simple unique patient identifier system is vital to label the patient, their medical notes, investigation requests/results and drug/blood product administration as the usual identifiers such as name, date of birth, previous hospital or national health service numbers may not be available for hours or days.

The continuum of trauma care should transition from damage control resuscitation to consideration of damage control surgery versus immediate definitive repair. Damage control surgery is an evolving philosophy that limits immediate surgical intervention to stopping bleeding, external stabilisation of major fractures and decontamination of wounds and/or body cavities. Consistent with this approach and in the setting of massive haemorrhage, in particular due to penetrating chest trauma, clam shell thoracotomy in the pre-hospital or hospital reception environment can be life saving. Following damage control surgery, patients are commonly transferred to ICU for physiological stabilisation and preparation for definitive surgery at the earliest opportunity. The decision to adopt a damage control strategy should be based upon the patient's physiology and not on a surgical outcome [20]. The patient may require a number of additional damage control surgical procedures. Daily multidisciplinary trauma rounds are essential to balance the competing demands for continuing physiological stabilisation with definitive surgical repair of injuries. The critical care team is central to the coordination of competing demands in the polytrauma patient, especially if the patient has significant brain and/or lung injuries. Returns to theatre should be coordinated such that multiple surgical specialties can operate simultaneously and thereby minimise the number of such episodes.

Spinal clearance

A robust and rapid spinal clearance protocol is essential to minimise immobilisation and its attendant complications. As seriously injured patients cannot fulfil the criteria for clinical clearance, early radiological clearance is essential. Performing spinal CT with planar reconstruction at the time of initial assessment is generally advocated as the best default approach. When the situation permits, an alternative or limited imaging approach that reduces the radiation dose can be employed. The best practice is to task the trauma reception team leader by ensuring that a radiological spinal clearance is achieved.

Additional intensive care requirements

Any ICU which regularly admits polytrauma patients must, in addition to standard ICU therapies, have the following capabilities:

- Continuous monitoring and management of patients with raised intracranial pressure, including rapid access to emergency CT and neurosurgical intervention.
- Optimal nursing care of patients requiring axial skeleton immobilisation for unstable spinal and/or pelvic injuries. This is facilitated by extra space around the bed to allow deployment of specialist equipment such as scoop stretchers with hoists. Such care often requires a higher than normal staff-to-patient ratio, for example, to facilitate frequent log rolling.
- Management of (multiple) pleural drains with access to high volume/low pressure suction systems.

- Monitoring of intra-abdominal pressure and management of intra-abdominal hypertension/ compartment syndrome including decompressive laparostomy.
- Optimal care of skeletal traction, external fixators, open wounds and negative pressure wound management systems.

In addition, there is anecdotal evidence to support the use of extra-corporeal cardio-respiratory support in severe trauma and, indeed from the biological plausibility standpoint, such patients are the most likely to benefit from this therapy. Accordingly, the ability to deliver such therapy and to do so on a regular basis, is probably desirable.

Unusual/specialist injuries – thermal, chemical and miscellaneous

The ability to decontaminate casualties from exposure to ionising radiation, chemical and biological agents is desirable/essential, depending upon the likelihood of one's ever receiving such casualties. Emergency departments must have protocols in place to deal with these situations and perform regular simulation training.

Trauma can occur in many different settings. For the same arguments that services for the severely injured be centralised, a smaller number of specialist units, such as those for burns, are required. Ideally these should be located within an MTC and have their own critical care capacity. If unfeasible, then a major trauma centre should develop an established relationship with their local unit(s).

Rehabilitation and discharge planning

Early and aggressive physical therapy is essential. This can be led and/or prescribed by specialist therapists but can be co-delivered by nursing and auxiliary staff. Early involvement of additional specialist therapists, as indicated, is similarly desirable. Identification of a key therapist who acts as a coordinator for each case is useful.

Early identification of and referral to the optimal discharge location from ICU is essential. This will depend upon the need for ongoing specialist surgical (and occasionally medical) management, the availability and location of local rehabilitation services including specialist services such as those for brain or spinal cord injury and the patient's usual address. A full neuropsychological assessment at the earliest practical opportunity, and a repetition as indicated by the patient's progress is essential. Provision for self referral back to support services is also vital. Facilitated access to legal and practical support services for both patients and their dependants is highly desirable [21].

The authors

Jonathan Ball, MD MRCP[1]
Rupert Pearse, MD FRCA[2]
Andrew Rhodes, FRCA FRCP[1]
Rui P. Moreno, MD, PhD[3]
   [1] Department of Intensive Care | St George's healthcare NHS Trust | London, UK
   [2] Intensive Care Unit | Royal London Hospital | Whitechapel, London, UK
   [3] Unidade de Cuidados Intensivos Polivalente | Hospital de Santo António dos Capuchos | Centro Hospitalar de Lisboa Central, E.P.E. | Lisbon, Portugal

Address for correspondence
   Andrew Rhodes
   General Intensive Care
   St George's Hospital
   London SW17 0QT, UK
   E-mail: andyr@sgul.ac.uk

References

1. Trauma: Who cares? A report of the National Confidential Enquiry into Patient Outcome and Death. 2007. http://www.ncepod.org.uk/2007report2/Downloads/SIP_report.pdf.
2. Giannoudis PV, Harwood PJ, Court-Brown C, Pape HC. Severe and multiple trauma in older patients; incidence and mortality. Injury 2009;40:362–7.
3. Gawande A. Casualties of War – Military Care for the Wounded from Iraq and Afghanistan. N Engl J Med 2004;351:2471–5.
4. Mock C, Lormand J, Goosen J, Joshipura M, Peden M. Guidelines for essential trauma care. Geneva: World Health Organization; 2004.
5. Stewart RM, Myers JG, Dent DL, et al. Seven hundred

fifty-three consecutive deaths in a level I trauma center: the argument for injury prevention. J Trauma. 2003 Jan;54(1):66–70.

6. Anderson ID, Woodford M, de Dombal FT, Irving M. Retrospective study of 1000 deaths from injury in England and Wales. BMJ 1988;296:1305–8.

7. Lansink KWW, Leenen LPH: Do designated trauma systems improve outcome? Current Opinion in Critical Care 2007;13:686–690.

8. Liberman M, Mulder DS, Jurkovich GJ, Sampalis JS. The association between trauma system and trauma center components and outcome in a mature regionalized trauma system. Surgery. 2005;137(6):647–58.

9. Chiara O, Cimbanassi S: Organized trauma care: does volume matter and do trauma centers save lives? Current Opinion in Critical Care 2003;9:510–514.

10. Nathens AB, Jurkovich GJ, Maier RV, et al. Relationship between trauma center volume and outcomes. JAMA. 2001;285(9):1164–71.

11. Nathens AB, Jurkovich GJ, Maier RV, et al. Relationship between trauma center volume and outcomes. JAMA. 2001;285(9):1164–71.

12. Durham R, Pracht E, Orban B, Lottenburg L, Tepas J, Flint L. Evaluation of a Mature Trauma System. Annals of Surgery: 2006;243:775–785.

13. Juillard C, Mock C, Goosen J, Joshipura M, Civil I: Establishing the Evidence Base for Trauma Quality Improvement: A Collaborative WHO-IATSIC Review. World Journal of Surgery 2009;33:1075–1086.

14. Hoff WSMD, Sicoutris CPC, Lee SYMD, Rotondo MFMD, Holstein JJMD, Gracias VHMD, Pryor JPMD, Reilly PMMD, Doroski KKDO, Schwab CWMD: Formalized Radiology Rounds: The Final Component of the Tertiary Survey. Journal of Trauma-Injury Infection & Critical Care 2004;56:291–295.

15. Lehmann R, Brounts L, Lesperance K, Eckert M, Casey L, Beekley A, Martin M: A Simplified Set of Trauma Triage Criteria to Safely Reduce Overtriage: A Prospective Study. Arch Surg 2009;144:853–858.

16. Jansen JO, Thomas R, Loudon MA, Brooks A: Damage control resuscitation for patients with major trauma. BMJ 2009;338:b1778.

17. Duchesne JC, Hunt JP, Wahl G, Marr AB, Wang Y-Z, Weintraub SE, Wright MJO, McSwain Jr. NE. Review of Current Blood Transfusions Strategies in a Mature Level I Trauma Center: Were We Wrong for the Last 60 Years? J Trauma 2008;65:272–8.

18. Kashuk JL, Moore EE, Johnson JL, Haenel J, Wilson M, Moore JB, Cothren CC, Biffl WL, Banerjee A, Sauaia A. Postinjury Life Threatening Coagulopathy: Is 1:1 Fresh Frozen Plasma: Packed Red Blood Cells the Answer? J Trauma 2008;65:261–71

19. Dawes R, Thomas GR: Battlefield resuscitation. Curr Opin Crit Care 2009;15:527–535.

20. Gawande A. casualties of war- military care for the wounded from Iraq and Afghanistan. New England Journal of Medicine 2004:351; 2471–5Eynon CA. what is the best outcome from severe head injury? Journal of the Intensive care Society. 2008;3:214–5.

21. Eynon CA. what is the best outcome from severe head injury? Journal of the Intensive care Society. 2008;3:214–5.

Maria Giulia Abate and Giuseppe Citerio

Special admission paths: acute brain injury

Clinical pathways (CP) have been defined as an optimal sequencing and timing of interventions performed by healthcare practitioners for a particular diagnosis. CPs are designed to improve the quality and value of patient care and to minimise delays and resource utilisation [1]. CPs are a recent trend in medicine through which multidisciplinary guidelines are developed for use in a defined patient population. The pathway establishes a framework from which further treatment decisions are derived and assist in coordinating patient care. CPs can thus improve overall quality of care without limiting physicians' decision-making capabilities.

Every acute condition offers the opportunity of developing special paths and, among others, traumatic brain injury (TBI) is an appropriate case for developing a CP.

TBI, in fact, is among the major causes of morbidity and mortality worldwide, principally among young populations and in low-income countries. Adequate management of head injury is complex and challenging, requiring the integration of expertise from several different specialties, i.e. a multidisciplinary team in the acute phase, consisting of neurointensivists, neurosurgeons, neuroanaesthesiologists and neuro-radiologists. Early treatment mainly focuses on the correction and/or avoidance of secondary insults [2] and optimisation of cerebral perfusion, oxygenation and metabolism [3]. Moreover, these patients often undergo long-lasting hospitalisation with frequent complications. As an example, Vitaz et al. [4] developed a multidisciplinary CP for the treatment of severe traumatic brain injury in their hospital. They managed a series of patients with a CP and compared the results with historical data. The authors divided the CP development into four phases:

- **Phase I:** Admission to the ICU with a standardised order sheet to ensure appropriate laboratory test, radiological scans, and consultations with specialists and, in addition, standardised protocols for ICP treatments.
- **Phase II:** Encoding of critical care management. In this stage authors refer to the AANS Brain Trauma Foundation's guidelines [5].
- **Phase III:** Focus on respiratory weaning with a standardised 'weaning protocol' driven by respiratory therapists. In this phase rehabilitation efforts were intensified.
- **Phase IV:** Preceded the discharge to rehabilitation facilities.

In the group of patients treated with a CP, a decreased length of stay in hospital (22.5 vs. 31 days, respectively) and in the ICU (16.8 vs. 21.2 days) and a reduction of length of ventilator support (11.5 vs. 14.4 days respectively) were reported. The use of a standardised clinical pathway resulted in estimated cost savings of $ 14,000 per patient.

Advances in acute brain injury management have taken place in the past decades [6]. These advancements are mainly due to:

- Progress in imaging technology
- The use of antibiotics and anticonvulsants
- New monitoring tools that allow recognition of secondary insults and derangements in brain physiology
- The introduction of guidelines such as Advanced Trauma Life Support (ATLS) and the Brain Trauma Foundation (BTF) guidelines
- The referral of patients with TBI to dedicated intensive care units with neurosurgical facilities driven by experts in neurosciences: the neurocritical care units (NCCU)

In this chapter we aim to focus on the two latter aspects: the application of guidelines in TBI and the need for treatment in neurosurgical hospitals and units managed by experts.

Guidelines

The Advanced Trauma Life Support (ATLS) guidelines describe in detail the specific skills, equipment and supplies needed to treat the immediately life-threatening injuries addressed in the initial evaluation and management. ATLS has systematised the organisation of trauma patients, promoting a uniform method of assessment, a clear order of priorities in resuscitation, the principle of 'do no further harm', an emphasis on the benefits of early surgical involvement in trauma care and, when needed, transfer to a trauma centre [7, 8]. Focusing on TBI, the American Association of Neurological Surgeons (AANS) and the Brain Trauma Foundation (BTF) guidelines summarise the best available evidence for TBI treatment in the pre-hospital [9] and in-hospital phase [5, 9].

Severely injured patients cannot be fully stabilised in the field. The definitive treatment of the intracranial lesion is always in the hospital setting.

The correct out-of-hospital path for brain-injured patients is a continuum that starts at the scene, with optimal stabilisation of ABCs and prompt transfer to a hospital with expertise and resources, thus *"getting the right patient to the right hospital at the right time"* [10].

The dilemma concerns the question of whether it is better to transfer the patient to the closer hospital or to the more specialised one. In real-life practice, traumatised patients can rapidly unstable, e. g. due to severe bleeding or hypoxia, and sometimes they need to be referred to the closest hospital if a comprehensive trauma centre with neurosurgery is too far. Once the patient is stable, he or she will be transferred to a hospital with neurosurgical capability and dedicated NCCU. In this condition, medical informatics networks and applications like remote imaging access and telemedicine may improve the efficiency and speed of treatments and avoid the risks of prolonged transport.

After the primary stabilisation at the scene, the latest edition of the BTF guidelines for pre-hospital management resolves the dilemma by stating that patients with head injury should be transported to a facility with:

- Immediate computed tomography (CT) scanner access
- Prompt neurosurgical care and the ability to monitor intracranial pressure (ICP)

In complex scenarios such as in major trauma, a limited number of structures have the capability to guarantee all the facilities needed (expert physicians, technology, the volume-related expertise). Hence the need arises to transport patients to reference hospitals, that is, to 'centralise' patients, mainly when affected by evolving lesions. In our region, we proposed the algorithm shown in Figure 1 to improve the clinical path of TBI patients. The correct out-of-hospital path starts at the scene, with an optimal stabilisation of ABCs and prompt transfer to a hospital with expertise and resources, i.e. "getting the right patient to the right hospital at the right time". The only exceptions to this general rule are:

- Unstable patient (severely hypotensive or/and severely hypoxic on the scene without response after advanced life support intervention)
- Very long distance to an adequate hospital with neurosurgery and ICU facilities

These patients could be urgently transported to a hospital without neurosurgery for resolution of the extracranial life-threatening conditions. A

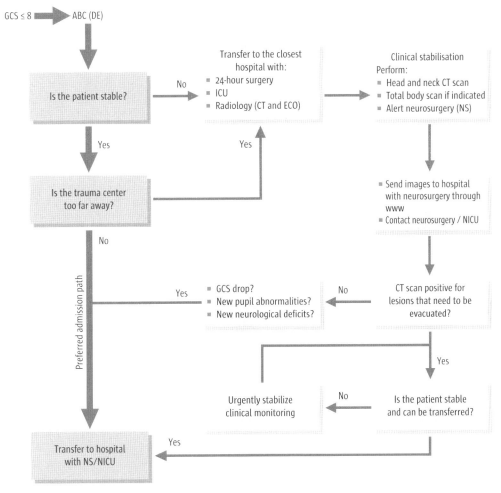

Fig. 1   Algorithm to improve the clinical path of TBI patients. See text for details.

stringent connection of this 'spoke' centre with the 'hub' of the system in all treatment phases, transmission of radiological images and clinical information to the neurosurgical/neuro-ICU and transfer of the severely ill patient as soon as possible, is the safest way to treat unstable severe TBI.

In a recent consensus paper of the NICEM section of the ESICM [11], we stated that "we recommend that all patients with severe TBI should be managed in specialised centres" and we strongly believe that this is the way to offer patients the best possibilities for having the best possible outcome, in relation to the primary damage.

Moreover, the BTF guidelines [5] state that "all regions should have an organized trauma care

system" and that "protocols are recommended to direct the Emergency Medical Service (EMS) personnel regarding destination decisions for patients with traumatic brain injury". For our region we reported on an analysis of hospitalisations for severe head injury covering a one-year period [12]. We demonstrated that the cases are scattered over many hospitals and we argue that to optimise the level of care for these patients, they must be referred to high-volume centers. The resulting centralisation of resources would improve the patients' level of care.

If the application of AANS guidelines has been shown to improve survival and functional outcome after severe head injury in high-income countries [13–19], optimal treatment of head injuries by these protocols requires some of the most expensive resources in the modern therapeutic armamentarium. It is unlikely that low- or even middle-income countries will be able to fully meet these guidelines. Recently, the World Health Organization (WHO) developed guidelines for worldwide essential trauma care [20], attempting to delineate the most effective diagnostic and therapeutic capabilities likely to be achievable at a reasonable and sustainable cost in low- and middle-income countries (see Fig. 2). It is acknowledged that full compliance with the AANS guidelines would be most desirable, but actually impossible to attain. Focusing on low-income countries, the resources needed for treating the patient have been graded as "basic, GP-staffed hospital, specialist hospital and tertiary level centre". Even in difficult healthcare conditions, some interventions are essential and desirable for offering the patient the possibility of best outcome after TBI, such as CT scan availability or ICP monitoring.

Hospital with neurosurgery and dedicated NCCU

Accordingly, the admittance path of patients with severe TBI (GCS ≤ 8, i.e. patients in coma) should identify the 'safest' place where to admit the patients, taking local circumstances into account. In the first hours and day after the trauma, identification and treatment of secondary insults (SI) is the aim of the therapeutic efforts. SIs occur in the hours and days following the primary injury and play a large role in the brain damage and death that result from TBI. Across the globe, preventing secondary brain damage in TBI patients poses an organisational and scientific challenge with respect to decision-making processes, patient assessment, neuroimaging and treatments. Patel et al. [22] prospectively analysed data collected from the Trauma Audit and Research Network database for a large number of patients (15,4231, thereof 22,216 with TBI) presenting between 1989 and 2003 in the UK. Patients with head injury had a ten-fold higher mortality and showed less improvement in the adjusted odds

Resources	Facility level			
	Basic	GP	Specialist	Tertiary
Recognize altered consciousness; lateralizing signs, pupils	E	E	E	E
Full compliance with AANS[1] guidelines for head injury	I	I	D	D
Maintain normotension and oxygenation to prevent secondary brain injury	D	E	E	E
Avoid overhydration in the presence of raised ICP[2] (with normal BP)	D	E	E	E
Monitoring and treatment of raised ICP	I	I	D	D
CT[3] scans	I	D	D	D
Burr holes (skill plus drill or other suitable equipment)	I	PR	D	E
More advance neurosurgical procedures	I	I	PR	D
Surgical treatment of open depressed skull fractures	I	PR	D	E
Surgical treatment of closed depressed skull fractures	I	I	PR	D
Maintenance of requirements for protein and calories	I	E	E	E

[1] AANS: American Association of Neurological Surgeons.
[2] ICP: Intracranial pressure.
[3] CT: Computerizes axial tomography.

Fig. 2   WHO guidelines for worldwide essential trauma care [from Mock C, Lormand JD, Goosen J, Joshipura M, Peden M. Guidelines for essential trauma care. Geneva, World Health Organization, 2004].
E: Essential; D: Desirable; PR: Possibly required; I: Irrelevant (not usually to be considered at the level in question, even with full resource availability). See text for details.

of death since 1989 than did patients without head injury. One third of patients with severe head injury were treated only in non-neurosurgical centres. This was associated with a 26% increase in mortality and a 2.15-fold increase (95% CI 1.77–2.60) in the odds of death adjusted for case mix compared with patients treated at a neurosurgical centre. This effect was present both in patients requiring and not requiring neurosurgical interventions. These data support the current guidelines, suggesting that treatment in a neurosurgical centre represents an important strategy in the management of severe head injury. Once the patient has been admitted to an intensive care unit, the process of care is not finished, but has only begun. In high-income countries, neurocritical care specialists can make the difference in terms of mortality and outcome when treating patients with head injury. The sum of expertise, specialisation, networks and high volume of activity are generally linked to better performance. The NCCU is important because it provides a focus for organisational development and structures for training and research. Specialised centres can enhance patient outcome through improved knowledge and expertise that comes with specialisation and the number of patients treated [23]. Many publications over recent years attest to the efficacy of protocol-driven neurocritical care in improving outcome in patients with TBI. Varelas et al. [24] analysed the impact of neurointensivist care on outcome in patients with TBI admitted to dedicated NCCUs. NCCU admission was associated with a 12% reduction of hospital length of stay, a 51% reduction in mortality rate and 57% greater odds of patients being discharged to their home.

Dedicated neurocritical care units (NCCU) can contribute to a better outcome for several reasons. Among them are:
1. Monitoring and treatment of intracranial hypertension
2. Option of additional brain physiology monitoring tools
3. Existence of volume/outcome relationship

Monitoring intracranial pressure

Despite the lack of data from randomised controlled trials to clarify the role of ICP monitoring in acute coma, a substantial body of evidence in the literature supports the benefits of intracranial pressure monitoring in patients with a severe head injury with clinical and radiological signs of intracranial hypertension [11].

ICP appears as an independent predictor of outcome in several studies, with values of 20–25 mmHg as a discriminatory factor between patients with potentially good or poor outcome [25].

In an interesting review of the literature, Treggiari [26] estimated the independent association between elevated ICP values or abnormal ICP patterns and mortality and neurological outcome in patients with TBI. They summarised the available data to identify critical thresholds of ICP and to explore whether sustained versus peak ICP values had a different prognostic meaning. In the studies evaluated, the overall mortality was 29.3%, 14.2% had poor neurological outcome (severely disabled [SD] or vegetative [V]) and 56.5% had good recovery (GR) or moderate disability (MD). In patients with an ICP < 20 mmHg, GR/MD was attained in 69% of the cases, whereas in patients with ICP values between 20 and 40, GR/MD was observed in 58%, and in 30% of patients with an ICP > 40 mmHg. The risk of having worse neurological outcome paralleled progressively higher ICP levels: The odds ratio (OR) for negative outcomes in patients with an ICP of 20–40 compared with cases with an ICP < 20 was 2.3 (95% CI: 1.37, 3.89), and the same OR comparison in TBI with an ICP > 40 was 4.1 (95% CI: 2.65, 6.29). This refractory ICP and response to treatment of raised ICP could be better predictors of neurological outcome than the absolute ICP value. This conclusion is a strong argument for monitoring and treating high ICP in TBI. It requires expertise and technology usually present in neuro-ICUs and a collaboration with neurosurgery due to the fact that roughly 50% of the cases require an intervention.

Patel and colleagues [27] in a recent retrospective analysis of 185 patients referred with the diagnosis of severe head injury have documented the potential benefits of protocol-driven therapies in a dedicated NCCU, delivered by specialist staff and aimed at intracranial pressure (ICP) and cerebral perfusion pressure (CPP) targets. Interestingly, such management may also benefit patients requiring no surgical therapy, some of whom may need complex therapeutic interventions.

The main findings of this retrospective study were essentially three:

1. Once protocol-driven therapies were instituted, there was a tendency to favourable outcome but not decreased mortality.
2. More patients treated in the NCCU had a good recovery that was statistically significant, with the greatest improvement in outcome evident in the reduction of the proportion of patients left severely disabled or in a persistent vegetative state ($p = 0.014$).
3. The referral and admission practice changed, since a larger proportion of patients not undergoing surgery was admitted in the NCCU era.

In light of these findings, the authors conclude that the presence of specialists in neurocritical care and protocol-driven therapy can lead to a significant improvement in outcome for patients with severe head injury [27].

Monitoring brain physiology

Brain physiology monitoring is a key element of current NCCU care. The goal of monitoring the injured brain is to detect harmful events before they cause irreversible damage. These methodologies, their advantages and pitfalls have been reviewed in a publication describing the NICEM consensus [11]. Many of the cerebral monitoring techniques currently available have drawbacks when considered in isolation; however, multimodality monitoring may facilitate a greater understanding of individual pathophysiology and allow for the delivery of tailored treatment strategies rather than strict adherence to universal physiological targets. Individualised treatment guided by multimodality monitoring has the potential to improve patient outcome after TBI [28]. Thus, different centres have developed different expertise, and different physicians today confidently use different tools. Multimodality monitoring could lead us toward an individually tailored, patient-specific approach.

Volume-outcome relationship

The volume-outcome relationship has been described in the literature mainly for surgical populations. However, studies in the ICU setting show the same relationship. This bears the potential for quality of care improvements [29, 30]. Most of the studies reporting a positive volume-outcome relationship included patients at very high risk of death (cardiac arrest, septic shock, and respiratory failure) with effect size varying among studies. The underlying mechanism builds on the clinical expertise gained from the high volume of patients treated for the same pathology, or increased volume leading to better outcome through selective referral whereby patients are sent to high quality physicians or hospitals. The studies concerning the volume-outcome relationship propose the criterion of regionalisation of care, which has already been associated with improved survival in trauma care. In other neurological emergencies, such as stroke, specialists can make the difference in terms of care [31].

Mauritz et al. [32] analysed a case series of 1,865 TBI patients admitted to 32 intensive care units. Among that population 58 % received ICP monitoring. The authors showed that there was a centre effect: Better outcome was associated to the number of patients treated per year.

Conclusion

The care of patients with TBI is a continuum from the prehospital phase to admission to a dedicated NCCU. To date, ATLS guidelines are a model for trauma treatment that is internationally acknowledged, along with the BTF guidelines.

Evidence emerging from the literature supports the hypothesis that being treated in dedicated centres with a high volume of patients, driven by specialists in neurocritical care, able to integrate the best knowledge available with appropriate monitoring tools, may positively affect outcome.

The authors

Maria Giulia Abate, MD[1]
Giuseppe Citerio, MD[2]
   [1]Medical staff | Neuroanaesthesia and Neurointensive Care | San Gerardo Hospital | Monza, Italy
   [2]Chief of Neuroanaesthesia and Neurointensive Care | San Gerardo Hospital | Monza, Italy

Address for correspondence
Giuseppe Citerio
Neurorianimazione
Anestesia e Rianimazione II
Ospedale San Gerardo
Via Pergolesi 33
20052 Monza (MI), Italy
E-mail: g.citerio@hsgerardo.org

References

1. Coffey RJ, Richards JS, Remmert CS, LeRoy SS, Schoville RR, Baldwin PJ. An introduction to critical paths. Qual Manag Health Care 2005;14:46–55.
2. McHugh GS, Engel DC, Butcher I, Steyerberg EW, Lu J, Mushkudiani N, Hernandez AV, Marmarou A, Maas AI, Murray GD. Prognostic value of secondary insults in traumatic brain injury: results from the IMPACT study. J Neurotrauma 2007;24:287–293.
3. Helmy A, Vizcaychipi M, Gupta AK. Traumatic brain injury: intensive care management. Br J Anaesth 2007;99:32–424. Vitaz TW, McIlvoy L, Raque GH, Spain D, Shields CB. Development and implementation of a clinical pathway for severe traumatic brain injury. J Trauma 2001;51:369–375.
5. The Brain Trauma Foundation. The American Association of Neurological Surgeons. The Joint Section on Neurotrauma and Critical Care. Trauma systems. J Neurotrauma 2000;17:457–462.
6. Keong NC, Gleave JR, Hutchinson PJ. Neurosurgical history: Comparing the management of penetrating head injury in 1969 with 2005. Br J Neurosurg 2006;20:227–232.
7. Driscoll P, Wardrope J. ATLS: past, present, and future. Emerg Med J 2005;22:2–3.
8. Kortbeek JB, Al Turki SA, Ali J, Antoine JA, Bouillon B, Brasel K, Brenneman F, Brink PR, Brohi K, Burris D, Burton RA, Chapleau W, Cioffi W, Collet e Silva Fde S, Cooper A, Cortes JA, Eskesen V, Fildes J, Gautam S, Gruen RL, Gross R, Hansen KS, Henny W, Hollands MJ, Hunt RC, Jover Navalon JM, Kaufmann CR, Knudson P, Koestner A, Kosir R, Larsen CF, Livaudais W, Luchette F, Mao P, McVicker JH, Meredith JW, Mock C, Mori ND, Morrow C, Parks SN, Pereira PM, Pogetti RS, Ravn J, Rhee P, Salomone JP, Schipper IB, Schoettker P, Schreiber MA, Smith RS, Svendsen LB, Taha W, van Wijngaarden-Stephens M, Varga E, Voiglio EJ, Williams D, Winchell RJ, Winter R. Advanced trauma life support, 8th edition, the evidence for change. J Trauma 2008;64:1638–1650.
9. Badjatia N, Carney N, Crocco TJ, Fallat ME, Hennes HM, Jagoda AS, Jernigan S, Letarte PB, Lerner EB, Moriarty TM, Pons PT, Sasser S, Scalea T, Schleien CL, Wright DW. Guidelines for prehospital management of traumatic

brain injury 2nd edition. Prehosp Emerg Care 2008;12 Suppl 1:S1–52.
10. Redmond AD. A trauma center for the United Kingdom. Ann Emerg Med 1993;22:1584–1588.
11. Andrews PJ, Citerio G, Longhi L, Polderman K, Sahuquillo J, Vajkoczy P. NICEM consensus on neurological monitoring in acute neurological disease. Intensive Care Med 2008;34:1362–1370.
12. Citerio G, Beretta L, Stocchetti N. Do we provide optimal care to patients with acute neurological injuries? Minerva Anestesiol 2010;76:155–156.
13. Stein SC, Georgoff P, Meghan S, Mirza KL, El Falaky OM. Relationship of aggressive monitoring and treatment to improved outcomes in severe traumatic brain injury. J Neurosurg 2009.
14. Faul M, Wald MM, Rutland-Brown W, Sullivent EE, Sattin RW. Using a cost-benefit analysis to estimate outcomes of a clinical treatment guideline: testing theBrain Trauma Foundation guidelines for the treatment of severe traumatic brain injury. J Trauma 2007;63:1271–1278.
15. Fakhry SM, Trask AL, Waller MA, Watts DD. Management of brain-injured patients by an evidence-based medicine protocol improves outcomes and decreases hospital charges. J Trauma 2004;56:492–499; discussion 499–500.
16. Arabi YM, Haddad S, Tamim HM, Al-Dawood A, Al-Qahtani S, Ferayan A, Al-Abdulmughni I, Al-Oweis J, Rugaan A. Mortality reduction after implementing a clinical practice guidelines-based management protocol for severe traumatic brain injury. J Crit Care 2009.
17. Rusnak M, Janciak I, Majdan M, Wilbacher I, Mauritz W. Severe traumatic brain injury in Austria VI: effects of guideline-based management. Wien Klin Wochenschr 2007;119:64–71.
18. Keris V, Lavendelis E, Macane I. Association between implementation of clinical practice guidelines and outcome for traumatic brain injury. World J Surg 2007;31:1352–1355.
19. Hesdorffer DC, Ghajar J. Marked improvement in adherence to traumatic brain injury guidelines in United States trauma centers. J Trauma 2007;63:841–847; discussion 847–848.
20. Mock C, Lormand JD, Goosen J, Joshipura M, Peden M. Guidelines for essential trauma care. Geneva, World Health Organization, 2004.
22. Patel HC, Bouamra O, Woodford M, King AT, Yates DW, Lecky FE. Trends in head injury outcome from 1989 to 2003 and the effect of neurosurgical care: an observational study. Lancet 2005;366:1538–1544.
23. Menon D. Neurocritical care: turf label, organizational construct, or clinical asset? Curr Opin Crit Care 2004;10:91–93.
24. Varelas PN, Eastwood D, Yun HJ, Spanaki MV, Hacein Bey L, Kessaris C, Gennarelli TA. Impact of a neurointensivist

on outcomes in patients with head trauma treated in a neurosciences intensive care unit. J Neurosurg 2006;104:713–719.

25. Czosnyka M, Balestreri M, Steiner L, Smielewski P, Hutchinson PJ, Matta B, Pickard JD. Age, intracranial pressure, autoregulation, and outcome after brain trauma. J Neurosurg 2005;102:450–454.

26. Treggiari MM, Schutz N, Yanez ND, Romand JA, Role of intracranial pressure values and patterns in predicting outcome in traumatic brain injury: a systematic review. Neurocrit Care 2007;6:104–112.

27. Patel HC, Menon DK, Tebbs S, Hawker R, Hutchinson PJ, Kirkpatrick PJ. Specialist neurocritical care and outcome from head injury. Intensive Care Med 2002;28:547–553.

28. Tisdall MM, Smith M. Multimodal monitoring in traumatic brain injury: current status and future directions. Br J Anaesth 2007;99:61–67.

29. Jones J, Rowan K. Is there a relationship between the volume of work carried out in intensive care and its outcome? Int J Technol Assess Health Care 1995;11:-762–769.

30. Pronovost PJ, Jenckes MW, Dorman T, Garrett E, Breslow MJ, Rosenfeld BA, Lipsett PA, Bass E, Organizational characteristics of intensive care units related to outcomes of abdominal aortic surgery. Jama 1999;281:1310–1317.

31. Organised inpatient (stroke unit) care for stroke. Cochrane Database Syst Rev 2007;17(4):CD000197.

32. Mauritz W, Steltzer H, Bauer P, Dolanski-Aghamanoukjan L, Metnitz P. Monitoring of intracranial pressure in patients with severe traumatic brain injury: an Austrian prospective multicenter study. Intensive Care Med 2008;34:1208–1215.

Ken Hillman, Jack Chen and Anders Aneman

The ICU without walls

Background

Intensive Care Medicine emerged as a specialty in its own right in the 1950s. Arguably, its beginnings were in Copenhagen during the poliomyelitis epidemic, when patients dying of respiratory failure were artificially ventilated [1]. As a ressult, mortality was reduced from around 80 % to 40 %. The same concept of life support was soon being used for other acute, potentially reversible disorders such as after major trauma or complex operative procedures, severe infections, neuromuscular failure, and serious cardiorespiratory failure. The techniques of life support have been refined but are based on the strategy first used in Copenhagen. Patients are supported with artificial ventilation; their cardiorespiratory function is supported with fluids, drugs and technology, and other bodily needs, such as feeding, are artificially delivered. During this period of total dependence, care has to be taken to prevent complications such as pressure areas, deep venous thrombosis and stress ulceration. A separate medical and nursing specialty has been built around developing and refining these skills. There are now separate national professional societies, textbooks, journals and conferences devoted to intensive care medicine.

The role of intensive care has expanded rapidly since the 1950s. As a result, the role of many other special-ties has also expanded. For example, many complex surgical procedures would not be possible without intensive care units (ICUs). More sophisticated care is also available to acute medical specialties such as cardiology; respiratory medicine; haematology; neurology; and gastroenterology. The level of intensive care provided in a hospital now determines the role of acute hospitals as much as the ICU is determined by the function of the hospital [2]. In fact, one could argue that the specialty of intensive care has become so successful that it may sometimes be employed inappropriately at the end of life (EOL).

Part of its emergence and success as a specialty is related to the fact that it developed within four walls, utilising techniques to create a new form of medicine, which, in turn, enabled other specialties to expand their own boundaries. The growth of intensive care was facilitated by doctors, nurses and other paramedic staff being able to develop special expertise and experience, shared through research and conferences. While other specialties such as cardiac surgery and neurosurgery maintain absentee landlord status in some units, most countries have now developed a separate specialty of intensive care medicine with separate accreditation and specific training requirements. It was within the shelter of the four walls of the ICU that the specialty was able to develop to its current status.

The plight of the seriously ill outside the walls of the ICU

Although the management of the seriously ill in ICUs has improved markedly over the last sixty years, the same cannot necessarily be said for at-risk patients in the remainder of the hospital, especially in the general wards of a hospital, where the monitoring of patients has changed little in the last 100 years. Patients still have vital signs measured in non-standardised ways, sometimes once every hour but often only once a day. In fact respiratory rate, one of the most important vital signs, may only rarely be measured [3, 4]. Serious adverse events in acute hospitals may occur in up to 17% of patients and approximately 70% are potentially preventable [5–7].

The impact of ischaemia and hypoxia

Even relatively small amounts of ischaemia and hypoxia can cause cellular dysfunction and damage, which can then eventually lead to multi-organ dysfunction [8]. When resuscitation is delayed, even if it is then delivered at supranormal levels, it is often not successful if significant ischaemia and hypoxia was present long before admission to the ICU [9–11]. On the other hand, when goal-directed therapy aimed at ischaemia and hypoxia is commenced at an earlier stage, patient outcome is improved [12]. This makes intuitive sense.

Factors affecting the outcome outside the four walls of the ICU

The importance of "lead-time bias" was recognised even as long ago as the 1980s [13, 14]. In this context the term referred to the poor outcome of patients admitted to ICUs, where treatment had been delayed for significant periods before the eventual admission to the ICU.

One of the great pioneers of intensive care medicine, Peter Safar, stated that "... the most sophisticated intensive care often becomes unnecessarily expensive terminal care when the pre-ICU system fails" [15] and fail it often does.

It has been clearly demonstrated that not only do many patients admitted to an ICU have serious abnormalities before their admission [16, 17]

but also their outcome is much worse [18, 19]. Up to 70% of all admissions to ICU from general wards have had many hours of unattended deterioration [20]. Hypotension was the most common factor, as well as tachycardia, tachypnoea, seizures and decreased level of consciousness. It is not surprising that a group of matched septic patients managed on general wards had a higher mortality than those initially managed in an ICU [21].

The changing role of acute hospitals

The changing nature of acute hospitals is increasingly resulting in an expansion of the role of intensive care beyond their four walls [22]. The changes are many and either directly or indirectly have led to a changing nature in the population of patients as well as a mismatch between patient needs and available resources. For some time there have been pressures on hospital beds to limit their number and their cost. The pressures have resulted in a reduction in the length of hospital stay. As a result of these changes the population of patients are now sicker, often with multiple co-morbidities, having more complex surgery and being subject to medications and interventions with higher risks.

While the population of patients is more at-risk, the resources available for their management outside environments such as ICUs has become increasingly inappropriate for matching the needs of patients. It remains common practice for patients to be admitted under a specialist surgeon or physician. This has many advantages. The admitting clinician is ultimately responsible for patient care. However, as specialisation in medicine has increased, other skills are lost. Even if the specialist, such as a neurologist, was once exposed to acute medicine, they would soon lose their skills as a result of not actively practising in the area but also not keeping up to date with developments. As a result, the neurologist may not necessarily have the appropriate skills to recognise serious illness, let alone to actively treat these patients. [22, 23].

Similarly, undergraduate education in acute medicine is deficient in the area of recognising at-risk patients and advanced resuscitation [24, 25]. And postgraduate training is mainly in the area of the chosen specialty and may not include appropriate exposure to advanced resuscitation training [22].

In summary, the population of patients in acute hospitals is now complex and includes many patients who are seriously ill. At the same time, there is a poor systematic, 24-hour cover in hospitals by staff with the appropriate skills and knowledge to adequately care for these patients [16, 17]. This crucial gap in the provision of services to the seriously ill is one of the key reasons for intensivists operating outside the four walls of their ICU.

Too little … too late

It was probably necessary for intensive care to originate and develop within the professional isolation of its four walls. However, this did not address the needs of the unfortunate patients elsewhere in the hospital who were not cared for by specialists in acute medicine and advanced resuscitation. The situation obviously varies between hospitals. A 100-bed hospital with a 60-bed ICU would obviously have less need to operate outside its four walls, compared to a 600-bed hospital with a 6-bed ICU. The latter ICU could only manage patients with severe multi-organ failure (MOF), often offering resuscitation at a late stage when MOF was inevitable. Ironically, if the same hospital did not operate an early resuscitation service across the whole hospital, many of its admissions would be as a result of poor resuscitation at an appropriate stage in the patient's deterioration [16, 20, 26]. Many patients who deteriorate on the general wards of a hospital may not even live to be admitted to an ICU. Over half of all patients without a 'do not attempt resuscitation' order (DNAR) have serious and potentially reversible abnormalities in their vital signs and observations in the 24 hours before their death [27]. Up to 80 % of all in-hospital cardiac arrests are also preceded by prolonged periods of serious abnormalities in vital signs [28–30]. In the past, the only systematic approach to serious illness was the cardiac arrest team [31].

Following the first descriptions of cardiopulmonary resuscitation [32, 33] in the late 1950s, cardiac arrests became the norm in most acute hospitals. However, the majority of patients requiring in-hospital cardiopulmonary resuscitation (CPR) die before hospital discharge [34]. Survival to discharge rates vary from 1 % [34] to around 14 % [35, 36]. There has been no improvement in these figures over the last 50 years in spite of enormous resources devoted to CPR in terms of education, research and clinicians' time. It has been estimated in the USA that it costs approximately US$ 400,000 per life saved to operate in-hospital CPR programmes [37].

There has been surprisingly little research or attention given to the circumstances of in-hospital cardiac arrests. In fact, most arrests do not occur unexpectedly or suddenly. Around 80 % of patients who have an in-hospital cardiac arrest have identifiable deterioration for many hours before the event [28]. In the same study, only 8 % of patients who arrested survived to hospital discharge. Other studies have identified similar potentially preventable antecedents prior to cardiac arrest [30, 38]. In contrast, patients rarely have a cardiac arrest or die a sudden and unexpected death in the ICU [39, 40]. In highly monitored situations such as ICUs, unexpected deterioration rarely occurs.

If the ICU were to expand its borders, it would seem logical to treat the seriously ill before deterioration rather than simply being involved in cardiac arrest teams, when the resource cost in maintaining the service is so high, when potentially preventable deterioration occurs long before they arrest, and when the outcome is so poor.

A broken system

While the standard of patient care in specialised units such as in the ICU is high, patients are managed in general wards much the same as they were over 100 years ago. Nurses record the so-called vital signs – pulse rate, blood pressure, respiratory rate and temperature – with widely varying frequency; anything from once an hour to only once a day with little evidence to support the ideal frequency rate [4, 41]. Moreover, the measurement of the respiratory rate is arguably the single most important predictor of adverse outcomes [26, 42–47]. And yet it is the most poorly documented [4, 42, 43, 48, 49].

Manual recording of vital signs on general wards is haphazard and inaccurate. What recordings are made are by nursing staff who are largely disengaged from the system. They passively record the vital signs with no standardised way of alerting the system of an at-risk deteriorating patient, apart from when a cardiac arrest occurs.

They may sometimes report abnormalities in vital signs to junior medical staff who themselves often have had little formal training in recognising and reacting appropriately to seriously ill patients [24, 25]. The problem can be exacerbated by the hierarchical system in medicine where problems are passed up through levels of seniority (see Fig. 1). Even when the acute resuscitation problem is referred to a senior clinician, they may not be available because of numerous commitments and they often lack comprehensive knowledge and practical skills in advanced resuscitation [31].

A new model of care

By the mid-1990s, a new concept of caring for the seriously ill across the whole hospital was established – The Medical Emergency Team (MET) [50, 51]. Usually organised by intensive care specialists operating out of ICUs, the system is simple in its construct. At-risk patients are identified early in the course of their deterioration, certainly before they have a cardiac arrest or die. This is achieved by specifying certain abnormalities in vital signs (pre-set levels of hypotension, tachycardia

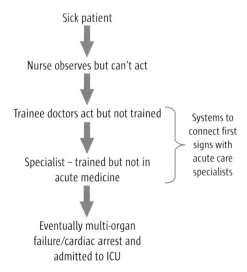

Sick patient

Nurse observes but can't act

Trainee doctors act but not trained

Specialist – trained but not in acute medicine

Systems to connect first signs with acute care specialists

Eventually multi-organ failure/cardiac arrest and admitted to ICU

Fig. 1   The failed hierarchy, pre-intensive care

and tachypnoea) as well as abnormal observations such as seizures, obstructed airway, a sudden decrease in the level of consciousness and, most importantly, staff concern: the so-called MET criteria [51, 52]. When these abnormalities occur, staff are empowered to immediately activate a response which includes those trained and experienced in all aspects of advanced resuscitation. The missing parts of patient safety in an acute hospital are now provided to at-risk patients; recognition of serious illness combined with an appropriate and rapid response to their needs.

This concept has now spread to many parts of the world, under many different names. The means of detecting at-risk patients and triggering criteria may be slightly different and the rapid response may involve different levels of expertise and seniority, but the basic concept, largely developed by intensivists, is now operating in many hospitals around the world.

Examples of variations include a Modified Early Warning Score (MEWS) [53]; the Outreach Strategy [54, 55]; the Patient At Risk Team (PART) [56]; and Condition C teams [57].

Do rapid response systems work?

In itself, this is an interesting question and one that is rarely asked of many system interventions. For example, the effect of cardiac arrest teams on mortality has never been tested and probably never will be. Apart from anything else, the randomisation of patients to have CPR or not would probably never be allowed by ethics committees. Similarly, no research ethics committee would allow the randomisation of seriously ill patients in the general wards of hospitals into a group which was allowed to have a cardiac arrest before resuscitation was commenced, as opposed to a group where they were recognised early and where appropriate resuscitation was commenced. Consequently, the evaluation of rapid response systems (RRSs), as they have become known, has concentrated on before and after or case control methodologies. Most have been positive: There has been a reduction in admissions to the ICU [58], and a reduction in cardiac arrest and/or death rates [59–63]. The largest study has been a cluster randomised study conducted in 23 Australian hospitals which showed a statistically significant

A

reduction in mortality rate in the MET hospitals compared to control hospitals [64] but no difference in the aggregate of unexpected deaths, cardiac arrests and admissions to the ICU [65]. A recent meta-analysis showed that RRSs were associated with a 34 % reduction in rates of cardiopulmonary arrests outside the ICU [66]. They also showed a significant reduction in cardiac arrest rates and hospital mortality in children where the system had been introduced. The reason that they did not show a reduction in adult hospital mortality may be related to the fact that they had not included the largest cluster randomised control trial which did show a reduction in hospital mortality in hospitals with a RRS [64].

There does not appear to be any argument that early intervention in critical illness is important. However, there remains the question of how to improve the monitoring of vital signs in patients on general wards; how to empower those working closest with patients in how to recognise and respond to at-risk patients; and exactly what skills are required to meet the needs of the deteriorating patient, no matter where they may be in a hospital. There is also the question of how to resource the ICU to enable it to perform activities outside the ICU, especially when the activities may compromise care within the ICU.

Other ways of working outside the walls of an ICU

There are many roles that intensivists are involved with outside their four walls (see Tab. 1):

- **High Dependency Units** – High dependency units (HDUs) take many forms: Some are operated mainly by nursing staff with the patient remaining under the admitting team, and in other forms; the HDU is an integral part of an ICU, with fully trained nursing and medical staff [67–70]. The level of acuity of patients is usually lower than that in an ICU, and the HDU aims at managing patients who are inappropriately managed on a general floor but not as demanding as a patient in an ICU. This type of step-down ward allows the intensivist to move outside the walls of the ICU but not to have the responsibility for directly caring for patients across the whole hospital. As with ICUs, there is very little data on the overall cost-effectiveness of HDUs but they make intuitive sense. Staff from the ICU may also be involved in systems of triage within a hospital, where patients are clustered according to level of illness rather than under admitting specialties.

- **Trauma** – Trauma systems provide an excellent systematic and standardised model for caring for seriously injured patients [71–74]. An ideal trauma system triages at the scene of the accident, rapidly transports the patient to a definitive site of care, triages the patient in the receiving section of the hospital, triggers a multi-disciplinary team to resuscitate and stabilise the patient, transfers the patient to an appropriate site of care within the hospital, tracks the patient through all phases of rehabilitation, and constantly measures the effectiveness of the system and adjusts it accord-

Tab. 1   Areas outside the four walls of ICU where intensive care clinicians are involved

High dependency areas
Establishing and being involved with systems to recognise and respond to deteriorating patients
Establishing being involved in systems to provide seamless and safe care across hospital networks
Transportation of the seriously ill
Involvement in resuscitation and care of trauma patients
Hospital consultations
Undergraduate education
Patient follow-up post-ICU discharge
Hospital, regional and national committees, and professional organisations

ingly to improve outcomes. Many intensivists are involved in the operation of such systems as part of their role outside the ICU.

- **Consultation Services** – Over and above the involvement of intensivists in MET and trauma systems, intensivists are often asked their opinion about patients by specialist colleagues in a hospital. The advice sought is often about whether the patient should be transferred to the ICU or if they are to remain on the ward, what would be the optimum way of managing them?
- **Research** – Many researchers from intensive care are interested in factors which may affect ICU outcomes that precede their admission, such as their level and type of illness and how delays in resuscitation affect outcomes. Similarly, researchers have been interested in factors around readmissions to ICU and outcomes after ICU, both in hospital and the problems encountered in the community.
- **Teaching** – There is probably a need for staff in intensive care to be more involved in increasing the skills of colleagues. This may reduce the burden of staff working in ICUs to be involved in resuscitation across the whole hospital. If the staff were adequately trained, it may mean that patients would be treated earlier and more appropriately by the admitting team with less reliance on staff from the ICU.

Management of patients at the end of life

Increasingly, intensivists are being ask to deliver end-of-life (EOL) care in ICUs [40, 75–77]. Most of these patients have active management either withdrawn or withheld. In fact, dying is the most common illness in the ICU with at least 20 % of Americans now dying in, or shortly after, having been in an ICU [78]. Managing the dying process in the ICU has become increasingly expensive and is a public health issue of great magnitude [79]. Many intensivists around the world have moved outside the four walls of their units and have provided valuable input into this important area.

Intensivists may be involved in EOL care at this time when, after assessing the patient, they explain that further management in an ICU has nothing to offer. The intensivist is, in fact, in this situation, helping to make the diagnosis of dying.

Possibly as a result of intensivist involvement, hospitals with RRSs have a higher incidence of patients being made DNAR than those hospitals without such a system [80].

Conclusion

The specialty of Intensive Care Medicine has come a long way since its modest beginnings in the 1950s. Intensive care is recognised as a separate medical and nursing specialty and has been responsible for ICUs becoming an integral part of all major acute hospitals. Increasingly, intensivists' skills are not only used within the four walls of their units but also for undergraduate and postgraduate teaching, health administration at local and national levels, research into factors outside ICUs which affect patient outcomes within the units, and also clinical involvement with deteriorating and seriously ill patients who are not necessarily within the four walls of the ICU at that point in time.

The authors

Ken Hillman, Prof.[1]
Jack Chen, Dr.[2]
Anders Aneman, A/Prof.[3]
[1]Professor of Intensive Care | University of New South Wales | Director | The Simpson Centre for Health Services Research (affiliated with The Institute of Health Innovation) | The University of New South Wales | Sydney, Australia
[2]Senior Research Fellow | The Simpson Centre for Health Systems Services (affiliated with The Institute of Health Innovation) | The University of New South Wales | Sydney, Australia
[3]Conjoint | The University of New South Wales | Sydney, Australia

Address for correspondence
Ken Hillman
Critical Care Services
Liverpool Hospital
Locked Mailbag 7103
Liverpool BC, NSW, 1871
Australia
E-mail: k.hillman@unsw.edu.au

References

1. Lassen HCA. A preliminary report on the 1952 epidemic of poliomyelitis in Copenhagen with special reference to the treatment of acute respiratory insufficiency Lancet 1953;1:37–41.
2. Hillman K. The changing role of acute-care hospitals. Med J Aust 1999;170:325–8.
3. Cretikos MA, Chen J, Hillman KM, Bellomo R, Finfer SR, Flabouris A, the MERIT study investigators. The effectiveness of implementation of the medical emergency team (MET) system and factors associated with use during the MERIT study. Crit Care Resus 2007;9(2):206–12.
4. Chen J, Hillman K, Bellomo R, Flabouris A, Finfer S, the MERIT Study Investigators for the Simpson Centre and the ANZICS Clinical Trials Group. The impact of introducing medical emergency team system on the documentations of vital signs. Resuscitation 2009;80(1):35–43.
5. Brennan TA, Leape LL, Laird NM Herbert L, Localio AR, Lawthers AG, et al. Incidence of adverse events and negligence in hospitalised patients. Results of the Harvard Medicine Practice Study I. N Engl J Med 1991;324(6):370–6.
6. Wilson RM, Runciman WB, Gibberd RW, Harrison BT, Newby L, Hamilton JD, et al. The quality in Australian Health Care Study. Med J Aust 1995;163:458–71.
7. Leape LL, Brennan TA, Laird N, Lawthers AG, Localio AR, Barnes BA, et al. The nature of adverse events in hospitalised patients. Results of the Harvard Medicine Practice Study II. M Eng J Med 1991;324(6):377–84.
8. Deitch EA. Multiple organ failure: Pathophysiology and potential future therapy. Ann Surg 1992;216:117–34.
9. Yu M, Takanishi D, Myers S, Takiguchi SA, Severine RMS, Nahidh H, et al. Frequency of mortality and myocardial infarction during maximizing oxygen delivery: a prospective, randomized trial. Crit Care Med 1995;23(6):1025–32.
10. Shoemaker WC, Kram HB, Appel PL, Fleming AW. The efficacy of central venous and pulmomary artery catheters and therapy based upon them in reducing mortality and morbidity. Arch Surg 1990;125(10):1332–8.
11. Haynes MA, Yau EH, Timmings AC, Hinds CJ, Watson D. Response of critically ill patients to treatment aimed at achieving supranormal oxygen delivery and consumption. Relationship to outcome. Chest 1993;103(3):886–95.
12. Rivers E, Nguyen B, Havstad S, Ressler J, Muzzin A, Knoblich B, et al. Early goal-directed therapy in the treatment of severe sepsis and septic shock. N Engl J Med 2001;345(19):1368–77.
13. Dragsted L, Jorgensen J, Jensen NH, Bonsing E, Jacobsen E, Knaus WA, et al. Interhospital comparisons of patient outcome from intensive care: Importance of lead-time bias. Crit Care Med 1989;17(5):418–22.

14. Bion JF, Edlin SA, Ramsay G, McCabe S, Ledingham IM. Validation of a prognostic score in critically ill patients undergoing transportation. Br J Med 1985;291:432–4.
15. Safar P. Critical care medicine–Quo Vadis? Crit Care Med 1974;2:1–5.
16. McQuillan P, Pilkington S, Allan A, Taylor B, Short A, Morgan G, et al. Confidential inquiry into quality of care before admission to an intensive care. Br Med J 1998;316:1853–6.
17. Garrad C, Young D. Suboptimal care of patients before admission to intensive care. Is caused by a failure to appreciate or apply the ABCs of life support. Br Med J 1998;316:1841–2.
18. Goldhill DR, Sumner A. Outcome of intensive care patients in a group of British intensive care units. Crit Care Med 1998;26:1337–45.
19. McGloin H, Adams S, Singer M. The quality of pre-ICU care influences outcome of patients admitted from the ward. Clin Intensive Care 1997;8:104.
20. Hillman KM, Bristow PJ, Chey T, Daffurn K, Jacques T, Norman SL, et al. Duration of life-threatening antecedents prior to intensive care admission. Intensive Care Med 2002;28:1629–34.
21. Lundberg JS, Perl TM. Wiblen T, Costigan MD, Dawson J, Nettleman MD, et al. Septic shock: An analysis of outcomes for patients with onset on hospital wards versus intensive care units. Crit Care 1998;26(6):1020–4.
22. Hillman KM. Reducing preventable deaths and containing costs: The expanding role of intensive care medicine. Med J Aust 1996;164:308–9.
23. Thwaites BC, Shankar S, Niblett D, Saunders J. Can consultants resuscitate? J Roy Coll Phys Lond 1992;26:265–7.
24. Harrison GA, Hillman KM, Fulde GW, Jacques TC. The need for undergraduate education in critical care. (Results of a questionnaire to year 6 medical undergraduates, University of New South Wales and recommendations on a curriculum in critical care). Anaesth Intensive Care 1999;27(1):53–8.
25. Buchman TG, Dellinger RP, Raphaely Rc, Todres ID. Undergraduate education in critical care medicine. Crit Care Med 1992;20:1595–603.
26. Goldhill DR, McNarry AF. Physiological abnormalities in early warning scores are related to mortality in adult inpatients. Br J Anaesth 2004;92(6):882–4.
27. Hillman KM, Bristow PJ, Chey T, Daffurn K, Jacques T, Norman SL, et al. Antecedents to hospital deaths. Internal Med J 2001;31:343–8.
28. Schein RM, Hazday N, Pena M, Ruben BH, Spring CL. Clinical antecedents to in-hospital cardiopulmonary arrest. Chest 1990;98(6):1388–92.
29. Franklin C, Matthew J. Developing strategies to prevent in-hospital cardiac arrest: Analyzing responses of physicians and nurses in the hours before the event. Crit Care Med 1994;22:244–7.

30. Kause J, Smith G, Prytherch D, Parr M, Flabouris A, Hillman K, for the Intensive Care Society (UK) and ANZICS CTG. A comparison of Antecedents to Cardiac Arrests, Deaths and EMergency Intensive care Admissions in Australia and New Zealand, and the United Kingdom – The ACADEMIA study. Resuscitation 2004;62(3):275–82.

31. Hillman K, Parr M, Flabouris A, Bishop G, Stewart A. Redefining in-hospital resuscitation: the concept of the medical emergency team. Resuscitation 2001;48:105–10.

32. Safar P, Escarraga EL, Elam JO. A comparison of the mouth-to-mouth and mouth-to-airway methods of artificial respiration with the chest-pressure arm-lift methods. New Engl J Med 1958;258:671–7.

33. Kouwenhoven WB, Jude JR, Knickerbocker GG. Closed-chest cardiac massage. JAMA 1960;173:1064–7.

34. Hershey CO, Fisher L. Why outcome of cardiopulmonary resuscitation in general wards is poor. Lancet 1982;i:31–4.

35. Tunstall-Pedoe H, Baily L, Chamberlain DA, Marsden AK, Ward ME, Zideman DA. Survey of 3765 cardiopulmonary resuscitations in British hospitals (the BRESUS study): methods and overall results. Br Med J 1992;304:1347–51.

36. Linko E, Koskinen PJ, Siitonen L, Ruosteenoja R. Resuscitation in cardiac arrest: An analysis of 100 successive medical cases. Acta Med Scand 1967;182:611–20.

37. Lee KH, Angus DC, Abramson NS. Cardiopulmonary resuscitation: What cost to cheat death? Crit Care Med 1996;24:2046–52.

38. Bedell SE, Deitz DC, Leeman D, Delbanco TL. Incidence and characteristics of preventable iatrogenic cardiac arrest. JAMA 1991;265:2815–20.

39. Manara AR, Pittman JAL, Braddon FEM. Reasons for withdrawing treatment in patients receiving intensive care. Anaesthesia 1998;53:523–8.

40. Keenan SP, Busche KD, Chen LM, McCarthy L, Inman KJ, Sibbald WJ. A retrospective review of a large cohort of patients undergoing the process of withholding or withdrawal of life support. Crit Care Med 1997;25:1324–31.

41. Zeitz K, McCutcheon H. Observations and vital signs: ritual or vital for the monitoring of postoperative patients? Appl Nurs Res 2006;19(4):204–11.

42. Hodgetts TJ, Kenward G, Vlachonikolis IG, Payne S, Castle N. The identification of risk factors for cardiac arrest and formulation of activation criteria to alert a medical emergency team. Resuscitation 2002;54(2):125–31.

43. Hudson A. Prevention of in-hospital cardiac arrest and formulation of improving patient care. Resuscitation 2004;60:113.

44. Constidine J. The role of nurses in preventing adverse events related to respiratory dysfunction Literature review. J Adv Nurs 2005;49(6):624–33.

45. Fieselmann JF, Hendryx MS, Helms CM, Wakefield DS. Respiratory rate predicts cardiopulmonary arrest for internal medicine patients. J Gen Intern Med 1993;8:354–60.

46. Goldhill DR. The critically ill: following your MEWS. Q J Med 2001;94:507–10.

47. Husum H, Gilbert M, Wisborg T, Van Heny Y, Murad M. Respiratory rate as a prehospital triage tool in rural trauma. J Trauma 2003;55(3):466–70.

48. McBride J, Knight D, Piper J, Smith GB. Long-term effect of introducing an early warning score on respiratory rate charting on general wards. Resuscitation 2005;65(1):41–4.

49. Dobbs P, Stubbins K, Leggott S, Adsetts D. A prospective audit of the incidence of physiologic monitoring in the 24 hours before a cardiac arrest in a district general hospital. Br J Anaesth 2002;89(2):353P.

50. Lee A, Bishop G, Hillman KM. Daffurn K. The medical emergency team. Anaesth Intensive Care 1995;23(2):183–6.

51. Hourihan F, Bishop G, Hillman KM, Daffurn K, Lee A. The medical emergency team: A new strategy to identify and intervene in high risk patients. Clin Intensive Care 1995;6(6):269–72.

52. Hillman KM, Bishop G, Lee A, Daffurn K, Bauman A, Crispin C, et al. Identifying the general ward patient at high risk of cardiac arrest. Clin Intensive Care 1996;7:242–3.

53. Stenhouse C, Coates S, Tivey M, Allsop P, Parker T. Prospective evaluation of a modified Early Warning Score to aid earlier detection of patients developing critical illness on a surgical ward. Brit J Anaes 2000;84(5):663.

54. Bright D, Walker W, Bion J. Clinical review: outreach – a strategty for improving the care of the acutely ill hospitalised patient. Crit Care 2004;8:33–40.

55. Scales DC, Abrahamson S, Brunet F, Fowler R, Costello J, Granton JT, et al. The ICU Outreach Team. J Crit Care 2003;18:95–106.

56. Subbe CP, Kruger M, Rutherford P, Gemmel L. Validation of a modified early warning score in medical admissions. Q J Med 2001;94(10):521–526.

57. Foraida MI, DeVita MA, Braithwaite RS, Stuart SA, Brooks MM, Simmons RL. Improving the utilization of medical crisis teams (Condition C) at an urban tertiary care hospital. J Crit Care 2003;18:87–94.

58. Bristow PJ, Hillman KM, Chey T, Daffurn K, Jacques TC, Norman SL, et al. Rates of in-hospital arrests, deaths and intensive care admissions: the effect of a medical emergency team. Med J Aust 2000;173:236–40.

59. Buist MD, Moore GE, Bernard SA, Waxman BP, Anderson JN, Nguyen TV. Effects of a medical emergency team on reduction of incidence of and mortality from unexpected cardiac arrests in hospital: preliminary study. Br Med J 2002;324:387–390.

60. Bellomo R, Goldsmith D, Uchino S, Buckmaster J, Hart GK, Opdam H, et al. A prospective before-and-after trial

of a medical emergency team. Med J Aust 2003; 179(6):283–9.

61. Priestley G, Watson W, Rashidian A, Mozley C, Russell D, Wilson J, et al. Introducing critical care outreach: a ward–randomised trial of phased introduction in a general hospital. Intensive Care Med 2004;30(7):1398–404.

62. Bellomo R, Goldsmith D, Uchino S, Buckmaster J, Hart G, Oppdam H, et al. Prospective controlled trial of effects of medical emergency team on postoperative morbidity and mortality rates. Crit Care Med 2004;32:916–21.

63. DeVita MA, Braithwaite RS, Mahidhara R, Stuart S, Foraida M, Simmons RL and members of the Medical Emergency Response Improvement Team (MERIT). Use of medical emergency team responses to reduce hospital cardiopulmonary arrests. Qual Saf Health Care 2004;13:251–4.

64. Chen J, Bellomo R, Flabouris A, Hillman K, Finfer S and the MERIT Study Investigators for the Simpson Centre and the ANZICS Clinical Trials Group. The relationship between early emergency team calls and serious adverse events. Crit Care Med 2009;37(1):148–53.

65. MERIT Study Investigators. Introduction of the medical emergency team (MET) system: a cluster-randomised controlled trial. Lancet 2005;365(9477):2091–7.

66. Chan PS, Jain R, Nallmothu K, Berg RA, Sasson C. Rapid response teams. A systematic review and meta-analysis. Arch Intern Med 2010;170(1):18–26.

67. Gerber DR. Structural models for intermediate care areas. one size does not fit all. Crit Care Med 1999;27:2321–2.

68. Cheng DCH, Byrick RJ, Knobel E. Structural models for intermediate care areas. Crit Care Med 1999;27:2266–71.

69. Vincent JL, Burchardi H. Do we need intermediate care units? Intensive Care Med 1999;25:1345–9.

70. Shakir T, Toosy N, Ridley SA. A survey of adult general high dependency units in the United Kingdom. Clin Intensive Care 1999;10(6):219–26.

71. West JG, Williams MJ, Trunkey DD. Woferth CC. Trauma systems. Current status – future challenges. JAMA 1998;259:3597–600.

72. Cales RH. Trauma mortality in Orange County: The effects of the implementation of a regional trauma system. Arch Emerg Med 1984;13:1–10.

73. Deane SA, Gaudry PL, Pearson I, Misra S, McNeil RJ, Read C. The hospital trauma team: A model for trauma management. J Trauma 1990;30:806–12.

74. Shackford SR, Hollingworth-Fridlung P, Cooper GF, Eastman AB. The effect of regionalisation upon the quality of trauma care as assessed by concurrent audit before and after institution of a trauma system: a preliminary report. J. Trauma 1986;26:812–20.

75. Prendergast TJ, Claessens MT, Luce JM: A national survery of end-of-life care for critically ill patients. Am J Respir Crit Care Med 1998;158:1163–7.

76. Wilson WC, Smedira NG, Fink C, McDowell JA, Luce JM. Ordering and administration of sedatives and analgesics during the withholding and withdrawal of life support from critically ill patients. JAMA 1992;267(7):949–53.

77. Sprung CL Cohen SL, Sjokvist P, Baras M, Bulow H-H, Hovilehto S, et al. End-of-life practices in European intensive care units: the Ethicus Study. JAMA 2003;290(6):790–7.

78. Angus DC, Barnato AI, Linde-Zwirble WT, Weissfeld LA, Watson RS, Rickett TBA, Tuberfeld GD on behalf of the Robert Wood Johnson Foundation End-of-Life Peer Group. Use of intensive care at the end of life in the United States: an epidemiologic study. Crit Care Med 2004;32:638.

79. Levy MM. Share decision-making in the ICU: entering a new era. Crit Care Med 2004;32(9):1966–8.

80. Chen J, Flabouris A, Bellomo R, Hillman K, Finfer S, The MERIT Study Investigators for the Simpson Centre and the ANZICS Clinical Trials Group. The medical emergency team system and not-for-resuscitation orders: Results from the MERIT study. Resuscitation 2008;79:391–7.

B. Structures, monitoring, and personnel

How to design a new ICU _____ 99
Michael Hiesmayr, Philipp G.H. Metnitz and Markus Haisjackl

Minimal structural requirements for ICUs and HDUs _____ 107
Patrick Ferdinande

Minimal training requirements for ICU physicians _____ 117
Armand R.J. Girbes, Albertus Beishuizen and Jan G. Zijlstra

Minimal training requirements for ICU nurses _____ 123
Ruth Endacott and Julie Scholes

Preparation and training of critical care pharmacists_____ 133
William E. Dager, Rob Shulman and Judith Jacobi

Requirements and standards for treating children in intensive care units (ICUs) _____ 143
Paolo Biban

Do we need specific cardiac (non-operative) ICUs? _____ 155
Elias Knobel, Marcia Makdisse and Marcos Knobel

Do we need specific neurocritical ICUs?_____ 167
Jorge Luiz da Rocha Paranhos, Gustavo Trindade Henriques-Filho and Odin Barbosa da Silva

Designing burn ICUs _____ 175
David M. Baron, Lars-Peter Kamolz and Philipp G.H. Metnitz

Design features of the ICU from the patient and family perspective _____ 181
Nils Theuerkauf, Ulf Guenther and Christian Putensen

Minimal standards for physiological monitoring in the intensive care unit_____ 191
Maurizio Cecconi, Lorenzo Spagnesi, Mark Hamilton, Rui P. Moreno and Andrew Rhodes

Medical work patterns: The impact on quality and burnout _____ 197
Dierk A. Vagts, Kristina Klöcker and Christian W. Mutz

Nursing work patterns_____ 205
Yên-Lan Nguyen, Sandrine Dray, Aude Soury-Lavergne and Bertrand Guidet

Physician extenders_____ 213
Maria Wittmann, Daniela Dewald and Christian Putensen

Organising the workflow in an ICU_____ 225
Hans U. Rothen

Evaluating staff performance in the ICU_____ 241
Armand R.J. Girbes and Jan G. Zijlstra

Michael Hiesmayr, Philipp G.H. Metnitz and Markus Haisjackl

How to design a new ICU

Fundamental changes in the perception of the task of an ICU are reality, with a focus on patient autonomy on the one hand and an emphasis on process orientation on the other. These seemingly contradictory elements, which from a historical perspective appear to be mutually exclusive, need to be formed into a functional unity. But this apparent contradiction may point toward a paradigm shift that holds new opportunities.

In this report about the design of an ICU we will focus on two perspectives and one outcome:

- Patient comfort & safety
- Embedding ICU processes within hospital processes
- Success of the ICU

The ICU of the future will increasingly focus on patient comfort and privacy. The medical environment of the patient has changed considerably in the last 30 years and patient autonomy is a fundamental right in a changing patient-agent relationship. This field was mainly considered from the personnel's perspective during a period in which most patients were sedated, ventilated and even paralysed. This type of patient today is seen only in about 10–25 % of cases; many are ventilated but not or only minimally sedated, and 50 % can communicate with respect to their needs, pain, discomfort, thirst and hunger. Thus, ICU organisation has to concentrate more and more on reactive patients. These patients need an appropriate environment to reduce long-term sequelae of intensive care treatment such as post-traumatic stress disorder or post-ICU depression.

How to feel well

Noise is usually much too high at 50–70 dB and far from the recommendation that daytime noise should not exceed 45 dB and nighttime noise should stay below 20 dB. Noise is associated with decreased attention, fatigue and may induce more aggressive behaviour.

Sound and images from a radio or television is appreciated by some patients but their capacity for prolonged attention is often limited. Thus the possibility of individual access to radio and TV is desirable but should only be used according to the patient's expressed preferences.

Light is a key factor for orientation in time. Thus sufficient access to natural light with a clear day and night distinction will probably be supportive. Of course, optimal bright light may be necessary for emergency situations or interventions, but individual lighting control for each patient is mandatory. Specialists in light design may even allow special atmospheres to be created with the available light sources. The patient's view of the interior very often is the ceiling of their room. In many instances, this ceiling is very technical and patients with delirium often experience stressful interpretations of these unfamiliar views.

Orientation in time and space is important for patients after critical illness. Simple measures such as a large clock and easily visible calendars may help. Another design feature could be that each room has characteristic elements, pictures, drawings displayed that can be remembered and easily recognised when awake.

A view of key elements in the exterior environment such as trees and open areas may benefit re-orientation. Some long-stay patients appreciate being brought outside the ICU to feel fresh air or the sun. Usually this is a challenging transport, with monitor and ventilator. Easy, same level access to a balcony or terrace on the sunny side of the building could be built and would certainly be widely accepted. Such exposure to the non-controlled environment has often been reported to give patients a sense of temporarily regaining autonomy.

Good protection of privacy while being treated or having visitors provides comfort but would also be respectful and better maintain the patient's dignity during his/her stay in the hostile environment of an ICU. The global task for us all is to promote **autonomy**, within the patient's individual limitations.

Much more so than in the past, the ICU of the future will see significant attention given to factors that improve the work environment and also benefit the patients.

Safety

Safety as a pivotal perspective covers many spheres within and around an ICU, the hospital and its interactions with its stakeholders. Safety in this regard has many dimensions and is not limited to direct patient interactions. It is a major paradigm shift which concerns staff, equipment, processes, environment, and societal issues. Considering the monetary expenditures of an ICU with up to 20 % of the hospital budget and 5 % of health expenditures, safety in a wider perspective and its impact must be investigated and new ideas created. The ICU being an embedded integral part

of a healthcare facility must link its actions with the overall strategy of the institution in all these dimensions centered around patients, admission and discharge as well as processes. On patient levels in each activity safety must be considered: What is the impact on patient safety and what might be the impact on staff? How safely are we dealing with waste, energy and water use? Can we construct an environmentally safe ICU? How can we reduce energy requirements? These considerations and intelligent solutions will contribute to a competitive advantage of the healthcare institution.

Patient safety

The patient's safety is improved when complications are prevented or their impact on outcome minimised. Impact minimisation in general means prompt and adequate reaction.

It is well known that the discrepancy between available resources, skills and knowledge and the needs of an individual patient has a major impact on post-ICU complications, mortality and readmission rate. This gap is much larger in wards than in adequately staffed intensive care units (see Fig. 1).

It is always important to consider that major resource deficits are more likely to appear at night and that workload in ICUs and wards may vary considerably during a day. An intensive care unit serving a large surgical population may have two peak workloads: the first when a number patients are discharged in the morning and the second when a number of patients are admitted in the early and late afternoon. The intensity of care for these patients will be at its maximum within the first 6–10 hours after admission. The future planning of human resources will certainly necessitate a smarter approach to day and night in intensive care units. Some of these fast-tracked patients may be ready for discharge at midnight but typically there will be no good receiving unit because normal wards often have very limited resources available at night.

The issue of care gaps after intensive care discharge in vulnerable patients needs real attention. The Austrian Center for Quality in Intensive Care (www.asdi.ac.at) has found within its network of 75 intensive care units that median

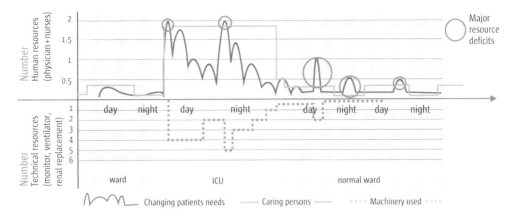

Fig. 1   Schematic representation of resource gaps in different structures of the hospital

post-ICU mortality is 33 % with a large variability between 5 and 55 % (see Fig. 2).

Single rooms versus open units

Optional single rooms for all patients are my choice for the future. Single rooms do not only promote privacy and allow individualised comfort but are also a safety factor. Single rooms have a favourable impact on the incidence of nosocomial infections and thus should be thought of as a preventive measure rather than an 'isolation' measure after the occurrence of an infection. One single room per 5–10 beds was traditionally considered sufficient.

Ideally you should plan a design where each patient area can easily be transformed into a single room. A large, transparent sliding door can increase the options to achieve a quiet environment,

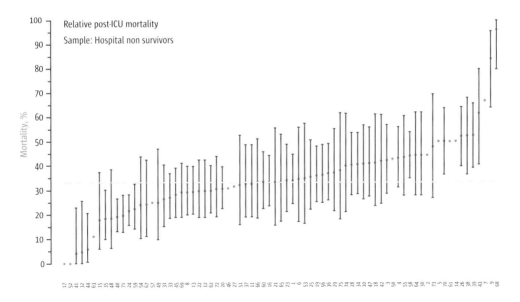

Fig. 2   Proportion of post-ICU mortality in relation to total hospital mortality in 75 Austrian intensive care units

noise protection and possibility for isolation without moving infected patients within the unit. The only advantage of open patient areas with many beds is easier overview for the nursing staff and help within 'shouting' distance. The disadvantages of the open area approach predominate. I think that an additional consideration should be that having a mix of open areas and isolation rooms may create large differences in patient care. Often nurses do not appreciate having to work in the isolated room, doctors tend to pass by or interact more rarely with these patients. Thus, one single style of room that permits isolation with little effort would be my preferred approach. Technical standards for rooms, air conditioning, and gas and power supply backups, are often governed by national laws that need to be adhered to carefully.

Distance & proximity

Duration of transport within the hospital is a safety factor for the patient and an important workload factor for the team. The smaller the distance from the partners sending patients (see Tab. 1) the shorter the duration of patient transport. The second group of distances should be those distances that need to be covered by patients during their ICU stay. Duration of transport with often limited monitoring and supporting technology as well as the risk of failure (power failure, gas failure, disconnections, alarm malfunction, distracted attention) at a distance from backup systems is the origin of transport-associated risk. Transports will necessitate specific technology such as transport ventilator and monitoring, which needs to be assessed.

Don't forget to plan and test how and on which path patients will be **transported** to radiology for special investigations like CT scans, angiography, etc., to the cath lab and to the operating theater. Often small elevators and narrow doors can be barriers to easy transportation.

The ICU staff often has the desire to give long-stay ICU patients a possibility to be brought **outdoors** to give these patients a positive, optimistic feeling. The final result of this analysis will be the possible location within the hospital. In addition, you will have obtained a common understanding of the expected function and possible constraints.

Workload reduction

All possible efforts should be undertaken to minimise the workload and to avoid unnecessary distractions particularly for nurses but also for doctors. At the stage of designing the ICU a central element would be the minimisation of walking distances between patients and central rooms. Rooms with frequent use should be close to patients, e.g. pharmacy and clean storage area, whereas storage for other, rarely used equipment may be located at a distance.

Unnecessary alarming is an enormous distraction. Alarming behaviour and the possibility to select different configurations is an important selection criterium for a monitoring device.

An electronic patient data management system (PDMS) should increase the precision of the documentation, increase patient safety and facilitate treatment and care planning. The essential components are the collection and display of data from various monitoring devices on one screen, a standardised ordering and recording system for medical and nursing treatment, a reminding system for treatments and examinations that may span several days as a minimum, a fluid balance documentation and calculation module, a module for documentation of clinical observations, a managing tool for notes, a module for recording

Tab. 1   Distance and barriers to safe transport to be evaluated

From	To & Back	To
Emergency department	Radiology (CT scan, MRI)	Intermediate care
Trauma unit	Cath lab	Surgical wards
Operating theatres	Operating theatres	
Interventional cardiology	Outdoor area	

of lab values, microbiology, etc. and, finally, the capacity to generate a smart printed summary that can accompany the patient at discharge from the ICU. The database should be sufficiently well structured to allow easy extraction of benchmarking, quality control and research data. Typically such a PDMS will support or even demand process standardisation. All data available in the hospital in an electronic format and necessary for proper patient care should be transferred electronically to the PDMS. A well-designed PDMS gives the nurse more time to work directly with the patient.

Don't forget

Space and rooms that are indirectly related to patient care are often too small or even missing. **Storage** space is necessary near the patient for daily care but also for disposables, machines and equipment not used. Non-communicating **clean and non-clean utility areas** are essential for structural infection control. A local **pharmacy** will always be necessary for clean and rapid drug and fluid preparation. A **laboratory** fulfilling the minimum requirements of determining blood gases, haemoglobin, serum electrolytes, glucose, lactate, and possibly point of care coagulation assessment, is necessary. Usually central lab response times are not short enough 24 hours a day to respond to intensive care needs. For all other measurements a central laboratory with a preferential path for intensive care patients is preferable.

A separate **office** for the nursing director and the doctors working on the unit needs to be planned and should be close enough to the central station to allow easy involvement in rapid decisions. The whole team should have a **staff lounge** for periods of rest. This area should be quiet and relaxing, allow the storage of personal items in lockers and permit food storage, preparation and eating. The intensivist in charge should have a centrally located individual room especially for the night period. A room that is able to accommodate the whole team present on a standard day should be available for **patient discussion and rounding** away from the patient with access to PDMS, PACS and all other regularly used electronic media. This room would also serve the purpose of **education**.

Relatives and family rooms are usually lacking and should be planned in any new ICU. The relatives' room should allow for waiting in a protected area before visiting a relative or friend or meeting with the treating team. An absolutely necessary **adjacent room** should be reserved for **communication and discussion** between the **ICU team and families** – for all types of news, and not just complicated or bad news. Having relatives in an ICU may be such a traumatic experience that the ICU should have the possibility to reduce this stress by way of a good, calm and consistent information policy.

At the planning stage the special needs of all **persons that collaborate and contribute** to the ICU team need to be considered. Their workplace requirements may be specific, and an area for interaction with others and for storing special devices may be necessary. Just think about physiotherapy, speech training, ergotherapy and dietetic counseling. The ICU team has mandatory personnel such as nurses, nursing aids and doctors, but also some desirable but not universally available persons, such as administrative personnel and secretaries to support documentation, or receptionists to manage visitors.

Embedding in hospital processes

Intensive care medicine has developed as a specialist entity that requires specific knowledge and abilities. Both elements have characteristics of economic ambivalence: They are essential for economies of scale or scope but also serve as the nucleus of professional identity, with transaction costs that may arise if the ICU is not fully embedded in the overall hospital processes.

Modern ICUs are considered an essential part of the course of treatment and care of severely diseased patients with arising treatment costs amounting to 10–20 % of total hospital costs. Thus economic issues will influence the planning of intensive care units. In an attempt to provide essentials for staffing and equipment, major intensive care societies published recommendations for minimal requirements for intensive care departments in 1997 and guidelines for intensive care unit design in 1995.

However, these recommendations provide only a static picture of the ICU – dynamics and an optimal fit between resourses and utilisation is what is called for now with hospital managers introducing knowledge gained from industry processes.

What will be design-related determinants of the overall success of an ICU?

- Integration
- Specialisation and segmentation
- Cooperation
- Connectivity
- Resource utilisation
- Process optimisation

The mission of the hospital and the contribution of the planned ICU to the success of the healthcare system both need to be clearly defined. What is the task of the ICU within the healthcare facility, what will be the likely load on the system and which input factors are required? Questions regarding interfaces and connectivity with partners are important for an optimal fit between workload, staff and equipment. Identification of the bottlenecks is essential for workflow optimisation and resource planning.

Quantify the expected patient flow through intensive care

An estimation of the actual needs and an estimation of future needs for intensive care services should be the basis for the design of an intensive care unit. It is generally assumed that 5–10 % of acute care beds should be available as intensive care beds. This rough figure must be adapted based on solid need estimates. The need must be derived from the patient flow in the hospital.

This estimation of the patient flow is driven by the hospital and its environment. The environment, on the one hand, is the population which typically uses this hospital with its demographic characteristics and professional environment, and on the other hand, it also consists of the other hospital facilities that serve the same population. The needs of a rural population may be much easier to estimate because the population is better defined than the needs of an urban population served by several hospitals simultaneously. In addition to the resident population, some hospitals may also have to consider moving populations, as well as dealing with seasonal variations created by travel and tourism.

The internal hospital perspective should include directly related partners such as 'intermediate care' or 'high dependency units'. The analysis should not stick with names of structures, since there is great variability in staffing, available technical infrastructure and actual functions between different structures. Structures dedicated to patients needing an increasing level of care or intensified level of surveillance based on the risk of changes in conditions necessitating prompt intervention may have different names in different countries. A categorisation into 3 categories depending on the available nursing, medical and technical resources has not been uniformly adopted. The task force of the European Society of Intensive Care Medicine has defined three levels of care. The highest proposed level of care (III) demands a 1/1 nurse/patient ratio and thus 6 full-time nurse equivalents (FTE) per intensive care bed run. In several countries, Austria being one example, the highest level ICUs in academic centres have a maximum of 4 FTE per bed, whereas in other countries like the UK it is common to have 7–8 FTE for an ICU bed and 4 FTE for a bed in a 'high dependency unit'. Another structure providing intensive care services specifically after surgery is the 'post-anaesthesia care unit'. The intensity of care may be similar to a high level intensive care unit but usually there are some limitations in the technical resources and accepted length of stay. Based on these disparities in terminology objective measures of activity should be used for planning and designing an ICU.

The typical sources for adult patients needing admission to intensive care units are:

- Emergency department
- Trauma unit
- Operating theatre
- Neurosurgery
- Cardiac surgery
- Transplantation services
- Interventional cardiology if no cardiac care unit is available
- Neurology if no stroke unit is available
- Any ward within the hospital, ideally via an outreach team

This list shows that the necessary intensive care resources will be highly dependent on the function of a given hospital within the healthcare system. Typical sources of patients should also be asked to state their perspectives on the development of the patient population. A general perspective is that length of stay in hospitals should decrease. Thus, patients with a low level of care will be discharged earlier to ambulatory care and therefore patients within the hospital will be more severely ill than in the past. This perspective has led countries like Australia to estimate that the need for intensive care resources will double within the next ten years.

Two developments can be foreseen. Firstly, there will be a centralisation of complex care into larger centres where the frequency of specific cases will be high enough to acquire and maintain a high level of expertise. Secondly, there will be a specialisation of intensive care within the larger centres to facilitate the care of relatively homogeneous patient groups. The size of individual intensive care units or subunits was ideally considered to be between 6–8 beds. This number will increase to 12–20 beds in the future. These larger units are slightly more complex to manage but offer more flexibility in resource allocation within the unit.

The destination of patients after the intensive care unit stay is the next element to consider. It is important to know exactly where patients can be discharged to. Availability and capacity of 'intermediate care units' or 'high dependency units' is the key to knowing how well patients have to be before they are discharged from the ICU.

Conclusion

An intensive care unit has the key function to facilitate an efficient and safe patient flow through an acute care hospital. Patients' best interest and well-being should be the primary focus. Patients deserve an appropriately designed environment for critical illness. The specific knowledge, technical skills and critical attitudes of the ICU team is the main resource. An adequate technological infrastructure is the tool for delivery of intensive care. Intensive care units do not fulfill their function if designed as independent structures, they need to understand themselves as a chain link in the process of acute care. Safety issues need to cover patient, personnel and institutionally focused aspects. Efficient resource use, consideration of environmental issues such as waste generation and disposal and economic think-

ing are of primary importance for safety in the area of intensive care medicine, which uses around 1 % of GNP. Inappropriate and inefficient design may jeopardise the performance of your ICU when economic constraints challenge the hospitals in the near future.

All design issues need to be thought and checked along an efficient patient flow. The second major intention must be support for fast recovery of autonomy. The possibility to promote even limited autonomy within the multiple constraint area of an ICU should be carefully addressed at the design stage of an ICU.

Appendix 1: The hard facts

The clear elements are the space typically required for each ICU bed and the technology that you will have to plan for your ICU.

Tab. 2   Basic requirements for each ICU bed

Space	15–20 m² (open)	20–25 m² (single room) + anteroom for isolation rooms
Oxygen	3	(near ventilator + both sides of the bed)
Compressed air	3	(near ventilator + both sides of the bed)
Suction	3	(both sides of the bed)
Power	16	(well distributed)
Data network	4	(monitor, PDMS, echocardiography/PACS) (1 reserve)
Ventilator	1	(consider NIV capacity)
Monitor	1	
PDMS	1	(Patient data management system)
ICU Bed	1	(select pressure sore-preventing technology)
Infusion pumps	4–8	(ideally grouped on a rack = less cables)
PN/EN pump	1/1	

(PDMS: patient data management system, PACS: picture archiving and communication system, NIV: non-invasive ventilation, PN: parenteral nutrition, EN: enteral nutrition)

Remark: Additional technology that is used for several patients and may sometimes be shared between several units includes: a cardioverter defibrillator, a portable X-ray device, an echocardiography machine with a trans-esophageal probe and a probe for identifying vessels for vascular access, several haemodiafiltration/haemofiltration/haemodialysis machines (1 for 2–3 ICU beds), an intra-aortic balloon pump (IABP) and an extra-corporeal membrane oxygenation device (ECMO). Not all technology is mandatory but should be considered depending on patient population and training.

The authors

Michael Hiesmayr, MD[1]
Philipp G.H. Metnitz, MD, PhD, EDIC, DEAA[2]
Markus Haisjackl, MD, MBA[1]
  [1]Division of Cardiac, Thoracic and Vascular Anaesthesia and Intensive Care | Medical University Vienna | Vienna, Austria

[2]Division of Anaesthesia, General Intensive Care and Pain Control | Medical University Vienna | Vienna, Austria

Address for correspondence
  Prof. Michael Hiesmayr
  Division of Cardiac, Thoracic and Vascular Anaesthesia and Intensive Care
  Medical University Vienna
  Währinger Gürtel 18–20
  1090 Vienna, Austria
  E-mail: michael.hiesmayr@meduniwien.ac.at

References

1. Ferdinande P. Members of the Task Force of the European Society of Intensive Care Medicine. Recommendations on minimal requirements for Intensive Care Departments. Intensive Care Medicine (1997) 23: 226–232.
2. Task Force on Guidelines. Recommendations for critical care unit design. Society of Critical Care Medicine. Critical Care Medicine. 1988; 16: 796–806.

Patrick Ferdinande

Minimal structural requirements for ICUs and HDUs

Setting up a new ICU (intensive care unit) or an HDU (high dependency unit) or re-engineering an existing unit is a once-in-a-lifetime experience for most ICU/HDU medical and nursing staff. This means that good or bad concepts may have an influence for a long time period on both patients (in terms of safety, stress, privacy and outcome) and on the working conditions for the staff and allied health personnel (e. g. provider burnout, human errors) working in this unit. Ergonomical principles must be included from the very beginning, although compromises sometimes have to be accepted (noise control versus alarm perception, patient privacy versus visibility). Structural requirements cannot be defined without a thorough analysis of the operational characteristics of the future unit. It is an occasion to query existing practices to create a momentum to implement new philosophies because function and structure go hand in hand.

The planning team

The process of designing a new ICU is both exciting and labor-intensive as every detail has to be anticipated. At some stages this may become a part-time or even full-time job. Ideally the planning team consists of a multidisciplinary group including the ICU medical staff, the head nurse, the architect, a representative of the hospital management and a chief operating engineer familiar with healthcare design as well as with state and local regulations. This planning team should be advised by a safety officer, the hospital infection specialist and representatives of referring medical and surgical departments in the hospital. Additional disciplines (pharmacy, physiotherapist, nutritional support team, logistics department) should provide their input in the planning stages at the appropriate time.

General floor plan and communications

The department consists of a geographically distinct entity in the hospital with controlled access. The through traffic of patients and provisioning not intended for the ICU should be avoided. Public and visitor traffic to the ICU should be separated from professional, patient and supply traffic. Wherever possible horizontal and short-distance connections with the operating theatres and emergency department are recommended, and a centrally located, keyed and oversized elevator for patient transport with priority for the

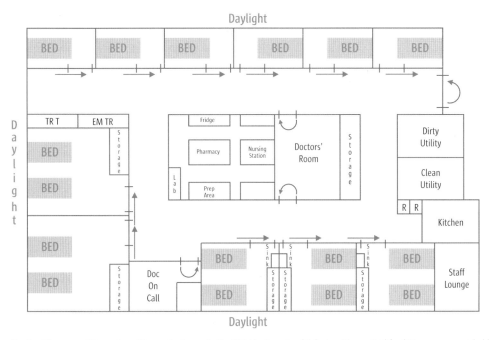

Fig. 1   The general floor plan of the patient area in the ICU: the "racetrack" design: The central facilities are surrounded by the patient areas (TRT: transport trolley; EMTR: emergency trolley; RR: restroom).

ICU assures the connection to referring and diagnostic departments (see Tab. 1). Proper evacuation routes and shelter in case of disaster must be planned in advance. The total surface area of the ICU is estimated to be roughly 2.5–3 times the total area devoted strictly to patient care. One of the most common mistakes is to underestimate the surface needed for non-directly patient-linked activities. Crucial at this point is to make appointments for future logistical arrangements (such as frequency and timing of provisioning) for sterile and non-sterile materials as this may affect the need for storage surface, stock size and turnover.

The best accepted concept for the general floor plan is the "racetrack" design (see Fig. 1) with a double corridor combining a daylight source in the patient areas at the outside with optimal patient visibility and short walking distances for the healthcare providers.

A special procedures/therapy room (approx. 35 sqm) may be optional for specific departments (burns, pacemaker implantation, etc.). All bedside facilities needed to continue monitoring and therapy of the patient should be provided in this area. High-intensity lighting and scrub-up sink are essential. It is adapted for unit-specific needs (radioscopy, angiography, etc.). When the ICU staff is also in charge of technical procedures in non-ICU hospitalised patients (e.g. catheter insertions) such a special procedure room may prove to be very useful.

Visual and auditive displays of alarm calls in the unit facilitate early intervention.

The size of the unit

An ICU should accommodate at least 6 beds [1, 2] but optimally 8 to 12 beds. Hospitals with several smaller units should be encouraged to rearrange these units into a single larger department to improve efficacy. On the other hand, a larger ICU may take the opportunity to create separate pathology-directed specialised functional subunits with 6–8 beds, sharing common functions (station laboratory, satellite pharmacy, etc.), administrative and logistical facilities. The size of

Tab. 1   Priority access for ICU to:

- the emergency department
- the operating theatres and postoperative areas
- the medical imaging department
- the laboratory
- the functional testing facilities
  (e.g. cath lab, endoscopy)

Depending on local arrangements easy access should be provided to:

The blood transfusion service, the hospital pharmacy, technical support services, the microbiology department, etc.

the unit is also influenced by the geographical and economic situation. On the other hand, a sufficient volume effect is also recognised to maintain a high quality standard of most activities (e. g. mechanical ventilation) [3, 4, 5].

The number of intensive care beds has to be calculated as a function of the type of hospital, admission of specific disease categories, elective surgical activity, the geographic location of the hospital, number of acute beds, etc.; the Hill-Burton formula (see Fig. 2) may be helpful. A survey of the international literature shows that an average of 5 % of hospital beds, and up to 10 % in university hospitals, are ICU beds. These numbers are indicative, as outpatient activity lead to a higher concentration of severely ill patients in the hospital [1, 6].

Standards for architecture, ICU staff and allied healthcare personnel have to be calculated for 100 % activity. In practice, only 75–80 % of the beds will be occupied if the occupancy rate is calculated on an hourly basis. This will allow to cope with the admission of major emergencies and to avoid premature discharges.

Separate ICU and HDU or a mixed ICU/HDU?

The choice to organise a mixed ICU/HDU or rather to opt for two separate units (ICU and HDU) can be made based on the following considerations: The bedside equipment has the least impact on ICU cost (in contrast to the staff salaries) [7]. In a mixed ICU/HDU all beds should be equipped at the highest level, otherwise "internal" moves to properly equipped beds will lead to problems related to the next reflection. Secondly, moving patients between separate units or internally between adequately equipped beds carries an obvious risk, induces loss of information, hampers continuity in management and creates an avoidable and unnecessary workload. Thirdly, a mixed ICU/HDU unit necessitates additional creativity to use the available manpower as efficiently as possible. On days with concentrated high activity some fully equipped beds may remain empty. Capacity calculation should then be performed based on available manpower and workload rather than on the number of equipped beds.

To assign a level of care and to decide whether a patient has to be admitted to an ICU or an HDU three levels of care (LOC) are proposed: III, II and I (see Tab. 2).

Tab. 2   Levels of care (LOCs)

LOC		Nurse/patient ratio	Nursing full-time equivalents per bed
III	ICU	1/1	6
II	ICU	1/2	3
I	HDU	1/3	2

Level of care LOC III (highest): ICU patients with or at risk of multiple (more than two) acute vital organ

$$\text{Calculated ICU capacity} = \frac{\text{number of admissions per year x average length of ICU stay (days)}}{365 \text{ x ideal occupancy rate (as fraction of 1)}}$$

e.g. ▪ Number of admissions per year   2000
      ▪ Average length of ICU stay   3 days
      ▪ Ideal bed occupancy rate   0.85 (= 85 % occupancy)

$$\text{Calculated ICU capacity} = \frac{2000 \times 3}{365 \times 0.85} = 19.3 \text{ ICU beds}$$

Fig. 2   The Hill-Burton formula: ICU capacity calculation

failures with an immediately life-threatening character. These patients will need organ support therapy such as haemodynamic support (at least two inotropic and/or vasoactive drugs in continuous infusion) plus respiratory assistance or continuous renal replacement therapy for a prolonged period of time.

Level of care LOC II (intermediate): ICU patients requiring monitoring and/or minor support of at least two acutely failing vital organ systems with a life-threatening character (e.g. respiratory assistance and continuous renal replacement therapy, respiratory assistance and one vasoactive drug in continuous intravenous infusion, etc.).

Level of care LOC I (lowest): Monitoring and minor support of only one vital organ system: HDU patients at risk of developing one or more acute organ failures necessitating close monitoring, patients recovering from one or more acute vital organ failures but whose condition is too unstable or when the nursing workload is too high or complex to be managed on a regular ward.

Several LOC can be integrated in the same ICD in a flexible structural organisation model [6, 8, 9, 10, 11, 12]. If, however, a separate ICU and HDU are planned, it is important to anticipate which activities will be deployed in the HDU (noninvasive ventilation or not, renal replacement or not) and to adapt the infrastructure accordingly. Experience teaches us that the range of therapeutic interventions conducted in HDUs is highly variable [13].

Patient area

The surface area for patient care is a minimum of 25 sqm for single rooms and 23 sqm per bed for shared rooms. The basic ground plan for single and shared rooms is rectangular with at least 2 metres of traffic area at either side of the bed. The doorways are wide enough and adequately positioned to allow a bed (with orthopedic traction, ECMO equipment, cot sides, etc.) to pass easily.

Single rooms are strongly recommended to minimise cross-contamination and the layout has to be adapted in such a way that conscious patients are not distressed by the acute problems (alarms, cardioversion, resuscitation, etc.) of other patients. Due respect for the privacy of the patients must be assured [14, 15], since a failure to do so may hamper their long-term outcome [16]. In isola-

tion rooms additional technical characteristics (i.e. negative pressure rooms) may be considered (airborne infections) [17]. The other option is to conceive an entire subunit as an isolation area with controlled access for pandemic infections. Two-bed rooms offer the added advantage of an enormous surface potential for the occasional patient with highly complex equipment (ECMO + CRRT + circulatory assistance + artificial ventilation, etc.).

Shared rooms (upper limit number of beds: 4) can fulfill a role in the ICU, provided that there are precautions to avoid cross-infection, to control noise and to assure patient privacy.

In the construction calculations the possible use of heavy-weight equipment (sophisticated hospital beds, mobile X-ray equipment, etc.) has to be anticipated.

The ratio of isolation to shared rooms should be in the range of 1–2 per 10 beds but may be higher [5–6, 10] in special departments (burn units, transplantation departments, infection units, etc.). Isolation rooms are optionally equipped with an anteroom of at least 3 sqm for hand washing, gowning and storage.

The instructions for isolation are clearly displayed at the entrance of each room.

The patient should be visible at all times to facilitate detection of status changes. This can be arranged from the central nursing station by analysing direct sightlines and angles during the design process or alternatively, as a second choice, by video camera. Patients should be oriented so that they can see the nurse but cannot see the other patients. Constant visual contact between nurse and patient may be achieved by large window openings, glass doors, etc. Nurses working bedside should have a view on neighbouring patients. All patient rooms have a daylight source. The position of the patient's bed should ideally also allow a direct view out of the external window. Outside windows can only be opened by releasing a safety lock.

Access to the patient is a top priority for intensive care. All sockets and service outlets should be distributed on both sides of the bed and arranged in such a way that there is minimal interference with nursing care. Adequate access to the head of the bed should also be provided for endotracheal intubation, resuscitation and central venous catheterisation. There are two options: first, the bed-head to the wall layout with the disadvantage of limited access to the patient's head in emergency situations (see Fig. 3), or second, the free-standing arrangement with one or two ceiling-mounted sta-lactite power columns. Although the second solu-tion is more expensive, it is to be recommended for optimal access to the head of the patient. Plug-in connections for pressurised gases should not be at eye level to avoid accidental injury. The use of fixed cabinets for storage in patient areas has largely been abandoned and replaced by a multi-functional trolley, reducing peripheral stocks and improving stock turnover. This concept also en-hances the cleaning and infection control process.

Ceiling-mounted patient lifting (and weigh-ing) systems have great ergonomic value as early mobilisation gains importance.

Access to the electronic patient file and hos-pital information systems is provided at each pa-tient bed. For patient use, access to IT communi-cation tools is worth considering.

Services in the patient area

Electricity: 16–20 grounded sockets divided over three isolated transformers are required per bed. Sockets on the same transformer have identical color codes. All sockets for vital support are on no-break circuits. Docking stations for infusion pumps and syringe drivers reduce the number of sockets needed. One socket for mobile radiol-ogy equipment per patient area. Wiring for IT applications should be provided.

Vacuum: Three outlets per bed, low vacuum type with keyed plug-in connections.

Oxygen: Four outlets with keyed plug-in con-nections per bed with flowmeter, two on each side of the bed.

Compressed air: Three outlets with keyed plug-in connections per bed (driving ventilators, gas mixing device for spontaneous breathing) and 1 flowmeter.

Tubing for facultative medical gas may be con-sidered, e.g. nitrous oxide, NO (with scavenging system and ambient pollution control).

Water supply: Minimum one hand basin, deep and wide enough to prevent splashing and equipped with elbow- or foot-operated taps, must be available for every patient care area to minimise the transfer of infection. Water sup-ply and sinks are positioned at the foot end of the bed. Self-sterilising heated traps are recom-mended. Hand drying facilities must be provid-

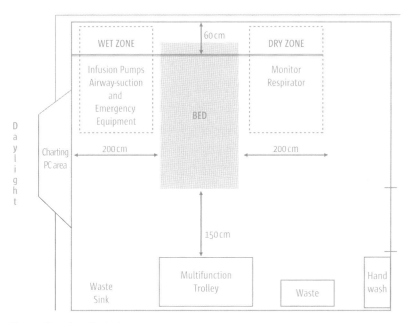

Fig. 3   Floor plan of a single room

ed. Hand disinfection facilities are provided in every patient room and anteroom at inviting and visible locations (entrance, head of the bed, doorways, ...). A dialysis tap and runoff may be considered in every room at a location where the dialysis tube does not interfere with regular traffic.

Central nursing station

The central nursing station allows direct and indirect (camera) visualization of the patient and it contains: Shelves for forms and library, a satellite pharmacy with central lockable drawer for narcotics or controlled dispenser, IT workstations, telephone, intercom and emergency call systems, satellite storage cabinets for sterile and non-sterile clean material, optional visual display with access to individual patient monitoring with alarm warning and a drug preparation area with adequate illumination.

The central station is equipped with air conditioning, adequate adjustable overhead lighting, a wall-mounted clock, hand basin, hand disinfection solution dispensers, writing and preparation counters. Worth considering is the need for a decentralised emergency lab for blood gas, electrolyte, lactate, glucose, hematocrite analysis in the central area. Adjacent to or incorporated within the nursing station a workplace for the attending intensivists is required. Enough individual work stations must be provided in order to facilitate workflow.

Storage

Sufficient storage space outside the patient area is essential. The storage room should be easily accessible for nursing and medical staff, at a maximum walking distance of 30 m from the patient area, ideally easy to approach both from the patient area and from the supply route.

Storage for consumables (5 sqm/bed) (satellite pharmacy, intravenous and dialysis fluids, enteral nutrition, sterile and non-sterile nursing material (linen, disposables), refrigerator for pharmaceuticals, refrigerator for temporary storage of blood and plasma products.

Storage for durable equipment (5 sqm/bed) for ventilators, dialysis machines, infusion pumps, back-up monitoring apparatus, drip stands, blood warmers, trolleys, suction units, mobile radiology and surgical equipment. Transport trolley attachable to the bed with transport monitor (ECG, invasive, non-invasive blood pressure monitoring, pulse oxymetry, respiration monitoring), transport ventilator and mobile suction unit. Defibrillator with rechargeable battery, adult and paediatric paddles, display and recorder. One anaesthesia trolley with scavenging system should be considered according to local needs. Only serviced equipment ready for use is stored in this space. This storage room should have a bench, electrical sockets, medical gas outlets, sinks and a wall rail.

Separate storage for emergency equipment centrally located
- Case with emergency drugs and equipment during transport of critically ill patients (1 for 6 beds)
- Pacemakers
- Crash cart with extended drug and resuscitation material and difficult airway equipment

Utility

Two completely separated spaces for clean (15 sqm) and dirty (25 sqm) utility rooms with separate access are necessary. The clean utility room is used for the storage of linen and assembling of sterile material.

One dirty utility room is used for the removal of soiled linen, waste, etc. It contains a clinical sink and hopper. A second dirty utility room for dismantling used equipment is desirable. The load on the dirty utility room will be reduced if individual patient rooms are equipped with bedpan cleaning equipment.

The utility rooms are air-conditioned. All air supplied to the dirty utility room is extracted. Removal of soiled items and waste should occur through a separate corridor.

Other important areas

Nurse's office

At least 20 sqm are provided as office space for the head nurse(s) with IT workstations, separate telephone extension, intercom, notice boards and alarm system for bedside calls.

Medical office

At least 20 sqm are provided as office space per physician with full-time activity in the department of intensive care medicine. It is equipped with a telephone, intercom and alarm registration on the department. A computer terminal with access to patient monitoring systems, laboratory and diagnostic departments is useful.

Secretariat

20 sqm for 8 intensive care beds

Staff lounge

A room of 30 sqm for 8 intensive care beds is needed as:
- Staff lounge with beverage bars, emergency code alarm system, intercom terminal and telephone extension
- Staff changing room, with lockers, showers and restrooms (M and F)

Physician on call bedroom(s)

15 sqm with bed, hand basin, shower, toilet, telephone, intercom terminal, alarmcode system, television. Access to daylight with opening window. Must be quiet.

Laboratory

15 sqm are provided as space for laboratory (point of care) purposes, allowing emergency examinations (blood gases, haemoglobin, haematocrit, glucose, lactate, serum electrolytes, etc.). Adequate bench space with at least 12 electrical points, sink, specimen refrigerator, intercom terminal, telephone. The central hospital laboratory can serve as an alternative if the service and communication lines are extremely quick.

Workshop

28 sqm are reserved as a technical workshop. Bench, shelves, sink, electrical outlets, oxygen, vacuum and compressed air are provided. This is used for minor repairs, adjustment, assembly and testing of equipment.

Kitchen

25 sqm for preparation of patients' special food and staff snacks. Microwave, refrigerator, sink, cooker, dishwasher. A separate kitchen in a relaxing environment for the staff members is desirable.

Reception area and relatives' rooms

10 sqm for 8 beds (1.5–2 chairs/bed) + 2 x 10 sqm for 8 beds (bed + shower) as sleep or rest cubicles for relatives are desirable. Intercom terminal, telephone, radio, restrooms for disabled persons, sink, TV plug, public telephone. It is desirable to have separate visitor and professional entrances to the unit.

Receptionist's office

10 sqm adjacent to the reception area for departments with more than 12 beds. Intercom terminal, telephone, computer terminal. The receptionist's office should be strategically located so that visitors must pass by the reception area for identification and notification by the receptionist or nursing staff.

Seminar room – multifunctional conference room

40 sqm for formal teaching, continuing education, discussion with other medical disciplines, will be equipped with seating, projection facilities, overhead, wall board, video equipment, air conditioning. The area must be adapted to the size of the department.

Interview room

15 sqm needed for interviews with patients' relatives

Cleaners' room (3–4 sqm for 8 beds)

Storage of cleaning equipment and materials. Housekeeping materials should not be used interchangeably with the public areas because of the possibilities of cross-contamination.

Corridors and floor coverings

Transport of patients to and from the ICD should ideally be separated from public corridors and visitor waiting areas to assure patient privacy and rapid and unobstructed patient transport. The corridors are wide enough (2.5 m) to allow unobstructed transport of patients with support equipment (intra-aortic balloon, circulatory assistance, transport, ventilator, etc.). Oversized keyed elevators are necessary.

The seamless floor covering is chemically inert, resistant to antiseptics and sound-absorbing. Special care is taken to avoid level differences. The floor coverings will allow heavy-wheeled equipment to be moved without difficulty.

Fire safety

Critically ill patients are extremely vulnerable not only to fire but also in terms of disruption of the life-supporting therapy. Fires affecting ICUs are rare. Still it is essential to make plans to prevent and to deal with fire. The basic principles of fire safety are avoidance of fire, compartmentalisation of fire, safeguarding of life and reduction of material damage. Each staff member must be familiarised with the emergency plan. Local regulations are usually available.

Control of the development of smoke and toxic gases can be achieved by containment (fire-resistant walls, ceilings, floors, doors), dispersal (natural or mechanical ventilation) and pressurisation of the patient areas (preventing entry of smoke)

Compartmentalisation and local fire control deserve attention in the early disaster stage. The individual patient area safety is of utmost importance.

An alternative route of escape and an adjoining safe space to move the patient should be provided. This space, equipped with oxygen administration, compressed air and electric facilities, should preferentially be on the same level of the building and protected from wind and rain. Both postoperative areas and emergency department may be used for this purpose.

Fire doors may be a hindrance to normal traffic and continuous visual inspection if maintained in a closed position. Automatic electromagnetic or electromechanical devices can be used to hold them open during normal operation.

Electrical wiring and piped gases must run in separate conduits. Service ducts containing piped gases must be suitably ventilated. Gas pipes must be tested for leakage before use.

Central services

Control switches, shut-off valves and monitoring (of gas pipe pressure) must be located adjacent to the unit where they can be operated by the staff in case of emergency. They must be clearly marked to indicate the type of service or part of the hospital supplied. Interruption of central services at intermediate points between the source and the unit should be made impossible.

All compressed medical gases should be supplied at the same pressure at all times to prevent cross-leakage in gas mixers. For safety reasons the floor plan of the unit with vital services is displayed in a visible place.

Electricity

220 V single-phase electrical supply with a single common earth and with all the outlets in the patient areas on the same phase are provided. Special care is taken to avoid electrical potential differences. The patient areas and central computers should be served by a maintained stand-by power source which is activated after a maximum of 5 seconds when the normal electrical current is interrupted. A separate circuit is required for emergency lighting, computers, ventilators and other sensitive equipment.

For computers, a back-up current source with separate, protected battery power is provided.

A circuit for non-vital purpose X-ray does not need to be backed up by a stand-by supply source.

Ventilation

All air should be 99 % filtered to a particle diameter of 5 microns. All rooms have air conditioning with adjustable ambient temperature, relative humidity between 40 % and 60 % and a choice of positive and negative pressure relative to the open area.

Air conditioning is also mandatory in:
- Rooms with heat-generating equipment (laboratory, computers, ...)
- Staff and conference rooms

Air changes should be six per hour in isolation rooms, other patient areas and staff rooms.

Active ventilation must be provided in restrooms, teaching rooms, laboratory and reception rooms.

Heating

Ambient temperature should be adjustable in:

Patient areas (individually adjustable) between	16–27°C
Staff rooms and open areas	18–21°C
Dirty utility	16–21°C
Storage rooms and cleaners' room	16–21°C

Communications

Provision should be made for easy and rapid communication within the unit and hospital systems which causes minimal auditive distress to patients and staff.

Lighting

Natural daylight with a view is essential for both patients and staff. The quality of the artificial lighting should approach daylight characteristics. Too much sunlight can be a hindrance and tinted glass may be needed. The view from adjacent wards or floors should be blocked. The artificial lighting consists of:
1. General illumination with dimming possibility
2. Indirect night illumination which allows for observation but does not disturb other patients
3. Reading lamp at each bed
4. Mobile operating theatre illumination
5. Instantaneously acting emergency lighting powered by a stand-by generator

Conclusion

Designing a new or adapting an existing ICU/HDU is a complex process. The concept exceeds the strictly architectural design elements. The integration of functional and operational aspects in the structural design is the only way to achieve a successful result. In most instances physicians and nurses feel unfamiliar with the process and end up with an unsatisfactory end product.

The process starts with an analysis and reengineering of the established practices and seeks new opportunities in a changing environment. Once this is done the structural requirements can be tailored according to the insights gained. The medical and nursing activity to be deployed in the unit interferes with almost all departments in the hospital, and their respective voice and contribution must be acknowledged.

The racetrack design concept of the unit is the preferred general layout. For patient and adjunctive areas the floor surface is of paramount importance as intensive care medicine will probably only become more complex in the future. Ergonomic considerations such as walking distances, patient visibility and patient lifting systems will not only contribute to patient safety and quality of care but also to the satisfaction of all caretakers. Due investment in IT technology is a reasonable choice, but whether telemedicine, artificial intelligence and other applications will claim their place by adding to the core business – namely excellent patient centred care – remains to be seen.

The author

Patrick Ferdinande, PhD, MD
Professor in Intensive Care Medicine
UZ Leuven, Campus Gasthuisberg
Intensive Care Unit
Herestraat 49
3000 Leuven, Belgium
E-mail: patrick.ferdinande@uz.kuleuven.ac.be

References

1. Bertolini G, Rossi C, Brazzi L, Radrizzani D, Rossi G, Arrighi E et al. The relationship between labour cost per patient and the size of intensive care units: a multicentre prospective study. Intensve Care Med 2003;29:2307–11
2. Jacobs R, Dawson D. Quality and efficacy decrease with decreasing number of beds. Hospital efficiency targets. Health Econ 2003;12:669–84.
3. Kahn JM, Goss CH, Heagerty PJ, Kramer AA, O'Brien CR, Rubenfield GD. Hospital volume and outcomes of mechanical ventilation. N Eng J Med 2006;355:41–50.
4. Lecuyer L, Chevret S, Guidet B, Aegerter P, Martel P, Schlemmer B et al. Case volume and mortality in haematological patients with acute respiratory failure. Eur Respir J 2008;32:748–54.

5. Pronovost PJ, Jenckes MW, Dorman T, Garrett E, Breslow MJ, Rosenfeld BA, et al. Organisational characteristics of intensive care units related to outcomes of abdominal aortic surgery. JAMA 1999;281:1310–17.

6. Wild C, Narath M. Evaluating and planning ICUs: methods and approaches to differentiate between need and demand. Health Policy 2005;71:289–301.

7. Flaatten H, Kvåle R Cost of intensive care in a Norwegian University hospital1997–1999. Critical Care 2003; 7:72–78

8. Iapichino G, Radrizzani D, Rossi C. Proposal of a flexible structural-organising model for the Intensive Care Units. Minerva Anesthesiol 2007;73:501–6.

9. American Thoracic Society (Medical Section of the American Lung Association). Fair allocation of Intensive Care Unit Resources. Am J Respir Crit Care Med 1997;156:1282–1301.

10. Dawson SM, Runk JA. Right patient? Right bed? A question of appropriateness. AACN Advanced Critical Care 2000;11:375–85.

11. Reis MD, Dinis MD, de Rijk A, Schaufeli W. Simplified therapeutic intervention scoring system: The TISS-28 items. Results from a multicenter study. Crit Care Med 1996;24:p64–73.

12. Pirret AM. Utilizing TISS to differentiate between intensive care and high-dependency patients and to identify nursing skill requirements. Intensive and Critical Care Nursing 2002;18:19–26.

13. Ridley SA. Intermediate care. Anaesthesia 1998;53:654–664.

14. Guises AP, Carayon P. Performance Obstacles of intensive care nurses. Nursing research 2007;56:185–194

15. Chaudhury H, Mahmood A, Valente M. Nurses perception of single-occupancy versus multioccupancy rooms in acute care environment. An exploratory comparative assessment. Applied Nursing Research 2006;19:118–125

16. Donchin Y, Seagull J. The hostile environment of the intensive care unit. Current Opinion in Critical Care 2002;8:316–20.

17. O'Connell N, Humphreys H. Intensive care unit design and environmental factors in the acquisition of infection. Journal of hospital infection 2000;45:255–262.

Armand R.J. Girbes, Albertus Beishuizen and Jan G. Zijlstra

Minimal training requirements for ICU physicians

Introduction

Medical training and education has changed tremendously over the last 10 to 20 years. The duration to become a fully trained medical specialist has been shortened and programmes have been condensed all over the world. In the UK, for example, the actual length of time allowed for training has been reduced by approximately half over the last two decades. Working hours for trainees have been reduced and more legal regulations on scheduling interfere with rota and exposure to patients during working hours. Moreover, medicine continues to increase in complexity, depth, and levels of intervention possible. All these changes necessitate the educational methods to compensate for the diminished exposure time to patients during training. Generally speaking, however, the efficiency of training has not kept pace with all these developments [1]. Medical training of students faces similar challenges, and new perspectives and approaches have been proposed [2]. Computer-centred training, and the use of information technology are, logically, new tools that can be utilised nowadays. Patient focus is retained in theoretical learning by means of a range of approaches to problem-centred learning using these electronic tools, e.g. virtual patients whose problems unfold over time. Computer-based programmes can be used to teach theory before actual practical exercise. Electronic curriculum programmes allow rapid access to information ('common blackboard') and quick turnaround of evaluation and messaging. The computer-based programmes also allow not only for an assessment of the students' knowledge, skills, attitudes and fitness for practice, but also for students themselves to appreciate their progress. All tutors, assessors, and students at any site can look at the curricular context of their own contribution. The clinical emphasis in new curricula is based on the perspective of the patient, and not on medical specialities.

In this chapter we will discuss the most important minimal requirements of the training of intensivists. Several features must be recognised is this respect: the entry criteria, the (total) duration of training, the institute where the training takes place, the competencies and curriculum vitae requirements of the trainers, and the competencies to be acquired by the trainee.

Transition in the training of medical specialists

In recent history a so-called guild system of apprenticeship-based training existed. The admission of trainees was arranged and regulated by the guild, i.e. the medical specialists/consultants, and the programme and curriculum, as well as the quality of training, were arranged and regulated internally, within the guild. The education was mainly based on work experience and the relationship between master and apprentice. The master was the role model for the trainee. In the past, training time was considerable and working hours were long. Exposure to patients therefore was long and continuity more or less ascertained by these extensive working hours. In addition, training time was expanded with advanced training programmes, e.g. on oncological surgery, or a focus on vascular surgery or on intensive care. In such a system the experience level is high when the former trainee enters a specialist job. However, this system will not work any longer since a change in mentality has occurred. Shorter working hours, part-time training, earlier acquisition of the final job and internationalisation have become a reality. Consequently, training needs to be more efficient, more effective and shorter and quicker. We are moving from a time-based apprenticeship to a competence-based apprenticeship. Knowledge, skills and attitude are the features that make a good doctor. The CanMEDS 2000 project (http://rcp-sc.medical.org/canmeds), which defines seven competencies, has tremendously changed the approach to physicians' training. Defining competencies means that they can be measured and therefore tested. With the training programme, the trainee will reach a higher level of specific competencies in due course. The level of expertise will start at "has knowledge of, describes" through "performs, manages or demonstrates under supervision" to "performs, manages or demonstrates independently". The next level is the ability to "teach and supervise others in the performance, management or demonstration". In order to obtain the competencies at the highest level, minimum requirements for the training of ICU physicians (in this chapter also referred to as intensivists) are necessary.

CanMEDS competencies

The Royal College of Physicians and Surgeons of Canada initiated an innovative framework for medical education called the CanMEDS framework of essential physician competencies. Fundamentally, CanMEDS is an initiative to improve patient care by making explicit the well-recognised abilities of highly skilled physicians. CanMEDS' focus is on articulating a comprehensive definition of the competencies needed for medical education and practice. Today, the CanMEDS model for physician competence is being adapted around the world, as well as in other professions.

Within the CanMEDS framework seven roles are distinguished. The pivotal role is, of course, that of the medical expert. But the other six roles are essential to being able to function as a medical expert: communicator, collaborator, health advocate, manager, scholar and professional. In the training programme of the VU Medical Center of Amsterdam, the role of the scholar has been slightly extended by underscoring its academic and scientific character. The scholar is thus called an "academic/university postgraduate". Additionally, the role of reflector has been explicitly added. The role of the reflector refers to the ability to reflect on one's own personal and professional performance to recognise one's own possibilities and limitations.

Intensive care training in Europe

In a major effort, with support from the European Society of Intensive Care Medicine (ESICM), Bion and the international team he created defined core competencies for an international training programme in intensive care medicine [3]. Little uniformity in training programmes for intensive care medicine exists even within Europe. The minimum duration of (additional) training in intensive care medicine varied among countries from 3 to 72 months [4]. Implicitly and explicitly, the minimum training requirements for ICU physicians thus vary grossly. Since intensive care is not a recognised speciality in most European countries, the speciality ownership varies. It is beyond doubt that these training programme variations in structure and process substantially impede the free movement of intensive care professionals/ICU physicians within Europe as intended by the European Union. Given the differences in training programmes and given the differences in ownership specialities for intensive care medicine, it is obvious that significant differences in the qualifications of intensivists exist, already within Europe and in countries closely linked to the ESICM (European Society of Intensive Care Medicine). Uniformity would be much easier if uniform (basic) requirements existed and intensive care medicine were recognised as a distinct speciality. The latter should not be considered an outrageous idea, since intensive care medicine nowadays concerns:

1. Well-identified patient groups, specifically to be treated by intensivists
2. Well-identifiable research directly related to intensive care medicine
3. Specific scientific journals on intensive care medicine
4. Additionally, in many European countries full professors in intensive care medicine have been appointed with a teaching commitment for intensive care medicine

These factors alone would and should be a sufficient incentive to make it a distinct medical speciality. As will be outlined below, other reasons exist related to attracting and holding young talented people to further develop intensive care medicine. In some countries the step of recognition of intensive care medicine as a separate entity has been made, although full European recognition by the UEMS (Union Européenne des Médecins Spécialistes) is probably still some distance away, because it is insufficiently realised that the existing rules impede one of the important aims of the European Union: the free movement of professionals. In Australia a major step forward was recently made with the formation of a new medical college, the College of Intensive Care Medicine of Australia and New Zealand, CICM (www.cicm.org.au).

Admission criteria for trainees

It is unrealistic to suppose that everyone, or any physician who just graduated, could become a good intensivist. Specific talents and personality traits are probably required, but the scientific foundation for arguing so is, to say the least, somewhat shaky. We select young colleagues for training positions in intensive care. However, there is little guidance for this process. We do not have good criteria for what makes a good intensivist. We know what we want to teach them, the

CanMEDS and CoBaTrICE or any other well-defined competencies. But we have no criteria to predict their trainability in these competences. Because we have only a poor description of what makes a good intensivist, we have no data as to which requisites are obligatory for an intensivist.

The same problem exists in medical education. The selection criteria for medical students are mainly based on the assumption that students who leave the training prematurely are not good prospective doctors. The critera are not based on which characteristics make a good doctor because we have only very poor definitions of what makes a doctor good. Motivation is generally believed to be an important factor. But we probably select those people that harmonise with our own personalities. This is probably why surgeons seem so much alike and why you can recognise an internist from a distance.

Duration of training

The required duration of additional training in intensive care medicine (ICM) to acquire the obligatory competencies will naturally depend on the competencies present at the start of the training. It is easy to imagine that a qualified internist will have other things to learn than a qualified anaesthesiologist or surgeon, pulmonologist or basic physician. Whereas internists will have a substantial gap in manual skills, e.g. central vascular access, airway management, chest drains and tracheotomy, anaesthesiologists will generally lack profound knowledge and skills in history taking, infectious diseases antibiotics, (internal) medical diseases and making differential diagnoses. All of them will probably have certain deficits in knowledge, or at least, experience, in specific ICM-related competencies such as, for instance, long-term mechanical ventilation. A recently updated (July 2009) Swiss postgraduate training programme in intensive care medicine has a total duration of 6 years [5]. In this training programme the non-specific part of the training varies between 2 and 3.5 years. This is, in fact, training in ICM-related specialities like anaesthesiology, internal medicine, (neuro-)surgery, pulmonology or neurology with the obligation to take at least 12 months of internal medicine and 12 months of anaesthesiology. The specific part of the training, lasting between 2.5 and 4 years, takes place in the intensive care unit. The British Intercollegiate Board for Training in Intensive Care Medicine (IBTICM) has defined a variable duration of the training programme. The factors related to programme duration are:

1. Progress made by any particular trainee
2. How much of the ICM programme is allowable for the programme in the speciality of primary appointment [6]

The trainee in intensive care will therefore, by completing the total programme, be acknowledged as a specialist in two areas (CCT = Certificate of Completion of Training), e.g. anaesthesiology and ICM. The duration of the ICM training programme varies between a minimum of 23 months and a maximum of 45 months. The IBTICM considers a total duration of 33 months as the most common duration. In many European countries and other countries linked to the ESICM, including the Netherlands and France, the duration of additional ICM training concurrently with or following a primary speciality is 24 months. However, it is of note that additional ICM training in certain countries can be as short as 3 months (Czech Republic and Spain). Most European and connected countries have a single training programme in ICM. Some countries have 2 or 3 different programmes, Germany topping the list with as many as 7 training programmes [4]. In Spain, the length of exclusively intensivist training is 60 months. The duration of the basic and advanced training programme in ICM in Australia and New Zealand is 72 months, according to the CICM [7].

The training institute

While everyone involved in ICM would agree that successful training in ICM could not be given at home, the standards for the institute where training takes place are not always obvious. And if these standards are defined, it is evident that they should be verified by an external visit, i.e. an audit. It is disappointing, however, to see that in many prominent – in terms of ICM – European countries such as France, Germany, Finland and Spain, according to a an international survey, this is not (yet) the case [4]. In countries like the UK,

Ireland, Italy, the Netherlands, Switzerland, and recently, Portugal, an external audit is part of the approval for training. The question arises which standards should be fulfilled. An important feature is sufficient exposure (where sufficient, again, is difficult to define precisely) to all patient groups. This means that in the training institute, patients with various diseases related to various specialities should be present, i.e. medical, surgery including traumatology, neurosurgery, neurology, and cardiac surgery. The volume of all these critically ill patients should be 'sufficient'. In the Netherlands it is defined that the ICU as a training institute should have at least 12 beds, with at least 3,000 days of mechanical ventilation and over 3,000 treatment days per year with admission of patients from all categories [8]. However, in Switzerland, for example, the minimum number of beds is 6 and 1,300 treatment days per year is considered sufficient for recognition as a (qualified) intensive care training institute, although in such an ICU where not all categories of patients are treated, the maximum time spent for training is 1 year, whereas trainees can spend the entire 3 years in an ICU where all categories of patients are treated [9]. Guidelines for the critical care environment in the USA have been described [10]. One could say that in terms of its structure and organisation the ICU should ideally be a 'role model' ICU for the trainees. Several requirements logically follow from this premise. A policy of quality assurance and control must exist, with an annual report and reporting on clinical performance, prevailing guidelines, continuous evaluation of medical performance with autopsy and complication conferences. An academic, evidence-based attitude exists in the entire department and participation in scientific research is the standard. Access to medical information must be outstanding. Consultation between medical and nurse staff on an executive level, daily bedside rounds with intensivists and nurses, and frequent, daily discussion between nurses and intensivists on patient care should all be arranged in a structured way. The equipment must be at the level of current standards. In terms of the medical and nursing team, it is required that sufficient qualified and dedicated staff is present '24/7' taking into account the number of patients. The director of the ICU is an intensivist. A system to keep family and patients well informed is mandatory for a good role model ICU, as well as an open and meticulous system to discuss end-of-life decisions. Apart from this 'hard' set of requirements, a very important characteristic must be present, although it is difficult to measure quantitatively: a good and warm climate for training. This is typically a feature that can only be identified by an external visit, an audit by peers. Therefore, we strongly believe that the training institution must be submitted to an audit to qualify as a training institute.

Training director

Although professional training of intensivists is teamwork, where the team includes all medical and nurse staff, the training director is the person responsible for the training programme. Commitment and competence are thus requirements. Therefore, the training programme director is a qualified intensivist with many years of experience, and is clinically active. The training director must have the skills, interest, authority and time to fulfil the role of instructor and training director. The instructor should be active in intensive care medicine on a national and international level and capable of conducting ICM-related research, substantiated by peer review publications. Importantly, as a physician the training director must perform well in all CanMEDS competencies. He or she should be a gifted and inspired teacher with high professional standards. The training director should also be submitted to an external audit, which can be done simultaneously with the audit of the intensive care training institute.

Presence of simulation centre with crisis resource management

Simulation provides safe and effective opportunities for learners at all levels to practice and acquire clinical skills needed for patient care. Simulation offers the possibility of standardisation and reproducibility. Therefore specific training can be done at any given moment, which is an advantage taking into account the reduced number of working and thus training hours of trainees. The intensive care environment is also

very suitable for virtual reality training. It is of note that not only relatively 'simple' skills like intubation, basic life support or chest drain insertion should be trained, but especially teamwork and communication during medical emergency situations (crisis resource management). Simulation is a powerful tool for the education of physicians and other healthcare workers at all levels. Although it cannot replace educational activities based on real patient care experiences, it is strongly believed that it significantly complements educational activities in ICM [11]. Those who think the evidence for the efficacy of simulation training, according to standard evidence-based medicine guidelines in terms of randomised trials, is insufficient, are referred to the simulation training of mechanics who train rapid tyre changes during Formula 1 races. In our view, access to simulation training should be considered a basic training requirement.

Additionally, training in conversation techniques, such as how to discuss end-of-life issues with patients and families, can be optimised with help from professional actors, thus creating an extra aspect of simulation training.

Portfolio and examination
During the training period regular (clinical) exams and mini clinical exams are taken. All interventions and results of the (mini) exams are recorded in the trainee's portfolio. The final examination is the European Diploma in Intensive Care, which contains both a written and clinical part.

Regulations
Regulations defining the course of the training, from entry until completion, must exist and be uniform. In general, the national intensive care society or other official body takes care of this.

Competencies of the intensivist

It is beyond the scope of this chapter to describe all competencies that trainees need to acquire to become good intensivists. Julian Bion and the international team he created developed, in a major effort and with the help of the European Society of Intensive Care Medicine (ESICM), definitions of "European" core competencies for intensive care: the CoBaTrICE Collaboration (Competency-Based Training programme in ICM for Europe [3]. Apart from the definition of competencies, the CoBaTrICE initiative has made teaching materials available on the web [12]. Training programmes from, among others, the UK, Australia and New Zealand, have described similar competencies. The reader is referred to recent publications on this subject [5–10, 13].

Conclusion

Minimal training requirements for ICU physicians are multifarious. It starts with the selection of the trainee. We cannot value sufficiently the importance to intensive care medicine as such to attract and keep young, talented people. These young, talented people will make the difference for intensive care medicine in the future with respect to achieving progress and improvement, for the sake of the patient. The demands for appropriate high-quality training involve a set of requirements for the training programme, the institute and equipment, the training director, and qualifications/competencies to be met by the trainee at the end of the programme. Most competencies are based on the CanMEDS set, with the addition of the CoBaTrICE set or, for example, the Australia/New Zealand set, Swiss or British set of well-defined competencies [5–7]. Although we are moving from a time-based apprenticeship to a competence-based apprenticeship, a minimal duration of training needs to be defined. Based on the empirical choices that have been made in several countries, it can be concluded that a minimal total postgraduate training time for an ICU physician/intensivist is between 5 and 6 years. In order to optimise the currently shorter duration of training, new educational technologies such as computer-based programmes and virtual reality simulation should be incorporated in the training programme of the 21st century.

The authors

Armand R.J. Girbes, MD, PhD[1]
Albertus Beishuizen, MD, PhD[2]
Jan G. Zijlstra, MD, PhD[3]
  [1]Professor in Intensive Care Medicine | Department of Intensive Care | University Hospital VU Medical Center | Amsterdam, The Netherlands
[2]Consultant in Intensive Care | Department of Intensive Care | University Hospital VU Medical Center | Amsterdam, The Netherlands
[3]Professor in Intensive Care Medicine | Department of Intensive Care | University Medical Center Groningen | Groningen, The Netherlands

Address for correspondence
Armand R.J. Girbes
Department of Intensive Care
University Hospital VU Medical Center
P.O. Box 7057
1007 MB Amsterdam, The Netherlands
E-mail: arj.girbes@vumc.nl

References

1. Stewart D. Medical training in the UK. Arch Dis Child 2003;88:655–658.
2. Howe A, Campion P, Searle J, Smith H. New perspectives-approaches to medical education at four new UK medical schools. BMJ 2004;329:327–332.
3. The CoBaTrICE Collaboration. Development of core competencies for an international training programme in intensive care medicine. Intensive Care Med 2006;32:1371–1383.
4. Barrett H, Bion JF. An international survey of training in adult intensive care medicine. Intensive Care Med 2005;31:553–561.
5. www.fmh.ch/files/pdf2/intensivmedizin_version_internet_f.pdf.
6. http://www.rcoa.ac.uk/ibticm/index.asp?InterPageID=62.
7. http://www.cicm.org.au/trainprogram.php.
8. www.cbo.nl/Downloads/111/rl_ic_2006.pdf.
9. www.sgi-ssmi.ch/fileadmin/user_upload/.../KAI_Reglement_071101_F.pdf.
10. Dorman T, Angood PB, Angus DC, Clemmer TP, Cohen NH et al. Guidelines for critical care medicine training and continuing medical eductaion. Crit Care Med 2004;32:263–273.
11. McGaghie WC, Siddall VJ, Mazmanian PE, Myers J. Lessons for continuing medical education from simulation research in undergraduate and graduate medical education. Chest 2009;135:62S–68S.
12. www.cobatrice.org.
13. Buckley JD, Addrizzo-Harris DJ, Clay AS, Curtis JR, Kotloff RM, Lorin SM et al. Multisociety task force recommendations of competencies in pulmonary and criticial care medicine. Am J Respir Crit Care Med 2009;180:290–295.

Ruth Endacott and Julie Scholes

Minimal training requirements for ICU nurses

Background

Why is it important to provide a minimum standard of education for ICU nurses? Specialist education is enshrined in the WHO definition of critical care nursing [1]: "The critical care nurse will have successfully completed specialist post-qualification education in critical care nursing, which builds upon initial generalist nursing education. This post-qualification education will allow the nurse to:

■ Meet the complex needs of critically ill patients
■ Achieve a well-developed knowledge base
■ Demonstrate specialist skills in both technological and caring dimensions
■ Develop the expertise to make sound and rapid clinical judgements
■ Recognize and deal with the ethical issues inherent in such an environment."

A minimum standard of education is important for a number of reasons:

1. Increase in standardisation across ICUs is a key element in the drive to improve patient safety [2]; standardised training is central to this process with studies demonstrating links between training and rates of adverse events [3, 4].

2. High rates of severe burnout syndrome have been reported in ICU nurses over past decades [5–8]. Strategies to reduce this include providing ongoing training.

3. There is evidence that education for ICU nurses varies across countries [9], hence it is important to set a minimal level of education and to provide ongoing training in order to maintain performance [10].

These drivers have been given added impetus in the wake of the H1N1 pandemic threat; the potential impact of this type of major event on ICUs is severe and preparations include retraining of nurses who have left the ICU and providing basic critical care training for ward nurses to provide a larger critical care nursing workforce [11]. This reinforces the need for training to be based in the local setting [10], removing the sense that it should be provided only in 'centres of excellence'. This shift would not only better prepare nurses for the real world in which they work but also integrate education and training into the local cultures such that it becomes the business of all clinicians, and improve the likelihood of smaller centres attracting and retaining a skilled ICU nursing workforce.

Education has been demonstrated to have an impact on patient outcomes, such as catheter-related bloodstream infections, across a range of settings [3, 4, 12]. Conversely, dissatisfaction with learning opportunities has also been linked to high nurse attrition rates [13].

Two levels of minimum training are described in this chapter: firstly, the minimum level required to allow the novice ICU nurse to provide safe and appropriate patient care within three months of commencing an ICU post and, secondly, the minimum level required for recognition as a specialist intensive care nurse. The World Health Organisation [1] suggests that such specialist education should commence after two years of ICU experience. The novice ICU nurse training may be provided as a concentrated block of education at the beginning of ICU employment or as a programme of training delivered part time over a longer period. Aside from the economic benefits, the latter approach also provides opportunities for learning at the bedside. The disadvantage is the temptation for the education programme to become lower priority when workload increases [14].

Developments in nursing practice

Increased co-morbidities and use of early intervention approaches to patient management [15] indicate the need for a differently trained nursing workforce. Two further developments in ICU nursing practice will have an impact on the minimal training required: firstly, the nature of interventions used and, secondly, the rapid decision-making required to ensure that patients receive timely care. To illustrate this point, the use of sedation in the ICU requires patients to be rousable rather than deeply sedated, requiring a different form of skilled nursing vigilance. In addition, the use of a nurse-implemented sedation protocol has been shown to decrease the rate of ventilator-acquired pneumonia (VAP) and the duration of mechanical ventilation in patients receiving mechanical ventilation and requiring sedative infusions with midazolam or propofol [16].

Care is frequently managed using care bundles (for example to prevent VAP, aid in weaning or prevent nosocomial infection). The care bundle approach aims to change the underpin-

ning philosophy of practice without dictating the precise nature of the intervention [17]. The bundling of interventions has been shown to be more effective than implementation of single interventions [18], particularly where multi-disciplinary teams are involved [19]. Many aspects of these bundles (for example, use of the 'head up' position and sedation holds in the VAP bundle) require implementation by nurses. To take another example, weaning from ventilation is now commonly started at higher FiO_2 [20]; this also has implications for nursing vigilance in coaching the patient and recognising weaning failure.

The increased emphasis on teamwork to deliver 'bundled' interventions has implications for novice and specialist training for ICU nurses. This is reflected both in the core standards required and learning environment, as discussed later in this chapter. Teamwork has also been demonstrated to reduce burnout; the quality of relationships between nurses and doctors has been found to influence levels of burnout in intensivists [21] and ICU nurses [8] whilst training in communication has been demonstrated to reduce burnout [22].

Differences in roles across countries

The scope of the ICU nurse role varies considerably across countries with differences in skills such as initiation of mask ventilation and cardiac massage, peripheral and arterial line insertion, pulmonary capillary wedge pressure measurements and weaning, use of physical and chemical restraint [23–25]. The involvement of nurses in end of life decision-making also varies significantly [26]. Further, whilst there may be international acceptance of the notion of critical care 'without walls' [27], this isn't necessary reflected in changes to practice, for example, nurse involvement in ICU outreach services. Alongside this variation in practice, comparison across 16 countries identified variation in access to specialist training [9, 23]. Perhaps not surprisingly, a number of papers have identified differences in ICU nurses' knowledge across countries [28–29].

A recent report on the global health workforce shortage [10] emphasised the need to not only grow the workforce in numbers but also ensure that clinicians have greater capacity to meet the needs of the population ('transformation of clinical capacity'). The potential impact of this for ICU nurses is a raising of the minimum standard of education in order to move towards an ICU nursing workforce able to, for example, implement care bundles. This also fits with the WHO goal that medical and nursing education should be set "in the context of the health system so that education, training, research and service delivery work in synergy not isolation" [10]. This raises the 'chicken and egg' conundrum of education and practice: Is the scope of nursing practice limited by the education provided or is education tailored to match nursing practice? No doubt the answer will vary from country to country; however, it is clear that the underlying message from the WHO reflects the latter goal.

Core skills for intensive care nurses

The expanding body of knowledge required for critical care practice means that determining what is 'essential' to inform core skills is contested. The WHO Europe Critical Care Nursing Competencies [1] (see Tab. 1) attempted to set these out. The list is comprehensive, based on the United Kingdom standards for specialist education [30] and delivered in seven modules, four of which addressed generic transferable skills. The emphasis was placed upon ensuring a minimum knowledge set with emphasis on competencies for life-long learning, capacity to effectively search the literature and critically appraise research evidence. In response to the WHO strategy, the European Federation of Critical Care Nursing Associations (EfCCNa) set out a position statement to endorse the importance of the critical care specialist training programme to 'equip nurses practically and theoretically to assume a growing number of responsibilities at specialist or advanced levels' so they might lead services based on protocols' [31]. Here we can see a tension emerge between the use of protocols to guide a repertoire of performance under prescribed conditions, often delegated by doctors [32] versus an aspiration that protocols might increase nursing autonomy and accountability [33]. The aspiration that these specialist programmes be delivered at master's or doctoral level indicates the complexity of knowledge for practice and a

determination to see specialist critical care nurses able to make discretionary judgments [31]. However, of note, these skills apply to the specialist, senior, advanced and consultant critical care practitioner [34]. Access onto these courses normally requires a minimum time of two years clinical experience in the field prior to undertaking the programme. This has resulted in intensive care units having to provide their own core skills framework to ensure fitness to practise as part of an induction programme for newly registered nurses. In response to this demand and the rising acuity of patient conditions in acute care, a specific branch of acute and critical care pre-registration nursing has been advocated [35]. However, increasingly registered nurses are supported by assistant practitioners and support workers, some of whom are entitled 'advanced'. Differentiating competencies and demarcating these for each level of practice further blurs what is core for whom, and at what depth this should be taught. Core skills can be divided between:

1. The operational aspects of practice e.g. admission and discharge, health and safety, legal and ethical issues
2. The core knowledge to inform practice, e.g. biopsychosocial sciences
3. Therapeutic aspects of care, e.g. technological support, care interventions, pharmacology, psychosocial support for patients and relatives
4. Effective team working (e.g. communication skills, inter-professional collaboration)

We suggest that these four areas of skill are central to practice both for novice and more experienced nurses. Programmes of education that are appropriate to the local policy, case-mix and skill-mix context, should be developed based on these four areas. Some aspects of these core skills lend themselves to the protocolised delegation of tasks to assistants and support workers, e.g. taking an arterial blood sample, or physiological recordings [36]. Thus we see the debates about delegation of medical tasks to nurses being replayed as qualified nurses delegate certain of their responsibilities to support workers [37].

Communication skills and team working are often promulgated as the core to effective working. Given the blurred boundaries stated above, this is not unsurprising. For example, many ICU errors are attributed to communication problems

Tab. 1   Critical Care Nurse Competencies [from WHO Europe Critical Care Nursing Curriculum. WHO European Strategy for Continuing Education for Nurses and Midwives 2003. Copenhagen, WHO Regional Office for Europe, 2003:7–8]

On completion of the course the critical care nurse will be competent to:
■ critically analyse theories relating to therapeutic communication suitable for use with an individual in crisis;
■ evaluate their own personal skills to identify their learning needs by reflecting upon the management of therapeutic communication with an individual in crisis;
■ appraise the physical, psychological, social and environmental issues that contribute to critical illness utilising appropriate epidemiological evidence;
■ examine current health promotion policies and their implications for critical care;
■ illustrate understanding of the physical, cognitive, emotional, behavioural and spiritual signs of burnout in a critical care setting;
■ assess the needs of patient and family regarding coping mechanisms in times of crisis;
■ complete nursing documentation accurately and in a timely fashion;
■ recognise signs of stress in self and others and promote the use of appropriate coping strategies;
■ apply the relevant communication skills to help the patient/family/multidisciplinary team mobilise effective coping strategies;
■ explore the potential consequences of the disease/condition with the patient and/or others with whom the patient wishes this to be discussed;
■ assess the health promotion needs of the critically ill patient and her/his family and/or carers;
■ appraise the diagnostic and monitoring requirements and management necessary to maintain homeostasis in the critically ill patient;
■ discuss the pharmacokinetics and pharmacodynamics of drugs used in the management of the critically ill patient utilising appropriate research based evidence;
■ explain the potential requirements and preparation of drug therapy for a critically ill patient;
■ assess the impact of multisystem disorders on the physiological condition of the critically ill patient;
■ interpret diagnostic/monitoring results and communicate their significance and possible consequences to relevant members of the multidisciplinary team;
■ illustrate safe and effective practice in the administration and disposal of drugs used in the care of the critically ill patient;
■ assess the effects of drug therapy and initiate action according to clinical unit protocol;
■ analyse management and leadership theories and demonstrate their application in professional practice;
■ analyse the concept of holism applied to critical care nursing;
■ reflect and critically evaluate their own practice in the application of an appropriate model of nursing;
■ analyse professional and legal issues in critical care and apply these to clinical practice;
■ apply knowledge of patient's rights in professional clinical practice;
■ apply knowledge of ethical theories and principles in the consideration of ethical dilemmas and their legal implications in clinical practice.

between nurses and doctors [38] and the root causes of adverse events are often interpersonal, especially communication-related [39–41]. This is significant as decreased professional collaboration is associated with higher moral distress in critical care nurses [42]; lack of recognition of one's own contribution by others, too much responsibility at times, making decisions alone were three stressors that could lead to stress and depression among intensivists [43].

As pressures increase for critical care practitioners to include societal threats such as pandemics, terrorism, changing climatic conditions, financial prudence in recession [44–46] that directly impact upon the surge capacity of critical care, practitioners are going to need additional personal resources to cope with these demands. The new and favoured personal capacity, is that of resilience.

Promulgated as the new strategy for emotion management in the workplace [47], resilience is seen as the way in which individuals can take responsibility for their own psychological and physical welfare and cope with the challenges of contemporary practice [48]. The notion of the resilient practitioner is not new and has been discussed in teaching and social work [49] and in counselling and psychotherapy [50]. Building upon and part of the positive psychology movement [51], the approach encourages individuals to maximise on their own resources and that of their immediate colleagues to recover, adapt and assimilate trauma [52]. The strategies advocated to enable people to foster resilience are set out in Table 2. The personal and professional sustaining activities assume that everyone has the autonomy, free will, independence and flexibility to adapt these strategies to their own situation. Of concern there is a risk that organisations need only take minimal responsibility for the emotions of their workers (at a level of risk management), and those who do not manage to exhibit resilience are somehow at fault, over-vulnerable or neurotic [47]. Therefore, although heralded as the new panacea, the strategies should be viewed with considerable caution and in due consideration of their limitations [52]. However, some of these interventions (see Tab. 2) might be useful along with other strategies to assist critical care practitioners to build effective teams and ensure effective communication.

Learning environment

In Europe it has been agreed that post-registration critical care education should be provided by

Tab. 2   Strategies for developing resilience

Sustaining the professional self	Sustaining the personal self
Engaging in meaningful work	Keep home fires burning
Focus on success and expertise	Nurturing the emotional self
Think long term (ideal and real)	Balance eating exercise rest and recreation
Develop plans toward the ideal	Time alone balanced with company
Actively seek to reduce organizational conflict – avoid the culture of blame	Self checks for signs of burn out
Build a professional 'greenhouse'	Collegiate checks for signs of burnout
Use the social capital of a Unit, (build trust, value reciprocity, and participation)	
Find points of commonality, use humour	
Know one's boundaries	
Articulate a problem	
Knowledge is power, help others	
Take strength in numbers	

the higher education sector or equivalent awarding body [31]. Emphasis is placed upon learning from practice with 50 % of any programme consisting of clinical learning opportunities [53]. Although a laudable philosophy, the level of supervision and mentorship provided by colleagues in clinical settings cannot be guaranteed, especially where the staffing ratio might prohibit direct supervision. As a consequence, there is a growing emphasis placed upon learning in skills laboratories and simulation environments where direct observation of performance can be assured. At the same time learners are encouraged to critically self-reflect to consciously gauge their own competence or incompetence. The portfolio as a tool to facilitate vigilant self-monitoring and record reflections of the students' learning journeys is advocated [31].

A number of approaches can optimise the likelihood of learning taking place from clinical practice. These include:

1. Making the learning 'real' by bringing contradictions from practice into the 'classroom' or through critical questioning in practice, illuminating new learning at the bedside
2. Using planned rather than serendipitous learning opportunities but also recognising potential learning experiences from everyday practice
3. Creating learning opportunities that create high intellectual interference (see examples in Fig. 1)
4. Using interprofessional team training [54] where feasible and appropriate
5. Using assessment as learning

Simulation is gaining in popularity as a proxy environment for clinical learning because:
- It is a useful in developing decision-making skills without risk to the patient [55]
- It is an environment that can provide 'amnesty' to address remedial error or discover omissions in the basic skill set and conversely it is an environment that can illuminate areas of good practice and build confidence [56]

However, the simulation environment also creates visibility, with personal attribution of er-

High intellectual interference

Higher order Q&A of 'hot' event	Direct observation with real time Q&A
	Nurse-led ward rounds
Reflective review of 'cool' event	
Student triggered teaching	
	Teaching reports
Amnesty: revisiting skills	
	Reviewing notes, x-rays, medications, observations

Classroom — *Bedside*

Unit based formal teaching sessions	
Assignments	Skills rehearsal
Book learning	
Student triggered Q&A	
	Working alone

Low intellectual interference

Fig. 1 Model to demonstrate learning opportunities in practice and the outcome on high or low intellectual interference [adapted from Scholes J, Endacott R. Evaluation of the effectiveness of educational preparation for critical care nursing London: English National Board for Nursing, Midwifery and Health Visiting, 2002]

ror that can lead to anxiety [57]; anxiety can also lead to diminished memory recall [58]. Poor performance can also be attributed to the lack of fidelity created by the simulated environment and unfamiliarity with the laboratory equipment. Despite these concerns, or indeed because of them, simulation has the potential to awaken discomforting contradiction, as the student discovers that what they thought they knew is faulty [59]. Careful facilitation and debriefing are essential to maximise experiential growth from these experiences [37]. Simulation scenarios drawn from real clinical problems with which the student is familiar increase the 'believability' in the case [54] and relevance for clinical practice. Simulation is also useful for training in teamwork [60] as well as skills in communication, cooperation and leadership [54]. However, it is suggested that the focus on non-technical skills should only come in when technical skills have been mastered, to reduce the cognitive load of having to learn technical and non-technical skills simultaneously [61].

Assessment reconsidered

Traditionally, summative assessment is undertaken to gauge whether learning has resulted from a training or educative intervention and is essential to ensure baseline competence. However, a more contemporary view is that assessment be considered a starting point to stimulate further learning [62], as ultimately this can transform performance [37]. Feedback from peers and supervisors is essential to inform goal-setting, critical self-reflection, and greater ownership of subsequent learning. As indicated earlier, portfolios are a favoured medium by which to collate feedback ranging from testimonials, assessment of competence, alongside critical self-reflective writing. Thus constructive criticism and feedback becomes something to embrace rather than fear because it informs professional development. This shift in thinking is essential as the dynamics of critical care practice demand reflexive practitioners capable of consciously monitoring their own competence.

Self-assessment can be assessment performed by a peer or colleague, if this has been actively pursued to gain appraisal to enhance perform-

ance. Assessment does not have to be limited to a single event under examination conditions, rather it can be generated within everyday encounters, exposing oneself to critical questioning and challenging discussion with peers. In this way learning is part of assessment and assessment part of learning. But not all questioning can create transformational learning. For example: The exploration of functional know-how to explore procedural knowledge by quizzing the student will not yield as much knowledge and insight as questions that seek an explanation of what and why something happened or the rationale behind clinical action. Further probing to explore hypothetical situations with increasing complexity increases the intellectual challenge of any question, while clinical anticipation represents the greatest intellectual challenge, demonstrating understanding of illness trajectories and clinical wisdom [63]. Importantly, this type of questioning takes place in practice and can often take the form of a purposeful professional dialogue that might not have been considered 'assessment'.

This type of shift in thinking about assessment and its possibility is important. We are increasingly seeing fewer of these types of conversations between students and their mentors. Therefore, assessment becomes an event, often artificial and discrete. Learning by working alongside an experienced colleague and having an ongoing dialogue about practice is rapidly becoming a dying art. We learn to question by being questioned, thus, with every generation of students under-exposed to this form of questioning we dilute the capacity to ask useful transformational questions.

This approach has another purpose. If we open ourselves to questions with the express purpose to learn from them (rather than consider ourselves assessed or confronted by them) it matters not who asks the question. Thus, we see learning potential in questions raised by patients and their families as much as those levelled by medical colleagues or other healthcare professionals. So who asks the questions is not as important as how the question is asked. This approach also helps us to reflect upon who should assess what, especially in critical care where competence is being assessed across a diverse range of activities, for example, to undertake delegated medical tasks through to non-technical skills.

It cuts through the debate as to whether nurses should assess nurses, or medical staff should assess delegated responsibilities. The reflective question is who is competent to ask competent questions that can ensure learning from assessment? It also ensures that we maintain the skill of open constructive professional debate to stimulate learning for generations of critical care practitioners to come. Assessment is no more a one-off stressful event, but part of professional self-monitoring and everyday reflexive learning from practice.

Conclusions

In this chapter we have outlined minimum standards of training and learning environment for novice and experienced ICU nurses, regardless of country. These standards apply to nurses managing critically ill patients in any location (for example obstetric unit, medical or surgical ward as well as ICU or HDU). However, in order to deliver the minimal training outlined in this chapter, there is a need to retain expert clinicians at the bedside to make the most of learning opportunities. Current trends in ICU practice, for example, increased emphasis on nursing interventions, suggest that training requirements will need to increase in the future, alongside greater empowerment for nurses in some countries [64].

The authors

Ruth Endacott, Prof.[1]
Julie Scholes, Prof.[2]
   [1]Professor of Critical Care Nursing | University of Plymouth UK and Monash University, Australia | Faculty of Health, Drake Circus, Plymouth
   [2]Professor of Nursing | University of Brighton | Centre for Nursing and Midwifery Research | Falmer, Brighton, UK

Address for correspondence
   Ruth Endacott
   Faculty of Health, Drake Circus
   Plymouth pl4 8AA, UK
   E-mail: ruth.endacott@plymouth.ac.uk

References

1. World Health Organisation. WHO Europe Critical Care Nursing Curriculum, 2003. Available at: www.euro.who.int/document/e81552.pdf.
2. Valentin A, Bion J. How safe is my intensive care unit? An overview of error causation and prevention. Curr Opinion Crit Care 2007; 13(6): 697–702.
3. Coopersmith CM, Zack JE, Ward MR, et al. The impact of bedside behavior on catheter-related bacteremia in the intensive care unit. Arch Surg 2004; 139:131–136.
4. Warren DK, Zack JE, Mayfield JL, et al. The effect of an education program on the incidence of central venous catheter-associated bloodstream infection in a medical ICU. Chest 2004; 126:1612–1618.
5. Soupious MA, Lawry K. Stress on personnel working in a critical care unit. Psychiatr Med 1987; 5: 187–98.
6. Sawatzky JA. Stress in critical care nurses: actual and perceived. Heart Lung 1996; 25: 409–17.
7. Chen SM, McMurray A. "Burnout" in intensive care nurses. J Nurs Res 2001; 9: 152–64.
8. Poncet MC, Toullic P, Papazian L, Kentish-Barnes N, Timsit JF, Pochard F et al. Burnout syndrome in critical care nursing staff. Am J Resp Crit Care Med 2007; 175: 698–704.
9. Baktoft B, Drigo E, Hohl M. A survey of critical care nursing education in Europe. Connect 2003; 2, 82–7.
10. World Health Organisation (WHO). Report on the WHO/PEPFAR planning meeting on scaling up nursing and medical education. Geneva 13–14 October 2009.
11. Department of Health. Critical Care Strategy: Managing the H1N1 flu pandemic. DH: London, September 2009. Available at: http://www.dh.gov.uk/prod_consum_dh/groups/dh_digitalassets/documents/digitalasset/dh_104973.pdf.
12. Coopersmith CM, Rebmann TL, Zack JE, et al. Effect of an education program on decreasing catheter-related bloodstream infections in the surgical intensive care unit. Crit Care Med 2002; 30:59–64.
13. Shields M, Ward M. Improving nurse retention in the National Health Service in England: the impact of job satisfaction on intentions to quit. J Health Econ 2001; 20: 677–701.
14. Endacott R, Scholes J, Freeman M, Cooper S. The reality of clinical learning in critical care settings: a practitioner:student gap? J Clin Nurs 2003; 12: 778–785.
15. Hasin Y, Danchin N, Filippatos GS, Hersa M, Janssens U, Leor J et al. Recommendations for the structure, organization, and operation of intensive cardiac care units. Eur Heart J 2005; 26:1676–1682.
16. Quenot JP, Ladoire S, Devouccoux F, Doise JM, Cailloid R, Cunin N et al. Effect of a nurse-implemented sedation protocol on the incidence of ventilator-associated pneumonia. Crit Care Med 2007; 35: 2031–36.

17. Haraden C. What is a bundle? http://www.ihi.org/IHI/ Topics/CriticalCare/IntensiveCare/ImprovementStories/ WhatIsaBundle.htm.

18. Cooke FJ, Holmes AH. The missing care bundle: antibiotic prescribing in hospitals. Int J Microb Agents 2007; 30:25–9.

19. Kollef M. SMART approaches for reducing nosocomial infections in the ICU. CHEST 2008; 134:447–56.

20. Adam S. Nursing and allied health professionals in ESICM: 25 years of limited progress. In: Kuhlen R, Moreno R, Ranieri M, Rhodes A (eds). 25 years of progress and innovations in intensive care medicine. (p359–368). Berlin: MWV, 2007.

21. Embriaco N, Azoulay E, Barrau K, Kentish N, Pochard F, Loundou A et al. High level of burnout in intensivists: prevalence and associated factors. Am J Respir Crit Care Med 2007; 175: 686–692.

22. Taormina RJ, Law CM. Approaches to preventing burnout: the effects of personal stress management and organizational socialization. J Nurs Manag 2000; 8: 89–99.

23. Depasse B, Pauwels D, Somers Y, Vincent J-L. A profile of European ICU nursing. Intens Care Med 1998; 24: 939–945.

24. Benbenishty J, DeKeyser Ganz F, Adam S. Differences in European critical care nursing practice: a pilot study. Intens Crit Care Nurs 2005; 21: 172–178.

25. Benbenishty J, Adam S. Physical restraint in European ICUs. Intens Care Med 2006; 32 (S1): S107.

26. Benbenishty J, Ganz FD, Lippert A, Bulow H-H, Wennberg E, Henderson B et al. Nurse involvement in end-of-life decision making: the ETHICUS study. Intens Care Med 2006; 32: 129–32.

27. Hillman K. Breaking the paradigm: the ICU without walls. In: Kuhlen R, Moreno R, Ranieri M, Rhodes A (eds). 25 years of progress and innovations in intensive care medicine. (p337–342). Berlin: MWV, 2007.

28. Labeau S, Vandijck D, Rello J, Adam S, Rosa A, Wenisch C et al. Evidence-based guidelines for the prevention of ventilator-associated pneumonia: results of a knowledge test among European intensive care nurses. J Hosp Inf 2009; 70: 180–185.

29. Labeau S, Vandijck D, Rello J, Adam S, Rosa A, Wenisch C et al. Centers for Disease Control and Prevention guidelines for preventing central venous catheter-related infection: Results of a knowledge test among 3405 European intensive care nurses. Crit Care Med 2009; 37: 320–323.

30. UKCC. Standards for specialist Education and Practice. London:UKCC, 1998.

31. European Federation of Critical Care Nursing Associations (EfCCNA). Position statement on post-registration critical care nursing education within Europe, 2004. Available at: www.efccna.org/downloads/ Position statement on education EfCCNa.pdf.

32. Lyon B. Getting back on track: nursing's autonomous scope of practice. Clin Nurse Spec. 2005;19(1):28–33.

33. Kingston ME, Krumberger JM, Peruzzi WT. Enhancing outcomes: guidelines, standards and protocols. AACN Clin Issues. 2000;11:363-374.

34. Department of Health and Skills for Health. The National Education and Competence Framework for Advanced Critical Care Practitioners. London, DH, 2008. Available at: http://www.dh.gov.uk/en/ Publicationsandstatistics/Publications/ PublicationsPolicyAndGuidance/DH_084011.

35. Scholes J, Freeman M, Gray M, Jasper M, Robinson D, Matthews Smith G, Miller C. Evaluation of Nurse Education Partnership. Final Report. 2004. Available at: www.brighton.ac.uk/inam/research/projects/ partnerships_report.pdf.

36. Sutton J, Valentine J, Rayment K. Staff views on the extended role of health care assistants in the critical care unit. Intens Crit Care Nurs 2004; 20, 249–256.

37. Scholes J. Developing Expertise in Critical Care Nursing Blackwell Publishing: Oxford, 2006.

38. Donchin Y, Gopher D, Olin M, Badihi Y, Biesky M, Sprung CL, Pizov R, Cotev S. A look into the nature and causes of human errors in the intensive care unit. Crit Care Med 1995; 23(2): 294–300.

39. Stein-Parbury J, Liaschenko J. Understanding collaboration between nurses and physicians as knowledge at work. Am J Crit Care 2007; 16: 470–7.

40. Pronovost PJ, Thompson DA, Holzmueller CG, Lubomski LH, Dorman T, Dickman F et al. Towards learning from patient safety reporting systems. J Crit Care 2006; 21:305–15

41. Williams R, Silverman R, Schwind C, Fortune JB, Sutyak J, Horvath KD et al. Surgeon information transfer and communication: factors affecting quality and efficiency ofinpatient care. Ann Surg 2007; 245: 159–71

42. Hamric AB, Blackhall LJ. Nurse-physician perspectives on the care of dying patients in intensive care units: collaboration, moral distress and ethical climate. Crit Care Med 2007; 35: 422–429

43. Coomber S, Todd C, Park G, Baxter P, Firth-Cozens J, Shore S. Stress in UK intensive care unit doctors. Br J Anaesth 2002; 89: 873–88.

44. Lawson R, Hawrylak M, Houghton S. Human Security for an Urban Century: Local Challenges, Global Perspectives. Netherlands: Springer, 2008.

45. Lyman B. Planning for surge capacity in HealthCare Services, Public Health Emergency Preparedness. California Department of Public Health 2009; Available at: www.healthyamericans.org/assets/files/ Lymanpresentation31909.ppt

46. Millard WB. With the Economy in the ICU, Pressure Increases on Emergency Departments. Ann Emerg Med 2009; 53: A19-A23.

47. Bolton S. Getting to the heart of the emotional labour process: a reply to Brovk. Work Employment and Society 2009; 23: 549–560.

48. Hodges L, Keeley A and Grier A. Professional resilience, career longevity and Parses Theory for Bacculaureate Education. Paper presented to Nursing Education Initiaitives: Sigma Theta Tau International 38th Biennial Conference, Indianapolis, US November 12–13, 2005.

49. Hendry LB. Survival in a marginal role: the professional identity of the physical education teacher Br J. Sociol. 1975; 26: 465–476.

50. Skovholt T M The resilient practitioner Burnout prevention and self care strategies for counsellors, therapists, teachers and health professionals. Allyn and Bacon: Boston, 2001.

51. Seligman M, Csikszentmihalyi M. Positive Psychology. An Introduction. American Psychologist 2000; 55: 5–14.

52. Scholes J. Coping with the professional identity crisis: is building resilience the answer? Guest Editorial. International Journal of Nursing Studies 2008; 45(2008) 975–978.

53. European Network of Nurses Organisations. Recommendations for a European Framework for Specialist Nursing Education. Paris, France: ENNO, 2000

54. Brattebo G. Training teamwork using simulation (pp93–101). In: Chiche J-D, Moreno R, Putensen C, Rhodes A (eds) Patient safety and quality of care in intensive care medicine. Berlin: MWV, 2009

55. McGaghie W, Issenberg S, Petrusa E, Sclese R. Effect of practice on standardised learning outcomes in simulation-based medical education. Medical Education 2006; 40: 792–97.

56. Kinsman L, Endacott R, Cooper S, Scholes J, Buykx P, McConnell-Henry T. Situational Awareness of Patient Deterioration in a Simulated Environment, Melbourne: Nurses Board of Victoria, 2009. Available at: http://www.nbv.org.au/web/guest/final-research-reports

57. Elstein AS, Bordage G. Psychology of Clinical Reasoning (p109–129) In: Dowie J, Elstein A. Professional Judgement: A reader in clinical decision making. Cambridge: Cambridge University Press, 1988.

58. Masters RSW. Knowledge, knerves and know-how: The role of explicit versus implicit knowledge in the breakdown of a complex motor skill under pressure. Br J Psych 1992; 83, 343–358.

59. Scholes J, Endacott R. Evaluation of the effectiveness of educational preparation for critical care nursing London: English National Board for Nursing, Midwifery and Health Visiting, 2002.

60. Sexton JB, Thomas EJ, Helmreich RL. Error, stress and teamwork in medicine and aviation: cross sectional surveys. BMJ 2000; 320:745–9

61. Reader T, Flin R, Lauche K, Cuthbertson BH. Nontechnical skills in the intensive care unit. Br J Anaesth 2006; 96:551–9

62. Cooper, D. Talk About Assessment: Strategies and Tools to Improve Learning. Toronto, ON: Thomson Nelson. Government of British Columbia, 2006.

63. Benner P, Hooper Kyriakidis P, Stannard D. Clinical Wisdom and Interventions in Critical Care: A Thinking-in-Action Approach. Philadelphia: Saunders, 1999.

64. Malloy DC, Hadjistavropoulos T, McCarthy EF, Evans RJ, Zakus DH, Park I, Lee Y, Williams J. Culture and organizational climate: nurses' insights into their relationship with physicians. Nurs Ethics 2009;16(6):719–733.

William E. Dager, Rob Shulman and Judith Jacobi

Preparation and training of critical care pharmacists

In many parts of the world, pharmacists have been utilized as an integral member of the critical care team. The system of training has evolved along parallel tracks in North America and the United Kingdom, and these serve as a model for training pharmacists elsewhere. This chapter will explore training considerations and preparation of pharmacists within varied practice settings.

Pharmacotherapy manager in the intensive care unit (ICU)

The critically ill patient frequently requires complex medication regimens where the potential exists for drug-drug and drug-disease related interactions. Co-morbid conditions and organ dysfunction require frequent reassessment of treatment regimens and constant adjustment to maintain the effectiveness of the therapy while avoiding adverse events. Baseline knowledge of optimal dosing may be limited as randomized, controlled trials used to determine the efficacy and optimal regimen of pharmacotherapeutic agents are not usually done in critically ill patients because of numerous confounding factors or their inability to provide informed consent. Other types of primary literature and case reports, along with extrapolation of data from other populations contribute useful knowledge to inform practitioners of potential treatments or risks. Pharmacists can focus on medication safety, since the risks associated with complex medication regimens are multiplied in critically ill patients. Clinicians who have the requisite background knowledge, skills and ability to focus on the pharmacotherapy component of patient management can offer valuable insights to individualized management plans to optimize patient outcome.

Literature supports the positive impact of the pharmacist in the critical care setting, describing improved clinical outcomes, and often with an associated financial benefit [1–4]. In response, health systems have created positions for pharmacists to meet demands for improved, cost effective and safe care. Common practice aspects are listed in Table 1.

Evolution and evidence supporting the pharmacist providing care in the ICU

In the United States (US), a shift in the type and scope of service provided by pharmacists began to occur in the mid-1960s. Instead of providing

Tab. 1 Examples of pharmacy services provided in critical care setting

Drug Information
Disease state management
Selective monitoring of a particular drug or drug class ■ Pharmacokinetic analysis of a drug regimen ■ Drug regimen management based on a measured pharmacodynamic response (i.e. anticoagulants)
Protocol or guideline development, implementation, and management
Admission and discharge medication history
Participation in patient rounds
Adverse medication reaction management
Cardiopulmonary resuscitation
Nutrition support

products to customers, their activities broadened to include patient-specific care with multi-professional interaction. Organizations such as the American Society of Health-System Pharmacists (ASHP) and the American Pharmacist Association (APhA) along with newer organizations including the American College of Clinical Pharmacy (ACCP) began to facilitate programs and legislative initiatives supporting the practice of "Clinical Pharmacy" and concepts such as "Pharmaceutical Care" [5].

Critical care pharmacist training

North America

Pharmacist training is incremental from the didactic and practical training in schools to formal experiential programs such as residencies to on-the job training and lifelong learning. Didactic training classes cover the basic sciences (anatomy, physiology, biology, microbiology, biochemistry, organic and physical chemistry) and applied sciences (pathophysiology, therapeutics). These courses do not need to be specific to pharmacy students, and joint training with other health-science students leads to important relationships that strengthen team concepts. Extensive instruc-

tion in pharmacognosy, pharmacodynamics, pharmacokinetics, and pharmacogenomics distinguishes pharmacists from many other healthcare providers. Pharmacists must also study business concepts, medication safety, communication, and team work. Students must be able to demonstrate competency with the core material to progress to the experiential phase of training. Interpretation and clinical application of knowledge is an essential skill for pharmacists to be successful. Students must demonstrate communication and problem-solving abilities. In the experiential phase of training, pharmacy students improve their teamwork skills and ability to direct the pharmacotherapy of individual patients or groups of patients. North American colleges of pharmacy award the Doctor of Pharmacy (Pharm.D.) degree after a total of 6 years of training (2 years pre-pharmacy and 4 years pharmacy training).

After school, pharmacists must pass an examination to obtain licensure to practice as a pharmacist, but additional training and certification often follows. Many pharmacists seeking hospital practice in the North American will receive training in general pharmacy practice areas in the post graduate year-1 (PGY1) and may focus on specialty areas in PGY2. These training programs are not required for practice, although a future training model may require residency preparation prior to hospital practice [6]. Advanced training programs or residencies, although in existence in the US since the 1930s evolved and expanded, with a full accreditation process put into place in 1962 by ASHP. Residency accreditation by ASHP is now provided in 15 subspecialties including critical care pharmacy, which is typically a PGY2 training program. At least 79 accredited post graduate year 2 critical care residency programs exist in North America. The accreditation process involves demonstration that the pharmacy department meets a high level of practice standard and the training program is well organized to enable the resident to meet the training goals and objectives [7]. At completion, the resident should be competent to practice at a level comparable to an experience practitioner.

The progressive expansion of education requirements and options were the result of a shift in pharmacy practice and increased demand for pharmacist services. Advancements in medical care and the related complexities, including the number of drugs choices and the creation of specialty practice environments within hospitals have increased the demand for specialists to provide efficient and optimal care. The concept of a multidisciplinary practice teams that includes pharmacists is rapidly becoming the standard instead of the exception [8]. For the critically ill patient, where the rapid delivery of optimal pharmacotherapy is vital, the need for pharmacist services is clear. Organizations such as the Society of Critical Care Medicine (SCCM), recognized pharmacists as a key member of the multi-professional management team along with other disciplines such as nurses and respiratory therapists [9]. The model for intensive care unit services and personnel was categorized into three levels (fundamental, desirable, and optimal) depending on available resources, and also described the key pharmacy services and personnel, with an emphasis on matching personnel to patient needs [10].

United Kingdom (UK)

The educational prerequisite for a pharmacy career in the United Kingdom is a four-year Master of Pharmacy degree. The coursework similarly covers a wide range of sciences, such as medicinal chemistry, pharmacognosy, pharmacology, biochemistry, pharmaceutics and pharmacy practice. This is followed by a one-year pre-registration training program for clinical experience. A registration exam is required for practice. The experiences within the National Health Service (NHS) are similar to North America, where a team approach is advocated. The basic-grade pharmacist experiences all aspects of pharmacy services for 1–2 years. Promotion to specialty practice can follow, with additional training and experience.

ICU pharmacist scope of practice

Pharmacy services must at least be basic/fundamental – ensuring prompt availability of drugs to patients – but at the same time should expand to more patient-specific/optimal models where pharmacists evaluate drug therapy needs and facilitate the design and achievement of complex drug regimens in areas with higher patient acuity.

North America

In 2000, ACCP and SCCM published an opinion paper defining the scope of critical care pharmacy services [11]. Three areas of pharmacy services were defined including fundamental, desirable and optimal (see Tab. 2). *Fundamental* activities involve the provision of basic services necessary for the safe provision of pharmacotherapy. This includes procuring, processing and distribution of the requested pharmacological regimen. Advanced pharmacy training is not essential for this role, although experience with and knowledge of the types of therapy used in critically ill patients is important to facilitate effective identification of drug therapy problems. *Desirable* activities describe the provision of more specialized, patient-focused functions necessary for the safe use of prescribed agents, including multidisciplinary rounds, medication history, education, and protocol development. *Optimal* activities reflect a more advanced practice model, where the pharmacist is fully integrated in to the multidisciplinary team, has specialized roles in research and education, and is dedicated or responsible for specific functions to maximize outcomes. The need for continuous patient care will typically require a team of pharmacy practitioners providing multiple levels of service that reflect the needs of the multi-professional team. An evaluation of the achievement of this practice model was done via survey [12]. A low response rate alters the ability to generalize the data but for those that responded, the majority of hospitals provided electronic medication records with allergy and drug interaction screening capabilities, and access to laboratory results with the pharmacy system. Pharmacists routinely provided drug information, intravenous compatibility information, prospectively evaluated medication orders and drug therapy, and intervened to improve care. Pharmacists also routinely provided education to other health professionals and pharmacy students and participated in drug-therapy related committees.

Tab. 2   Three levels of pharmacist activities [with kind permission from Springer Science + Business Media: Intensive Care Medicine, The impact of critical care pharmacists on enhancing patient outcomes, 29, 2003, p. 696, Kane SL, Weber RJ, Dasta JF]

Activity	Definition [a]	Description
Fundamental	A pharmacist dedicated to critical care services whose activities are vital to the safe provision of pharmaceutical care	■ Evaluates patient drug regimens based on the pharmaceutical care model and assesses their efficacy ■ Provides nutritional care ■ Prevents and documents ADEs and medication errors ■ Provides written communication of recommendations ■ Monitors pharmacokinetics ■ Provides drug information ■ Educates other healthcare professionals ■ Participates in reports for accrediting agencies, institutional committees, and programs
Desirable	In addition to fundamental activities, includes more specialized critical care pharmacotherapeutic services	■ Participates in patient care rounds ■ Maintains knowledge of primary literature ■ Reviews medication history ■ Educates through didactic/ experiential teaching ■ Aids in preparing protocols and critical care pathways ■ Contributes to research and medical writing
Optimal	In addition to fundamental and desirable activities, includes an integrated, specialized, and dedicated model of critical care which aims to optimize pharmacotherapeutic outcomes through the highest level of teaching, research and pharmacotherapy practices	■ Facilitates patient/ family discussions about treatment ■ Provides accredited educational sessions ■ Reports results of his/her independently initiated/collaborated clinical, pharmacoeconomic, and outcomes research to the medical community through lectures and publications ■ Develops post-doctoral training programs

[a]   It is not expected that these activities are performed on a daily basis to every patient

National health service pharmacists

In the UK, The Pharmacy Advanced And Consultant Level Framework (ACLF) was developed to describe and support the skills required for advanced levels of practice up to and including NHS Consultant level working [13]. The ACLF consists of 34 behavioural competencies consolidated into six clusters namely: expert professional practice, building working relationships, leadership, management, education, training and development and research and evaluation.

The ACLF is organized so that clinical pharmacists are able to locate their current level of practice classification in terms of 'foundation', 'excellence' and 'mastery' and each cluster has descriptions of attainment relating to these clusters. Typically a rotational clinical pharmacist practices at the 'foundation' level in the dispensary, the manufacturing unit, medicines information, and general and specialist wards. An advanced practitioner meets the definition of 'excellence' level and a consultant pharmacist practice meets the definition of a 'mastery' level of practice. The concept of the NHS 'consultant pharmacist' was developed in England in 2005 to provide access to recognizable, high quality care for patients, to achieve strategic engagement of pharmacy in specialist care, to create the opportunity for a new kind of relationship with higher education and to promote a form of expert practice unconstrained by traditional boundaries of institution [14]. Typically, consultant pharmacists spend 50 % of their time in direct clinical care.

Within critical care the generic competencies have been refined to be more specifically applicable to a critical care pharmacist with the document New Ways of Working – Adult Critical Care Specialist Pharmacy Practice [15]. Here there is a clear description of what activities a critical care pharmacist should be involved with at various levels of practice. It provides two important functions, firstly to map one's level of practice, and secondly to view practical examples of how to progress to the next level or to overcome weaknesses.

Critical care disease-state knowledge

The requisite knowledge of a critical care practitioner has been outlined in both North America and the UK. North American critical care pharmacist residency training standards define the goals, outcomes, objectives, skills, and disease knowledge areas required for practice [6]. Trainees will not be exposed to patients with all potential disease-related problems, and this document outlines topics for additional reading and discussion. In addition, specialty practice areas may require additional education, either formal or self-directed for competent practice. Completion of formal critical care residency training at a site accredited by the ASHP is accompanied by the awarding of a certificate of completion.

In the UK, critical care knowledge areas are partially defined in New Ways of Working – Adult Critical Care Specialist Pharmacy Practice [15]. This was further expanded in the Critical Care Syllabus Foundation and Excellence Level written by the UK Clinical Pharmacist Association (UK-CPA) Critical Care Group [16]. Here knowledge is defined as what should be known at 'foundation' and 'excellence' levels and furthermore what knowledge is unique to critical care 'specialist'

and 'core' knowledge areas that generalist and other specialty pharmacists should also know. The curriculum has been classified in a body function systems approach and a small section is included in Table 3. Armed with a competencies and knowledge, practitioners have a 'roadmap' to self-improvement, and this critical care core curriculum describes the "Expert professional practice" cluster of the ACLF.

Universally, a successful critical care pharmacist must be able to incorporate specific therapeutics with disease and diagnostic knowledge to meet the needs of a complex patient. Many sources of this information have been published, in addition to information available in pharmacotherapy textbooks [17–20]. The critical care clinician must also have the ability to create innovative solutions when necessary and relay the necessary information to other providers in a concise manner. To create and deliver such solutions, the provider needs to have an understanding of the "big picture" so that their contribution fits the overall needs of the patient. Pharmacists should take caution with less-integrated, focused management approaches where only one aspect of drug therapy is considered. For example, the dose of a drug may be correctly adjusted using serum concentrations, but it may also be the incorrect agent or interact to neutralize the effects of separate, more critical agents. Thus, training should provide a focus on understanding the big picture, an understanding of what other clinicians are doing, what is involved in invasive procedures, and how it can impact subsequent management approaches.

The pharmacotherapy specialist should understand how diagnostic studies are done including the benefits and downfall of the information. Examples include an understanding of how the pharmacotherapy plan should be modified for heart failure using an ejection fraction as a guide to cardiac output and reduction in drug clearance, knowing how end-diastolic volume is a component of that cardiac output, and how positive pressure ventilation can further influence those parameters. Medications may be used in the operating room that continue to influence patient responses post operatively. After coronary bypass graft surgery, hypertensive urgencies may require some adaption secondary to issues in the surgical site. Heparin that was administered may

Tab. 3   Example of a section of the UKCPA Critical Care Syllabus Foundation and Excellence [16]

Understands and applies methods of sedation management	Specialist (S) or Core (C)	Foundation (F) Excellence (E)
Knows the differences between classes of commonly used sedative agents used in the management of a level 2 (or below) patient	C	F
Knows the differences between classes of commonly used sedative agents used in the management of a level 3 patient	S	F
Knows the basic pharmacology and pharmacokinetics of sedative agents in a level 2 (or below) patient	C	F
Can describe the basic pharmacology and pharmacokinetics of sedative agents in a level 3 patient	S	F
Know the common uses of sedative agents in critically ill patients	S	F
Can describe the key monitoring parameters for the use of sedative agents in a level 2 (or below) patient	C	F
Can describe the key monitoring parameters for the use of sedative agents in a level 3 patient	S	F
Can provide details of national or international guidelines that include the use of sedative agents in a level 3 patient	S	F
Knows the differences between a broad range of sedative agents used in critically ill patients	S	E
Knows the pharmacology and pharmacokinetics of a broad range of sedative agents used in critically ill patients	S	E
Know the different uses of a broad range of sedative agents	S	E
Can describe and critique different monitoring parameters for the use of sedative agents in critically ill patients	S	E
Can outline the evidence base around current concepts and debates in sedation	S	E

rebound and re-establish anticoagulation and bleeding after the administration of protamine. Cardiac output may be transiently diminished post operatively, gradually recovering over several days. Response to drug therapy during this time may occur at lower doses, but as organ systems recover, lead to diminished responses. The clinician who understands this, and adjusts the dosing regimen in anticipation of the patient's needs instead of reacting to situations later will be more capable of meeting the overall care needs. Other examples include being able to weigh whether an observation is related to a drug, or some other factor such as differentiating when thrombocytopenia is secondary to a drug or related to margination on endovascular grafts or balloon pump access.

Credentialing

North America

To demonstrate broad knowledge of pharmacotherapy, a certification exam is also an option after 3 years of practice experience or completion of a residency. The Board of Pharmaceutical Specialties (BPS) was created in 1976 with a goal to "improve health through recognition and promotion of specialized training, knowledge, and skills in pharmacy, and board certification of pharmacists". Pharmacists who are Board Certified in Pharmacotherapy (BCPS) have passed a written examination of knowledge in disease-states, pharmacotherapy, and literature evaluation [21]. The exam is offered once a year, and administered in multiple nations. Board certification is for 7 years, at which time the exam can be re-taken, or a rigorous education program completed. Additional certification programs, such as diabetes or anticoagulation management, are also available to pharmacists, although current training areas are focused on outpatient management of chronic diseases. Maintenance of certification requires completion of continuing education modules and testing. There is no specific credentialing process for critical care practitioners beyond the BCPS process.

United Kingdom

The first steps taken in the UK were to identify a method to assess critical care pharmacists. A pilot documentation has been undertaken [22] which it is hoped will be replicated nationally and internationally within critical care and in other areas of pharmacy practice. The process is intentionally generic and tests against the competencies and the knowledge syllabus previously described [15, 16]. Components of the evaluation include development of practice portfolios, observational assessment, peer review, performance on case-based discussion and patient interactions.

Practice portfolios are collections of representative documents, intended to illustrate the variety and depth of activities performed throughout an individual's professional career. It was deemed essential that the portfolio provide evidence of the candidate's *level* of practice, and be directly mapped onto the ACLF matrix of competencies (see Tab. 4) [15]. A *viva voce* evaluates the practice portfolio in order to explore, to corroborate or to refute the presented evidence

therein, and to help establish the true level of capability of the candidate.

Observation of practice is another component of the certification. Observation provides real-time evidence of the candidates approach, attitude and application of in-practice competencies. It allowed an accurate view to be formed of the candidates "hands-on" competencies as compared with predominantly document-led work presented in the practice portfolio. Pharmacists are members of multidisciplinary teams (MDT), and much of the work a candidate undertakes is within the MDT. A broader viewpoint on the candidate's usual performance is obtained from a multi-professional perspective by asking other workplace colleagues to locate the candidate across all six competency domains [23, 24].

Case-based discussions (CbD) are designed to assess clinical decision-making and the application or use of relevant knowledge in the care of patients appropriate to the candidate's own clinical speciality. The candidate has time to prepare for the evaluation prior to it, and the main focus of the evaluation is the candidate's prioritisation and proposed management of pharmaceutical issues uncovered in the preparation time. A mini-clinical evaluation exercise (CEX) was originally developed in the US by the American Board of Internal Medicine. Under the Modernising Medical Careers structure, junior doctors use the mini-CEX (and case-based discussions) to evaluate their practitioner/patient interactions, and specifically to evaluate skills, attitudes and behaviours of the practitioner in question. These are also used in pharmacist evaluation. The clinical assessments are hosted at a reference site in order to support consistency and to make the assessment process more cost-efficient.

Tab. 4   Practice portfolio components

1. An executive summary and overview allowing quick reference of portfolio contents

2. Details of the candidate's practice role, including a *curriculum vitae,* current job description, job plan and organogram for the candidate's post, together with an illustrative outline of the critical care pharmacy service

3. A self-assessment using the ACLF-style matrix [14].

4. A range of documents put forward as evidence by the candidate to be illustrative of their level of practice (breadth, scope and complexity) to support the self assessment in point 3 here.

5. Other evidence or reports of formal peer reviews conducted by appropriate evaluators.

The review panel considers each candidate and assigns a location for each of the 6 competency clusters of the ACLF as determined by each method (patient based assessment, wider peer assessment and portfolio/*viva voce* examination). An overall "practice level location" matched to the ACLF criteria (foundation, excellence or mastery) is assigned for each of the 6 main clusters by the panel, who also notes particular points of commendation, developmental needs and any other professional development issues required for the purposes of feedback. The panel gives feedback on the credentialing process against the evaluation criteria, including a timeline for re-application for evaluation if the panel decided that this would be in the candidate's best interest for continued development.

Mentoring

New practitioners in critical care may benefit from a relationship with a more experienced mentor [25, 26]. These individuals may practice in other sites, and networking in professional organizations assists with the development of relationships. Mentors may also come from various disciplines including physicians and nurses. They may be co-workers, established experts for a given discipline, other critical care practitioners or non-critical critical care related personal. Identifying and developing mentors is vital to the success of a training experience. A mentor should have a grasp of what the critical care pharmacist needs, and provide the necessary input. Such mentors should be allowed time and flexibility to successfully provide the necessary mentoring. Successful mentors can provide creative approaches that adapt to each mentee's strengths and weaknesses to achieve training goals. To accomplish this, programs which train mentors should be developed. A mentor should provide guidance in handling daily challenges in the critical care setting including development of necessary skills, problem solving, making judgment decisions, approaches to positive interactions and effective communication with other ICU practitioners, time management and task prioritizations of tasks. Mentees should consider the importance of supporting their mentors to free up their time to provide the education sought.

Specialty practice

Unique populations of critical care patients are typically clustered in specialized units. These populations demand additional education and training by pharmacists to understand the use of specialized medications or treatments that are specific to that population. Various age groups (e.g. neonates, paediatric, geriatrics), transplant patients, other immunodeficient patients and organ-system disruption (e.g. burns, neurologic injury, cardiovascular disease) all require additional expertise, beyond the basic critical care knowledge. Specialized settings such as the emergency department or the operating room also require specialized knowledge and skills. Pharmacists will continue to expand practice into these and other areas as the need for economical and efficient drug therapy expertise grows. Professional development programs will need to expand to meet these needs.

Description of the scope of practice will need to expand along with these changing practice models. The challenge remains to advance practices worldwide with consideration of existing levels of practice. National and international organizations can facilitate and motivate practitioners to create change.

Application in other settings

The UK and North American perspective on critical care pharmacist assessment distinguishes between the individual critical care pharmacist's competence and knowledge and the pharmacy service that is delivered to the critical care unit. In any setting, a very competent ICU pharmacist who has insufficient time available relative to the size of the unit will not be able to deliver higher level activities. In England, the department of health defined national guidelines of requirement for critical care pharmacists in 2003. They stated that a specialist critical care pharmacist should be an integral part of the critical care team and that units should fund at least 0.1 specialist clinical pharmacist per ITU bed or per two HDU beds [27]. The additional time commitment needed for the new requirements for medicine reconciliation across the interfaces of care and other new programs may require reassessment of staffing ratios [28]. The next phases of work will be to roll-out the credentialing process. This will be followed by the development of a strategy for ICU pharmacists to meet the competencies and knowledge that has been defined. Finally, a tool which is suitable for peer review of the critical care pharmacy service rather than the individual pharmacist, and which can establish national standards will need to be developed.

Some European countries have less well-established, routine presence of clinical pharmacists attached to medical specialties in general. Resources and laws allowing expanded practice may also be limiting factors. In these settings, the pharmacist has a more limited role with a focus on the supply function. These countries need to embark on a process of development of their clinical pharmacists and to fully integrate them into critical care multidisciplinary team, so that the teams can benefit from the unique contribution that a specialized, experienced pharmacist can make. New programs can utilize existing practice standards and models. Training sites will need to be developed, and interested practitioners should be encouraged to seek experience and mentorship at established sites. Many pharmacists around the world have taken advantage of this format, and effectively raised practice standards within their home countries. There is a need for closer international collaboration between pharmacists from countries with more developed roles, in order to support colleagues wishing to develop their own roles.

The authors

William E. Dager, Pharm.D.,
    BCPS, FCSHP, FCCP, FCCM, FASHP[1]
Rob Shulman, BscPharm (Hons),
    MRPharmS, DHC(Pharm)[2]
Judith Jacobi, Pharm.D., BCPS, FCCM, FCCP[3]
    [1] Pharmacist Specialist | University
    of California | Davis Medical Center |
    California, USA
    [2] Lead Pharmacist | Critical Care |
    University College Hospitals NHS
    Foundation Trust | London, UK
    [3] Pharmacist Specialist | Critical Care |
    Methodist Hospital | Indianapolis, IN, USA

Address for correspondence
Judith Jacobi
Critical Care Pharmacist
Methodist Hospital
1701 N. Senate Blvd.
Indianapolis, IN, 46052 USA
E-mail: jjacobi@clarian.org

References

1. Kopp BJ, Mrsan M, Erstad BL, Duby JJ. Cost implications of and potential adverse events prevented by interventions of a critical care pharmacist. Am J Health-Syst Pharm 2007;64:2483–7.
2. Leape LL, Cullen DJ, Clapp MD, et al. Pharmacist participation on physician rounds and adverse drug events in the intensive care unit. JAMA 1999;282:267–270.
3. McLaren R, Bond CA: Effects of pharmacist participation in intensive care units on clinical and economic outcomes of critically ill patients with thromboembolic or infarction-related events. Pharmacotherapy 2009;29:761–768.
4. McLaren R, Bond CA, Martin SJ, Fike D. Clinical and economic outcomes of involving pharmacists in the direct care of critically ill patients with infections. Crit Care Med 2008; 36:3184–89.
5. Hepler CD, Strand LM. Opportunities and responsibilities in pharmaceutical care. Am J Hosp Pharm 1990;47:533–543.
6. Murphy JE, Nappi JM, Bosso JA, et al. American College of Clinical Pharmacy's 1 vision of the future: postgraduate pharmacy residency training as a prerequisite for direct patient care practice. Pharmacotherapy 2006;26:722–33.
7. http://www.ashp.org/s_ashp/docs/files/accreditation/RTP_ObjCriticalCare032608.doc, accessed 5/1/2010.
8. Horn E, Jacobi J. The critical care clinical pharmacist: Evolution of an essential team member. Crit Care Med 2006;34:S46-S51.
9. Brilli RJ, Spevitz A, Branson RD, et al. Critical care delivery in the intensive care unit: Defining clinical roles and the best practice model. Crit Care Med 2001;29:2007–2019.
10. Haupt MT, Bekes CE, Brilli RJ, et al. Guidelines on critical care services and personnel: Recommendations based on a system of categorization of three levels of care. Crit Care Med 2003;31:2677–2683.
11. Rudis MI, Brandl KM, et al. Position paper on critical care pharmacy services. Crit Care Med 2000;28:3746–3750.
12. McLaren R, Devlin JW, Martin S, et al. Critical care pharmacy services in United States hospitals. Ann Pharmacother 2006;40:612–8.
13. Advanced to Consultant level Framework. CoDEG (Competency Development and Evaluation Group) 2009

[accessed 09 04 10]; Available from: URL:http://www.codeg.org/fileadmin/codeg/pdf/ACLF.pdf.

14. Barnett N. 'Consultant pharmacist' – what does it mean? Hospital Pharmacist 2008;15:34.

15. Young K., Farrell J., McKenzie C., Tomlin M., Borthwick M., Forrest R. et al. New Ways of Working – Adult Critical Care Specialist Pharmacy Practice. Department of Health and United Kingdom Clinical Pharmacy Association 2005 [accessed 20 01 10]; Available from: URL: http://www.dh.gov.uk/en/Publicationsandstatistics/Publications/PublicationsPolicyAndGuidance/DH_4113862.

16. Shulman R, Offord R, Thacker M, Whelan G. Critical Care Syllabus Foundation and Excellence Level UKCPA Critical Care Group. UKCPA 2009 [accessed 20 01 10]; Available from: URL:http://www.ukcpa.org/docs/Critical%20Care%20Syllabus%202009.pdf.

17. Erstad BL. A primer on critical care pharmacy services. Ann Pharmacother 2008;42:1871–81.

18. Erstad BL, Jordan CJ, Thomas MC. Key articles and guidelines relative to intensive care unit pharmacology. Pharmacotherapy 2002;22:1594–610.

19. Erstad BL, Martin SJ, Brophy GM, et al. Key articles and guidelines relative to intensive care unit pharmacology — 2004. Pharmacotherapy 2005;25:585–610.

20. Erstad BL, Brophy GM, Martin SJ, et al. Key articles and guidelines relative to ntensive care unit pharmacotherapy: 2009 update. Pharmacotherapy 2009;29:1228–8 69.

21. http://www.bpsweb.org/specialties/pharmacotherapy.cfm, accessed May 1, 2010.

22. Borthwick M., Thacker M, Shulman R, Offord R, Thacker M, McRobbie D et al. Developing a Credentialing Process using Multi-source evaluation tools for Advanced Level Practice. Pharmaceutical Journal (submitted) 2010.

23. Patel J, West D, Bates IP, Eggleton A, Davies G. Early experiences of the mini-PAT (Peer Assessment Tool) amongst hospital pharmacists in South East London. International Journal of Pharmacy Practice 2009; 17:123–126.

24. Patel J, Sharma A, West D, Bates IP, Davies JG, Abdel-Tawab R. Is there a place for the mini Peer Assessment Tool (PAT) among general level pharmacists working in secondary care? Clinical Pharmacist 2009;1(S1).

25. Haines ST. The mentor-protégé relationship. Am J Pharm Ed 2003;67:82–4.

26. Sauer KA, Hepfinger CA, Wilhardt MS, Sahni S, Weber EW, Koontz R. Pharmacy research mentoring. Am J Health-Syst Pharm 2004 Dec 1;61:2552–6.

27. Critical Care Programme MC. Allied health professional and healthcare Scientists Critical care Staffing Guidance Intensive Care Society Standards Committee. 2003.

28. National Institute for Health and Clinical Excellence and National Patient Safety Agency. Technical patient safety solutions for medicines reconciliation on admission of adults to hospital. 2008.

Paolo Biban

Requirements and standards
for treating children in intensive care units (ICUs)

Introduction

In the last two decades, paediatric intensive care has become a particularly specialised area, transcending the boundaries of paediatric anaesthesia, paediatric medicine, critical care and emergency medicine. It has progressively developed into a sub-specialty in its own right, not simply as an extension of paediatric anaesthesia or a scaled-down version of adult intensive care [1–4].

Paediatric intensive care may be defined as care for medically unstable or critically ill children mostly requiring constant monitoring, nursing, continual respiratory support, complex surgical procedures, or other complicated intensive interventions. In general, paediatric intensive care units (PICUs) deliver intensive care to children up to adolescence, whilst intensive care of newborn and premature babies is usually conducted by neonatologists in the neonatal ICU. In some centres, however, newborns requiring paediatric surgery or cardiac surgery are routinely cared for in the paediatric intensive care unit in the postoperative phase [5]. Some national health authorities and hospitals have policies of delivering children's services up to the age of 18 years, whereas others assume that 14- and 16-year-olds are already adults. In the older age range, some adolescents may feel out of place in a PICU, which often admits predominantly very young children, while others feel out of place in an adult ICU, which may contain a large number of elderly patients [5]. Thus, sensitivity to their particular emotional, educational and family needs is required.

Although there are commonalities in the care given to critically ill children and adults, several aspects do distinguish paediatric from adult critical care. Indeed, children have special health needs because they are physically and emotionally different from adults and they need constant care and support from their parents. Furthermore, the relative immaturity may affect their physiological, anatomical, functional, developmental and psychological status, creating greater vulnerability to various adverse influences. Critically ill children admitted to PICUs represent an extremely heterogeneous patient population, showing a highly varied range of illnesses and continually changing pathophysiology, from infancy to adolescence. Among PICU patients, children with profound disabilities constitute a special category of patients, where the expectations of families are changing dramatically [6]. Indeed, therapeutic options are increasingly offered for extending the duration of life for children suffering from conditions that will ultimately be fatal. For instance, children with neuromuscular disorders and chronic respiratory disease are often provided with non-invasive or invasive respiratory support. However, the financial burden of carers and equipment for "technology-dependent children" is quite relevant. In fact, many of these children will have multiple admissions to intensive care prior to being established in a home ventilation programme. Many will require prolonged intensive care as a result of pulmonary infection, aspiration and episodes of acute on chronic respiratory failure. Children with severe cerebral palsy, gross neuro-developmental delay, intractable seizures and severe scoliosis are often admitted to paediatric intensive care either as a result of acute episodes or following surgical procedures, such as gastrostomy or orthopaedic surgery [6].

These and other rare life threatening illnesses, which are peculiar for the paediatric age, underline that clinical experience may play an important role in assuring good quality of care and determining a better outcome.

Indeed, many deaths can be prevented with optimal specialized paediatric care [7]. Mortality of paediatric patients with respiratory failure or head injury is lower in hospitals that provide tertiary-level paediatric intensive care than in those which do not [8]. Apparently, the difference in mortality increases as the severity of illness or injury increases [8]. Furthermore, the presence of a paediatric critical care specialist supervising care leads to lower severity-adjusted mortality for illness and injury in PICUs [9, 10].

Levels of care for critically ill children

Critically ill children need different levels of care depending on the nature and severity of their illness. However, a wide consensus on what constitutes a PICU is still lacking. Indeed, the patient characteristics and delivery of paediatric intensive care may vary significantly in different medical centres.

Some countries, such as the USA and UK, have defined specific levels of care, while others have informal or no systems for classification. The American Academy of Pediatrics has defined PICU levels and sub-levels of care based primarily on availability of specialized equipment and staff [11]. Differently, in Europe many PICUs often include both intensive and step-down or intermediate care.

In 1993, as a result of a consensus report of critical care experts, the concept of level I and level II PICUs was established in the USA [11]. Within such organization, the highest quality of paediatric critical care is provided by a level I PICU, capable to offer multidisciplinary definitive care

for a wide range of complex, progressive, medical, surgical, and traumatic disorders, occurring in paediatric patients of all ages.

In general, level I PICUs in the USA are located in major medical centres or within children's hospitals and have a full complement of medical and surgical subspecialists, including paediatric intensivists. Even though level I PICUs should provide care to the most severely ill patient population, level II PICUs are often considered an appropriate alternative to the transfer of all critically ill children to a level I PICU. This occurrence may be caused by many factors, including geographic and transport limitations, insufficient availability of level I PICU beds or lack of trained paediatric intensivists. Actually, level II PICUs may be necessary to provide stabilization of critically ill children before transfer to another centre or to avoid long-distance transfers for disorders of less complexity or lower acuity. However, each level II unit must have a well-established communications system with a level I unit, to allow for timely referral of patients who need care that is not available in the level II PICU. Specifications for level I and II PICUs have been recently revised by Rosenberg et al. [12].

In Europe the classification and organization of PICUs may vary considerably in different countries, in terms of size, administration, personnel, physical characteristics, drugs, equipment and types of specialised care provided. In the UK, the Paediatric Intensive Care Society (PICS) has recently updated the documents of paediatric intensive care standards, in which four distinct levels of care and patient dependency are defined, ranging from level I, which refers to high-dependency care, when a child may simply require closer observation and monitoring, to level 4, which refers to the highest level of intensive care, set for children requiring the most intensive interventions, such as extracorporeal life support (see Tab. 1) [13].

Regionalization of paediatric critical care

High-quality care does require adequate continuous staff training and maintenance of their practical experience, particularly in specialties looking after complex and heterogeneous patient categories. These requirements are unlikely to be

Tab. 1   Levels of care and patient dependency (clinically based) according to the UK Paediatric Intensive Care Society.
[Modified from "Appendices to Standards for the care of critically ill children", by a Multidisciplinary Working Group
of the Paediatric Intensive Care Society. Version 3.1, January 2010 [13].]

Level 1 — High Dependency Care
(requiring nurse to patient ratio of 0.5:1 or 1:1 if in a cubicle)

Close monitoring and observation required but not requiring acute mechanical ventilation. Examples would also
include the recently extubated child who is stable and awaiting transfer to a general ward; the child undergoing
close post-operative observation with ECG and pulse oximetry and receiving oxygen. Children requiring long term
chronic ventilation (with tracheostomy) are included in this category, as are CPAP and non-invasive ventilation.

The dependency of a level 1 patient increases to level 2 if the child is nursed in a cubicle.

Level 2 — Intensive care
(requiring nurse to patient ratio of 1:1)

The child requiring continuous nursing supervision who is usually receiving advanced respiratory support, i.e
intubated and ventilated or receiving BiPAP.

Also the unstable non-intubated child, for example some cases with acute upper airway obstruction who may be
receiving nebulised adrenaline.

The dependency of a level 2 patient increases to level 3 if nursed in a cubicle.

Level 3 — Intensive care
(requiring nurse to patient ratio of 1.5:1)

The child requiring intensive supervision at all times who needs additional complex therapeutic procedures and nursing.
For example, unstable ventilated children on vasoactive drugs and inotropic support or with multiple organ failure.

The dependency of a level 3 patient increases to level 4 if nursed in a cubicle.

Level 4 — Intensive care
(requiring a nurse to patient ratio of 2:1)

Children requiring the most intensive interventions such as particularly unstable patients, level 3 patients managed
in a cubicle, those on ECMO, and children undergoing renal replacement therapy.

available in small units with few admissions and
insufficient variation in case mix. Indeed, early
observations of an inverse relationship between
patient volume and outcomes suggest that regionalization may improve patient care quality
[14]. Studies documenting improved outcomes
from increased patient volume have led some researchers to speculate that volume will become
the proxy indicator for quality in health care and
will result in the reorganization of systems to reflect this emphasis [15].

Volume–outcome relationships have been
studied in a number of different settings, including neonatology and paediatric cardiac surgery,
and have generally documented improved outcomes from greater volume [16–21]. In addition,
several studies support the view that the most
important element of paediatric intensive care

service is the skills and experience of the medical and nursing staff, again suggesting that the
services should be centralized [22, 23].

Some of the earliest work supporting regionalized care for critically ill children were related
to trauma [24, 25]. Hulka et al. compared outcomes of injured children in the States of Washington and Oregon during two time periods, one
when neither state had a state-wide trauma system and the other when only one of the states
had such a system [25]. They found that the risk
of death in severely injured children was similar
before the implementation of the trauma system
but, after implementation, was significantly better in the state with a trauma system (mortality
OR, 0.68; $p = 0.019$) [25]. More recent studies
have compared tertiary trauma care provided at
adult versus paediatric facilities. Researchers at

the University of Pittsburgh found that children treated at paediatric trauma centres had better outcomes than children treated at adult trauma centres [26]. In 1997, Pearson et al. looked specifically at the effect of regionalization in paediatric critical care, comparing severity-adjusted ICU mortality in children in a region of Australia, which has centralized paediatric critical care, to that of a region of the United Kingdom, which does not centralize [27]. Even though incidence of ICU admission rates was similar in the two regions, they observed a higher mean length of stay and a severity-adjusted mortality odds ratio of 2.1 (95% CI, 1.4–3.2) in the region without centralized care [27].

In 2000, a specific task force assembled by the American Academy of Pediatrics (AAP] and the Society of Critical Care Medicine (SCCM) concluded that evidence supporting regionalized care for critically ill children was sufficiently strong to recommend its implementation [28, 29].

Detailed discussion of the importance of regionalization of critical care services has been provided by the American College of Critical Care Medicine and the American Academy of Pediatrics [30]. Recent studies in paediatric critical care have confirmed improved outcomes at high-volume centres. Tilford et al. studied over 11,000 admissions in 16 paediatric ICUs and found a severity adjusted odds ratio of 0.95 per 100 patients admitted per year as well as a decreased length of stay in high-volume units [21]. In another large multicentre study, involving 32 paediatric ICUs, high-volume units showed lower severity-adjusted mortality as well as shorter lengths of stay and higher efficiency compared to low-volume units [31].

Location and size of PICUs

In general, all critical care areas should be in close proximity in order to share core support services [13]. Thus, PICUs should be easily accessible to elevators and located within the vicinity of all major interacting departments, such as high dependency units, operating and recovery rooms, cardiac catheterisation laboratory, emergency department, laboratories, radiological and other diagnostic units, as well as the ambulance or helicopter access.

Conversely, an "ideal" size valid for any PICU cannot be recommended, this being dependent on several different factors and variables, for instance those related to the size of the population to be served, the geographical location and the connection facilities, the presence of concomitant critical care services or special units in the same hospital or in the same region (i.e. adult cardiac ICUs serving also children), the presence of highly-specialised medical specialties attracting complex patients. Additionally, distinct clinical admission and discharge criteria can have a significant impact on the number of beds needed [13].

PICUs smaller than six beds may become highly uneconomic, and also have scarce throughput for the medical and nursing staff to maintain the necessary skills. Very large units, however, are often difficult to manage unless they are divided into specialised sub-units. For these reasons a unit of between 8 and 16 beds may be preferable, albeit the present situation may vary considerably in Europe, even within the same country. Nonetheless, design systems offering maximum size flexibility are the most advantageous, allowing step-up and step-down facilities as the patient mix changes, thus addressing the potential need to expand services to accommodate increased demand, such as during the winter season.

Layout and design

Recommendations about PICUs' design have been released by many different entities in Europe and overseas, such as the Society of Critical Care Medicine in 1996, the Committee on Hospital Care and Pediatric Section of the Society of Critical Care Medicine in 1993, the UK Intensive Care Society in 1997 (Standards for Intensive Care Units) and the American Academy of Pediatrics in 2004 [12].

More recently, detailed information on the specific design and engineering requirements for critical care areas, with costs information, schedules of accommodation and room layouts, have been provided in the UK, in Health Building Note 57 [32]. Further information may be found in the proof version of UK PICS standards 2010, now available for consultation [13]. Nonetheless, each unit will have to comply with local regulations concerning building, medical engineering, health and safety issues.

In most cases, similarly to adult ICUs, the essential accommodation for a PICU consists of the patient care areas and management base, reception area, equipment and consumables storage areas, utility rooms, laboratory, procedure room, workshop, cleaner's room, on-call physicians' bedroom, staff sitting room and kitchen, toilets, showers, and relatives' facilities. Access to the PICU should be monitored to maintain patient and staff safety and confidentiality. Other accommodation required include a seminar room, computer room and offices for medical, nursing and secretarial staff.

The design of a PICU should aim to create a critical care environment facilitating the work of health care professionals, in order to achieve the best patient outcome. Such an environment will lead to improved health and developmental outcomes for infants and greater family and staff satisfaction. When designing a new paediatric intensive care unit it would be important to ensure that the new facility best meets the needs of the children and families whom the unit serves [33].

Several distinct room types are required within the PICU, including isolation rooms and separate rooms for linens and equipment. A separate room for family counselling is necessary for private discussions between the staff and the family [12].

An adequate space per PICU bed should be allowed, according to local regulations [12, 13]. The head of each bed should be rapidly accessible for emergency airway management. Electrical power, oxygen, medical compressed air, and vacuum outlets sufficient in number to supply all necessary equipment should meet local requirements. In most cases, 12 or more electrical outlets and a minimum of two compressed air outlets, two oxygen outlets, and two vacuum outlets will be necessary per bed space. Reserve emergency power and gas supply (oxygen, compressed air) are essential. All outlets, heating, ventilation, air conditioning, fire safety procedures and equipment, electrical grounding, plumbing, and illumination must adhere to appropriate local and national codes [12]. Notably, pertinent rules and policies may vary extensively throughout Europe.

Family-centred care in PICUs

Infants and children are admitted to the paediatric intensive care unit for a variety of reasons. This experience can be particularly distressing for them and for their families. Not surprisingly, the presence of parents has been shown to be beneficial to children, both physiologically and psychologically. When faced with a PICU admission, parents may suffer the unfamiliar and potentially threatening environment of an intensive care unit. As shown in neonatal and paediatric ICUs, these parents often encounter challenges to the development of their parenting roles, with potential long lasting effects even on family functioning [34–38]. The inability to help, hold, care for the child, protect the child from pain, and share the child with other family members are primary sources of stress. Disruption of the parent-child relationship may cause more stress to parents than the actual physical PICU environment itself, and by supporting parents in pursuing their parenting role, whenever possible, this stress can be reduced.

In paediatric intensive care most children may be unable to express their needs and experiences. In this perspective the principles of family-centred care mandate incorporation of parents in daily care [39]. The central foundation of family-centred care in paediatrics is that the child's family is a constant and is comprised of the most important people in the child's life. Families, specifically parents, provide children support, comfort, and reassurance during times of stress. A respecting of that role is central to family-centred care. In all paediatric settings, parents are increasingly encouraged and even expected to be actively involved in the care of their children. Likewise, parents have this expectation of themselves. This approach to health care leads intuitively to better health outcomes, and greater patient and family satisfaction [40].

The needs of parents with a child in the PICU must not be ignored. Resident accommodation for at least one parent for each child must be available at the bedside, allowing the parents to stay as long as they feel is necessary. The Institute for Family-Centered Care of the American Academy of Pediatrics describes family-centred care as being guided by several principles, which are listed in Table 2 [34].

Tab. 2 Core principles of family-centred care [reproduced with permission from Pediatrics, 112, 691-696, © 2003 by the AAP].

1. Respecting each child and his or her family

2. Honouring racial, ethnic, cultural, and socioeconomic diversity and its effect on the family's experience and perception of care

3. Recognizing and building on the strengths of each child and family, even in difficult and challenging situations

4. Supporting and facilitating choice for the child and family about approaches to care and support

5. Ensuring flexibility in organizational policies, procedures, and provider practices so services can be tailored to the needs, beliefs, and cultural values of each child and family

6. Sharing honest and unbiased information with families on an ongoing basis and in ways they find useful and affirming

7. Providing and/or ensuring formal and informal support (e.g., family-to-family support) for the child and parent(s) and/or guardian(s) during pregnancy, childbirth, infancy, childhood, adolescence, and young adulthood

8. Collaborating with families at all levels of health care; in the care of the individual child; and in professional education, policy making, and program development

9. Empowering each child and family to discover their own strengths, build confidence, and make choices and decisions about their health

Intensive care professionals are increasingly concerned about patient and family-centred care and are more prone to involve family members in the care of the patient. Staff who are appropriately trained in the care of children and adolescents will recognise the need for parental involvement, ensuring that open access is available for parents and siblings to visit and be involved in their child's care. Clinical practice guidelines on family-centred care in intensive care units has been recently issued by a task force of the American College of Critical Care Medicine [41].

Equipment

Standard and more sophisticated equipment are both essential because of the nature of work carried out in modern PICUs. Life-saving, therapeutic, and monitoring equipment, in particular drugs for resuscitation and advanced life support, according to international guidelines, should be present or immediately available for any patient in the PICU. Detailed lists of drugs, equipment and devices have been published elsewhere [12, 42]. Portable equipment will include an emergency trolley provided with different sizes of blades, laryngoscopes, cuffed and uncuffed tracheal tubes, Magill forceps, suction catheters,

oropharyngeal and nasopharyngeal airways, neonatal and paediatric laryngeal mask airways and a portable mechanical ventilator. In addition to standard apparatus, other specific items for children that should be on hand include paediatric sized blood pressure cuffs, a defibrillator with paediatric paddles and pacing capabilities, thermometers to identify extremes of hypothermia and hyperthermia, heating and cooling devices, transthoracic pacer with paediatric pads, devices for accurately weighing patients, cribs and paediatric beds with easy head access, transport monitor with paediatric sensors, central catheters for vascular access, intraosseous needles, catheters for arterial access, high-precision infusion pumps, different sized thoracostomy tubes, surgical trays for vascular cut-downs, open chest procedures, cricothyroidotomy, and emergency tracheostomy. Equipment for neonatal and paediatric flexible bronchoscopy should also be available.

Mechanical ventilators suitable for neonatal and paediatric patients of all sizes, providing the most updated modes of ventilation, should be available in any PICU, together with pulse oximeters and transcutaneous oxygen monitors, end-tidal and transcutaneous CO_2 monitors. The minimal number of ventilators will depend on the size of the unit and the patient case-mix. At the bedside, PICU monitors should have the capability for ongoing monitoring heart rate, arrhythmias, respiratory rate, oxygen saturation, end-tidal CO_2, temperature, invasive and non-invasive blood pressure, central venous and intracranial pressure, as needed [12]. Depending on the level of intensive care required, more sophisticated monitoring systems and more complex therapeutic options may be required, such as life support techniques [43, 44].

Medical and nursing staffing

One of the most important attributes of a PICU is its high medical and nursing staff needs. The level of staffing has to be appropriate to the severity and the case mix of the unit. Indeed, successful management of the unit also depends very much on collaboration of many disciplines with good medical and nursing leadership. Administration of a multidisciplinary PICU requires a director who should either be a paediatrician, paediatric anaesthetist or both. The medical director should be trained in one of the above major clinical specialities with expertise in the care of sick children requiring advanced skills in life-support techniques such as ventilation. The director should also have adequate organisational and managerial skills, as well as a commitment to training of junior medical staff and to organising clinical research. In addition, the director should count on an appropriately trained and credentialed medical personnel in the PICU, plus a nursing staff which should be dedicated to the care of the critically ill infant and child. A nurse manager with substantial paediatric experience is essential for any PICU. The senior nurse should have had several years of experience in paediatric intensive care and have sound managerial skills. In 1985, the American Board of Pediatrics recognized the subspecialty of paediatric critical care medicine and set criteria for subspecialty certification. In 1990, the Residency Review Committee of the Accreditation Council for Graduate Medical Education completed its first accreditation of paediatric critical care medicine training programs. In 1986, the American Association of Critical Care Nurses developed a certification program for paediatric critical care, and in 1999, a certification program for clinical nurse specialists in paediatric critical

care was initiated. In this regard, the situation in Europe is quite variable. In the UK, the Intercollegiate Committee for Training in Paediatric Intensive Care Medicine was established in 1993, with the aim to provide guidance on the training required by anaesthetists, paediatricians or paediatric surgeons willing to practice paediatric intensive care [45, 46]. For nurses, a report prepared under the auspices of the NHS Chief Nursing Officer, 'Bridge to the Future', was published in 1997, addressing the issues of standards, education and workforce planning. The key nursing standards determined that one children's nurse with an intensive care qualification should be present at the bedside in PICU throughout every 24-hour period [47]. Post-graduate courses on paediatric intensive care nursing are now offered at various university nursing departments, linked to regional PICUs. In addition to postgraduate PIC nurse training, courses in the advanced practice of PIC have been developed. The health care teams of some units are now supported by advanced nurse practitioners and nurse consultants.

Caring for critically ill children in adult ICUs

Children looked after in specialist paediatric ICUs in tertiary hospitals seems to have a lower mortality than children in mixed adult and paediatric units in district hospitals [8]. As a consequence, the Australian National Health and Medical Research Council has issued statements advocating that critically ill children should not be cared for in adult units apart from for short periods or prior to retrieval [48]. Furthermore, children should not be admitted to adult wards as they are not only more emotionally vulnerable than adults, but also have different needs requiring alternative equipment, techniques and staff skills [49].

However, there is no worldwide consensus as to where children requiring intensive care should be admitted. Although desirable, it may not be possible to have individual PICUs in all referral hospitals, so that many countries have to find a balance between available PICUs and adult units with some paediatric commitment. Most adult units are staffed and run by anaesthetists, who are often lacking an adequate paediatric training to enable them to manage the complete age range of children requiring intensive care. Equally important is the lack of trained paediatric nurses in the adult units.

In a recent multicentre study, Cogo et al. compared the outcome of 1265 children admitted to 124 adult intensive care units in Italy, between 2003 and 2007, with that of 1533 children admitted to 26 Italian paediatric intensive care units between 1994 and 1995 [50]. Risk of ICU mortality was assessed with the Pediatric Risk of Mortality score (PRISM) in both study and historical control groups. The standard mortality ratios were similar in the two paediatric groups, suggesting that quality of care provided nowadays to children admitted to adult ICUs in Italy is similar to that provided by Italian PICUs 10 years earlier. Given that Italian PICUs may well have improved the level of care in the same period, these results, if confirmed, suggest a better quality of care for children admitted to PICUs as compared to adult ICUs. However, due to some methodological limitations, further studies will have to confirm such interesting findings.

Even if intensive care is provided within the setting of the adult unit, the specific and special needs of children and their parents make it essential that they are managed within an area separated from the principal unit. In fact, the presence of adult patients is reported to increase parents' distress. Scothern et al. found that such parents would not want to exchange the general intensive therapy unit for an environment that offered less expertise or technology, but would appreciate children being nursed in separate areas, away from the more distressing adult patients [51]. Similarly, adult patients and their relatives are often distressed to observe small children undergoing invasive therapies, and are disturbed by the noise that children can make [33].

Standardization of equipment with other departments, specifically emergency department, operating rooms, paediatric wards and delivery room, may ensures to the ICU a safe minimum level of equipment and ready reserves. A mobile trolley for emergencies, with drawers clearly labelled and containing key equipment for different paediatric sizes, should be always on hand. A paediatric booklet with recommended drugs, dosages and calculations, a 'Broselow' tape and an emergency drug box should be immediately available, as well as a ventilator at the ready, in anticipation of a paediatric emergency. Diversional therapy such as toys, television, tapes, puzzles and books, plus facilities for the parents to stay overnight may be quite functional.

Transport of critically ill children

Although the treatment of critically ill children is improved by transfer to a tertiary PICU, it is important that these patients are adequately resuscitated before secondary transport to avoid any deterioration in their condition.

Inter-hospital transport can provoke clinical deterioration in unstable patients and can be particularly hazardous in critically ill children. For such reasons, many centres are convinced that the most satisfactory way to transfer children requiring intensive care is for the referral unit to send out a paediatric critical care retrieval team. Indeed, there is evidence that the number of adverse events that occur during an ICU transfer may be minimized by the use of specialist teams [52, 53]. The purpose of retrieval is to transfer the child to a PICU safely and efficiently with minimal risk. The team therefore goes quickly to the referring hospital, performs on-site assessment and stabilisation of the child, and institutes appropriate monitoring and treatment. In effect this brings the benefits of the PICU to the child. Thereafter, except for rare circumstances, return to the tertiary unit should only be undertaken once the child's condition is stabilised. In fact, recent data have confirmed that time spent undertaking intensive care interventions early in the course of patient illness at the referring hospital does not worsen patient outcome, suggesting that the "scoop and run" model can be safely abandoned in inter-hospital transport [54].

Any paediatric transport service should be available on a 24-hour basis to retrieve critically ill children from referring hospitals. All transfers should be accomplished by appropriately trained and equipped staff, ideally provided by a PICU or by a dedicated retrieval service. The retrieval team should be equipped to care for children of different ages. Drugs and equipment should be checked in accordance with local policies [13]. The retrieval service should have written guidelines covering arrangements for transfer of parents.

Wherever possible, parents should be given the option to accompany their child during the transfer. The retrieval service should have a written policy on reporting of clinical incidents. This policy should ensure that, where appropriate, clinical incidents are reported to the governance arrangements of both the host organisation and referring hospital. The retrieval service should produce an annual report summarising activity, compliance with quality standards, and clinical outcomes. This report should be shared with referring hospitals. Finally, the retrieval service should offer an education/training programme for referring hospitals covering assessment, resuscitation, stabilisation and maintenance of critically ill and injured children prior to the arrival of the retrieval service [13].

Conclusions

Paediatric critical care medicine is a complex area that is constantly developing. The role of the paediatric critical care physician has evolved from that of a postoperative adjunct to that of the true intensivist of today, working in multidisciplinary ICUs which care for children with a whole spectrum of critical illnesses. The assessment and management of critical illness and injury in paediatric patients requires specialized training and experience. The steadily evolving technology and continuous introduction of new medications and devices makes paediatric critical care even more challenging for healthcare providers, who have to stay up to date and acquire both new skills and knowledge while simultaneously caring for the sickest of patients. Notably, in areas where specialized paediatric emergency and critical care are not available, the outcome of paediatric critical illness and injury appears to be adversely affected. Thus, centralisation of paediatric intensive care into a limited number of tertiary units seems preferable to unrestricted fragmented care in adult intensive care units or paediatric wards which lack staff specially assigned to paediatric intensive care. In addition, the quality of care provided in PICUs may be positively affected by the implementation of clinical guidelines and by the observance of modern standards and requirements. Indeed, the PICU environment is a very complex organization with many different services, which requires a suitable design and a well organized administrative structure, to enable the team to care for the patient, in a safe and effective way, with a family-centred approach. The PICU

should be perceived as the place where the sickest child receives the best possible care by comforting and skilled doctors and nurses, who are able to address many of the patient's as well as the family's concerns, with the aim to promote optimal outcomes.

The author

Paolo Biban, MD

Director, Division of Paediatrics
Neonatal and Paediatric Intensive Care unit
Major City Hospital
Azienda Ospedaliera Universitaria Integrata Verona
Piazzale Stefani 1
37126 Verona, Italy
E-mail: paolo.biban@ospedaleuniverona.it

References

1. Downes JJ. Development of pediatric critical care medicine – How did we get here and why? In: Wheeler DS, Wong HR, Shanley TP. Science and practice of pediatric critical care medicine. London: Springer Verlag, 2009.
2. Vidyasagar D, ed. Progress in Pediatric Critical Care. Critical Care Clinics 1992;8:1–228.
3. Downes JJ. The historical evolution, current status, and prospective development of pediatric critical care. Crit Care Clin 1992;8:1 22
4. Orlowski JP, ed. Pediatric Critical Care—A New Millennium. Pediatr Clin N Amer 2001;48:553–814.
5. National Coordinating Group on Paediatric Intensive Care (1997) Paediatric intensive care: a framework for the future. Department of Health, London. http://www. dh.gov.uk/en/Publicationsandstatistics/Publications/ PublicationsPolicyAndGuidance/DH_4005760. Accessed May 2010
6. Duncan AW. The burden of paediatric intensive care: an Australian and New Zealand perspective. Paediatr Respir Rev. 2005;6:166–73.
7. Ramenofsky M, Luterman A, Quidlen E, Riddick L, Curreri PW. Maximum survival in pediatric trauma: the ideal system. J Trauma 1984;24: 818–823.
8. Pollack MM, Alexander SR, Clarke N, Ruttimann UE, Tesselaar HM, Bachulis AC. Improved outcomes from tertiary center pediatric intensive care: a statewide comparison of tertiary and nontertiary care facilities. Crit Care Med 1991;19:150–159.
9. Pollack MM, Cuerdon TC, Patel KM, Ruttimann UE, Getson PR, Levetown M. Impact of quality-of-care factors on pediatric intensive care unit mortality. JAMA 1994;272:941–946.

10. Pollack MM, Katz RW, Ruttimann UE, Getson PR. Improving the outcome and efficiency of intensive care: the impact of an intensivist. Crit Care Med 1988;16:11–17.

11. American Academy of Pediatrics, Committee on Hospital Care and Pediatric Section of the Society of Critical Care Medicine. Guidelines and levels of care for pediatric intensive care units. Pediatrics 1993;92:166–175.

12. Rosenberg DI, Moss MM. Guidelines and levels of care for pediatric intensive care units. Pediatrics 2004;114:1114–1125.

13. Standards for the care of critically ill children. London: Paediatric Intensive Care Society; 2010. http://www.ukpics.org/images/stories/pics_documents/pics%20standards%204th%20edn%20v2%2020100707.pdf

14. Luft HS, Bunker SJ, Enthoven A. Should operations be regionalized? An empirical relation between surgical volume and mortality. N Engl J Med 1979;301:1364–1369.

15. Van Etten P. Camelot or common sense? The logic behind the UCSF/Stanford merger. Health Aff 1999;18:143–148

16. Dudley RA, Johansen KL, Brand R, Rennie DJ, Milstein A. Selective referral to high-volume hospitals: estimating potentially avoidable deaths. JAMA 2000; 283:1159–1166.

17. Phibbs CS, Bronstein JM, Buxton E, Phibbs RH. The effects of patient volume and level of care at the hospital of birth on neonatal mortality. JAMA 1996;276:1054–1059.

18. Mayfield JA, Rosenblatt RA, Baldwin LM, Chu J, Logerfo JP. The relation of obstetrical volume and nursery level to perinatal mortality. Am J Public Health 1990;80:819–823.

19. Hannan EL, Racz M, Kavey RE, Pediatric cardiac surgery: the effect of hospital and surgeon volume on in-hospital mortality. Quaegebeur JM, Williams R. Pediatrics 1998;101:963–969.

20. Spiegelhalter DJ. Mortality and volume of cases in pediatric cardiac surgery: retrospective study based on routinely collected data. BMJ 2002;324:261–263.

21. Tilford JM, Simpson PM, Green JW, Lensing S, Fiser DH. Volume-outcome relationships in pediatric intensive care units. Pediatrics 2000;106:289–294.

22. Groeger JS, Strosberg MA, Halpern NA, Raphaely RC, Kaye WE, Guntupalli KK, et al. Descriptive analysis of critical care units in the United States. Crit Care Med 1992;20:846–863.

23. Pollack MM, Cuerdon TC, Getson PR. Pediatric intensive care units: results of a national survey. Crit Care Med 1993;21:607–613.

24. Haller JA, Shorter N, Miller D, Colombani P, Hall J, Buck J. Organization and function of a regional pediatric trauma center: does a system of management improve outcome? J Trauma.1983;23:691–696.

25. Hulka F, Mullins RJ, Mann NC, Hedges JR, Rowland D, Worrall WH, et al. Influence of a statewide trauma system on pediatric hospitalization and outcome. J Trauma 1997;42:514–519.

26. Potoka DA, Schall LC, Gardner MJ, Stafford PW, Peitzman AB, Ford HR. Impact of pediatric trauma centers on mortality in a statewide system. J Trauma 2000;49:237–245.

27. Pearson G, Shann F, Barry P, Vyas J, Thomas D, Powell C, et al. Should pediatric intensive care be centralised? Trent versus Victoria. Lancet 1997;349:1213–1217.

28. Consensus report for regionalization of services for critically ill or injured children. Council of the Society of Critical Care Medicine. Crit Care Med 2000;28:236–239.

29. American Academy of Pediatrics. Committee on Pediatric Emergency Medicine. American College of Critical Care Medicine. Society of Critical Care Medicine. Consensus report for regionalization of services for critically ill or injured children. Pediatrics 2000;105:152–155.

30. American College of Critical Care Medicine, Society of Critical Care Medicine: Critical care services and personnel: Recommendations based on a system of categorization into two levels of care. Crit Care Med 1999;27:422–426.

31. Ruttimann UE, Patel KM, Pollack MM. Relevance of diagnostic diversity and patient volumes or quality and length of stay in pediatric intensive care units. Pediatric Crit Care Med 2002;1:133–139.

32. Facilities for critical care, 2005. London, UK, NHS Estates, Document Health Building Note 57 (HBN 57).

33. de Courcy-Golder K. A strategy for development of paediatric intensive care within the United Kingdom. Intensive Crit Care Nurs 1996;12:84–89.

34. American Academy of Pediatrics Committee on Hospital Care. Family-centered care and the pediatrician's role. Pediatrics 2003;112:691–696.

35. Carter MC, Miles MS, Burford TH, Hassanien RS. Parental environmental stress in paediatric intensive care units. Applied Nursing Research 1985;4:181–188

36. Cox P Children in critical care: how parents cope. British Journal of Nursing 1992;1:764–768.

37. Heerman JA, Wilson ME, Wilhelm PA. Mothers in the NICU: outsiders to partners. Pediatr Nurs 2005;31,176–200.

38. Lupton D, Fenwick J. "They've forgotten that I'm the mum" constructing and practicing motherhood in special care nurseries. Social Sci Med 2001;53,1011–1021.

39. Latour JM, van Goudoever JB, Hazelzet JA. Parent satisfaction in the pediatric ICU. Pediatr Clin N Am 2008;55:779–790.

40. Latour JM, van Goudoever JB, Duivenvoorden HJ, van Dam NAM, Dullaart E, Albers MJIJ, et al. Perceptions of parents on satisfaction with care in the pediatric intensive care unit: the EMPATHIC study. Intensive Care Med 2009;35:1082–1089.

41. Davidson JE, Powers K, Hedayat KM, Tieszen M, Kon AA, Shepard E, et al. Clinical practice guidelines for support of the family in the patient-centered intensive care unit: American college of critical care medicine task force 2004–2005. Crit Care Med 2007;35:605–622.

42. Standards for the care of critically ill children. London: Paediatric Intensive Care Society; 2010. http://www. ukpics.org/images/stories/pics_documents/2010picsst andardsappendicesproof.doc Accessed June 2010

43. Fiser RT, Morris MC. Extracorporeal cardiopulmonary resuscitation in refractory pediatric cardiac arrest. Pediatr Clin N Am 2008;55:929–941.

44. Huang SC, Wu ET, Chen YS, Chang CI, Chiu IS, Wang SS, et al. Extracorporeal membrane oxygenation rescue for cardiopulmonary resuscitation in pediatric patients. Crit Care Med 2008;36:1607–1613.

45. Macrae DJ. The burden of paediatric intensive care: a perspective from the UK and Ireland. Paediatr Respir Rev 2005;6:154–159.

46. The Intercollegiate Committee for Training in Paediatric Intensive Care Medicine ICTPICM). http://www.rcoa.ac. uk/index.asp?PageID=37.

47. "A Bridge to the Future" Report of the Chief Nursing Officer's Taskforce. Department of Health, London, 1997.

48. National Health and Medical Research Council. Management of seriously ill children in adult intensive care units. Report of the 94th Session of the Council. Canberra: Commonwealth of Australia, 1982.

49. Department of Health. Welfare of children and young people in hospital. HMSO, London,1991.

50. Cogo PE, Poole D. Codazzi D, Boniotti C, Capretta A, Langer M, et al. Outcome of children admitted to adult intensive care units in Italy between 2003 and 2007. Intensive Care Med. 2010 May 20. [Epub ahead of print]

51. Scothern GC, Jones S, MacFadyen U. Young children in a general intensive therapy unit. Care Crit Ill 1992;8: 208–209.

52. Edge WE, Kanter RK, Weigle CG, Walsh RF. Reduction of morbidity in interhospital transport by specialized pediatric staff. Crit Care Med 1994;22:1186–1191.

53. Orr RA, Felmet KA, Han Y, McCloskey KA, Dragotta MA, Bills DM, et al. Pediatric specialized transport teams are associated with improved outcomes. Pediatrics 2009;124:40–48.

54. Borrows EL, Lutman DH, Montgomery MA, Petros AJ, Ramnarayan P. Effect of patient- and team-related factors on stabilization time during pediatric intensive care transport. Pediatr Crit Care Med 2010 May 6. [Epub ahead of print].

Elias Knobel, Marcia Makdisse and Marcos Knobel

Do we need specific cardiac (non-operative) ICUs?

Introduction

Intensive Care Units (ICU) are hospital units designed for the treatment of patients who present with severe or potentially severe organic dysfunction. Because these patients have a variety of clinical demands, ICUs have had to specialise into medical, surgical, and specialty ICUs (e.g., cardiac ICU, respiratory ICU, etc.), and step-down units in order to provide distinct levels of care. A hospital may have stand-alone sub-speciality ICUs, one general ICU, or no ICU at all, depending on its size and type: public, private, community, or teaching hospital.

Although ICUs share many characteristics, their structure, organisation, and the way care is delivered are not standardised. The same is also true for the different specialised ICUs. As a consequence, medical, surgical, and cardiac critical care units have been denominated by different names and have been differently established across hospitals and health systems worldwide (see Tab. 1) [1]. In this text, the term Cardiac Intensive Care Unit (CICU) refers to a unit for treating non-surgical cardiac patients.

History and evolution of intensive care units and cardiac intensive care units

ICUs were created following the polio epidemics of the 1950s. In the beginning they were merely seen as an expansion of the postoperative recovery rooms that had been created following World War II. Respiratory paralysis caused by polio was the main driver for the development of mechanical ventilation and consequently for the establishment of long-term intensive care units (ICUs), which resulted in reduced mortality. Around the same time, patients who had cardiovascular conditions were being admitted to small cardiac intensive care units (CICUs). The first CICU de-

Tab. 1 Commonly used ICU denominations and target population (data from [1])

Target population	Denomination
Medical patients	Medical ICU
Surgical patients	Surgical ICU
Non-surgical cardiac patients	Cardiac ICU (CICU)
	Coronary care unit (CCU)
Surgical cardiac patients	Cardiothoracic ICU
	Cardiovascular ICU
	Thoracic ICU

scription was suggested by D. J. Julian in 1961 to the British Thoracic Society [2]. Soon after, following the publication of the landmark study by Killip and Kimball in which the authors confirmed the role of the CICU as a beneficial tool in the management of patients with acute myocardial infarction (AMI), the first CICU was established in the United States [3]. Their study was crucial in showing the benefits of CICUs over a regular ward setting in early identification and treatment of potentially life-threatening arrhythmias, which in turn resulted in survival benefits for high-risk cardiac patients. Further studies also showed that specially equipped units that were staffed by personnel trained in critical care led to a significant reduction in arrhythmia-related mortality [4].

Despite some controversy regarding their cost-effectiveness, CICUs continued to be implemented and developed, and were considered to be one of the most important advances in the care of acutely ill cardiac patients [5].

At the time, the CICUs evolved faster than ICUs did, probably due to the higher morbidity and mortality of AMI patients and to the advent of modern technologies of bedside rhythm monitoring, defibrillators, new cardiopulmonary assist procedures, and pacemakers [6, 7].

During the 1970s, great interest and considerable efforts were directed into improving the knowledge of critical care medicine regarding its pathophysiological processes, treatments, and outcomes. As a consequence, specialty journals, training and qualification programmes dedicated to intensive care emerged and critical care medicine became a separate medical specialty.

At the same time, great progress was being obtained in the treatment of cardiovascular diseases. For instance, reperfusion strategies for AMI evolved from thrombolytic therapy to primary angioplasty and stenting, while advances in low cardiac output syndrome management, mechanical circulatory assistance devices, postcardiac transplant care, and more recently postpercutaneous valve implant care took place. As a consequence, the CICUs that were initially seen as merely clinical observation units to treat potential complications of AMI evolved into specialised units to treat a wider range of cardiac conditions. Almost 50 years later, current CICUs turned out to be strikingly different than the prototypical CICUs of the 1960s.

However, population aging and its associated co-morbidities such as acute and chronic sequelae of nonfatal AMI, plus the epidemics of obesity and the metabolic syndrome, as well as complications of intravascular and implantable devices, have all increased patient susceptibility to critical illness. These factors represent new challenges for CICU personnel, as most units are staffed with cardiologists who are not trained in critical care medicine. On the other hand, the majority of ICUs are staffed with intensivists who have only a limited knowledge of cardiology [8, 9].

The process of care in ICUs

ICUs may be organised in various ways. They may be "closed" units in which care is provided by an ICU-dedicated multi-professional team that controls all aspects of patient care, "hybrid or transitional" units that are managed by a certified intensivist and where care is delivered as a consequence of a co-management between the ICU staff and private physicians, or "open" units where patients remain under the care of their admitting physicians who assume full clinical responsibility, and which may or may not offer the support of an intensivist who works as a consultant on ICU cases [10].

The process of care in the ICU is typically a horizontal one and both its organisation and its management structure must take into account its fundamental features.

The patient who presents a specific type of pathology needs to be directed to the right place at the right time in order to receive the appropriate treatment. One of the major challenges of ICUs is to reduce delay in assisting patients so that the patient treatment is not compromised [11]. All hospitals should determine the level of critical care services they are able to provide and these should be aligned with their mission, goals, and local needs (see Tab. 2) [12].

Better management of the whole process is crucial for providing a better assistance and for that the ICU needs, besides adequate technology resources, to rely on a well-trained and qualified staff that has clinical knowledge and is able to treat specific pathologies. The recommendations for the structure, organisation, and operation of CICUs published by the European Society of Cardiology Working Group on Acute Cardiac Care in 2005 are summarised in Table 3 [13].

Trends in CICU care delivery

The CICU environment has changed dramatically in the last decades due to population aging, and because of the increased prevalence of concomitant chronic illnesses.

Trends in patient characteristics

In most ICU and CICU settings, a consistent male-to-female ratio of 3:2 has been observed among admitted patients [14, 15]. Recently published data, from a study that included nearly 30,000 patients admitted to a large, academic CICU over nearly two decades, showed a progressive increase in mean age and in the proportion of female patients admitted to a CICU [16]. This trend follows the same pattern observed for the prevalence of cardiovascular disease among male and female individuals. Female presence in CICUs is expected to continue to increase as the population ages.

Trends in co-morbidity pattern of cardiac ICU patients

Along with CICU patient aging, a significant increase in non-cardiovascular critical illness prevalence has been observed in CICUs over time, including acute renal failure, respiratory failure, chronic kidney disease, pneumonia, sepsis/septic shock, gastrointestinal bleeding, and multiorgan failure (see Fig. 1) [16]. Besides the increase in prevalence, the severity of co-morbid illnesses, measured according to the Charlson Comorbidity Scores, has increased significantly over time as well (mean score raised from 1.8 ± 1.6 to 2.3 ± 1.8, $p < .001$), which suggests that patients currently admitted to CICUs are more severely ill than they were in the past decades [17].

Tab. 2   Definitions of levels of care according to the Task Force of the American College of Critical Care Medicine of the Society of Critical Care Medicine, 2003 (data from [12]).

Level of care	Characteristics
I	■ Comprehensive critical care centres for a wide range of disorders ■ Continuous availability of sophisticated equipment, specialized nurses, and physicians with critical care training ■ Support services: pharmacy services, respiratory therapy, nutritional services, pastoral care, and social services
II	■ Centres able to provide comprehensive critical care but unable to provide critical care for specific areas of expertise (e.g., cardiothoracic surgery, neurosurgery, and trauma). ■ Criteria for transfer patients should be specific and readily available to hospital personnel in order to avoid delays in definitive care
III	■ Centres able to provide initial stabilization of critically ill patients but have limited ability to provide comprehensive critical care ■ Basic services for stabilizing, monitoring, and treating critically ill patients should be available such as ECG, arterial pressure, central venous pressure and transcutaneous oxygen monitoring; equipment to maintain the airway and to ventilate, to resuscitate and support haemodynamically unstable patients; beds with removable headboard and adjustable position, specialty beds; adequate lighting for bedside procedures; suction; hypo/hyperthermia blankets; scales; temporary pacemakers, and temperature monitoring devices. ■ Detailed transport policies and expertise in the transport of patients are essential for these centres ■ Telemedicine-driven ICU care should be considered

Tab. 3   European Society of Cardiology recommendations for the structure, organization and operation of intensive and intermediate CICUs (data from [13]). (For abbreviations, see below.)

	Intensive CICU	Intermediate CICU
Patients	STEMI (first 24 h) or complicated AMI (> 24 h) High-risk unstable ACS patients Life-threatening arrhythmias High-risk unstable post-PCI patients Unresolved acute pulmonary oedema Patients in need of haemodynamic monitoring Acute complications of heart transplant Massive pulmonary embolism	Intermediate risk ACS patients First stages of recovery from AMI Uncontrollable cardiac insufficiency Unresponsive to regular oral therapy Need of medical therapy adjustment or invasive cardiac investigations or procedures (EPS, cardiac catheterization, pacemaker/defibrillators implants, etc).
Beds	Recommended formula (use the highest value): 4 to 5 beds for each 100,000 inhabitants 10 beds for every 100,000 ER visits per year	1:3 is the desired ratio of beds between CICU and the intermediate CCU
Equipment	Monitoring unit ≥ 2 ECG channels, invasive pressure channel, non-invasive BP monitor, and SaO_2 metre. Additional basic parameters (available in ≥ 50 % of beds: 5 ECG channels, 2 additional haemodynamic channels, end tidal CO_2, non-invasive cardiac output, and thermometer	Monitoring unit ≥ 2 ECG channels, invasive pressure channel, non-invasive BP monitor, and SaO_2 metre
	Central monitoring and analysing Station ≥ 1 ECG lead from each patient, relevant haemodynamic and respiratory data Slave monitors Working stations for retrospective analysis	Central monitoring and analysing Station ≥ 1 ECG lead from each patient, relevant haemodynamic and respiratory data Working stations for retrospective analysis
	Additional equipment 4 to 6 volumetric pump/automatic syringe per bed 1 mechanical respirator (including CPAP system) every 2 beds 1 IABP consol every 3 beds 1 pacemaker/defibrillator apparatus every 3 beds 1 to 2 external pacemaker every 6 to 8 beds 3 to 4 VVI and 1 DDD temporary pacemakers every 6 to 8 beds 1 blood clot metre (ACT) 1 glucose level measurement kit 1 mobile echocardiography machine X-ray fluoroscopy	Additional equipment Volumetric pump/automatic syringe per bed External pacemaker/defibrillator every 6 to 8 beds Glucose level measurement kit
Staff	Department Head	Department Head
	Certified cardiologist trained and accredited as an acute cardiac care specialist and with further training in general critical care medicine.	Certified cardiologist

	Intensive CICU	Intermediate CICU
	Physicians	Physicians
	First 6 beds: 1 physician every 3 beds. > 6 beds: 1 physician every 4 beds. On-duty physician always present in the unit On-call physician always available for consultation and assistance	First 12 beds: 1 physician every 6 beds > 12 beds: 1 physician every 8 beds
	Nurses	Nurses
	Daytime: ≥ 1 nurse per 2 beds Night shift: ≥ 1 nurse per 3 beds A head nurse with authority and responsibility for the appropriateness of nursing care Only registered nurses should be employed (≥ 75 % with completed formal intensive care training, including formal cardiology training) plus further training once in at least 5 years in general ICU.	Daytime: ≥ 1 nurse per 4 beds Night shift: ≥ 1 nurse per 6 beds
	Additional staff	
	Full time secretary and nurse assistant Part time dietician, computer expert, ventilation technician, social worker, physiotherapist, porters, and cleaners	
Construction	Independent ward in the hospital	Up to 2 to 3 patients per room
	Separate room for each patient ≥ 1 single bedroom with isolation Central nurse station Procedure room (X-ray, heavy monitoring, IABP) Dialysis facility Electrical equipment with emergency feeding and continuity apparatus	
Other areas	Staff rooms, meeting room, family waiting room, office, store room	

ACS = acute coronary syndrome; AMI = acute myocardial infarction; BP = blood pressure; DDD = dual-chamber pacemaker;
ECG = electrocardiogram; EPS = electrophysiological study; ER = emergency room; IABP = intra-aortic balloon pump;
PCI = percutaneous coronary intervention; VVI = ventricular demand inhibited pacemaker; STEMI = ST elevation myocardial infarction

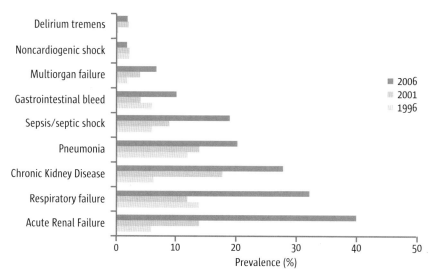

Fig. 1   Trends in CICU co-morbidities [modified from Katz JN, Turer AT, Becker RC. Cardiology and the critical care crisis: a perspective. J Am Coll Cardiol 2007;49:1279–82]

Trends in the rate of cardiac complications of non-cardiac ICU patients

Cardiac arrhythmias, myocardial dysfunction, and peri-operative myocardial infarction are the most common cardiac complications among critically ill non-cardiac patients. The incidence of atrial fibrillation following non-cardiac thoracic surgery and non-thoracic general surgery may reach 15 and 10 %, respectively [18]. As for the incidence of perioperational AMI, it may vary between 1 and 3 % in low-risk patients to almost 40 % in patients with previous coronary artery disease. Decompensated heart failure, which is the most frequent cardiac complication in surgical patients, may occur after major surgeries in 1 to 6 % of the cases and in 6 to 25 % in patients with previous cardiomyopathies (ischemic or valvular problems) [19]. Therefore, the intensivist must be able to handle such complications and rely on the support provided by cardio intensivists in order to confirm the patient diagnosis. The support of the cardio intensivist is also needed for treatment decisions for more severe patients or those who are resistant to the initial treatment.

Trends in outcomes

As mentioned at the beginning of this text, an important contribution of the study by Killip and Kimball [3] was to show the advantage of CICUs over a regular ward setting in the treatment of AMI, and especially in the early identification and treatment of potentially life-threatening arrhythmias, resulting in survival benefits for high-risk cardiac patients. Later, Quinn and collaborators [4] showed that specially equipped units staffed with critical-care-trained personnel led to a significant reduction in arrhythmia-related mortality.

In 2004, an evaluation of the impact on clinical outcomes of admission to a CICU, compared to an ordinary ward, used discharge data of 181,049 heart disease admissions from Italian hospitals (Lazio). The evaluation revealed a significantly lower risk of death in patients admitted directly to CICUs for AMI (OR = 0.57), acute coronary syndromes (OR = 0.55), and arrhythmias (OR = 0.56) [20]. More recently, an analysis by Katz and collaborators showed that in-hospital and CICU mortality remained relatively stable between 1989 and 2006 and presented only a modest actual decrease over time after adjusting for age, sex, and race, despite the substantial changes in patient characteristics (increase in co-morbidities in particular), diagnoses, and procedures observed over time [17].

Intensivist and cardiologist training and performance

CICU patients who used to be more stable and have less organic dysfunction have progressively moved into a pattern of increased patient complexity similar to that observed in general ICUs. ICU physician staffing varies widely and the challenge posed by the current situation is the imminent shortage of physicians trained in critical care medicine who are able to meet such demands. Additionally, CICU cardiologists nowadays need to expand their training in critical care medicine in order to be able to adequately manage a wider range of co-morbidities and clinical complications.

Back in 2002, one of the authors of this text (Knobel, E.) was one of the founders and first head of the Study Group on Intensive Care and Cardiology ("GETIC" – Grupo de Estudos em Terapia Intensiva e Cardiologia), which worked as a branch of the Brazilian Society of Cardiology and aimed to provide continuing medical education on critical care medicine applied to patients with acute cardiac diseases. The group

also provided training on the cardiologic aspects of critically ill patients. Such initiatives, as well as the abbreviated critical care rotations that are part of the cardiovascular disease fellowship training programme, are important and have contributed to increasing the critical care skills of cardiologists. Nevertheless, they have not turned cardiologists into intensivists, but remain cardiologists with a special interest in critical care and who are able to assist the critically ill cardiac patients who are admitted to the CICU.

According to the American Board of Internal Medicine, training requirements for cardiologists seeking critical care certification must include at least 12 months of appropriately supervised clinical activity directly related to the care of critically ill patients and in cases of dual certification (critical care medicine/cardiovascular disease), the minimum time required in clinical training is 30 months (see Tab. 4) [21].

In regard to staffing strategies, the best setup for ICU/physician specialty (intensivists versus cardiologists trained in critical care medicine versus non-intensivists) in relation to patient outcomes remains controversial. Although a number of studies have consistently shown that better patient outcomes are obtained when patients are treated by critical care specialists, more recent studies have shown otherwise. A systematic re-

Tab. 4   American Board of Internal Medicine (ABIM) training requirements for specialists in cardiovascular disease seeking critical care certification (data from [21])

Criteria for admission to the critical care medicine examination
▪ Three years of accredited fellowship training in cardiovascular disease, including the care of patients in critical care units
▪ Certification by ABIM
▪ One year of accredited clinical fellowship training in critical care medicine.

Training requirements
▪ Training in critical care medicine must include at least 12 months (up to one month vacation allowed)
▪ For dual certification (critical care medicine/cardiovascular disease), the minimum total full-time training is 30 months.

Procedural requirements
▪ Airway management and endotracheal intubation
▪ Ventilator management and non-invasive ventilation
▪ Insertion and management of chest tubes, and thoracentesis
▪ Advanced cardiac life support (ACLS)
▪ Placement of arterial, central venous, and pulmonary artery balloon flotation catheters
▪ Calibration and operation of hemodynamic recording systems
▪ Proficiency in use of ultrasound to guide central line placement and thoracentesis is strongly recommended.

view of 17 studies showed that ICUs with a high-intensity staffing strategy (a mandatory intensivist consultation or closed ICU in which care is entirely directed by the intensivist) were associated with lower hospital mortality in 94 % of studies (RR for mortality = 0.71, 95 % CI 0.62–0.82), lower ICU mortality in 93 % of studies (RR for mortality = 0.61, 95 % CI 0.50–0.75), reduced hospital length of stay (LOS) in 77 % of studies, and reduced ICU LOS in 78 % of studies [22]. More recently, an analysis based on data from over 100,000 ICU patients surprisingly revealed higher mortality rates among patients managed by intensivist specialists as compared to those managed by other physicians. The authors explained the results as being due to the confounding effects of unrecognised or unmeasured contributors to illness severity. The authors also considered the possibility that the intensivists' greater use of procedures might have led to more complications, with increased morbidity and mortality [23].

As for the care of critical cardiac patients, previous studies have shown that patients with acute coronary syndromes receive better outcomes and a higher probability of receiving effective medical therapy and interventional procedures when patients were treated by cardiologists [24, 25].

A recent study evaluated the association between specialty ICU care and hospital mortality and ICU LOS in a diverse population of 84,182 patients with six different diagnoses (AMI among them) in 124 ICUs (35 % admitted to a general ICU, 57 % to the ideal specialty ICU, and 8 % to a non-ideal specialty ICU). Patients were admitted to a specialty ICU either because it was the right specialty ICU for their diagnosis (ideal specialty ICU; e.g., AMI, CICU) or because the right specialty ICU was full or unavailable (non-ideal specialty ICU). The results failed to demonstrate any survival or LOS benefit of specialised units compared to general ICUs, but risk-adjusted mortality was significantly greater for patients admitted to non-ideal specialty ICUs [26]. The general ability of ICUs in treating underlying conditions common to critically ill patients may play an important role on performance even when dealing with specific conditions. On the other hand, when critically ill patients presenting specific conditions were treated in the ideal specialised unit, their outcome was as good as that of general ICU.

ICU and CICU management issues

Both intrinsic and extrinsic factors influence ICU structure and organisation. The size and other characteristics of the population that use the service are the main determinants of ICU type and capacity. Therefore, an ICU located in an area where emergency cases are frequent must have a structure distinct from one in which elective surgeries are more common or cardiovascular diseases predominate. On the other hand, changes in health-care reimbursement rules and insurance coverage may also impact ICU structure and distribution of critically ill patients. Depending on the demand for ICU beds, stand-alone units may be necessary, such as a neurointensive care unit (NICU), trauma intensive care unit (TICU), or cardiac ICU (CICU). The existence of a unique multispecialty ICU for treating critically ill patients rather than multiple separate subspecialty units has a great impact on hospital resource allocation and cost rationalisation strategies. Multispecialty units lead to reduced duplication of expensive technologies and staff.

Another issue involved with the hospital decision on structure and resource allocation is the existence of high-dependency care units (HDCU) such as post-anaesthesia care units, intermediate care, or step-down units. Table 5 shows five common CICU models that are available to care for the critically ill cardiac patients, and that differ from each other in structure, organisation, function, and type of staff.

From an economic perspective, despite possible benefits, specialised critical care units consume high levels of resources, while costs are expected to continue to increase as new technologies and procedures become available. On the other hand, demand for CICU beds varies substantially over time, which compromises the efficiency in using the resources, especially human resources, which represent a major cost factor in this setting.

In a retrospective cohort study that compared clinical outcomes of intermediate-risk patients hospitalised either in a coronary care unit or in an intermediate coronary care unit, the use of interventional procedures (coronary angiography, angioplasty, and coronary artery surgery), the incidence of myocardial infarction, length of stay, and mortality did not differ between groups.

Tab. 5   CICU models to attend critically ill cardiac patients

Type of CICU	Characteristics
CICU inside the ICU	CICU works as a subunit area under the command and control of the multispecialty ICU. Usually, dedicated beds intended for cardiac patients may be used for other patients in cases of volume peaks. An on-duty cardiologist should always be present in the unit, but this seldom occurs worldwide.
CICU adjacent to ICU	CICU is separate but located adjacent to multispecialty ICU.
	Critically ill cardiac patients which are presented with multiple co-morbidities are often transferred to the ICU.
CICU integrated to ICU	A separate CICU works integrated with a multispecialty ICU. Critically ill cardiac patients are admitted to an ICU and stay there for the first 24 hours and then are transferred to CICU once they stabilize. More stable patients may be admitted directly to the CICU. Cardiologists must be available to support patient care while patient is in the general ICU.
Stand-alone CICU	CICU is totally independent from the multispecialty ICU. Duplication of equipment and staff is required. Cardiologists working in such units must have been trained in critical care medicine.
Universal bed care	Patients stay in the same room during hospitalization with the appropriate level of care brought to them. Facility design, organization, equipment and staff must be able to accommodate all critical care needs of the CICU patient from admission to recovery, including telemetry, space for ambulation and family visitation.

The only difference was that patients admitted to the intermediate coronary care unit represented a lower cost. This indicates that intermediate CCUs are a cheaper and safer alternative for intermediate-risk patients [27] and that CICUs should be saved for high-risk patients.

During our 32 years of experience heading the Critical Care Unit of Hospital Israelita Albert Einstein in São Paulo, Brazil, from 1972 to 2000 all patients with AMI were first admitted to the ICU. The average length of stay of these patients admitted to the ICU with AMI was one day. After this period, stable patients were moved to the general intermediate care unit for monitoring and/or telemetry and vigilance.

After the creation of a specific intermediate coronary care unit in 2003, only cardiac patients with hemodynamic instability and/or severe arrhythmias were admitted to a specific cardiac unit located inside the ICU. Otherwise, patients were admitted directly to the intermediate coronary care unit [28]. Of note is the fact that during the whole period all cardiologists who integrated the critical care team were qualified and held a certificate on general intensive care. The inverse situation was also true; i.e., intensivists were qualified and trained to manage cardiac disturbances of critically ill patients. This situation certainly contributed to the good quality of the care delivered in this critical care unit department.

Benefits and drawbacks of a separate CICU

CICUs are the most common type of specialty intensive care unit and serve a purpose different than that of an ICU. In general, CICU patients are less critically ill, have fewer co-morbidities and less organic dysfunction, require more monitoring than therapeutic interventions, and benefit from a quiet and lower-stress environment [29]. The creation of a separate CICU usually requires a large investment in equipment and staff, which represents higher costs. Additionally, there is always the risk that the CICU may be underused. On the other hand, multispecialty ICUs allow greater efficiency in resource allocation. They also allow consistency in the application of evidence-based critical care and ensure standards of care for patients with multiple co-morbidities and complications [30].

Nosocomial infections are a major concern that leads to complications in 25 to 33 % of the patients admitted to ICUs. The most common nosocomial infections are pneumonia related to mechanical ventilation, intra-abdominal infections following trauma or surgery, and bacteremia derived from intravascular devices [31]. On the other hand, CICU patients are less vulnerable to acquire nosocomial infections than patients admitted to multispecialty ICUs, mainly because of the lower rates of invasive device usage [32, 33]. Besides that, the stressful ICU environment imposed by constant staff activity, various beeping machines, and alarms constantly going off makes it difficult for cardiac patients to rest adequately, and this may predispose patients to ICU syndrome or psychosis [34]. CICUs tend to be a less-stressful environment, allowing more privacy for both patient and family. Tables 6 and 7 show the main benefits and drawbacks of multispecialty ICU and separate CICU.

When is a stand-alone CICU to be created

The major factors involved in the decision to create a stand-alone CICU to provide specialised critical care to a subset of cardiac patients who experience an acute event, are local patient demand followed by market differentiation (or positioning). High-volume ICUs (with over 40 beds) tend to specialise primarily on the basis of disease prevalence, level of staff specialisation

Tab. 6   Main benefits of multispecialty ICU and separate CICU

	ICU	CCU
Quality of care	▪ Usually staffed by physicians trained in critical care medicine ▪ Optimization and uniformization of critical care medicine processes of care ▪ Better handling of comorbidities and multiorgan dysfunction	▪ Overly specialized staff in cardiac care ▪ Processes focused on cardiac conditions allowing better coordination of care and implementation of guidelines. ▪ Up-to-date knowledge easier to maintain ▪ Lower risk of nosocomial infections ▪ Less stressful environment
Management issues	▪ Lower operational costs due to convergence of different specialties that allows staff and equipment sharing enhancing efficiency ▪ Better optimization of volume levels	▪ Marketing differentiation ▪ Lower levels of diagnostic diversity may facilitate diagnostic coding and reimbursement

Tab. 7   Main drawbacks of multispecialty ICU and separate CICU

	ICU	CCU
Quality of care	▪ Less focused process of care ▪ More difficult to be kept up-to-date on all subspecialties protocols and guidelines ▪ Intensivists not used to handle disease-specific conditions – demands cardiologist support for the decision making process ▪ Increased cross-infections among seriously ill patients ▪ Noisy and stressful environment	▪ Cardiologists not adequately trained in critical care medicine in most units ▪ Tendency to fail of standardization of critical care across different specialized units
Management issues	▪ Potential to lose patients who value specialized cardiac care ▪ More complex administrative structure	▪ Focused care for a limited range of critically ill patients leads to lower efficiency in resources use ▪ Lowers hospital ability to handle volume peaks

required, and predictability and similarity of recovery patterns. Based on these criteria, CICUs tend to be among the first specialties to become a separate unit. Hospitals with smaller demand for ICU beds may consider building a CICU as part of a comprehensive cardiac centre in order to be recognised in the market for a certain specialty and thereby gain a share in the market. In this case, peaks of volume may be a concern, especially when units are not adjacent, and this limits their flexibility [35].

Conclusion

In summary, a lot has been written about the care delivered in the various types of critical care unit. Nevertheless, little and controversial information exists on the most efficient and appropriate overall design, structure, functionality, cost-effectiveness, and outcomes of such units. It is not clear whether a separate stand-alone CICU is more beneficial than a general ICU. Based on our experience, we conclude that to provide better care for critically ill cardiac patients, the quality of the caring processes and the participation of an integrated multi-professional team that is trained in critical care medicine are more important than the structure or location of the critical care unit.

Each hospital must define its structure based on volume, disease prevalence, and marketing strategies (which may consider patient and family satisfaction, proximity to the catheterisation laboratory, marketing differentiation, etc.). Because of the high costs involved in building and sustaining unique critical care units, patient demand should be the primary consideration when deciding whether or not to open a separate CICU. Published literature does not support the assumption that such investments will improve patient outcomes. Nevertheless, once hospital managers have decided to create a stand-alone CICU, they must keep in mind that this should not compromise the quality of general critical care of critically ill cardiac patients who present multiple non-cardiac complications.

This can only be achieved if the CICU is staffed with specially trained cardiologists who hold dual certification in both cardiology and critical care medicine. On the other hand, the care of critically ill cardiac patients that is delivered in a general ICU by intensivists must receive the support of cardiologists in order to ensure that timely and appropriate evidence-based cardiac strategies are offered to patients. There is an urgent need for well-designed studies that produce scientific evidence on this unresolved issue and that may guide hospitals in their future decisions.

The authors

Elias Knobel, MD, PhD, MACP, FAHA, FCCM[1]
Marcia Makdisse, MD, MSc, PhD[2]
Marcos Knobel, MD[3]
[1] Director emeritus and founder of the ICU | Hospital Israelita Albert Einstein | São Paulo, Brazil | Associate Professor of Medicine | Federal University of São Paulo | São Paulo, Brazil
[2] Head of Cardiology | Hospital Israelita Albert Einstein | São Paulo, Brazil
[3] Medical Coordinator – Coronary Care Unit | Hospital Israelita Albert Einstein | São Paulo, Brazil

Address for correspondence
Elias Knobel
Hospital Israelita Albert Einstein
Av. Albert Einstein 627/701
CEP 05651-901 Morumbi
São Paulo, Brazil
E-mail: knobel@einstein.br

References

1. Kelley MA, Angus D, Chalfin DB, Crandall ED, Ingbar D, Johanson W, et al. The critical care crisis in the United States: a report from the profession. Chest. 2004;125(4):1514–17.
2. Julian DG. Treatment of cardiac arrest in acute myocardial ischemia and infarction. Lancet 1961;ii:840–4.
3. Killip T, Kimball JT. Treatment of myocardial infarction in a coronary care unit. A two year experience with 250 patients. Am. J. Cardiol. 1967;20(4):457–64.
4. Quinn T, Weston C, Birkhead J, Walker L, Norris R. Redefining the coronary care unit: an observational study of patients admitted to hospital in England and Wales in 2003. QJM. 2005;98(11):797–802.
5. Braunwald E. Evolution of the management of acute myocardial infarction: a 20th century saga. Lancet. 1998;352(9142):1771–4.
6. Mangan B. Structuring cardiology services for the 21st century. Am. J. Crit. Care. 1996;5(6):406–11.
7. Khush KK, Rapaport E, Waters D. The history of the coronary care unit. Can J Cardiol. 2005 Oct;21(12):1041–5.

8. Valente S, Lazzeri C, Sori A, Giglioli C, Bernardo P, Gensini GF. The recent evolution of coronary care units into intensive cardiac care units: the experience of a tertiary center in Florence. J Cardiovasc Med (Hagerstown). 2007;8(3):181–7.

9. Katz JN, Turer AT, Becker RC. Cardiology and the critical care crisis: a perspective. J. Am. Coll. Cardiol. 2007;49(12):1279–82.

10. Joint Commission on Accreditation of Healthcare Organizations. Organizational Models and Patient Care in the ICU. In: Joint Commission Resources, Inc. (JCR). USA, 2004, pp 50–5.

11. Eagle KA, Goodman SG, Avezum A, Budaj A, Sullivan CM, López-Sendón J. Practice variation and missed opportunities for reperfusion in ST-segment-elevation myocardial infarction: findings from the Global Registry of Acute Coronary Events (GRACE). Lancet. 2002;359(9304):373–7.

12. Haupt MT, Bekes CE, Brilli RJ, Carl LC, Gray AW, Jastremski MS, et al. Guidelines on critical care services and personnel: Recommendations based on a system of categorization of three levels of care. Crit. Care Med. 2003;31(11):2677–83.

13. Hasin Y, Danchin N, Filippatos GS, Heras M, Janssens U, Leor J, et al. Recommendations for the structure, organization, and operation of intensive cardiac care units. Eur. Heart J. 2005;26(16):1676–82.

14. Cullen DJ, Keene R, Waternaux C, Kunsman JM, Caldera DL, Peterson H. Results, charges, and benefits of intensive care for critically ill patients: update 1983. Crit. Care Med. 1984;12(2):102–6.

15. Le Gall JR, Brun-Buisson C, Trunet P, Latournerie J, Chantereau S, Rapin M. Influence of age, previous health status, and severity of acute illness on outcome from intensive care. Crit. Care Med. 1982;10(9):575–7.

16. Katz JN, Turer AT, Becker RC. Cardiology and the critical care crisis: a perspective. J. Am. Coll. Cardiol. 2007;49(12):1279–82.

17. Katz JN, Shah BR, Volz EM, Horton JR, Shaw LK, Newby LK, et al. Evolution of the coronary care unit: clinical characteristics and temporal trends in healthcare delivery and outcomes. Crit. Care Med. 2010;38(2):375–81.

18. August C, Clinical and Echocardiographic Correlates of Symptomatic Tachydysrhythmias After Noncardiac Thoracic Surgery. 1995;108:349–54.

19. Sprung J, Abdelmalak B, Gottlieb A, Mayhew C, Hammel J, Levy PJ, et al. Analysis of risk factors for myocardial infarction and cardiac mortality after major vascular surgery. Anesthesiology. 2000; 93(1):129–40.

20. Saitto C, Ancona C, Fusco D, Arcà M, Perucci CA. Outcome of patients with cardiac diseases admitted to coronary care units: a report from Lazio, Italy. Med Care. 2004;42(2):147–54.

21. Critical Care Medicine Policies. Available at: <http://www.abim.org/certification/policies/imss/ccm.aspx#special>. Accessed February 26, 2010.

22. Pronovost PJ, Angus DC, Dorman T, Robinson KA, Dremsizov TT, Young TL. Physician staffing patterns and clinical outcomes in critically ill patients: a systematic review. JAMA. 2002;288(17):2151–62.

23. Levy MM, Rapoport J, Lemeshow S, Chalfin DB, Phillips G, Danis M. Association between critical care physician management and patient mortality in the intensive care unit. Ann. Intern. Med. 2008;148(11):801–9.

24. Schreiber TL, Elkhatib A, Grines CL, O'Neill WW. Cardiologist versus internist management of patients with unstable angina: treatment patterns and outcomes. J. Am. Coll. Cardiol. 1995;26(3):577–82.

25. Jollis JG, DeLong ER, Peterson ED, Muhlbaier LH, Fortin DF, Califf RM, et al. Outcome of acute myocardial infarction according to the specialty of the admitting physician. N. Engl. J. Med. 1996;335(25):1880–7.

26. Lott JP, Iwashyna TJ, Christie JD, Asch DA, Kramer AA, Kahn JM. Critical illness outcomes in specialty versus general intensive care units. Am. J. Respir. Crit. Care Med. 2009;179(8):676–83.

27. Calvin JE, Klein L, VandenBerg E, Parrillo JE. The intermediate CCU admission: a preliminary study. Heart Dis. 2001;3(1):18–23.

28. Cheng DC, Byrick RJ, Knobel E. Structural models for intermediate care areas. Crit. Care Med. 1999;27(10):2266–71.

29. Draper EA, Wagner DP, Knaus WA. The use of intensive care: a comparison of a university and community hospital. Health Care Financ Rev. 1981;3(2):49–64.

30. Takala, J. Organisation of intensive care. In 25 years of progress and innovation in Intensive Care Medicine, Kuhlen R, Moreno R, Ranieri M and Rhodes Q, eds, MWV, Berlin, pg 343–50, 2007.

31. Eggimann P, Pittet D. Infection control in the ICU. Chest. 2001;120(6):2059–93.

32. Richards MJ, Edwards JR, Culver DH, Gaynes RP. Nosocomial infections in coronary care units in the United States. National Nosocomial Infections Surveillance System. Am. J. Cardiol. 1998;82(6):789–93.

33. National Nosocomial Infections Surveillance (NNIS) System Report, data summary from January 1992 through June 2004, issued October 2004. Available at http://www.cdc.gov/ncidod/dhqp/pdf/nnis/2004NNISreport.pdf.

34. McGuire BE, Basten CJ, Ryan CJ, Gallagher J. Intensive care unit syndrome: a dangerous misnomer. Arch. Intern. Med. 2000;160(7):906–9.

35. The Advisory Board Company. Lesson #6 – Minimize Specialization to Maximize Efficiency. In: Hospital of the future, The Advisory Board Company. USA, 2007, pp 26–7.

Jorge Luiz da Rocha Paranhos, Gustavo Trindade Henriques-Filho
and Odin Barbosa da Silva

Do we need specific neurocritical ICUs?

Introduction

Although intensive care medicine (ICM) is a new medical specialty, it has for many years been modifying the scenario and evolution of many nosological entities and changed the history of medicine.

Since the appearance of the iron lungs for prolonged ventilatory support in 1928, introduced by Drinker and Shaw [1], later used in the treatment of patients who were victims of the poliomyelitis epidemic in the 50s, until the more recent 2009 pandemic influenza caused by the A H1N1 virus, intensive treatment has improved the prognosis and reduced morbidity and mortality of patients, with technological advances both in terms of diagnosis as well as monitoring and therapy. Therefore, throughout this period of improvements, the natural history of many diseases has been modified in a number of different medical areas.

Many infectious diseases have become easier to treat with intensive care support. AIDS would have resulted in many more victims if immunocompromised patients did not receive adequate support for severe sepsis, patients with *pneumocystis* pneumonia (PCP) were not mechanically ventilated or if carriers of neurotoxoplasmosis did not receive the necessary neurocritical care.

Accidental tetanus, described since the time of Hippocrates, had a drastic reduction of mortality since the critical care treatment was established as it is nowadays. In several series of cases the lethality ranges from 30 to 50%, being the lethality of Brazil in 2004 of 31.05% [2], while in the state of Pernambuco (northeast of Brazil), in the period between 1998 and 2004, it was 12.6% [3] – mainly to the fact that the treatment was exclusively carried out in an Intensive Care Unit (ICU) specialised in infectious diseases, with a well trained team and with specific protocols.

Even human rabies has become today a disease to be treated in intensive care units. The first national protocol for the treatment of this disease was established in Brazil in Recife-PE (Protocol of Recife), after the therapeutic success with cure and recovery of a patient based on a treatment that was originally described in the United States of America (Protocol of Milwaukee). This was the third case of cure in the world [4, 5].

Among critically ill patients suffering from hematologic diseases, specialised ICU treatment seems to considerably improve the prognosis, especially because it allows faster access to the intensive support of a trained and experienced medical team. Studies show that the mortality rate of those hematological patients increases significantly when they develop complications from the initial disease itself or secondary diseases to the treatment, such as bone marrow aplasia, sepsis, respiratory insufficiency and acute renal insufficiency requiring dialysis therapy. Data from Brazilian specialised units show a coefficient of specific ICU mortality of 50.9 % between 2004 and 2007 in São Paulo (University of São Paulo – USP), and of 47.9 % between 2005 and 2008 in Recife (Haematology Hospital of Pernambuco – HEMOPE).

In cardiology it was not any different. In 1907, Heinrich Dräger developed and patented a resuscitation device that was activated by compressed air or oxygen. In the 30s, Poulton and Barack introduced a respiratory system by continuous positive airway pressure to treat cardiogenic acute pulmonary oedema. Coronary units (CU) were only created at the beginning of the 60s, initially only for patients with myocardial infarction (MI). These became units of reference for the treatment of patients with many other cardiocirculatory complications, led by skilled professionals in clinical, interventionist and surgical cardiology – with well-established protocols written by international societies such as the American Heart Association [6].

In the 50s, mortality of patients with MI was of nearly 30 %, and it was twice this amount in cases of cardiogenic shock. With the advent of ICUs, and later the CUs, this mortality fell almost by half, essentially because of better control of arrhythmia. In the 80s there was a drastic reduction in mortality during the acute phase of MI with the use of fibrinolytics. After this, with the new processes of percutaneous intervention, invasive (and minimally invasive) haemodynamic monitoring, increasingly more specific titrated drugs, surgery with less risk and more advanced technology, the death incidence in patients with MI reached the current 6 to 10 %.

Neurointensivism

Patients with acute neurological diseases are basically subject to two types of injuries:
1. Primary injury, for which we can often act only with preventive measures, such as the adequate treatment of systemic arterial hypertension and *diabetes mellitus*, dietary control and medication for dyslipidaemia, and the campaigns against smoking, alcohol consumption and traffic accidents (the exception to this is the treatment with fibrinolytics in the initial hours of a stroke and neurosurgical interventions)
2. Secondary injury, situations that are potentially preventable and treatable by adequate medical treatment

These secondary lesions are responsible for most of the deaths of neurocritical patients, and could be avoided through proper monitoring and periodical evaluations for early diagnosis and treatment of these complications. Thus, the concern with the prevention and rapid and effective treatment of complications such as hypoxia, hypotension, hyperthermia, dysglycaemia and seizures, among others, can save many lives. Clearly, treating such patients in a unit that has expertise in neurocritical diseases makes this task easier. Therefore, there is a great need today for specialised teams to monitor and carry out quick diagnosis and treatment. But this concern is not a new one. In the middle of the 20th century, Europe was devastated by the poliomyelitis epidemic, mentioned above, and big wards were created to offer negative pressure ventilatory support and intensive care nursing – initially in Denmark, but later also in countries such as England, Germany and France and then throughout the continent. Treatments in these units were carried out by teams coordinated by pulmonologists and neurologists, becoming perhaps the first neurological intensive care units [7].

In the following decades, advances occurred in anaesthesiology, particularly for neurosurgery, generating demand for postoperative units. However, since at that time there was no advanced technology, a large proportion of those neurocritical patients died or had severe sequelae, which did not stimulate the creation of specialised units.

However, in the 80s, neurology and neurosurgery scientists started to invest more in patient diagnosis and therapy, and thus the first specialised units emerged, encompassing postneurosurgical patients, as well as clinical patients with strokes, seizures, encephalitis and neuromuscular diseases.

Currently, the neurointensive care units use a multidisciplinary approach, with teams formed by nurses, physiotherapists and phonoaudiologists trained to deal with the particularities of neurocritical patients; and the doctors in this area have a wider view of intensive medicine, not only related to the framework of the neurological case itself, but also and particularly on the principles of haemodynamic monitoring, mechanical ventilation, management of invasive methods of treatment of multiple organ dysfunctions, and pathophysiologic knowledge – all that can cause a secondary injury in a neurocritical patient.

Therefore, by the current level of knowledge, a neurointensivist doctor must have all this wide-ranging, complex training, aside from knowing about the physiology of intracranial pressure, cerebral maetabolism, cerebral blood flow, post-operative care in neurosurgery and the multisystemic complications affecting acute neurological patients. This kind of preparation is more commonly found among intensivist doctors than in other specialties, which allows them to become neurointensivist doctors more easily than the neurologists and neurosurgeons themselves.

Finally, it is important to be conscious of the necessity to treat particular patients as a team, to better face the pathophysiologic complexity and the potential complications of each case. This team effort must always be stimulated by and composed of clinical neurologists, neurosurgeons and neurointensivists, all exchanging knowledge and contributions with each other with the common aim to reduce mortality and sequels in patients [8].

Are there advantages in having specialised units in neurointensivism?

There is no doubt that having doctors specialised in intensive care medicine in the ICU is important. Studies show that units with intensivist doctors present lower mortality, better resource allocation with lower costs, and also shorter length of stay than the units without permanent doctors or without specialists [9].

Clearly, patients with a severe neurological condition could be adequately treated in general intensive care units not necessarily specialised in neurointensivism. However, well-defined and strictly followed protocols are more easily implemented in specialised units, as it has already been observed in specialised CUs and ICUs in other areas.

This also is the case in neurocritical units. Studies involving patients suffering traumatic brain injury (TBI) show reduction in ICU mortality from 20 % to 13.5 %, and hospital mortality from 24.5 % to 20.8 % after the routine use of measures defined through protocols guided by evidence-based medicine [10]. Other studies also show that teams which follow strict conduct protocols on severe neurological patients, with more aggressive monitoring and treatment methods, achieve better results in terms of morbidity and therefore of quality of life [11, 12, 13].

A paper by Diringer and Edwards showed that patients with intracerebral haemorrhage have 3.5 times higher mortality when they are admitted and managed in a general ICU, in relation to a neurointensive specialised unit [14], since here the protocols are followed more rigorously. Moreover, aside from these cases, in many other situations the neurological intensive care units can make a significant difference in terms of prognosis.

Up-to-date monitoring of neurocritical patients is an extremely complex task. Aside from ventilation, haemodynamic and metabolic monitoring techniques, commonly used for any critically ill patient in the ICU, many other techniques are essential in the management of these patients in particular. These vary from the necessity to carry out a more aggressive general monitoring, with capnography, invasive haemodynamic monitoring and more rigorous maetabolic evaluation exams, such as arterial and venous gasometry, lactate, glucose and sodium levels and core temperature; to monitoring techniques for intracranial pressure (ICP) and cerebral perfusion pressure (CPP), brain temperature, jugular bulb saturation and the global cerebral oxygen extraction, brain oxygen pressure, cerebral blood flow evaluation by transcranial Doppler, laser Doppler fluxometry, fluxometry by thermal diffusion and xenon clearance, electroencephalography, sequential neuro-imaging monitoring and brain tissue metabolism analysis by microdialysis, among others.

It is well known that for all monitoring methods the evaluation in itself does not change the prognosis; instead, it is the speed and efficiency in changing the clinical management after the data is provided that can do this. This is classically known for the haemodynamic variables obtained by the Swan-Ganz catheter, as well as for the monitoring of ICP and CPP, as described by authors who found an increase of favourable outcomes from 40.4 % to 59.6 %, by proper handling of ICP and CPP monitoring, among other cares, in traumatic brain injury patients [12]. In specialised units such monitoring methods are more frequently used than in general ICUs. Also, control routines and therapeutic measures are more effective as a result of the analysis of the data.

In relation to the specific techniques for neurointensive monitoring, specialised units provide better conditions to acquire and update them than general units, and they can offer better training to the professionals involved in the treatment.

Aside from the techniques mentioned above, clinical, surgical and intensive neurological management and treatment has been modified in recent years with a significant impact on the recovery of these critically ill patients.

Patients with ischaemic stroke until recent years had a poor prognosis in terms of sequels and quality of life. Beginning in the 70s, stroke units began to appear throughout the world, the true precursors of the neurointensive care units that we have nowadays. In 1995, it was established that the use of intravenous thrombolysis in the first three hours of cerebral ischaemia carries a benefit for the patient in terms of recovery – reducing by 30% the number of individuals dependent on care after three months. It is necessary to treat 10 cases to have this beneficial effect in one patient (NNT) [15]. More recent studies show the same efficacy when the intravenous thrombolysis is performed up to four and a half hours after the start of the event, extending the therapeutic window to carry out an intra-arterial thrombolysis (after an angiography) to up to six hours [16]. Moreover, other techniques have been described to expand the therapeutic possibilities, such as mechanical intravascular thrombolysis and ultrasound thrombolysis.

Among victims of haemorrhagic stroke, both patients with intracerebral haematoma and subarachnoid haemorrhage (SAH) have had benefits from neurointensive management.

It is well known that an intracerebral haematoma is the kind of stroke which most likely leads to death and functional incapacity. Up to 52% of patients die in the first month, only close to 38% survive the first year, and only 20% present independent physical and intellectual activities six months after the event. Classically, the factors determining poor prognosis are age over 75 years, arriving with a Glasgow Coma Scale less than nine, having a volume of supratentorial haematoma greater than 10 ml and infraten-

torial haematoma greater than 3 ml, an interval between bleeding and surgery – when indicated – longer than eight hours, and early rebleeding, which occurs in up to 38% of cases in the first hours of the initial episode. Nevertheless, some authors suggest that admission to a non-specialised ICU is also a factor which contributes to a poor prognosis, and that when a patient is treated in a neurointensive unit, the favourable impact is significant with respect to mortality, morbidity, length of hospital stay and costs [14, 17].

SAH also is a condition which leads to considerable morbidity and mortality. Up to 15% of patients die before receiving medical attention, 40 to 50% die within 30 days after the event, and of the survivors nearly half are left with severe sequelae. The two major neurological complications, aside from the multisystemic dysfunction that can occur in these patients, are rebleeding, which occurs in up to 20% of patients in the first two weeks of treatment when the aneurysm is not treated by surgery or interventional radiology – with a mortality of nearly 50% among these patients –, and cerebral vasospasm, the leading cause of morbidity and mortality in patients who survive the bleeding events, which appears symptomatically in up to 36% of patients [18].

For rebleeding prevention, aside from the definitive treatment of the aneurysm which caused the SAH, the main strategy is rigorous control of the arterial pressure with well-defined objectives for patients before and after treatment of the aneurysm. As was mentioned before, protocols are better followed and practised when they are conducted in specialised units, but this specific type of management can equally be done in general ICUs [18].

Vasospasm requires specific diagnostic and therapeutic procedures. Monitoring with transcranial Doppler, measurement of ICP and CPP, of haemodynamic parameters and haematimetry, aside from sodium and magnesium levels, among other things, are determinant factors in the prevention and early diagnosis of ischaemia by low cerebral blood flow. Rigorous protocols must be followed and aggressive therapeutic measures taken in the face of a vasospasm diagnosis, whether clinical or endovascular. Therefore, patients with SAH must be treated in multidisciplinary services with trained and specialised teams, which theoretically results in a more effective practice of the procedures of this complex protocol.

Some authors suggest that patients submitted to neurosurgery for the treatment of ruptured cerebral aneurysm have a significantly lower mortality when treated in units that have access to multidisciplinary specialised care [19, 20], while others show a greater cost-effectiveness in the treatment of patients with SAH classified as clinically more severe (Hunt-Hess IV and V) through more aggressive and rigorous management protocols [21].

As for patients who suffer cardiac arrest, nearly 44 % survive initially, 30 % will be alive after 24 hours, 13 % after one month and 6 % after six months. It is estimated that only 15 % of resuscitated patients are discharged from hospital. Of those who survive the initial insult and do not wake up after resuscitation measures, nearly 98 % will not regain consciousness if they have a score lower than five in the Glasgow Coma Scale 48 hours after the arrest [22].

In recent years, based on the knowledge that the cerebral damage happens not only during the arrest, but also after resuscitation, many therapeutic procedures have been described to minimise hypoxic brain injury, such as adequate maintenance and control of arterial pressure, control of glucose, sodium and body temperature, as well as adequate haemodynamic support, ventilation and nutrition. Moreover, it has been shown that the induction of mild hypothermia leads to an increased survival in six months, with an NNT of seven [23], and a reduction of functional limitations in these individuals, with an NNT of four to six [24]. This is due to the fact that this strategy has many beneficial effects for the central nervous system, such as reduction of cerebral oxygen consumption, suppression of chemical reactions related to the reperfusion injury, reduction of free radical reactions and release of intracellular calcium, modulation of apoptosis and of the inflammatory response, and the protection of lipoprotein membranes.

Some studies have shown that there are many reasons for not adhering to therapeutic hypothermia after cardiac arrest – among them the technical difficulty of carrying it out was cited. In fact, the whole protocol is complex and must be instituted quickly, which requires training, organisation and a multidisciplinary specialised team in dedicated units [25].

Also, as mentioned before, a specialised team is necessary to attend to patients with TBI. This type of injury has an incidence of 200,000 cases per year in the United States, which represents nearly one case every seven minutes, with one death every five minutes. It is the most significant cause of death in more than 50 % of trauma victims, the third leading cause of death in all age groups and the second for central nervous system disorders. There are an estimated 500,000 deaths annually by TBI in the world, 10 % occurring in Brazil, and for each death there are three patients with permanent neurological sequelae.

However, mortality has been reduced in recent years, firstly because of improvements in pre-hospital care, and secondly because of the protocols of care in emergency departments and ICUs. Aside from the data mentioned earlier, which reflect better results in terms of morbidity and mortality of TBI victims when treated under rigorous protocols, it is important to also highlight the study of Varelas et al. [26], which demonstrated a significant improvement in outcome of patients – with a reduction of the length of hospital stay and an increased number of patients who were released from the hospital – after being treated in specialised units led by a neurointensivist.

Finally, specialised neurointensive units also allow a more adequate training of the multidisciplinary teams involved in the care and encourage new professionals who are interested in pursuing this path to a new professional specialty, stimulating the creation of educational programmes aimed at improved practices and more focused studies, which are extremely important today in defining the best therapy to be provided to neurological patients.

The specialty, neurointensivism

In spite of the fact that the existence of units for neurointensive patient care does not currently obligate the presence of specialists in the area, in the last decade some steps were taken towards the recognition of this expertise. An important step was the acceptance in the United States by the United Council of Neurological Subspecialties (UCNS) of a new subspecialty dedicated to neurointensive care [27]. Medical training standards were created and a period of 2 years was established of which one year must comprise continuous work in an ICU. Moreover, the programme coordinator must dedicate at least 50 % of his/her medical activities to intensive care [28]. Fellowships are also available in several European countries [29].

The Neurocritical Care Society was founded in the United States in 2002, with the mission of promoting better quality of care for neurointensive patients, professional collaboration, research, training and education focused on this particular sort of patient – with an annual congress taking place since 2003 [30].

In Brazil, there are many intensive care units with considerable experience in the treatment of severe neurological diseases, although they are not exclusively dedicated to this sort of patient. However, a few essentially neurointensive units have opened in recent years. The professionals who work in these units are mainly specialists in intensive care medicine with training in neurointensivism, and receive support from neurosurgeons and clinical neurologists.

Conclusion

Specialised intensive therapy units for neurological patients seem to offer better diagnostic, therapeutic and monitoring support for neurocritical patients, in many cases reducing both mortality and the number of incapacitating neurological sequelae. These units offer better quality of life after hospital release, optimise investments and costs, and shorten hospital stay [31].

However, some authors also describe that a better prognosis is associated with the rigid protocols that must be followed, particularly when practised in larger units, where practical action and the reproducibility of these techniques increasingly improves the experience of these professionals.

Therefore, it is recommended that the creation of specialised units be stimulated in tertiary clinical centres with a high volume of neurological critical care patients, whereas in places that receive fewer patients with this characteristic at least one neurointensivist must be present in the team – the other professionals undergoing neurointensive care training on a regular basis. In both cases, multiprofessional and technological support must be available so that the best possible specialised diagnostics, monitoring and treatment are offered to patients.

The authors

Jorge Luiz da Rocha Paranhos, MD[1]
Gustavo Trindade Henriques-Filho, MD[2]
Odin Barbosa da Silva, MD[3]
[1] Intensive Care Medicine | Santa Casa da Misericórdia | São João del Rey-MG, Brasil
[2] Intensive Care Medicine | Hospital Santa Joana | HEMOPE | Hospital Universitário Oswaldo Cruz| Recife-PE, Brasil
[3] Intensive Care Medicine | Hospital Santa Joana | HEMOPE | Hospital da Restauração | Recife-PE, Brasil

Address for correspondence
    Jorge Luiz da Rocha Paranhos
    Intensive Care Medicine
    Santa Casa da Misericórdia
    Avenida Tiradentes 389
    36397–346 São João del Rey-MG, Brasil
    E-mail: jorgeparanhos@uol.com.br

References

1. Arregue D. Fisioterapia em terapia intensiva: resumo histórico da ventilação mecânica, 2009. [Online] Available on the internet: http://fisioterapiaemterapiaintensiva.blogspot. com/2009/05/resumo-historico-da-ventilacao-mecanica. html. Accessed in March 2010.
2. Ministério da Saúde. Departamento de Vigilância Epidemiológica. Secretaria de Vigilância em Saúde. Tabela de casos confirmados de tétano acidental. Brasil, 1990–2007, 2009 [Online]. Available on the internet: http://portal.saude.gov.br/portal/arquivos/pdf/casos_ conf_tetano_acidental.pdf. Accessed in March 2010.
3. Miranda-Filho DB et al. Tendência temporal do tétano acidental no período de 1981 a 2004 em Pernambuco com avaliação do impacto da assistência em unidade de terapia intensiva sobre a letalidade. Rev Soc Bras Med Trop, 2009; 42(1):54–7.
4. Ministério da Saúde. Departamento de Vigilância Epidemiológica. Secretaria de Vigilância em Saúde. Protocolo de tratamento de raiva humana no Brasil – Protocolo de Recife. 2009. [Online]. Available on the internet: http://portal.saude.gov.br/portal/arquivos/ pdf/protocolo_tratamento_raiva_humana.pdf.Accessed in March 2010.
5. Henriques-Filho GT et al. Treatment of human rabies following vampire bat bite using the modification of Milwaukee Protocol – Recife-Pernambuco, Brazil, 2009. MMWR (in press).

6. Julian DG. The history of coronary care units. Br Heart J, 1987; 57(6):497–502.

7. Ropper AH. Neurological intensive care. Ann Neurol 1992; 32:564–569.

8. Rincon F, Mayer SA. Neurocritical care: a distinct discipline? Curr Opin Crit Care, 2007; 13:115–21.

9. Pronovost PJ, Angus DC, Dorman T, et al. Physician staffing patterns and clinical outcomes in critically ill patients: a systematic review. JAMA, 2002; 288:2151–62.

10. Clayton TJ, Nelson RJ, Manara AR. Reduction in mortality from severe head injury following introduction of a protocol for intensive care management. Br J Anaesth, 2004; 93:761–7.

11. Elf K, Nilsson P, Enblad P. Outcome after traumatic brain injury improved byan organized secondary insult program and standardized neurointensive care. Crit Care Med, 2002; 30:2129–34.

12. Patel HC, Menon DK, Tebbs S, et al. Specialist neurocritical care and outcome from head injury. Intensive Care Med, 2002; 28:547–53.

13. Bulger EM, Nathens AB, Rivara FP, et al. Management of severe head injury: institutional variations in care and effect on outcome. Crit Care Med, 2002; 30:1870–6.

14. Diringer MN, Edwards DF. Admission to a neurologic/neurosurgical intensive care unit is associated with reduced mortality after intracerebral haemorrhage. Crit Care Med, 2001; 29:635–640.

15. The National Institute of Neurological Disorders and Stroke rtPA Stroke Study Group. Tissue plasminogen activator for acute ischemic stroke. NEngl J Med. 1995; 333:1581–1587.

16. Hacke W, Kaste M, Bluhmki E, Brozman M, Dávalos A, Guidetti D et al. Thrombolysis with alteplase 3 to 4,5 hours after Acute ischemic Stroke. NEngl J Med. 2008; 359:1317–1329.

17. Mirski MA, Chang CW, Cowan R. Impact of a neuroscience intensive care unit on neurosurgical patient outcomes and cost of care: evidence-based support for an intensivist-directed specialty ICU model of care. J Neurosurg Anesthesiol, 2001; 13:83–92.

18. Réa-Neto A, Maciel FMB, Paranhos JLR, Silveira RR, Plotnik R. CITIN – Curso de Imersão em Terapia Intensiva Neurológica. AMIB, 2006.

19. Solomon RA, Mayer SA, Tarmey JJ. Relationship between the volume of craniotomies for cerebral aneurysm performed at New York state hospitals and in-hospital mortality. Stroke, 1996; 27:13–17.

20. Berman MF, Solomon RA, Mayer SA, et al. Impact of hospital-related factors on outcome after treatment of cerebral aneurysms. Stroke, 2003; 34:2200–7.

21. Wilby MJ, Sharp M, Whitfield PC, et al. Cost-effective outcome for treating poor-grade subarachnoid hemorrhage. Stroke, 2003; 34:2508–11.

22. Pereira JCRG. Care of patient resuscitated from cardiac arrest. Rev Bras Ter Intensiva, 2008; 20(2).

23. The Hypothermia after Cardiac Arrest Study Group. Mild therapeutic hypothermia to improve the neurologic outcome after cardiac arrest. N Engl J Med, 2002; 346:549.

24. Treatment of comatose survivors of cardiac arrest with induced hypothermia. Bernard SA, Gray TW, Buist MD, et al.N Engl J Med 2002; 346: 557–63.

25. Bernard SA, Buist M. Inducer hypothermia in critical care medicine: a review. Crit Care Med, 2003; 31:2041–51.

26. Varelas PN, Eastwood D, Yun HJ, et al. Impact of a neurointensivist on outcomes in patients with head trauma treated in a neurosciences intensive care unit. J Neurosurg, 2006; 104:713–9.

27. Mayer SA, Coplin C, Chang C, et al. Program requirements for fellowship training in neurological intensive care: United Council for Neurologic Subspecialties guidelines. Neurocritical care 2006; 5:166–171.

28. Mayer SA, Coplin WM, Chang C, et al. Core curriculum and competencies for advanced training in neurological intensive care: United Council for Neurologic Subspecialties guidelines. Neurocritical care 2006; 5:159–165.

29. Wijdicks E.F.M. The Practice of Emergency and Critical Care Neurology. Oxford University Press Inc. New York, 2010.

30. Neurocritical Care Society – http://www.neurocriticalcare.org. Accessed in march 2010.

31. Menon D. Neurocritical care: turf label, organizational construct, or clinical asset? Curr Opin Crit Care, 2004; 10:91–3.

David M. Baron, Lars-Peter Kamolz and Philipp G.H. Metnitz

Designing burn ICUs

Introduction

With new discoveries and growing knowledge, intensive care medicine is a steadily evolving field. The increasing flow in research results has created the need for specialization in many areas. Especially burn care has undergone substantial changes over the last decades. Various studies have been conducted, and novel aspects have evolved in the care of severely burned patients. New procedures, new technology, and new protocols in the treatment of severely burned patients have generated a demand for specialists and specialized centres to provide optimal care for these patients [1, 2].

Most burns can be managed outside of burn centres. The American Burn Association has defined specific criteria for referral of patients to specialized burn centres [3] (see Tab. 1). A burn intensive care unit (ICU) is an important part of a burn unit or burn centre. It must be predominantly used to treat patients with burn injuries or patients with skin disorders, major wounds, or other problems requiring treatment similar to that of burn patients [3]. Burn ICUs should be incorporated into hospitals of maximal care and should be easy to reach by emergency teams via ground and air and accessible at any time. Several requirements need to be met before severely burned patients can be treated sufficiently and will be discussed in this chapter.

Infrastructure for the ICU

Equipment

Monitoring [1, 4]

Patients admitted to a burn ICU should be monitored according to the severity of their burns and concomitant trauma.

The need for both non-invasive and invasive monitoring devices (see Tab. 2) should be evaluated on a daily basis.

Mechanical ventilation [5, 6]

Most patients admitted to burns ICUs require mechanical ventilation (MV), which means that any burn ICU must be equipped with standard ICU ventilators. The recommendation is one ventilator per ICU bed + one for reserve + one for emergency admissions.

In case these ventilators do not support demand-CPAP, external CPAP devices should be available.

Ideally, all ventilators should have the possibility to be moved around, in order to accompany

Tab. 1 Burn centre referral criteria [adapted from ABA/ACS. Guidelines for the operation of burn centres.
J Burn Care Res 2007;28(1):134–141]

1.	Partial-thickness burns greater than 10 % of the body surface area
2.	Burns that involve the face, hands, feet, genitalia, perineum, or major joints
3.	Third-degree burns in any age group
4.	Electrical burns, including lightning injury
5.	Chemical burns
6.	Inhalation injury
7.	Burn injury in patients with pre-existing medical disorders that could complicate management, prolong recovery, or affect mortality
8.	Any patients with burns and concomitant trauma (such as fractures) in which the burn injury poses the greatest risk of morbidity or mortality. In such cases, if the trauma poses the greater immediate risk, the patient's condition may be stabilized initially in a trauma centre before transfer to a burn centre.
9.	Burned children in hospitals without qualified personnel or equipment for the care of children
10.	Burn injury in patients who will require special social, emotional, or rehabilitative intervention

Tab. 2 Monitoring

Non-invasive	Invasive
Non-invasive blood pressure	Arterial blood pressure
ECG	Central venous blood pressure
Pulse oxymetry	Pulmonary blood pressure
Urinary output	Thermodilution-based cardiac parameters
Temperature measurement	Intra-cranial pressure
Weight measurement	Intra-abdominal pressure
Hepatic ICG clearance	

the patient into the OR, the bath or other diagnostic and therapeutic interventions. If this is not available for all ventilators, then dedicated transport ventilators should be present. The recommendation is to have at least one transport ventilator for four ICU beds.

For cases with severe inhalation trauma and ARDS, supportive therapy (kinetic therapy, extracorporeal membrane oxygenation) should be available at least in the hospital.

Renal replacement therapy (RRT) [7]

Depending on the extent of the burns and pre-existing pathologies, several patients develop acute renal failure, often requiring haemo-dialysis. Therefore renal replacement therapy devices have to be available. The recommendation is to have at least one RRT machine for every three to four ICU beds.

Heating devices [8]

A sound skin barrier is prerequisite for proper thermo-regulation, making severely burned patients prone to a decrease of core temperature, especially during dressing changes and surgery [9]. Consequences are dysfunctions of the coagulatory and metabolic system, as well as delayed wound healing. Heating devices are thus specifically needed on burn ICUs. Currently, there exist different methods to heat patients:

- Laminar airflow heaters are the current standard of care. They allow for a proper heating of the room around the patient. Recommendation is to have 50 % of ICU beds equipped with laminar airflows.
- If laminar airflows are not available, other devices might be used to heat patients, including elevation of the room temperature, intravascular catheter devices etc.

Emergency equipment

As within every ICU, defibrillators and cardiac emergency carts must also be readily available at burn ICUs, especially since lightning victims and patients involved in high-voltage-accidents in particular tend to develop cardiac arrhythmias.

Other equipment

Additionally, a blood gas analyser should be available at every burn ICU. It must be able aside standard blood gas measurements to measure carboxy-haemoglobin (to rule out CO intoxication).

A bronchoscope should be on hand as a diagnostic and interventional tool.

An ultrasound-imaging device should be part of every burn ICU.

Space allocation

When designing burn ICUs, space allocation and strategic positioning are key factors.

- Each patient should have his own room, thus reducing the possibility of cross-contamination. Regardless of that fact, ICUs should be designed in accordance with the most up-to-date hygienic standards.
- In addition to the space needed for the patient's rooms, more space is required as storage area. All necessary medications have to be readily available, some of it requiring storage in refrigerators.
- Moreover, infusions, lines, materials for dressing changes, and catheters have to be stocked on the ICU.
- Space needs to be allotted for medical equipment and corresponding expendable materials.

- It is advisable to assign a separate meeting room for rounds.
- Finally, a central base, a lounge, and an on-call-room have to be included in the plan, which is not different from that of other ICUs.

Additional facilities

Primary care room

To triage incoming patients, a separate room should be available to apply primary care.

This room should be big enough to enable a smooth working process of the whole burn care team. Standard facilities for this room include a ventilator, a patient monitor, bronchoscopy and emergency equipment (intubation ready).

Additionally shower and tub to clean incoming patients have to be available. This must be a special device with integrated hygienic filters to prevent contamination of the burned skin area.

Operating room

It is advisable to have an operating room (OR) adjacent to the ICU in case the patient requires immediate surgical procedures such as escharotomy or fasciotomy.

This OP should have the possibility to be heated up, in order to prevent cooling of the severely burned patients during operations.

Transport time and distance between OR and ICU bed should be short.

Skin bank

Also a skin bank should be located close to or within the burn ICU or within the burn centre.

Tub room

- After skin-graft transplantation, scabs tend to form on the wounds. They can be removed more easily after first bathing the patient.
- Since mobility of most patients is limited, devices are needed to transport them from

their bed to the tub room. The tub itself has to be positioned in order that there is enough space around it for nurses and doctors to attend to the patient.

- Additional space is needed for monitoring devices and respiratory machines.

Due to the disintegrated skin-barrier it is easier for microbes to translocate into the blood [10]. Since the immune system of severely burned patients is compromised, infections of wounds and blood are common. Thus it is important to apply strict hygiene standards already in the planning phase of a burn ICU to decrease the risk of infection and contamination.

Infrastructure in the hospital

A burn ICU should be imbedded in a hospital of maximal care where specialists from several necessary disciplines are available for consultation (see Tab. 3). Even though the skin represents the primary injury, all organ systems can be affected during the course of hospitalization as a result of the inflammatory reaction caused by the burn. In addition to monitoring devices discussed earlier in this chapter, diagnostic tools need to be on hand 24 hours a day.

Tab. 3 Specialties which should be available for consultation [adapted from ABA/ACS. Guidelines for the operation of burn centres. J Burn Care Res 2007;28(1):134–141]

Indispensable	Important	Necessary
Anaesthesiology	Cardiology	Neurosurgery
General surgery	Gastroenterology	Obstetrics/ gynaecology
Infectious disease	Haematology	Pathology
Ophthalmology	Neurology	Psychiatry
Otolaryngology	Urology	
Paediatrics	Trauma/ Orthopaedic surgery	
Radiology		

First of all, a laboratory has to be within reach of the burn ICU to analyse blood samples immediately. Especially in the early stages, organ failure can develop very quickly, thereby requiring frequent examination of blood parameters.

Since surgeries involve large areas of the skin and can lead to major blood loss and require transfusion of blood products, a transfusion medicine facility should also be part of the burn trauma centre.

Another important diagnostic discipline is radiology. A mobile X-Ray, a CT scan and a MRI scan should also be available at all time.

Staffing

ICU Directors

Every burn ICU requires at least one board certified intensive care physician and a board certified plastic surgeon, both with experience in burn traumas. Together they should form the leadership of the ICU in a cooperative manner.

Physicians

Generally, staffing standards for burn ICUs are not different from other ICUs in that they require a physician present on the ICU 24 hours/7 days a week. However, due to the fact the critically ill burned patients need, alongside intensive care treatment, also frequent observation and intervention from plastic surgeons, both disciplines need to be available.

Due to the fact that staffing requirements for ICU are different between different countries, no rules can be given here. However, ideally a specialized intensivist and a specialized plastic surgeon should be specifically available for the burn ICU 24 hours/7 days a week.

Nursing staff

Certified nursing staff is one of the most important factors for a successful ICU. Severely burned patients demand more care than most other patients, and nurses are the ones spending most time with the patients. A nurse manager should be administratively responsible for the burn centre. As for patient/nurse ratio there should be a system in place to determine daily staffing needs.

Other staffing

During the course of the ICU stay body weight and muscle strength of the patients decrease. Due to the burns and surgeries, they also develop scars and stiff joints. Rehabilitation and physiotherapy play an important role in the reintegration into society. Most severely burned patients have to re-learn simple processes such as walking and eating. Specially trained physiotherapists and nutritionists help them to deal with these problems and to regain the ability to perform basic and also more complex movements. Recommendation is to have one physiotherapist specifically for the burn ICU.

Another important factor for a successful rehabilitation is taking care of the patient's psychological needs. On one hand psychologists help the patients to process the mental trauma imposed by the burns. On the other hand, they assist to provide the motivation needed by burn victims to successfully complete the difficult tasks of reintegration and rehabilitation.

Continuity of care programme

Beside the burn ICU, there has to be a step down and normal ward (for patients after transfer from the ICU or for patients with smaller burns, which require surgery) in the hospital. These wards have to be experienced in and equipped for treating burn patients (e.g. tub room).

Moreover there is a need for a specialized outpatient clinic, which will take of the burn patients after discharge or in case of smaller burns, which requires no hospital admission and no surgery. The outpatient clinic is also responsible for the planning of future rehabilitative and reconstructive needs.

Educational Program

The burn ICU should have an educational program for the medical staff. Residents of both disciplines should rotate on the burn ICU.

Research Program

The burn ICU should participate in basic, clinical or health science research and should demonstrate ongoing involvement in burn-related research

Conclusions

To design a burn centre, meticulous planning is required. Patients will only have a favourable outcome when doctors, nurses, and other members of the hospital work together as a team. Constant cooperation between the different members of the burn team is necessary to provide optimal care for burned patients.

The authors

David M. Baron, PhD[1]
Lars-Peter Kamolz, PhD, Assoc. Prof.[2]
Philipp G.H. Metnitz, MD, PhD, EDIC, DEAA[1]
[1] Department of Anaesthesiology | General Intensive Care and Pain Medicine | Medical University Vienna | Vienna, Austria
[2] Division of Plastic and Reconstructive Surgery | Department of Surgery | Medical University Vienna | Vienna, Austria

Address for correspondence
Philipp G.H. Metnitz
Department of Anaesthesiology
General Intensive Care and Pain Medicine
Medical University Vienna
Währinger Gürtel 18–20
1090 Vienna, Austria
E-mail: philipp@metnitz.biz

References

1. Latenser BA. Critical care of the burn patient: the first 48 hours. Crit Care Med 2009;37:2819–2826.
2. White CE, Renz EM. Advances in surgical care: management of severe burn injury. Crit Care Med 2008;36:318–324.
3. ABA/ACS. Guidelines for the operation of burn centres. J Burn Care Res 2007;28(1):134–141.
4. Pizano LR, Davies J, Corallo JP, Cantwell PG. Critical care and monitoring of the pediatric burn patient. J Craniofac Surg 2008;19:929–932.

5. Dries DJ. Key questions in ventilator management of the burn-injured patient (first of two parts). J Burn Care Res 2009;30:128–138.

6. Dries DJ. Key questions in ventilator management of the burn-injured patient (second of two parts). J Burn Care Res 2009;30:211–220.

7. Chung KK, Lundy JB, Matson JR, Renz EM, White CE, King BT, Barillo DJ, Jones JA, Cancio LC, Blackbourne LH, Wolf SE. Continuous venovenous hemofiltration in severely burned patients with acute kidney injury: a cohort study. Crit Care 2009;13:R62.

8. Demling RH, Perea A, Maly J, Moylan JA, Jarrett F, Balish E. The use of a laminar airflow isolation system for the treatment of major burns. Am J Surg 1978;136:375–378.

9. Ross FP. Christiano AM. Nothing but skin and bone. J Clin Invest 2006;116:1140–1149.

10. Segre JA. Epidermal barrier formation and recovery in skin disorders. J Clin Invest 2006;116:1150–1158.

Nils Theuerkauf, Ulf Guenther and Christian Putensen

Design features of the ICU from the patient and family perspective

In recent years, with advances in survival of critically ill patients, critical care physicians and researchers have begun to focus on long-term outcome of ICU survivors and quality of care [1–4]. Considerable attention is now devoted to patients and families, and concepts of family-centred critical care are being developed.

Concerning the organisation and management of intensive care medicine, different design features of the ICU and the quality of medical care have substantial influence on how patients and their relatives experience critical care medicine.

Patient's perception of the ICU

Both the critical illness and intensive care therapy expose patients to enormous physical and psychological stress. Early work concerning this subject was performed by DeMeyer (1967), who was the first to give a description of the patient in the ICU and how features of the intensive care unit relate to the stress experienced by the patient [5]. Since then, several studies have documented both the nature and impact of the stress experienced by ICU patients. The ICU Environmental Stressor Scale (ICUESS) was introduced and validated by Ballard [6] in 1981 and has been used in different studies evaluating the stressors of ICU patients [6–8].

By means of the ICUESS, Novaes et al. found "having pain", "being unable to sleep", "having tubes in nose or mouth", "not having control of oneself", "being tied down by tubes" and "having no explanations about treatment" to be the major stress factors ICU patients are subjected to [7]. Interestingly, there is a great discrepancy between the perception and evaluation of the patient's stress among groups. Several studies consistently observed that the experience of stress factors in the ICU differed significantly between patients on one hand side, and families or healthcare staff on the other. Of note, there was little correlation between the reports given by the patient and those given by healthcare team members [8–10]. "Pain" and "sleeping disturbances" were consistently considered to be major stress factors by all three groups, which underlines the importance to monitor and control for pain and to re-establish a natural circadian rhythm. The perception of "loss of self-control", "suffering from physical restraints" and "lack of communication and information", however, differed significantly between patients and healthcare staff [8].

Communication with the patient by means of direct address, writing and physical contact, reorientation with regard to locality, time, person and treatment, raising hope and relieving fear and anxiety, information about healthcare status, illness and treatment by use of simple, comprehensible and positive speech may be useful to reduce stress originating from these issues and thus ought to be the main features outlining the interaction with critically ill patients.

Post-ICU depression and post-traumatic stress disorder (PTSD)

In a recently published systematic review of psychiatric morbidity in patients discharged from the ICU, the point prevalence of a clinician-diagnosed depressive disorder was found to be 33 % [11]. Evaluation of risk factors for the occurrence of post-ICU depressive disorders excluded "age", "gender" and "severity of illness at admission" to be of importance, whereas "early post-ICU depressive symptoms" were found to be a strong risk factor for subsequent depressive disorders [11]. In contrast to a previously published systematic review in survivors of acute respiratory distress syndrome [12], "length of stay in the ICU" and "duration of sedation" were not verified to be risk factors for the occurrence of post-ICU depressive symptoms. Post-ICU depressive disorders exert a substantial influence on the health-related quality of life [13] and post-ICU morbidity. Further research will identify risk factors to allow for specific therapeutic intervention.

Estimates of the prevalence of post-traumatic stress disorder (PTSD) in ICU patients have been reported to be as high as 63 % [14]. A systematic review published in 2006 confirmed "increased length of stay in the ICU and/or in the hospital and/or increased length of mechanical ventilation", "greater levels of sedation and/ or neuromuscular blockade", "female gender", "younger age", "presence of delusional memories" and a "prior mental health history" to be associated with the occurrence of PTSD in patients discharged from the ICU [15]. As with the phenomenon of post-ICU depressive symptoms, continuing research with regard to PTSD in different populations of ICU patients will convey information on the prevalence and nature of this

condition to allow for the conceptualisation of possible therapeutic interventions.

The role of the family

As a consequence of the underlying disease, delirium and medical care, ICU patients are often incapacitated and therefore cannot make decisions themselves [16, 17]. Less than 5 % of ICU patients retain decision-making capacity when medically treated in the ICU, and only about 10 % have prepared advance directives [18]. Thus, family members and next of kin receive full information on the patient's diagnosis, prognosis and treatment and often become involved in discussions with ICU physicians about the goals of care. They frequently must represent patients' values and treatment preferences in a series of further discussions to act as surrogate or be a participant in the decision-making process [19]. Consequently, there appears to be a high proportion of family members suffering from stress-related psychological disorders that should direct our attention as attending clinicians to the patient's family. 50 to 70 % of family members of ICU patients experience symptoms of anxiety, depression and post-traumatic stress disorders [20–22], and there is evidence of a correlation between these symptoms and deficiencies in effective communication between family members and the ICU healthcare team [22].

Communication with family members

Informing patients' relatives is an obligation to physicians and, just as much, crucial in improving the effectiveness of communication between family members and the healthcare team [23] and in meeting family needs [24]. In our experience, family members of critically ill patients frequently are more afflicted with the patient's uncertain destiny than the patients themselves. They often feel a substantial need for information on the health status, prognosis and therapeutical measures, which are frequently felt not to be completely satisfied (see below) [25]. Every member of the ICU staff should bear in mind that having a family member in the ICU does not only mean a vital threat to a beloved one's life, but also puts the relatives themselves in a crucial phase of their life. Likewise, premorbidly deranged intra-familiar structures often experience a sharp accentuation during critical illness of a family member.

A growing number of publications on the issue of quality improvement and outcome assessment in critical care medicine demonstrate that there is consistent dissatisfaction of ICU patients' family members with both the communication with physicians and the interaction between families and healthcare providers [26]. The complexity and complicacy of the family-physician interaction has been impressively illustrated in a study performed by the 'famille en réanimation' FAMIREA workgroup. Comprehension of both content and dimension of the diagnosis, prognosis and treatment as communicated in a family-physician conference has been shown to be inadequate in half of the families of ICU patients [25]. Another study conducted by White et al. found that clinician-family communication commonly did not meet basic standards of informed decision-making [27].

Measuring family satisfaction

Several validated instruments are available for measuring the quality of care delivered to patients and families in the ICU. The most extensively evaluated tool is the 14-item *Critical Care Family Needs Inventory* developed by Nancy Molter and the Society for Critical Care Medicine [28, 29]. Another instrument to measure family satisfaction in the ICU is the Critical Care Family Satisfaction Survey, consisting of a 20-item questionnaire [30]. More recently, the *Family Satisfaction in the ICU Survey* (FS-ICU) was developed and validated for assessing family satisfaction in the ICU by Daren Heyland [31]. The FS-ICU consists of two conceptual sections. The first part contains 18 items focusing on satisfaction with overall care, the second part assesses satisfaction with the process of decision-making (16 items). In a multiple-centre study published in 2002, Heyland and coworkers measured levels of family satisfaction with critical care provided in the ICU in six centres across Canada and identified

1. "completeness of information received",
2. "respect and compassion shown to the patient and family members", and

3. "the amount and level of health care provided to the patient"

as key variables correlating most with high degrees of satisfaction [26]. Thus, studies on the issue of family needs and family satisfaction consistently emphasize the need for personal information and communication provided by a healthcare team delivering honest, loyal, and unequivocal information in a timely and regular fashion [24, 26].

An evidence-based approach to communication

Several published reviews and articles have reported on distinct methodological approaches aiming at improving family-physician communication in the ICU in general care [32] and in end-of-life care [33–36].

In an evidence-based approach to communication between families and physicians, Curtis and White summarised specific features of family-physician conferences that have been found to be associated with a higher degree of family satisfaction and with a better quality of communication [37]. They found:

- Clinicians spending more time listening and less time talking [38]
- Having a private place for family communication
- Consistent communication by all members of the healthcare team [22]
- Assurances that the patient will not be abandoned prior to death [39, 40]
- Assurances that the patient will be comfortable and will not suffer [41]
- Support for a family's decisions about care, including support for family's decision to withdraw or not to withdraw life support [41]
- Empathic statements [42] (acknowledging the difficulty and sadness of having a critically ill loved one, the difficulty of surrogate decision-making) associated with improved family experience [37]

Further, investigators evaluated and identified important, commonly missed opportunities during ICU family conferences, including the opportunity to listen and respond to family members' questions, to acknowledge and respond to family emotions, to address basic principles of palliative care and to assure non-abandonment by clinicians [39, 40].

Some of these findings have been summarised in the "VALUE mnemonic", consisting of the five features "value", "acknowledge", "listen", "understand" and "elicit" [37]. In an interventional study conducted by Lautrette et al. in 2007, the introduction of a strategy in the ICU using this mnemonic has been found to improve clinician-family communication and to significantly reduce family symptoms of anxiety, depression, and post-traumatic stress disorder 3 months after the patient's death [21].

The process of decision-making

When the patient becomes incompetent due to illness or medical treatment, family members are an important source of information about the patient's wishes and treatment preferences [37]. With regard to the relationship and interaction between physicians and patients and their surrogates, respectively, three main distinct concepts of decision-making may basically be differentiated:

1. "Parentalism", in which the physician makes the decision with little or no input from the family
2. "Informed choice", in which the physician provides all relevant medical information but withholds his or her opinion, leaving the decision to the family
3. "Shared decision-making", in which the physicians and family members share their opinions and jointly reach a consented decision [37]

There are great differences in the process of decision-making within Europe and between Europe and North America. This may be reflected numerically by the rates of patients' deaths following the decision to withhold or withdraw treatment and by the frequency by which admission to the ICU is refused [43]. These discrepancies in the ethical practice of end-of-life decisions may be founded in individual, professional, societal, cultural and religious differences. In the United States, respect for the autonomy of each patient is paramount and limiting life support is both ethically and legally justified under the principle of autonomy and self-determination. US law grants each patient with decision-making capac-

ity the right to refuse medical treatment, including life-sustaining therapies [44]. Every clinician is obliged to respect this right. When patients become incompetent and cannot make decisions for themselves, decisions are made on their behalf by surrogates, using either the "substituted judgement standard" or the "best interests standard" [44]. "Shared decision-making" has been supported by the three American professional critical care societies and has been affirmed by the American College of Critical Care clinical practice guidelines for support of the family during patient-centred critical care [45].

In contrast, in Europe there has been a paternalistic way of decision-making. Despite differences in the 'autonomous' American and 'paternalistic' European approach, both the United States as well as European countries have in recent years moved towards the principle of "shared decision-making". This principle has been endorsed in a joint consensus conference statement issued by five North American and European critical care societies in 2003 [46]. A "shared decision" is characterised in this statement as a decision in which "responsibility for decisions is shared jointly by the treating physician and the patient's family" [46].

End-of-life decisions

Epidemiological studies from the United States have shown that 20% of all patients die in an ICU [47] and this number is expected to grow further in the future. Although it is now generally accepted that there is no difference between withholding and withdrawing a medical treatment from the ethical standpoint [48, 49], there are significant differences between individuals, ICUs, hospitals and countries with regard to both frequency and mode by which end-of-life decisions are met and accomplished [50, 51]. For instance, reported rates from European countries on withdrawing/withholding therapy in ICU patients range from 41% in Sweden [52], 53% in France [53] to 82% in the United Kingdom [54]. Interestingly, withdrawal of therapy appears to be more common in northern than in southern Europe, as has consistently been shown in several surveys and studies comparing ethical practices across Europe [50, 51].

Along these lines, there are major differences as to who decides in the process of end-of-life care [43]. An Italian study published in 2003 reported that 82% of end-of-life decisions were made by the medical team with 56% of physicians claiming never to involve the patient, even if competent [55]. In Spain, families were not involved in 28% of the cases [56], whereas in France 56–83% of family members were not involved [53, 57]. In an ethics questionnaire published 20 years ago, Vincent et al. observed that in Italy, Greece and Portugal decisions were made by the physician alone, whereas in the United Kingdom and Switzerland the whole ICU staff was commonly involved in the process of decision-making [51].

Communicating and proceeding in end-of-life decisions

Despite ongoing advances in clinical practice and scientific research having led to improved outcomes in critically ill patients, too often sustaining or further escalating therapy, technological or medical support translates not into improvement, but prolongs suffering and delays an inevitable death [58]. Several studies reported that families want to be involved in the process of end-of-life decisions [59] and several national critical care societies emphasise the importance of such involvement of patients and families [45, 46]. In a longitudinal survey of a random sample of 8,000 individuals in France, the FAMIREA workgroup found that up to 85% of respondents prefer a surrogate decision-maker to be involved in the process of critical care decision-making [60]. Another study from the same group showed support for family involvement by 85% of nurses and 90% of physicians in the ICU setting [61].

Several limitations in surrogate decision-making have been addressed:

1. The key ethical principle of autonomy actually determines the patient as the ultimate decision-maker.
2. The majority of patients is unable to decide on their own [18].
3. Surrogates often fail to accurately meet patients' wishes [62].
4. Only the attending physician can assess illness and prognosis of the patient, and is ultimately responsible for the patient's care in the ICU.

Mostly, therefore, neither the patient, nor the surrogate, nor the physician can be the *single* decision-maker. In their consensus statement covering life support and end-of-life care in the ICU, a shared approach to decision-making has been advocated by a conference of international critical care societies [46].

It often appears unbearable for family members to accept the burden of responsibility associated with end-of-life decisions. Therefore, while the decision how to proceed and how to implement the decision made must be a medical one [49], we interpret the role of the family in the process of "shared decision-making" as one of guiding and directing decisions on behalf of the patient as the patient's surrogate, attempting to express either previously mentioned or presumed wishes of the patient [63]. Thus, the purpose of a shared decision is to reach consensus on a process that is in accordance with the patient's wishes while providing comfort and support to both the patient and the family [46].

Healthcare professionals are assigned to convey the perception of such end-of-life decisions to the family as a change in the goal of therapy, namely the transition from curative to palliative care, rather than thinking in terms of limitation, withholding or withdrawal of treatment [43]. To provide best possible comfort and care to both the patient and the family and to make the dying process as comfortable as possible to all participants, we feel that it is paramount in end-of-life care to involve family members, to enable them to comprehend and agree with the process of shared but guided decision-making. The responsibility must be taken by the care-giver team, but must be in accordance with the patient's wishes as represented by the family [49]. It must be avoided to leave the family behind with the feeling that they have decided on the death of their loved one. A shared but guided decision-making process must give family members the opportunity to cede responsibility for difficult decisions to physicians [37].

In a valuable paper published in 2008, Curtis and White suggested a three-step approach to patient- and family-centered decision-making, emphasising the need for a regular reassessment of the family's preference for their role in the process of decision-making and a subsequent adaption of the communication strategy between an autonomous, paternalistic and shared decision-making process [37]. Sharing the decision-making process means for the healthcare providers not only to be responsive to the family's needs and competence (which may change over time and during the course of critical illness) [37], but to move horizontally between the process of 'shared' decision-making in the middle, and the 'autonomous' decision-making process on the one and the 'paternalistic' approach on the other side. Most notably, the family's needs, demands and capabilities are heterogeneous. This has been emphasised only recently, as it has been shown that there is considerable variation in family members' views about whether or not clinicians should give recommendations regarding withdrawal or withholding of life support in critically ill patients, with a little more than half of the families (56%) preferring such a recommendation, while 42% of families did not [64].

Again, we want to emphasise two aforementioned aspects of communication in end-of-life care, namely the identification of missed opportunities [39], and the affirmation of non-abandonment [40]. Exploring the patient's preferences and wishes in family-physician conferences and the appropriate impact of the patient's perspective on decision-making is one of the most commonly missed opportunities in critical care medicine [39]. Further along these lines, it is paramount to reassert that limitation, withholding or withdrawal of life-sustaining therapy does not mean to withhold or withdraw care, and that the dying patient will not be abandoned [33, 40].

Despite ongoing advances in critical care medicine, too little is known about the incidence and risk factors for post-ICU depression, post-traumatic stress disorders and about quality of life after discharge from the ICU. With aging societies and a growing number of critically ill patients and patients surviving the ICU, more scientific efforts must be made to facilitate therapeutic intervention, to reduce risk-factors for long-term sequelae not only in ICU patients, but also in their families.

Conclusion

From the patient's perspective, ICU caregivers must acknowledge, identify and minimise ICU-related stressors and risk factors for post-ICU depressive symptoms and ICU-related stress disorders. Defining a team performance framework by establishing an institutional concept for patient- and family-centered critical care medicine may be a first step to raise healthcare members' awareness of this issue and to build a foundation for such patient- and family-centered intensive care. The introduction of systemic performance questionnaires to gauge family satisfaction may be helpful to identify deficiencies in medical care and will identify amendable points in the daily practice of ICU care.

Education of healthcare team members in communication skills, translation of communication skills into daily practice by means of checklists, guidelines or mnemonics and the regular performance of healthcare team conferences will improve the quality of ICU care. The use of family information leaflets improves communication between family members and ICU caregivers.

ICU physicians must be aware of different or changing attitudes of families towards decision-making in critical and end-of-life care. Family conferences and communication within the healthcare team constitute a dynamic process and one of learning, and the healthcare team should be responsive to patients' and families' requirements and capacities and must be flexible during the process of decision-making while caring for their patients.

The authors

Nils Theuerkauf, MD
Ulf Guenther, MD, DESA, EDIC
Christian Putensen, Prof., MD
   Dept. of Anaesthesiology & Intensive Care
   Medicine | University Hospital | Bonn,
   Germany

Address for correspondence
   Nils Theuerkauf
   Department of Anaesthesiology & Intensive
   Care Medicine
   University Hospital
   Sigmund-Freud-Str. 25
   53105 Bonn, Germany
   E-mail: nils.theuerkauf@ukb.uni-bonn.de

References

1. Broomhead LR, Brett SJ. Clinical review: Intensive care follow-up–what has it told us? Crit Care 2002 Oct;6(5):411–7.

2. Dowdy DW, Eid MP, Sedrakyan A, Mendez-Tellez PA, Pronovost PJ, Herridge MS, et al. Quality of life in adult survivors of critical illness: a systematic review of the literature. Intensive Care Med 2005 May;31(5):611–20.

3. Dowdy DW, Eid MP, Dennison CR, Mendez-Tellez PA, Herridge MS, Guallar E, et al. Quality of life after acute respiratory distress syndrome: a meta-analysis. Intensive Care Med 2006 Aug;32(8):1115–24.

4. Hopkins RO, Jackson JC. Long-term neurocognitive function after critical illness. Chest 2006 Sep;130(3):869–78.

5. DeMeyer JA. The environment of the intensive care unit. Nurs Forum 1967;6(3):262–72.

6. Ballard KS. Identification of environmental stressors for patients in a surgical intensive care unit. Issues Ment Health Nurs 1981 Jan;3(1–2):89–108.

7. Novaes MA, Aronovich A, Ferraz MB, Knobel E. Stressors in ICU: patients' evaluation. Intensive Care Med 1997 Dec;23(12):1282–5.

8. Novaes MA, Knobel E, Bork AM, Pavao OF, Nogueira-Martins LA, Ferraz MB. Stressors in ICU: perception of the patient, relatives and health care team. Intensive Care Med 1999 Dec;25(12):1421–6.

9. Carr JA, Powers MJ. Stressors associated with coronary bypass surgery. Nurs Res 1986 Jul;35(4):243–6.

10. Ross SE, MacKay RC. Postoperative stress. Do nurses accurately assess their patients? J Psychosoc Nurs Ment Health Serv 1986 Apr;24(4):16–22.

11. Davydow DS, Gifford JM, Desai SV, Bienvenu OJ, Needham DM. Depression in general intensive care unit survivors: a systematic review. Intensive Care Med 2009 May;35(5):796–809.

12. Davydow DS, Desai SV, Needham DM, Bienvenu OJ. Psychiatric morbidity in survivors of the acute respiratory distress syndrome: a systematic review. Psychosom Med 2008 May;70(4):512–9.

13. Wells KB, Stewart A, Hays RD, Burnam MA, Rogers W, Daniels M, et al. The functioning and well-being of depressed patients. Results from the Medical Outcomes Study. JAMA 1989 Aug 18;262(7):914–9.

14. Schelling G, Briegel J, Roozendaal B, Stoll C, Rothenhausler HB, Kapfhammer HP. The effect of stress doses of hydrocortisone during septic shock on posttraumatic stress disorder in survivors. Biol Psychiatry 2001 Dec 15;50(12):978–85.

15. Jackson JC, Hart RP, Gordon SM, Hopkins RO, Girard TD, Ely EW. Post-traumatic stress disorder and post-traumatic stress symptoms following critical illness in medical intensive care unit patients: assessing the magnitude of the problem. Crit Care 2007;11(1):R27.

16. Appelbaum PS, Grisso T. Capacities of hospitalized, medically ill patients to consent to treatment. Psychosomatics 1997 Mar;38(2):119–25.

17. Grisso T, Appelbaum PS. Comparison of standards for assessing patients' capacities to make treatment decisions. Am J Psychiatry 1995 Jul;152(7):1033–7.

18. Cook DJ, Guyatt G, Rocker G, Sjokvist P, Weaver B, Dodek P, et al. Cardiopulmonary resuscitation directives on admission to intensive-care unit: an international observational study. Lancet 2001 Dec 8;358(9297):1941–5.

19. Azoulay E, Pochard F. Communication with family members of patients dying in the intensive care unit. Curr Opin Crit Care 2003 Dec;9(6):545–50.

20. Azoulay E, Pochard F, Kentish-Barnes N, Chevret S, Aboab J, Adrie C, et al. Risk of post-traumatic stress symptoms in family members of intensive care unit patients. Am J Respir Crit Care Med 2005 May 1;171(9):987–94.

21. Lautrette A, Darmon M, Megarbane B, Joly LM, Chevret S, Adrie C, et al. A communication strategy and brochure for relatives of patients dying in the ICU. N Engl J Med 2007 Feb 1;356(5):469–78.

22. Pochard F, Azoulay E, Chevret S, Lemaire F, Hubert P, Canoui P, et al. Symptoms of anxiety and depression in family members of intensive care unit patients: ethical hypothesis regarding decision-making capacity. Crit Care Med 2001 Oct;29(10):1893–7.

23. Way J, Back AL, Curtis JR. Withdrawing life support and resolution of conflict with families. BMJ 2002 Dec 7;325(7376):1342–5.

24. Azoulay E, Pochard F, Chevret S, Lemaire F, Mokhtari M, le G, Jr., et al. Meeting the needs of intensive care unit patient families: a multicenter study. Am J Respir Crit Care Med 2001 Jan;163(1):135–9.

25. Azoulay E, Chevret S, Leleu G, Pochard F, Barboteu M, Adrie C, et al. Half the families of intensive care unit patients experience inadequate communication with physicians. Crit Care Med 2000 Aug;28(8):3044–9.

26. Heyland DK, Rocker GM, Dodek PM, Kutsogiannis DJ, Konopad E, Cook DJ, et al. Family satisfaction with care in the intensive care unit: results of a multiple center study. Crit Care Med 2002 Jul;30(7):1413–8.

27. White DB, Braddock CH, III, Bereknyei S, Curtis JR. Toward shared decision making at the end of life in intensive care units: opportunities for improvement. Arch Intern Med 2007 Mar 12;167(5):461–7.

28. Harvey MA, Ninos NP, Adler DC, Goodnough-Hanneman SK, Kaye WE, Nikas DL. Results of the consensus conference on fostering more humane critical care: creating a healing environment. Society of Critical Care Medicine. AACN Clin Issues Crit Care Nurs 1993 Aug;4(3):484–549.

29. Molter NC. Needs of relatives of critically ill patients: a descriptive study. Heart Lung 1979 Mar;8(2):332–9.

30. Wasser T, Pasquale MA, Matchett SC, Bryan Y, Pasquale M. Establishing reliability and validity of the critical care family satisfaction survey. Crit Care Med 2001 Jan;29(1):192–6.

31. Heyland DK, Tranmer JE. Measuring family satisfaction with care in the intensive care unit: the development of a questionnaire and preliminary results. J Crit Care 2001 Dec;16(4):142–9.

32. Vincent JL. Communication in the ICU. Intensive Care Med 1997 Oct;23(10):1093–8.

33. Curtis JR, Patrick DL, Shannon SE, Treece PD, Engelberg RA, Rubenfeld GD. The family conference as a focus to improve communication about end-of-life care in the intensive care unit: opportunities for improvement. Crit Care Med 2001 Feb;29(2 Suppl):N26–N33.

34. Curtis JR, Wenrich MD, Carline JD, Shannon SE, Ambrozy DM, Ramsey PG. Understanding physicians' skills at providing end-of-life care perspectives of patients, families, and health care workers. J Gen Intern Med 2001 Jan;16(1):41–9.

35. Curtis JR, Engelberg RA, Wenrich MD, Nielsen EL, Shannon SE, Treece PD, et al. Studying communication about end-of-life care during the ICU family conference: development of a framework. J Crit Care 2002 Sep;17(3):147–60.

36. Levy MM. End-of-life care in the intensive care unit: can we do better? Crit Care Med 2001 Feb;29(2 Suppl):N56–N61.

37. Curtis JR, White DB. Practical guidance for evidence-based ICU family conferences. Chest 2008 Oct;134(4):835–43.

38. McDonagh JR, Elliott TB, Engelberg RA, Treece PD, Shannon SE, Rubenfeld GD, et al. Family satisfaction with family conferences about end-of-life care in the intensive care unit: increased proportion of family speech is associated with increased satisfaction. Crit Care Med 2004 Jul;32(7):1484–8.

39. Curtis JR, Engelberg RA, Wenrich MD, Shannon SE, Treece PD, Rubenfeld GD. Missed opportunities during family conferences about end-of-life care in the intensive care unit. Am J Respir Crit Care Med 2005 Apr 15;171(8):844–9.

40. West HF, Engelberg RA, Wenrich MD, Curtis JR. Expressions of nonabandonment during the intensive care unit family conference. J Palliat Med 2005 Aug;8(4):797–807.

41. Stapleton RD, Engelberg RA, Wenrich MD, Goss CH, Curtis JR. Clinician statements and family satisfaction with family conferences in the intensive care unit. Crit Care Med 2006 Jun;34(6):1679–85.

42. Selph RB, Shiang J, Engelberg R, Curtis JR, White DB. Empathy and life support decisions in intensive care units. J Gen Intern Med 2008 Sep;23(9):1311–7.

43. Thompson BT, Cox PN, Antonelli M, Carlet JM, Cassell J, Hill NS, et al. Challenges in end-of-life care in the ICU: statement of the 5th International Consensus Conference in Critical Care: Brussels, Belgium, April 2003: executive summary. Crit Care Med 2004 Aug;32(8):1781–4.

44. Truog RD, Campbell ML, Curtis JR, Haas CE, Luce JM, Rubenfeld GD, et al. Recommendations for end-of-life care in the intensive care unit: a consensus statement by the American College [corrected] of Critical Care Medicine. Crit Care Med 2008 Mar;36(3):953–63.

45. Davidson JE, Powers K, Hedayat KM, Tieszen M, Kon AA, Shepard E, et al. Clinical practice guidelines for support of the family in the patient-centered intensive care unit: American College of Critical Care Medicine Task Force 2004–2005. Crit Care Med 2007 Feb;35(2):605–22.

46. Carlet J, Thijs LG, Antonelli M, Cassell J, Cox P, Hill N, et al. Challenges in end-of-life care in the ICU. Statement of the 5th International Consensus Conference in Critical Care: Brussels, Belgium, April 2003. Intensive Care Med 2004 May;30(5):770–84.

47. Angus DC, Barnato AE, Linde-Zwirble WT, Weissfeld LA, Watson RS, Rickert T, et al. Use of intensive care at the end of life in the United States: an epidemiologic study. Crit Care Med 2004 Mar;32(3):638–43.

48. Withholding and withdrawing life-sustaining therapy. This Official Statement of the American Thoracic Society was adopted by the ATS Board of Directors, March 1991. Am Rev Respir Dis 1991 Sep;144(3 Pt 1):726–31.

49. Vincent JL, Berre J, Creteur J. Withholding and withdrawing life prolonging treatment in the intensive care unit: a current European perspective. Chron Respir Dis 2004;1(2):115–20.

50. Sprung CL, Cohen SL, Sjokvist P, Baras M, Bulow HH, Hovilehto S, et al. End-of-life practices in European intensive care units: the Ethicus Study. JAMA 2003 Aug 13;290(6):790–7.

51. Vincent JL. Forgoing life support in western European intensive care units: the results of an ethical questionnaire. Crit Care Med 1999 Aug;27(8):1626–33.

52. Nolin T, Andersson R. Withdrawal of medical treatment in the ICU. A cohort study of 318 cases during 1994–2000. Acta Anaesthesiol Scand 2003 May;47(5):501–7.

53. Ferrand E, Robert R, Ingrand P, Lemaire F. Withholding and withdrawal of life support in intensive-care units in France: a prospective survey. French LATAREA Group. Lancet 2001 Jan 6;357(9249):9–14.

54. Turner JS, Michell WL, Morgan CJ, Benatar SR. Limitation of life support: frequency and practice in a London and a Cape Town intensive care unit. Intensive Care Med 1996 Oct;22(10):1020–5.

55. Giannini A, Pessina A, Tacchi EM. End-of-life decisions in intensive care units: attitudes of physicians in an Italian urban setting. Intensive Care Med 2003 Nov;29(11):1902–10.

56. Esteban A, Gordo F, Solsona JF, Alia I, Caballero J, Bouza C, et al. Withdrawing and withholding life support in the intensive care unit: a Spanish prospective multi-centre observational study. Intensive Care Med 2001 Nov;27(11):1744–9.

57. Pochard F, Azoulay E, Chevret S, Vinsonneau C, Grassin M, Lemaire F, et al. French intensivists do not apply American recommendations regarding decisions to forgo life-sustaining therapy. Crit Care Med 2001 Oct;29(10):1887–92.

58. Levy MM. Evaluating our end-of-life practice. Crit Care 2001 Aug;5(4):182–3.

59. Sjokvist P, Nilstun T, Svantesson M, Berggren L. Withdrawal of life support–who should decide? Differences in attitudes among the general public, nurses and physicians. Intensive Care Med 1999 Sep;25(9):949–54.

60. Azoulay E, Pochard F, Chevret S, Adrie C, Bollaert PE, Brun F, et al. Opinions about surrogate designation: a population survey in France. Crit Care Med 2003 Jun;31(6):1711–4.

61. Azoulay E, Pochard F, Chevret S, Arich C, Brivet F, Brun F, et al. Family participation in care to the critically ill: opinions of families and staff. Intensive Care Med 2003 Sep;29(9):1498–504.

62. Coppolino M, Ackerson L. Do surrogate decision makers provide accurate consent for intensive care research? Chest 2001 Feb;119(2):603–12.

63. Sulmasy DP, Terry PB, Weisman CS, Miller DJ, Stallings RY, Vettese MA, et al. The accuracy of substituted judgments in patients with terminal diagnoses. Ann Intern Med 1998 Apr 15;128(8):621–9.

64. White DB, Evans LR, Bautista CA, Luce JM, Lo B. Are physicians' recommendations to limit life support beneficial or burdensome? Bringing empirical data to the debate. Am J Respir Crit Care Med 2009 Aug 15;180(4):320–5.

Maurizio Cecconi, Lorenzo Spagnesi, Mark Hamilton, Rui P. Moreno
and Andrew Rhodes

Minimal standards for physiological monitoring in the intensive care unit

Introduction

The derivation of the word 'to monitor' is from the Latin infinitive monēre – to observe, to keep under review, to measure or test at intervals, especially for the purpose of regulation or control, to warn. DeVita et al. [1] defined monitoring as, 'the ongoing assessment of a patient with the intention of

1. detecting abnormality, and
2. triggering a response if an abnormality is detected.'

The European Society of Intensive Care Medicine (ESICM) PACT module on health technology assessment [2] states that 'in the absence of an alarming system, or when the detection of an abnormality did not result in specific staff actions, the act of merely assessing a patient and recording the findings was defined as 'observation', and was not considered 'monitoring''.

Context

The intensive care unit (ICU) is a part of the hospital where the sickest patients are grouped together in order to utilize the human and technical resources in a more cost-effective and efficient way. Consequently, the ICU must be able to provide the necessary technical and human skills and competencies, in quantity and quality, in order to deliver the most appropriate care to patients with established or imminent critical illness, with the aim of improving their outcome (quantity and/or quality of life). A major component of this care package is the monitoring of the patients' vital status – as evaluated by a series of physiological and laboratory parameters – in order to forewarn of impending problems and to follow disease progression and to allow for sensible therapeutic titration (see Tab. 1). This chapter will make some suggestions as to what levels of monitoring should be available in any ICU

Tab. 1   Reasons for physiological monitoring

To ensure safety
To forewarn of future crises
To diagnose specific problems
To determine the physiological status
To follow disease progression
To select and titrate therapy
To detect points for preventive or proactive intervention

which has to manage complex critically ill adult patients. Given their specificities, we will not address the particular methods and techniques of neonatal and paediatric intensive care. The suggestions will also not cover patients in other ward settings, in the operating department or accident and emergency setting, in the pre-hospital setting or those required during the intra and inter-hospital transport of the patient with any critical illness. These will by definition require different standards and modalities that will depend on the skill base and case mix relevant to that area.

Reference to the world of evidence-based medicine

It is perhaps unfortunate that there is no strong evidence base behind the use of physiological monitoring. Indeed the studies that have been performed have often been disappointingly negative. Pulse oximetry, as an example, has perhaps been the best studied of the available monitoring systems. In 2007, the Cochrane group published a meta-analysis of the available studies which have attempted to answer the question of whether routine pulse oximetry alters outcome if used for perioperative monitoring [3]. They concluded that pulse oximetry can detect hypoxaemia and related effects, thus reducing the number of desaturation episodes; however, there was no evidence that it affected outcome. Also, as a trigger to detect earlier the need for intensive care admission several investigators, such as Taenzer et al. demonstrated, it may result in a reduced need for rescues and for intensive care unit transfers [4, 5] Perhaps this should not be a surprise given the low incidence rate of complications having a direct impact on mortality, however the necessary point to understand is that a monitoring system in itself is only as good as the technology behind it and can only impact on a patient's outcome if combined with a sensible clinician (of whatever profession is involved) and a treatment modality that will in itself improve the patients condition. In other words it is nonsensical to say that pulse oximetry (or pulmonary artery catheterization) [6] is not beneficial; they are both warranted in particular circumstances, so long as the medical team are willing, and able, to act on the information derived [7]. However, its use to drive therapy has not been fully explored in all circumstances; for example in cardiac arrest scenarios, its use has been demonstrated to improve neurological outcomes [8]. It is quite obvious that any monitor is able to track the dying process; the key point is that for a monitor to be useful it must provide information to clinicians at a stage where intervention can arrest physiological decline and thus improve patients' outcomes.

Reference to the world of anaesthesia

The necessity for good standards of physiological monitoring has long been recognized in the field of anaesthesia, particularly within the operating theatre department. In recent years, many national and international groupings have published standards of monitoring that must be adhered to (minimal standards) for safe anaesthetic practice. These include recommendations from the American Society of Anesthesiologists (ASA) in 1986 [9], the World Federation of Societies of Anesthesiologists (WFSA) in 1992 [10], the Italian Society of Anaesthesia, Analgesia and Intensive Care Medicine (SIAARTI) in 1994 [11], the Association of Anaesthetists of Great Britain and Ireland AAGBI (2007) [12], and more recently the Canadian Society of Anesthesia [13]. These recommendations can be used to develop some consensus as to the standards that should be applicable to ICU settings. If we consider that for an anaesthetized patient (often healthy patients having procedures under general anaesthesia or deep sedation) there are now clear standards as to what should be the minimal levels of monitoring. Even for procedures and in outpatient settings, it seems illogical that there is no clear guidance for the monitoring of critically ill patients who are by definition sicker and in need of closer observation. A remarkable example of this fact is the heterogeneous use of mandatory end-tidal CO_2 monitoring in ventilated patients, which is almost universally mandatory in the operative theatre, but much less often recommended or even used in the more severe ventilated patients in the ICU.

Standards for physiological monitoring in the ICU

A number of key principles need to be understood when generating universal (or near-universal) standards for physiological monitoring in the ICU setting. These should include:

1. **Staffing levels** (covered in a separate chapter). Physiological monitoring systems are only as good as the training and expertise of the staff that looks after and utilizes them. It is vital that all staff can understand the technical pitfalls and limitations of the devices and the appropriate course of action to transform the acquired data into knowledge in regard to the patient's condition and also in the necessary actions. Without adequate and safe numbers of nurses and doctors that conduct a timely and appropriate action when a deviation is detected, monitoring will always be a waste of time and money.

2. **Ability to alert staff.** All monitoring systems need to be able to alert healthcare professionals when there is an underlying problem that is at a level likely to be critical to that patient's outcome [14, 15]. These alarms need to be able to be configured for specific patient circumstances but must also be able to alert staff that there is a problem even when they are not at the immediate bedside. It is beyond the scope of this chapter to review the abundance of data that describe how an alarm must sound and how to best set it to avoid the frequent false positive events that lead to the 'boy crying wolf' scenario, but the alarm configuration is very important for the system to be robust in a complex and difficult environment.

3. **When to monitor.** All critically ill patients need a minimum level of monitoring, however some require the use of complementary or additional modalities that depend on their specific diagnosis, circumstances and typology. We can therefore split the levels of monitoring up into those that need to be applied to all ICU patients that must be in an ICU (either for intensive monitoring or for intensive therapy), those who remain unstable or are at risk of deteriorating, and those that are not mandatory but are optionally dependent on the situation. A good example of an optional monitoring modality would be intra-cranial pressure monitoring [16]. This is obviously important for a sub group of neurological critical care patients but would be completely irrelevant for a routine patient with bronchopneumonia. The same is true for other techniques, such as intra-abdominal pressure monitoring.

Physiological monitoring

There are a number of monitoring systems available that can be configured for the ICU patient. On the whole they can be split into those systems that are necessary to monitor the patient and those that are designed to monitor the equipment that are used to support the patient and the environmental conditions in which the patient is cared for. We will not describe in detail in this chapter the equipment monitoring devices or the characteristics of the environment. These include such parameters as the rate of microbial colonization of certain devices for instance air conditioners or humidifiers, the quality of air and other medicinal gases, electrical characteristics of the support systems, gas pressures, calibration coefficients and pump functions. We will focus on the devices designed to monitor the patients' physiological status.

All monitoring systems must be designed so that they can be seen easily and reviewed from a distance. Nowadays this means that they must incorporate a bright high definition screen that is designed with a colouring system that provides sufficient contrast and clarity to be visible in the changing light conditions of an ICU. All devices must be designed to an appropriate level of electrical safety, to ensure that no patient is put into danger in case of malfunction or even in the event of human error [17, 18].

In 1997, Ferdinande on behalf of a task force of the European Society of Intensive Care Medicine (ESICM) described a set of European recommendations for monitoring an ICU patient. They split the patients up into three levels of care, and these include level one being the lowest level of severity (high-end ward care), and level three the highest [19]. The monitoring systems were then described as being essential, desirable and/or optional for each category (see Tab. 2 and 3). Although these recommendations are now almost 15 years old, and a major revision is underway (and which should be presented in October 2010) most of these are still relevant to current practice.

Whichever device is chosen, a number of key principles should be adhered to for that technology [20]. These devices should be accurate, reproducible, have a rapid response time, be continuous, relatively operator independent, easy to

Tab. 2   Suggestions for monitoring systems as split by the level of care which patients are receiving: the lowest level of severity or high-end ward care (1), level 2 (2), and the highest level (3), and as to whether they are essential (E), desirable (D) or optional (O). [Modified from 19]

Monitoring system	Levels of care		
	1	2	3
Modular systems	E	E	E
Uniformity with OR, ED	D	D	D
Trending capability	D	E	E
Visible and audible alarms	E	E	E
Unobstructed comfortable viewing	E	E	E
Networking capability	D	D	D
Simultaneous display 4-waveforms and selected digital values for:			
1. Electrocardiogram	E	E	E
2. Arterial pressure	E	E	E
3. Central venous pressure	E	E	E
4. Multi-purpose pressure channel (e. g. pulmonary artery catheter, intra cranial pressure)	O	D	E
5. Temperature (central/cutaneous)	E	E	E
6. Pulse oximetry	E	E	E
7. Capnography	D	E	E
8. Continuous monitoring of ventilation	D	E	E
9. Endotracheal cuff monitoring	E	E	E
11. Non invasive arterial pressure monitoring	E	E	E
12. Cardiac output and derived values	D	E	E
13. Volumetric monitoring of circulation	O	O	O
14. Alarm recording and hard copy	D	E	E

Tab. 3   Suggestions for additional monitoring systems split by the level of care that patients are receiving and as to whether they are Essential, Desirable of Optional. [Modified from 19]

Additional monitoring	Levels of care		
	1	2	3
Oximetry of inspired gases	D	E	E
Pulmonary function	O	D	D
Mixed/central venous saturation	O	D	D
Arrhythmia detection	O	D	D
Electronic urine output measurement	D	D	D
ST-T wave analysis	D	D	D
Patient weighing systems	D	E	E
Indirect calorimetry	O	O	O
Point of care analysis systems			
1. Arterial blood gas analysis	D	E	E
2. Electrolyte monitoring	D	D	E
3. Blood sugar monitoring	E	E	E
4. Lactate monitoring	D	E	E
10. Intra-abdominal pressure monitoring	O	D	E

use, cost-effective and associated with no additional morbidity. Of course no monitor fulfils all of these standards completely, but all of them should be consistent with most standards. Nowadays, the capability to integrate the information between the different devices in a unique or central, user-customisable display, able to integrate triggers for action and protocols is also more and more desirable.

Conclusion

All critically ill patients require their physiological status to be monitored, continuously (or as much as possible), with a high level of accuracy and almost 100 % safety. The most important part of any monitoring package is the clinical team that is driving the care package and using the information to transform data into knowledge and knowledge into action – whether preventive or corrective. The specific monitoring modalities used are described in this chapter and can be split into those that are mandatory and those that are context-dependent.

The authors

Maurizio Cecconi, MD MD(UK)[1]
Lorenzo Spagnesi, MD[1]
Mark Hamilton, MRCP FRCA[1]
Rui P. Moreno, MD, PhD[2]
Andrew Rhodes, FRCA FRCP[1]
  [1]General Intensive Care | St George's
  Hospital | London, UK
  [2]Unidade de Cuidados Intensivos
  Polivalente | Hospital de Santo António
  dos Capuchos | Centro Hospitalar de Lisboa
  Central, E.P.E. | Lisbon, Portugal

Address for correspondence
  Andrew Rhodes
  General Intensive Care
  St George's Hospital
  London SW17 0QT, UK
  E-mail: andyr@sgul.ac.uk

References

1. DeVita MA, Smith GB, Adam SK, Adams-Pizarro I, Buist M, Bellomo R, Bonello R, Cerchiari E, Farlow B, Goldsmith D, Haskell H, Hillman K, Howell M, Hravnak M, Hunt EA, Hvarfner A, Kellett J, Light-hall GK, Lippert A, Lippert FK, Mahroof R, Myers JS, Rosen M, Reynolds S, Rotondi A, Rubulotta F, Winters B. "Identifying the hospitalised patient in crisis" – a consensus conference on the afferent limb of rapid response systems. Resuscitation; 81:375–82.

2. Jerome Cockings MJ, Carl Waldmann. Health Technology Assessment, an ESICM Multidisciplinary distance learning programme for intensive care training. PACT ESICM 2010.

3. Tanner J. Cochrane reviews-pulse oximetry for monitoring. Br J Perioper Nurs 2002;12:430.

4. Eichhorn JH. Pulse oximetry monitoring and late postoperative hypoxemia on the general care floor. J Clin Monit Comput 1998;14:49–55.

5. Taenzer AH, Pyke JB, McGrath SP, Blike GT. Impact of pulse oximetry surveillance on rescue events and intensive care unit transfers: a before-and-after concurrence study. Anesthesiology;112:282–7.

6. Vincent JL, Pinsky MR, Sprung CL, Levy M, Marini JJ, Payen D, Rhodes A, Takala J. The pulmonary artery catheter: in medio virtus. Crit Care Med 2008;36:3093–6.

7. Pinsky MR, Vincent JL. Let us use the pulmonary artery catheter correctly and only when we need it. Crit Care Med 2005;33:1119–22.

8. Balan IS, Fiskum G, Hazelton J, Cotto-Cumba C, Rosenthal RE. Oximetry-guided reoxygenation improves neurological outcome after experimental cardiac arrest. Stroke 2006;37:3008–13.

9. ASA. Standards for basic anesthetic monitoring http://www.asahq.org/. 2005.

10. [The 2008 international standards for a safe practice of anesthesia]. Anesteziol Reanimatol 2009:4–10.

11. SIAARTI. [Recommendations for basic monitoring of patients during anesthesia. Gruppo di Studio SAARTI per la Sicurezza in Anestesia e Terapia Intensiva]. Minerva Anestesiol 1997;63:267–70.

12. AAGBI. Recommendations for standards of monitoring during anaesthesia and recovery http://www.asahq. org/. 2007.

13. Merchant R, Bosenberg C, Brown K, Chartrand D, Dain S, Dobson J, Kurrek M, LeDez K, Morgan P, Penner M, Shukla R. Guidelines to the Practice of Anesthesia Revised Edition 2010. Can J Anaesth;57:58–87.

14. Critical alarms and patient safety. ECRI's guide to developing effective alarm strategies and responding to JCAHO's alarm-safety goal. Health Devices 2002;31:397–417.

15. Korniewicz DM, Clark T, David Y. A national online survey on the effectiveness of clinical alarms. Am J Crit Care 2008;17:36–41.

16. Rickels E. [Monitoring intracranial pressure. Indication, limits, practice]. Anaesthesist 2009;58:398–404.

17. Valentin A, Capuzzo M, Guidet B, Moreno R, Metnitz B, Bauer P, Metnitz P. Errors in administration of parenteral drugs in intensive care units: multinational prospective study. BMJ 2009;338:b814.

18. Valentin A, Capuzzo M, Guidet B, Moreno RP, Dolanski L, Bauer P, Metnitz PG. Patient safety in intensive care: results from the multinational Sentinel Events Evaluation (SEE) study. Intensive Care Med 2006;32:1591–8.

19. Ferdinande P. Recommendations on minimal requirements for Intensive Care Departments. Members of the Task Force of the European Society of Intensive Care Medicine. Intensive Care Med 1997;23:226–32.

20. Shephard JN, Brecker SJ, Evans TW. Bedside assessment of myocardial performance in the critically ill. Intensive Care Med 1994;20:513–21.

Dierk A. Vagts, Kristina Klöcker and Christian W. Mutz

Medical work patterns: The impact on quality and burnout

Over the last decades the character of intensive care units has changed dramatically from more or less 'intermediate care' units with a high emphasis on nursing and medical observation to medically highly specialised units with highly professional, multi-professional and interdisciplinary teams with a high focus on medical treatment including very expensive devices.

While nurses have been used to a full-shift rota on intensive care units nearly from the beginning, doctors quite often were not especially dedicated to this part of their work. Partially because they experienced working in the operating theatre or on the normal ward as more exciting, partially because intensive care medicine was regarded as an evil necessity. Hence, covering the intensive care unit during on-calls at night or on weekends interrupted the continuity of caring for patients and implicated 'stand-still' of therapy and just maintenance of the status quo.

Today, intensive care medicine uses about 20 % of financial resources of a hospital while it provides only about 5 % of hospital beds. Because in Europe the need for intensive care beds will increase over the next decades due to demographic changes (growing number of old patients with multimorbidity and, for example, further developments in cancer surgery), it seems reasonable to optimise workflows, structures and work patterns to reduce costs and maintain or – even better – to improve the quality of care.

However, we do not know very much about the impact of doctors' full shift rotas or the structure of ward rounds on the quality of information transfer and treatment. We do not know whether 8- or 12-hour shifts are favourable regarding work performance and transfer – or should we say, reduction of the loss – of information, and we do not know which work patterns are superior regarding life-long engagement in intensive care medicine and safeguarding against burnout.

The impact of full shift, partial shift or on-call systems

We know that fatigue reduces performance, and failure of attention may lead to increased clinical errors. 20 to 25 hours without sleep reduce psychomotor performance equivalent to a blood alcohol concentration of 0.1 %. Furthermore, permanent night shifts have an impact in the form of increased adverse health effects and impairment of learning. Hence we have to reduce night work shifts to an absolute maximum of 7 shifts per month and provide enough time for recovery.

However, little is known about the impact of work patterns on doctors' quality of work or life. Most studies available were conducted with nurses. But because nurses traditionally have been used to more restricted work patterns than doctors, transfers or results must be considered only with great caution.

Rogers (2004) found that the risks of making an error were significantly increased when work shifts were longer than twelve hours, when nurses worked overtime, or when they worked more than forty hours per week [41, 42].

The risk of errors occurring began to increase when shift durations exceeded 8.5 hours and became significant when they exceeded 12.5 hours. Since the errors in this study were relatively rare, probably this study lacked sufficient power to detect the effects for exceeding 8.5 hours of work.

In a different study Mills and co-workers found that probed performance tests reveal that nurses working twelve-hour simulated shifts make more frequent errors on grammatical reasoning tasks and medical record reviewing [31].

Regarding work-life balance and job satisfaction, Zboril-Benson revealed that nurses who worked 12-hour shifts expressed lower job satisfaction than nurses working 8-hour shifts [55].

In summary, longer work duration increased the risk of errors and near errors and decreased nurses' vigilance. These findings support the Institute of Medicine recommendations [24] to minimise the use of 12-hour shifts and at least to limit nurses' working hours to no more than 12 consecutive hours within a 24-hour period [45], even if these 12-hour shifts are very popular [40, 27].

Very interesting research results on mitigating the adverse effects of fatigue in aviation, transportation, military and industry have emerged over the last years, which have been implemented in some Japanese companies already, but scepticism remains in conservative areas like medicine: Planned naps as a fatigue countermeasure during night shifts can improve the safety of patients and staff. Implementing such an innovative measure requires a new approach to work design, new logistic structures and a new attitude towards improving work patterns [18, 47].

However, for nearly 10 years now the recommendation for an eleven-hour interruption of activity exists as a 'rest for safety', especially after a night-call or shift. Several studies had shown links between excessive work hours and occurrence of medical incidents related to fatigue. The tiredness resulting from sleep deprivation and disturbances in circadian rhythms is a cumulative phenomenon erased by a period of rest. In spite of a large individual variability, tiredness increases anxiety scores, irritability, depression and impairs cognitive performance. The concept of 'prophylactic' rest considers that a person cannot begin work rested if he or she did not sleep at least 5 hours the previous night, or 12 hours during the previous 48 hours.

Another important aspect of the 'rest for safety' concept is the long-term prevention of potential pathologies in medical staff, particularly burnout syndrome. Night calls in particular are considered most stressful. The psychological stress related to anticipation and the night-time context causes measurable cardiovascular disturbances, for example, in anaesthesiologists. Shift-work sleep disorders may induce gastric ulcers, heart attacks, metabolic syndrome, depression and accidents related to somnolence. Long-duration work hours, accompanied by sleep deprivation, may double the risk of car accidents in junior physicians. However, taking the necessary rest is not shown to be synonymous with a decrease in the efficiency of patient care, but the danger of limited information transmission should be counteracted with an optimisation of staff requirements and organisation.

In this regard, ageing and shortage of doctors is another emerging problem [32].

The impact of work patterns on burnout

Burnout syndrome associated with stress has been documented in healthcare professionals in many specialties. To define burnout syndrome exactly would exceed the scope of this chapter by far. However, speaking of burnout in this chapter describes a psychological term for the experience of long-term exhaustion and diminished interest. Psychologists Herbert Freudenberger and Gail North have theorised that the burnout process can be divided into 12 phases, which are not necessarily followed sequentially, nor necessarily are relevant in any sense, or exist other than as an abstract construct. A compulsion to prove oneself by working harder, neglecting one's own needs, displacing conflicts (the person does not realise the root cause of the distress), revising of values (friends or hobbies are completely dismissed), denying emerging problems (cynicism and aggression become apparent), withdrawing (reducing social contacts to a minimum, becoming walled off; alcohol or other substance abuse may occur), leads to behavioral changes becoming obvious to others, to inner emptiness, depression, and burnout syndrome.

The intensive care unit is a highly stressful environment. Yet little is known about burnout syndrome in critical care nursing staff and even less in the case of intensive care doctors.

Factors which promote burnout syndrome in nursing staff are futile efforts to improve a patient's status over a long period [28].

Quite often organisational mishaps like excessive overtime, a bad working atmosphere, heavy workload and number of off-days and scheduling practice (number of night shifts per month, extended periods between non-working weeks, night shift the day before the survey) are important factors for the development of burnout syndromes [20, 34]. Other factors are conflicts with patients and critical relationships with other staff members and seniors.

Systemic problems might contribute to this situation as well: imprudent and aggressive strategies of treatment, unacceptable consumption of resources in the public health system, incompetent behaviour of doctors in regard to communication with patients and relatives, doctors ignoring patients' advance directives, inaccessible and divergent aims of treatment between relatives and doctors [22], confrontation with the 'end-of-life situation', complex technologies, the daily challenge of treating critically ill patients, and daily confrontation with pain, suffering, agony and death [23].

But individual personality plays an important role as well: People who are over-motivated in the beginning have a greater risk of developing burnout syndrome than people with a normal level of motivation [9].

A pyramid scheme has been described by Bakker [6] for the propagation of burnout syndromes within a peer group by "talking about it". And last but not least, there are differences between the sexes [36].

Hence, early recognition of burnout as a result of prolonged stress and frustration among intensive care staff will contribute to better professional behaviour.

About one-third of ICU nursing staff has severe burnout syndrome. Areas for improvement include conflict prevention, participation in ICU research groups, and better management of end-of-life care. Organisational structure changes in the work environment can improve healthcare quality for critically ill patients, but these changes need to include appropriate staffing for nurses and physicians to guarantee that no staff member is working more than 4 night shifts in a row, and not more than a maximum of seven per month for a restricted period of time.

However, interventional studies are needed to investigate these potentially preventive strategies.

The impact of memory and ward round structure on information transfer

Technical developments in intensive care medicine provide many new parameters and information about the patients. Over recent years we have experienced a tremendous condensation of the workload due to a reduction in length of stay, treatment of more patients per doctor in the same time, extended communication with patients, relatives and inside the multidisciplinary and multiprofessional team and due to an increasing number of multimorbid patients. Hence, during handover and ward rounds physicians are confronted with a very high number and denseness of new information every day [48]. But the question is whether the human brain is really capable of processing this flood of information, or if this exceeds the natural boundaries of human concentration and memory?

Studies have shown that most transfer of information takes place from doctor to doctor by direct communication instead of using information from written or electronic charts [11]. Even in hospitals with computer-based patient data information systems 50 % of information transfer happens by direct verbal communication [44].

However, communication is variable and prone to different influences, like hierarchic structures, stress, or a busy environment [30].

Another source of error in communication is that it relies on the physiology and functioning of the human brain.

Information transfer becomes insufficient if it exceeds the cognitive capacity of the human brain [37]. By exceeding the capacity of the human brain we induce a reduction of attention and oblivion, which may result in further mistakes [38]. 50 % of adverse events in the hospital are associated with inadequate communication [7], and communication deficits are the most important reason for increased hospital mortality [52].

Recent research projects mainly dealt with the interaction between doctors and patients [57, 58, 59] or doctors and nurses [1, 56, 61, 62]. Unfortunately, there is a lack of knowledge about communication between doctors, and especially in intensive care units, one of the most vulnerable areas in the hospital.

Our own research group has analysed the transfer of information between doctors in an 18-bed ICU at a university hospital. We conducted a prospective, observational study to examine the capability of the human brain to process the flood of information during an ICU ward round. The question was whether traditional structures of ward rounds exceed the natural limits of human concentration and memory [60].

The information transfer and process of our ward rounds was analysed with the help of video recordings. A total of 8 24-hour ward round cycles were recorded, each consisting of 4 consecutive ward rounds within one day in a full shift system. In the beginning of each cycle clinically relevant information of 5 patients was established and standardised. This predetermined information served as the default value to detect information loss throughout the 24 hours. Of these five patients, 2 were chosen from the beginning (randomly chosen from patients 1–4 of the ward round), one from the middle (randomly chosen from patients 8–11) and 2 from the end (randomly chosen from patients 16–18) of the ward round, in order to find fluctuations in the physicians' ability to concentrate and memorise information throughout the ward round. Except for the physician initially passing over the information, the rest of the ward round members did not know which patients would be evaluated in the end. To test the physicians' memory they were asked to fill out a questionnaire on 10 clinically important issues immediately after the ward round. All the information asked for had been mentioned during the ward round.

The results were very interesting and alarming at the same time: During the first ward round an average of 15 items of information were given per patient. Of these only 11 (75 %) were transferred to the second ward round. During the third ward round only 8 (52 %) of these pieces of information were passed on and slightly more than 8 (54 %) during the fourth. A major loss of information over 24 hours could be discovered for clinically relevant information.

However, we could detect a difference between patients who had always been visited and revisited at the beginning of a ward round and those who had been visited at the end of each ward round:

For those patients discussed in the beginning of the ward round 70 % of the information was passed on during the course of 24 hours. For those discussed in the middle only 55 % and for the later patients only 39 % of the initial information was passed on, even though the average time needed for each patient remained the same throughout the whole ward round (about 5 minutes per patient). This shows that towards the end of the ward round the physicians' ability to concentrate decreased and the density of information lessened. This study shows that the structure of the ward round as organised up until now – visiting all patients in an 18-bed ICU with the complete team of doctors from the current and the following shift – needs to be reconsidered.

Three facts of brain physiology and cognitive psychology need to be considered when planning ICU ward rounds:

Ebbinghaus' learning and forgetting curve [19]: After a number of repetitions, Ebbinghaus would attempt to recall the items on the list. It turned out that his ability to recall the items improved as the number of repetitions went up, rapidly at first and then more slowly, until finally the list was mastered.

To test retention, Ebbinghaus practised a list until he was able to repeat the items correctly two times in a row. He then waited varying lengths of time before testing himself again. Forgetting turned out to occur most rapidly soon after the end of practice, but the rate of forgetting slowed as time went on and fewer items could be recalled.

Roughly speaking, one hour after learning items human beings are able to remember only 50 % of these items. From the 2nd to the 31st day the loss of memory is only 5 % [33].

Ability to keep attention: Broadbent described a theory of perception and communication where attention regulates the input of information to the human brain (bottleneck) [8]. This theory is still the basis for research on perception, attention, and information transfer [1]. People are not able to process all information which is acting on them simultaneously. Attention helps to focus and select information by way of two mechanisms: target-controlled attention or stimulus-induced attention. Stimulus-induced attention works through sudden appearance, loudness, or special colours or effects [54].

Human memory: According to Attkinson and Shiffrin, human memory consists of three storage areas: sensory memory, short-term and long-term memory.

Sensory memory recalls stimuli from the environment for 2 seconds or less, hence expanding the availability of information for processing in the brain for a short time [54].

Short-term memory is a temporary resource, which can store information for 10 to 15 seconds. Miller described in 1956 that the human brain is only capable of processing 7 (± 2) items simultaneously (the 'magical number seven'). 'Chunking' – grouping items of information into bigger structures, which are called chunks – can increase the capacity of short-term memory [29].

Another possibility to increase short-term memory capacity is the concept of rehearsing. Repeating items in the mind is helpful for retaining this information in memory. Otherwise the information is lost over time. Repetition transfers information from short-term to long-term memory [3].

Another mechanism of losing information from memory is by displacing and replacing old information with new information [39].

Long-term memory items can quite often be recalled for an entire lifetime.

Its capacity seems to be unlimited, and it characterises our world [54]. Professional experience and recalling 'older' – and similar – cases is part of this long-term memory, which differentiates short-term memory more precisely [4, 5]. The working memory consists of a central executive and a phonological loop, a visuospatial sketchpad and an episodic buffer. The central executive is responsible for regulating attention, generating conclusions and decision-making [33].

The working memory is not an anatomic structure, but more a process which integrates new information and previous knowledge from experience to focus on solving an actual problem [54].

Serial position effect: If humans are asked to remember items from a list of unconnected words, they will be able to recall especially the first and the last items. This phenomenon is called serial position effect. The increased ability to recall items from the beginning of a list is called primacy effect, the ability to recall items from the end is called recency effect [33]. The theory of Atkinson and Shiffrin has been proven by many studies [43, 21, 35].

Why did we focus on this subject in our chapter?

The knowledge about cognitive psychology explains why we are losing so much information during our daily ward rounds. Experienced consultants wonder why young residents cannot keep all the important information in mind. But the key to improving the transfer of information during ICU ward rounds is to restructure our routine ward rounds.

Ideally, from the cognitive psychological point of view, every young resident (doctor in training) should not care for more than 6 to 7 ICU patients.

A routine daily ICU ward round should be restructured in such a way that consultants supervise a direct handover from junior doctors for no more than 7 patients. The handover should happen within a small team (e.g. consultant, 2 junior doctors, nurse) to minimise distraction of all participants and to focus on the relevant information. Handover should take no longer than 30 minutes for 6 patients, as the attention of all participants decreases after this time. In a larger unit (e.g. 18 beds) this structure should be implemented three times.

Summary

Medical work patterns are important for the quality of treatment for three reasons:

The organisational structure of an ICU can influence the satisfaction of nurses and doctors with their work (in regard to burnout syndrome of staff), reduce tiredness after night shifts or long working hours (in regard to attention and medical errors) and improve conveyance of medical concepts (in regard to loss of information during ward rounds). However, these conclusions are mainly transferred from studies with nursing staff. Further investigations focusing on doctors are desirable.

The authors

Dierk A. Vagts, MD, PhD, MSc., DEAA, EDIC[1,2,3]
Kristina Klöcker[3]
Christian W. Mutz, MD[3,4]
[1]Consultant Anaesthetist | Intensive Care Medicine, Emergency Medicine, Palliative Care | Head of Department of Anaesthesiology and Intensive Care Medicine | Emergency Medicine, Pain Therapy, Palliative Care | Hetzelstift Hospital Neustadt/Weinstraße | Neustadt, Germany
[2]Senior lecturer | University of Rostock, Germany
[3]Department of Anaesthesiology an Intensive Care Medicine | University of Rostock, Germany
[4]Consultant Anaesthetist | Department of Anaesthesiology and Intensive Care Medicine | Emergency Medicine, Pain Therapy, Palliative Care | Hetzelstift Hospital Neustadt/Weinstraße | Neustadt, Germany

Address for correspondence
Dierk A. Vagts
Department of Anaesthesiology and Intensive Care Medicine
Hetzelstift Hospital Neustadt/Weinstraße
Stiftstraße 10
67434 Neustadt/Weinstraße, Germany
E-mail: dierk.vagts@uni-rostock.de

References

1. Anderson JR. Kognitive Psychologie. Heidelberg 2007. Springer-Verlag.
2. Alvarez G, Coiera E. Interruptive communication patterns in the intensive care unit ward round. Int J Med Inform 2005;74:791–796.
3. Atkinson RC, Shiffrin RM. Human memory: A proposed system and its control processes. In: Spence KW, Spence JT. The psychology of learning and motivation. New York 1968;2:249. Academic Press.
4. Baddeley AD, Hitch GJ. Working memory. In: Bower GA. Recent advances in learning and motivation. New York 1974;8. Academic Press.
5. Baddeley AD. Exploring the central executive. Q J Exp Psychol A. 1996; 49: 5–28.
6. Bakker A, Arnold B, Le Blanc, Pascale M, Schaufli, Wilmar B. Burnout contagion among intensive care nurses. J Adv Nurs. 2005; 51: 276–287.
7. Bhasale AL, Miller GC, Reid SE, Britt CB. Analysing potential harm in Australian general practice: an incident-monitoring. Med J Aust. 1998; 169: 73–76.
8. Broadbent D. Perception and communication. London 1958. Pergamon Press.
9. Bühler K-E, Land T. Burnout and personality in extreme nursing: an empirical study. Arch Neurol Psychiatr 2004;155:35–42.
10. Coiera E. When Conversation is better than computation. J Am Med Inform Assoc. 2000;7:277–286.
11. Covell DG, Uman GC, Manning PR. Information needs in office practice: are they being met? Ann Intern Med. 1985;103:596–599.
12. Craik FI. Levels of processing: past, present … and future? Memory 2002;10:305–318.
13. Craik FI, Lockhart RS. Levels of processing: A framework for memory research. Journal of Verbal Learning and Verbal Behavior 1972;11:671–684.
14. Craik FI, Tulving E. Depth of processing and the retention of words in episodic memory. Journal of Experimental Psychology 1975;104:268–294.
15. Crowder RG. Principles of Learning and Memory. Hillsdale 1976. Erlbaum.
16. Čubrillo-Turek M, Urek R, Turek S. Burnout Syndrome – Assesment of a stressful Job among Inetnsive Care Staff. Coll. Antropol. 2006;30:131–135.
17. Daneman M, Carpenter PA. Individual differences in working memory and reading. Journal of Verbal learning and Verbal Behavior 1980;19:450–466.
18. Driskell JB, Mullen B. The Efficacy of Naps as a Fatigue Countermeasure: A Meta-Analytic Integration. The Journal of the Human Factors and Ergonomics Society 2005;47:360–377.
19. Ebbinghaus H. Über das Gedächtnis. Leipzig 1885. Dunker.
20. Embriaco N, Papazian L, Kentish-Barnes N, Pochard F, Azoulay E. Burnout syndrom among critical care healthcare workers. Curr Opin Crit Care 2007;13:482–488.
21. Glanzer M, Cunitz AR. Two Storage mechanisms in free recall. Journal of verbal learning and verbal behaviour 1966;5:351–360.

22. Gutierrez, Karen M. Critical Care Nurses' Reception of and Responses to Moral Distress. Dimens Crit Care Nurs. 2005;24:229–241.

23. Hurst S, Kopelin-Baucum S. A Pilot Study Relating to Hardiness in ICU Nurses. Dimens Crit Care Nurs. 2005;24:97.100.

24. Institute of Medicine. Keeping patients aafe: Transforming the work environment of nurses. Washington, DC 2004: National Academies Press.

25. Lehto J. Are executive function test dependent on working memory capacity. The Quarterly Journal of Experimental Psychology 1996;49A:29–50.

26. Lloyd-Jones, N. Stress und Burn-out-Syndrom in der Intensivpflege. In: Millar, Brian, Burnard, Philip (Hrsg): Intensivpflege – High-touch und High-tech, Psychosoziale, ethische und pflegeorganisatorische Aspekte. Bern 2002. Huber.

27. McGettrick KS, O'Neill MA. Critical care nurses – perceptions of 12-h shifts. Nursing in Critical Care 2006;11:188–197.

28. Meltzer LS, Huckabay LM. Critical Care Nurses' Perception of Futile Care and its Effect on Burnout. Am J Critical Care 2004;13:202–208.

29. Miller GA. The Magical Number Seven, Plus Or Minus Two. Psychol Rev 1956;63:81–97

30. Miller S. Conversation: A History of a Declining Art. New Haven 2006. Yale University Press.

31. Mills ME, Arnold B, Wood CM. Core 12: A controlled study of the impact of twelve-hour scheduling. Nursing Res 1983;32:356–361.

32. Mion G, Ricouard S. Rest for safety: which stakes? Ann Fr Anesth Reanim 2007;26:638–648.

33. Parkin AJ. Erinnern und Vergessen – Wie das Gedächtnis funktioniert und was man bei Gedächtnisstörungen tun kann. Bern 2000. Huber.

34. Poncet MC, Toullic P, Papaziani L, Kentish-Barnes N, Timset J-F, Pochard F, Chevret S, Schlemmer B, Azoulay E. Burnout Syndrome in Critical Care Nursing Staff. Am J Respir Crit Care Med 2007;175:698–704.

35. Postman L, Phillips LW. Short term temporal changes in free recall. Q J Exp Psychol. 1965;17:132–138.

36. Raggio B, Malacarne P. Burnout in Intensive Care Unit. Minerva Anestesiol 2007;73:195–200.

37. Reason JT. Managing the risks of organizational accidents. University of Michigan 1997.

38. Reason JT. Safety in the operating theatre – Part 2: Human error and organisational failure. Qual Saf Health Care 2005;14:56–61.

39. Reitmann JS. Mechanisms of forgetting in short-term memory. Cognitive Psychology 1971;2:185–195.

40. Richardson A, Dabner N, Curtis S. Twelve-hour shift on ITU: a nursing evaluation. Nursing in Critical Care 2003; 8:103–108.

41. Rogers AE, Hwang W-T, Scott LD, Aiken LH, Dinges DF. The working hours of hospital staff nurses and patient safety. Health Affairs 2004;23:202–212.

42. Rogers AE, Hwang W-T, Scott LD. The effects of work breaks on staff nurse performance. JONA 2004;34:512–519 (The Journal of Nursing Administration)

43. Rundus D. Analysis of rehearsal processes in free recall. Journal of Exp Psychol. 1971;89:63–77.

44. Safran C, Sands DZ, Rind DM. Online medical records: a decade of experience. Methods Inf Med. 1999;38:308–312.

45. Scott LD, Rogers AE, Hwang W-T, Zhang Y. Effects of critical care nurses' work hours on vigilance and patients' safety. Am J Crit Care 2006;15:30–37.

46. Singh R, et al.: Disability and rehabilitation 2006;28:1299–1300.

47. Smith-Coggins R, Howard S, Mac D, Wang C, Kwan S, Rosekind M, Sowb Y, Balise R, Levis J, Gaba D. Improving alertness and performance in emergency department physicians and nurses: The use of planned naps Ann Emerg Med 2006;48:596–604.

48. Specht M. Intensivmedizin. Stuttgart 2007. Georg Thieme Verlag. 392–395.

49. Sternberg S. High-speed scanning in human memory. Science 1966;153:652–654.

50. Tang P, Jaworski MA, Fellencer CA, Kreider N, La Rosa MP, Marquardt WC. Clinical information activities in diverse ambulatory care practices. Proc AMIA Annu Fall Symp. 1996:12–16.

51. Waters GS, Caplan D. The measurment of verbal working memory capacity and its relation to reading comprehension. Q J Exp Psychol A 1996;49:51–75.

52. Wilson RM, Runciman WB, Gibberd RW, Harrison BT, Hamilton JD. The Quality in Australian Health Care Study. Med J Aust. 1995;163:458–471.

53. Woloshynowych M, Davis R, Brown R, Vincent C. Communication patterns in a UK emergency department. Ann Emerg Med 2007;50:407–413

54. Zimbardo PG, Gerrig RJ. Psychologie. München 2004: Pearson Studium.

55. Zboril-Benson LR. Why nurses are calling in sick: The impact of health-care restructuring. Can J Nursing Res 2002;33:89–107.

56. Cadogan MP, Franzi C, Osterweil D, Hill T. Barriers to effective communication in skilled nursing facilities: differences in perception between nurses and physicians. J Am Geriatr Soc 1999;47:71–5.

57. Dowsett SM, Saul JL, Butow PN, Dunn SM, Boyer MJ, Findlow R, Dunsmore J. Communication styles in the cancer consultation: preferences for a patient-centred approach. Psycho-Oncology 2000;9:147–56.

58. Evans K, Hind T. Getting the message across. Nurs Times 1987;83:40–2.

59. Frederikson LG. Exploring information-exchange in consultation: the patients' view of performance and outcomes. Patient Educ Couns 1995;25:237–46.

60. Klöcker K, Schindler N, Schindler AW, Vagts DA. Information transfer during ICU ward rounds – analysis under cognitive psychological aspects. ESICM Wien 2009; Intensive Care Med 2009;35:S111.

61. Larson E, Hamilton HE, Mitchell K, Eisenberg J. Hospitalk: an exploratory study to assess what is said and what is heard between physicians and nurses. Clin Perform Qual Health Care 1998;6:183–9.

62. Van Ess Coeling H, Cukr PL. Communication styles that promote perceptions of collaboration, quality, and nurse satisfaction. J Nurs Care Qual 2000;14:63–74.

Yên-Lan Nguyen, Sandrine Dray, Aude Soury-Lavergne and Bertrand Guidet

Nursing work patterns

Critical care nurses have a central role in critical care delivery, particularly in ensuring quality decisions and promoting team synergy [1]. Whereas critical care demand is increasing in developed countries due to aging of the population, we are currently faced with a major problem: the shortage of critical care nurses. If the provision of trained staff is lower than the nursing requirement, it leads partly to insufficient time for clinical procedures, inadequate training, errors and nosocomial infections [2].

Nursing work in the intensive care units (ICUs) is characterized by a high level of work-related stress, heavy workload, sleep deprivation, limited rest and high risk of severe burnout syndrome [3]. Nursing work patterns such as the lengths of shifts vary across hospitals and within countries. The aim of this chapter is to discuss the methodological limitations of current studies on shift lengths, and to describe the impact of two-shift and three-shift models on patients and staff-centred outcomes (see Tab. 1).

Analysis of the literature

There are many studies which have been published on the effects of shift length (most often 8 hours versus 12 hours) on quality of patient care and nurse outcomes, but most of them suffer from major limitations. The majority of them are at least 10 years old and only a minority of them are focused on critical care nurses. Unfortunately, the methodological quality of the majority of these projects is relatively poor [4].

The design most commonly used is observational (cross-sectional or before-after studies). To our knowledge, no randomized-controlled study has been published recently. The definitions of main outcomes (quality of patient care and nurse outcomes) are not standardized. They also vary among studies, and this does not allow any comparisons to be made. The quality of patient care may be defined by either patient recovery, errors or near errors, mortality or length of stay. Nurse outcomes may be defined by job satisfaction, well being, physical complaints, psychological complaints (stress and emotional exhaustion), fatigue or drug and alcohol consumption. There is a failure to control results with additional factors which may influence main outcomes such as individual factors (e.g. years of experience, nurse-patient ratio, rotating shifts), quality of working relations (e.g. relations with physicians or with head-nurses) or structural factors (e.g. workload, work place climate, presence

Tab. 1   Comparison between two-shift lengths models

	8 hours	12 hours
Advantages	**At the patient level:**	**At the patient level:**
	Better follow-up of patient care Trustful relationship with patients and their families Increased participation in end-of-life discussions More efficient work	Better continuity of care (theoretical): better cooperation between nurse teams, between nurses and physicians
	At the nurse level:	**At the nurse level:**
	Less fatigue More likely to have contact with nurse chairman and nurse clinician More likely to have a familial life and leisure during working days	Planning and prioritizing patient care is easier Increased job satisfaction Decreased emotional exhaustion Satisfaction with free time: more likely to have leisure, sportive activities Increased self-estimated quality of life Reduction of sleep and gastro-intestinal disorders
		At the manager level:
		Good recruitment strategy (young nurses) Good retention strategy (less turn-over) Planning is easier to do Decreased number of caregivers to hire
Drawbacks	**At the patient level:**	**At the patient level:**
	Discontinuity of care (theoretical) Increased complications, re-interventions and ICU admissions rates Increased ICU length of stay	Decreased direct nursing care activities Increased non care activities Increased risk of errors if sleep deprivation
	At the nurse level:	**At the nurse level:**
	Increased risk of sleep disorders	± stress ± fatigue ± emotional exhaustion Increased risk of struggling to remain awake and drowsy driving if sleep deprivation associated Less performance (older nurses) Health complaints Greater use of cigarettes and alcohol Decreased contact between staff and nurse chairman and nurse clinician
	At the manager level:	
	Difficulties to do the planning Increased number of caregivers to hire	

of information technology). There is a lack of data on the case mix of patients treated which may influence the level of workload (e.g. complex or unstable patient versus stable patient). Finally no study has compared different kind of units (e.g. surgical versus mixed ICU) or different settings (e.g. academic versus community hospital, or urban versus non-urban). Indeed, ease on travel to work influences quality of life and is likely to be shorter in an urban setting.

Randomized-controlled studies with critical care nurses are needed to compare the two models. Unfortunately, carrying out such a project is apparently difficult for a couple of reasons. First, as previously seen, the choice of the main outcomes might be not so easy. It could involve either patient-centred criteria (see Tab. 2) or nurses-centred criteria (see Tab. 3). Among patient criteria, ICU mortality and morbidity, even when not specific, seem to be the best patient quality care outcomes. ICU mortality is easy to measure but the difference between the two models is likely to be small and the study might lack enough power to detect an existing difference. ICU morbidity (including the rate of medications errors, ulcer complications, patient falls, nosocomial infections and tight glucose control) is likely to be more sensitive but suffers from reporting bias. The measure of patient recovery is not standardized and does not allow comparisons. ICU length of stay is less relevant and is dependent on too many factors that outweigh critical care organization. Among all nurse outcomes' measures currently used, all are relevant but some of them lack a standardized measure or fail to control individual, team or structural factors (e.g. mean workload, presence of a safety culture). The questionnaire named the "Culture, Organization and Management in Intensive Care" (COMIC) might be a useful tool to evaluate nurse outcomes [5]. Indeed, the questionnaire evaluates organizational performance (organizational learning and change, communication, coordination, problem solving management, skills developed in the relation patient/caregiver) through cultural values (team satisfaction, people-security orientation, task-security orientation), individual well being (burning out, job satisfaction) and structural factors (mean workload per day, occupation rate, length of stay, age, years of experience, physician nurse-bed, unit size). Data were collected through answers of 1000 ICU personnel to a COMIC questionnaire [5]. Organizational performance was assessed through a composite score related to five dimensions: coordination and adaptation to uncertainty, communication, conflict management, organizational change and organizational learning, skills developed in relationship with patients and their families. The organisational performance score differed among ICUs. Some cultural values were negatively correlated with a high level of organizational performance suggesting improvement potential. Several individual and structural factors were also related to the quality of ICUs organization, including absence of burnout, older staff, satisfaction to work and high workload (p < 0.02 for each). Secondly, the voluntary participation of nurse staff might be difficult to obtain. Indeed, nurses might be reluctant to participate in worrying about their family lives. Thirdly, the schedule organization might be difficult particularly if there is the necessity to hire more caregivers. Finally, in order to be sure that the two groups are going to be similar, a large participation is necessary.

Studies with better methodological quality are needed [4]. However, conducting such a study might be challenging due to difficulties related to the definition of the main outcome or the participation of nurse staff.

Patient-centred outcomes

Three-shift model

Spending more days weekly in the unit increases the probability of nurses having a better follow-up of patient care, building a trustful relationship with patients and their families, and participating in end-of-life discussions (which occurred more often during daily rounds). All of these factors may contribute to reducing the risk of a severe burnout syndrome [3]. The 8-h shift model might be associated with more efficient work. Reid et al. found that nurses working 8 h spent more time in direct nursing care activities (particularly at the end of their shift) and less time in non care activities in comparison to those working 12 h [6].

On the other hand, the three-shift model might be associated with poor outcomes. Bollschweiler et al. found that in surgical ICUs organized by surgeons, a three-shift model (for physicians) was associated with a greater risk of complications, re-interventions, readmission to ICU and a longer ICU length of stay [7]. To our knowledge, this is the only study which looked at those outcomes among critically ill patients. These results might not be applicable to ICUs organized by intensivists or medical ICUs. The reasons for the lack of benefit of a three-shift model remain unknown. One hypothesis might involve

Tab. 2   Criteria for measuring patient quality of care

Patient quality of care	Advantages	Drawbacks
ICU-mortality	Relevant Easy to measure	Not specific Difference of ICU mortality between the two-shift models might be small
ICU-morbidity: Medications errors Ulcer complications Patients falls Nosocomial infections Tight glucose control	Relevant Might lead to quality improvement projects	Not specific Reporting bias
Patient recovery	Relevant	Not specific Measure not standardized Time of follow up? (6 months, 1 year?)
ICU length of stay	Less relevant Easy to measure	Not specific Difficulties to adjust to some organizational factors such as number of hospital beds available

the discontinuity of care partly due to the lack of time for nurse-to-nurse handoff at the end of the shift, or the number of daily handoffs (three rather than two).

Two-shift model

On one hand, the continuity of care is likely to be more efficient in a two-shift model. Indeed, the number of hand-offs is reduced (two rather than three per day) which might lead to a decreased risk of loss of information between caregivers. A 12-h shift is likely to enhance the communication and cooperation between medical and paramedical teams which might contribute to reduce conflicts between caregivers. Indeed, physicians working in the ICU are also divided into two teams: day and shift teams.

On the other hand, there is no study showing that communication is improved in a two-shift model. Although the prevalence of conflicts and good communication are linked, a recent multi-centre observational study showed that the number of hours worked per shift in the ICU did not influence the prevalence of conflicts [8]. Nurses working in 12-h shifts rarely work more than three consecutive days weekly, leading to a

reduced participation in discussions on patient end-of-life care. Such communication gap between nurses and medical staff might lead to conflicts and severe burnout syndrome [3, 8]. Also, nurses working only on night shifts are more likely to be excluded of professional teaching sessions occurring during the day. Therefore, such a schedule might not lead to an improvement in nurse-physician relationship [9]. Also, the benefits of continuity of care might be counterbalanced by a reduction of direct nursing care activities during the shift. Indeed, an American study found that a 12-h shift was associated with both a reduction in direct nursing care activities and an increased rate of non care activities [6]. Such a schedule might not lead to an improvement in any nurse-physician relationship [9]. Finally, the risk of error is increased by a factor of 2 to 3 when the shift length is greater than 12 h and 30 min [10, 11].

Staff-centred outcomes

Three-shift models

The main advantage is to preserve a family life. A recent French study showed that nearly one third of nurses working on an 8-h night shift has three

Tab. 3   Criteria for measuring nurse outcomes

Nurse outcomes	Advantages	Drawbacks
Well being	Relevant Existing standardized measure (EQ5D, SF36)	Not specific Reporting bias
Physical complaints (musculoskeletal complaints)	Relevant	Not specific Reporting bias No standardized measure Does not reflect health
Psychological complaints (stress and emotional exhaustion)	Relevant	Not specific Reporting bias No standardized measure Does not reflect health
Fatigue	Relevant	Not specific Reporting bias No standardized measure
Drug and alcohol use		Less relevant Not specific Reporting bias No standardized measure
Job satisfaction	Relevant	Not specific Reporting bias No standardized measure
Intention to quit	Relevant	Not specific Reporting bias
Burnout syndrome	Relevant Standardized measure (Maslach Burnout Inventory)	Not specific
Absenteeism, turn-over	Easy to measure	Not specific

or more children [12]. Indeed, such rotation allows them to be with their children before and after school. Then, another French survey showed that the three-shift model allows nurses to have more leisure during working days but this was not associated with a better self-estimated quality of life [13].

On the other hand, permanent night shifts or rapidly rotating shifts lead to sleep disorders [12, 14, 15]. Another drawback of a three-shift model is the need to hire an increased number of caregivers, which might be difficult in this period of shortage of health care professionals. Planning organization is more complex particularly if nurses do not want to rotate between morning, afternoon and night shifts. A French study found that three quarters of the nurses working on 8-h shifts suffered from schedule-frequent changes [13].

Two-shift model

Planning and prioritizing patient care is likely to be easier [16]. The effect of 12-h shift on stress, emotional exhaustion and job satisfaction remain unclear [4, 6, 11, 13, 17]. An explanation might be the failure to control personal characteristics such as nurses' ages. Indeed, Reid et al. found that the performance on a simulated 12-h shift rotation was influenced by age, younger caregivers performing better [18]. Another confounding factor might be the nurse to patient ratio. An American study found that in a surgical ICU, a nurse to patient ratio of less than two is associated with increased post-operative complications, increased length of stay and increased health care costs [19]. In comparison to older studies, recent published data show that nurses working on 12-h shift have the perception of an increased self-performance, an increased job satisfaction, and a decreased emotional exhaustion [11]. In a British survey, less than 10 % of nurses working on 12-h shifts had difficulties to concentrate at work [16]. A French study revealed that a two-shift model was associated with a similar level of fatigue and a reduction of sleep and gastro-intestinal disorders [12].

Several studies showed that nurses working in 12-h shifts have a better quality of life [12, 13, 16]. An easiness of travel to work, an increased number week-ends and days off, the possibility to have a social life, as well as the increased ability to read and to practice sport might partly explain these results [12, 13, 16]. At the manager level, recruitment and retention of young nurses as well as the organization of the timetable are all easier [11]. Also, the number of caregivers to hire is reduced.

On the other hand, the effects of a 12-h shift on stress, emotional exhaustion and job satisfaction remain controversial [17]. Reid et al. reported lower performance of older nurses (median 43.9 years old versus 21.2 years old) during a simulated 12-h shift rotation [18]. Some studies reported increased health complaints (musculoskeletal disorders, sleep disorders) and an increased consumption of drugs and alcohol [20–22]. An Australian study found that both shift length and sleep loss were predictors of the ability to remain awake at work, and consequently these were both predictors of errors and drowsy driving [22]. An American study showed that a shift length of longer than 12.5 h increased the risk by 1.5 to 2.4 of drowsiness or episodes of sleep [23]. An increased number of days off per week might lead to a deterioration of the relations between nurse staff, nurse chairman and nurse clinician [9]. A two-shift rotation might not be associated with greater career satisfaction [17]. At the manager level, the absenteeism rate is unlikely to be reduced in a two-shift rotation [11]. Finally there is no data on the cost-effectiveness of 12-h shift.

Conclusion

There is currently insufficient evidence to recommend a particular shift length model. ICU organizational performance is influenced by several factors (e.g. burnout level, satisfaction at work) that are directly correlated to the nurses' shift length model [5]. Therefore, choosing the shift-length model that best fits patients and staff-centred outcomes might contribute to improve ICU performance. Further studies with critical care nurses and standardized outcomes measures are definitely needed.

The authors

Yên-Lan Nguyen, MD, MPH[1]
Sandrine Dray, RN[2]
Aude Soury-Lavergne, RN[3]
Bertrand Guidet, MD[1,4,5]
[1] Assistance Publique | Hôpitaux de Paris | Hôpital Saint-Antoine | Service de réanimation médicale | Paris, France
[2] Service de réanimation médicale | Centre Hospitalier Universitaire de Marseille | France
[3] Service de réanimation polyvalente | Centre Hospitalier Universitaire de Lille | France
[4] Inserm, Unité de Recherche en Épidémiologie Systèmes d'Information et Modélisation (U707) | Paris, France
[5] UPMC Université Paris VI

Address for correspondence
Yên-Lan Nguyen
Service de Réanimation Médicale
Hôpital Saint-Antoine
Assistance Publique des Hôpitaux de Paris
184, rue du Faubourg Saint-Antoine
75571 Paris Cedex 12, France
E-mail: YenlanFr@aol.com

References

1. Propp KM, Apker J, Zabava Ford WS, Wallace N, Serbenski M and Hofmeister N. Meeting the complex needs of the health care team: identification of nurse-team communication practices perceived to enhance patient outcomes. Qual Health Res 2010;20(1):15–28.
2. Tarnow-Mordi WO, Hau C, Warden A, and Shearer AJ. Hospital mortality in relation to staff workload: a 4-year study in an adult intensive-care unit. Lancet 2000;356(9225):185–9.
3. Poncet MC, Toullic P, Papazian L, Kentish-Barnes N, Timsit JF, Pochard F, Chevret S, Schlemmer B, and Azoulay E. Burnout syndrome in critical care nursing staff. Am J Respir Crit Care Med 2007;175(7):698–704.

4. Estabrooks CA, Cummings GG, Olivo SA, Squires JE, Giblin C, and Simpson N. Effects of shift length on quality of patient care and health provider outcomes: systematic review. Qual Saf Health Care 2009;18(3):181–8.

5. Minvielle E, Dervaux B, Retbi A, Aegerter P, Boumendil A, Jars-Guincestre MC, Tenaillon A, and Guidet B. Culture, organization, and management in intensive care: construction and validation of a multidimensional questionnaire. J Crit Care 2005.;20(2):126–38.

6. Reid N., Robinson G, and Todd C. The quantity of nursing care on wards working 8- and 12-hour shifts. Int J Nurs Stud 1993;30(5):403–13.

7. Bollschweiler E, Krings A, Fuchs KH, Pistorius G, Bein T, Otto U, Muhl E, Backes-Gellner U, and Holscher AH. Alternative shift models and the quality of patient care. An empirical study in surgical intensive care units. Langenbecks Arch Surg 2001.;386(2):104–9.

8. Azoulay E, Timsit JF, Sprung CL, Soares M, Rusinova K, Lafabrie A, Abizanda R, Svantesson M, Rubulotta F, Ricou B, Benoit D, Heyland D, Joynt G, Francais A, Azeivedo-Maia P, Owczuk R, Benbenishty J, de Vita M, A. Valentin, A. Ksomos, S. Cohen, L. Kompan, K. Ho, F. Abroug, A. Kaarlola, H. Gerlach, T. Kyprianou, Michalsen A, Chevret S, and Schlemmer B. Prevalence and factors of intensive care unit conflicts: the conflicus study. Am J Respir Crit Care Med 2009.;180(9):853–60.

9. Mills ME, Arnold B, and Wood CM. Core-12: a controlled study of the impact of 12-hour scheduling. Nurs Res 1983.;32(6):356–61.

10. Rogers AE, Hwang WT, Scott LD, Aiken LH and Dinges DF. The working hours of hospital staff nurses and patient safety. Health Aff (Millwood) 2004;23(4):202–12.

11. Stone PW, Du Y, Cowell R, Amsterdam N, Helfrich TA, Linn RW, Gladstein A, Walsh M, and Mojica LA. Comparison of nurse, system and quality patient care outcomes in 8-hour and 12-hour shifts. Med Care 2006.;44(12):1099–106.

12. Estrin-Behar M, and Bonnet N. Travailler de nuit en 8, 10 ou 12 heures à l'hôpital. Arch. mal. prof., Masson ed. 2000.;402–416.

13. Barrau-Baumstarck K, Rebeschini E, Dalivoust G, Durand-Bruguerolle D, Gazazian G, and Martin F. [Shiftwork and quality of life among critical care nurses and paramedical personnel]. Presse Med 2009;38(3):346–53.

14. Poissonnet CM, and Veron M. Health effects of work schedules in healthcare professions. J Clin Nurs 2000;9(1):13–23.

15. Garde AH, Hansen AM, and Hansen J. Sleep length and quality, sleepiness and urinary melatonin among healthy Danish nurses with shift work during work and leisure time. Int Arch Occup Environ Health 2009;82(10):1219–28.

16. Richardson A, Turnock C, Harris L, Finley A, and Carson S. A study examining the impact of 12-hour shifts on critical care staff. J Nurs Manag 2007;15(8):838–46.

17. Hoffman AJ, and Scott LD. Role stress and career satisfaction among registered nurses by work shift patterns. J Nurs Adm 2003.;33(6):337–42.

18. Reid K, and Dawson D. Comparing performance on a simulated 12 hour shift rotation in young and older subjects. Occup Environ Med 2001;58(1):58–62.

19. Amaravadi RK, Dimick JB, Pronovost PJ, and Lipsett PA. ICU nurse-to-patient ratio is associated with complications and resource use after esophagectomy. Intensive Care Med 2000;26(12):1857–62.

20. Trinkoff AM, and Storr CL. Work schedule characteristics and substance use in nurses. Am J Ind Med 1998;34(3):266–71.

21. Lipscomb JA, Trinkoff AM, Geiger-Brown J, and Brady B. Work-schedule characteristics and reported musculoskeletal disorders of registered nurses. Scand J Work Environ Health 2002;28(6):394–401.

22. Dorrian J, Tolley C, Lamond N, van den Heuvel C, Pincombe J, Rogers AE, and Drew D. Sleep and errors in a group of Australian hospital nurses at work and during the commute. Appl Ergon 2008;39(5):605–13.

23. Scott LD, Rogers AE, Hwang WT, and Zhang Y. Effects of critical care nurses' work hours on vigilance and patients' safety. Am J Crit Care 2006;15(1):30–7.

Maria Wittmann, Daniela Dewald and Christian Putensen

Physician extenders

Introduction – what are physician extenders?

A physician extender is a non-physician providing medical services on behalf of, or in conjunction with, a leading physician. He is specially trained and certified to provide basic medical services under the supervision of a licensed physician. Physician extenders may order tests and make referrals related to the patient's medical needs; the most common groups of physician extenders are nurse practitioners (NP) and physician assistants (PA).

Historical development

In the 17th century, Feldshers, originally German military medical assistants, were introduced into Russian armies by Peter the Great to provide medical care. 1803 in France "Officiers de Sante" were introduced by Rene Fourcroy to help alleviate health personnel shortages in the military and civilian sectors.

In the 1960s, China trained more than 1.3 million "barefoot doctors" to improve the delivery of health care. Due to a nationwide shortage of doctors in primary care in the mid-1960s a new cadre of providers of medical care was developed in the United States to address the short-

age and uneven distribution of primary care physicians. The official origin of nurse practitioners (NPs) took place when the first class of NPs graduated at the University of Colorado in 1965. To expand the delivery of quality medical care, in 1965 Dr. Eugene Stead of the Duke University Medical Centre in North Carolina initiated the first formal physician's assistant program, now called the Physician's Associate Program [1, 2]. He selected Navy corpsmen who received considerable medical training during their military service and during the war in Vietnam but who had no comparable civilian employment. He based the curriculum of the physician assistants (PA) program in part on his knowledge of the fast-track training of doctors during World War II.

Shortly after establishing the first physician assistants, studies have been conducted to investigate the need for physician extenders and to evaluate the quality of their work. Extensive studies of "what physician extenders do" in practice have been published since 1969. In January 1969 a task delegation questionnaire was used to compare physician extender practices in seven primary care-orientated sites [3].

In July 1969 a study was performed, documenting the expectations of physicians towards the physician extenders [4]. In 1973 a survey was performed to measure physician attitudes towards delegating responsibility in North Carolina, where 52 % of the physicians declared that they had approved of the concept but would not hire a NP, whereas only 34 % of the respondents would hire a NP [5]. The quality of the work of physician extenders was evaluated in 1973 from Fine and Silver, who compared the quality of diagnostic and therapeutic processes for PAs with that of physicians. Concurrence of diagnosis was found in 91.6 percent of the examined cases [6].

As of today there are over 120,000 practicing NPs in the United States. Close to 6,000 new NPs are prepared each year at over 325 colleges and universities. There are approximately 68,100 practicing PAs (in January 2009). Approximately 12,470 students are currently enrolled in over 140 PA programs.

Recently, several countries have become interested in adapting the concept of physician assistants to their needs. In the United Kingdom interest in the concept is increasing, as shown by the call by the NHS and the Royal College of Physicians for an early start of pilot projects [7].

The physician extenders concept in different countries

For physician extenders there is a wide diversity in the different countries concerning the occupational title, the responsibilities and the legislation.

United States

In the US, the most common types of physician extenders are PAs and NPs.

Physician assistants (PAs) are health professionals licensed to practice medicine with physician supervision. PAs perform a comprehensive range of medical duties, from basic primary care to high-technology specialty procedures. PAs often act as first or second assistants in major surgery and provide pre and post-operative care.

In some rural areas where physicians are in short supply, PAs serve as the primary providers of health care, conferring with their supervising physicians and other medical professionals as needed and as required by law. PAs can

be found in virtually every medical and surgical specialty. According to the 2008 census report of the American Academy of Physician Assistants, PAs practise in family and general medicine (25.9 percent), general surgery and surgical subspecialties (25.1 percent), general internal medicine and its subspecialties (15.6 percent), emergency medicine (10.5 percent) and other areas of medicine. The PA's responsibilities depend on the type of practice, his or her experience, the working relationship with physicians and other health care providers, and state laws.

Their education requires a bachelor's degree, plus two to three years of additional training that results in a relevant master's degree. PAs are accredited by the Accreditation Review Commission on Education for the Physician Assistant (ARC-PA). A Physician Assistant National Certifying Exam (PANCE) has to be absolved.

Nurse practitioners (NPs) have completed a registered nursing degree as a part of a bachelor's degree, plus a master's degree. A NP may be certified in a specialty area, such as family health, oncology, or paediatrics. They can serve as a patient's regular healthcare provider, and may diagnose, order tests, develop treatment plans and write prescriptions. Most NPs work in collaboration with a physician. They are accredited through several organizations, including the American Academy of Nurse Practitioners.

The NP generally completes a two year master's level course after a four year registered nurse degree program [8]. They mainly work semi-autonomously in association with individual doctors, but an increasing number works in hospitals. They seem to be well accepted by both doctors and patients.

Both NPs and PAs have similar pathways following graduation. They are licensed to practice in all States under the supervision of a practicing physician and must abide by the governing rules of the State and the medical organizations therein. They can prescribe medications including narcotics; they carry malpractice insurance and are recognized for payment by Medicare and Medicaid. Both groups have national organizations – The American Academy of Physician Assistants and the American Academy of Nurse Practitioners. Both NPs and PAs have progressed into specialty and subspecialty areas of medicine. In intensive care units (ICUs), intensivists provide care only to a minority of ICU patients in the United States [9].

Canada

The first physician extenders have been employed by the Canadian Forces (CF) over 50 years ago. In 1984 the first class of "Physician Assistants" graduated from the Canadian Forces Medical Services School at Borden Ontario [10] . They are generally acknowledged as the first formally trained PAs in Canada. In October 1999 the Canadian Academy of Physician Assistants (now the Canadian Association of Physician Assistants, CAPA) was formed. In 2003 military PAs gained legislative changes allowing them to work in the civilian world after retirement. Each jurisdiction in Canada has its own regulation for Physician Assistants. Most are trying to develop their own programs with different admission requirements. Physician Assistants can be certified by the CAPA. The University of Manitoba started the first Physician Assistant Education Program for Graduate students in 2008. As of January 2010, Canada will have four physician assistant education programs.

England

The National Health Service (NHS) faces a serious shortage of medical doctors. The NHS Plan stated that staffing constraints, rather than lack of funding, posed the greatest threat to NHS modernisation. One option for improvement is to introduce a new group of staff – PAs, to function between fully trained doctors and nurses [11, 12]. Initially, U.S.-trained PAs worked in a pilot project in Sandwell and West Birmingham [13]. Later the University of Birmingham was approached by a local primary care organisation to develop an own training program for medical care practitioners (MCP), the new physician assistant equivalent for the UK. Afterwards, in 2004 a pilot project started to develop the new role of primary care MCPs. The National Competence and Curriculum Framework Steering Group formally constituted in 2004, and its task was to develop practical guidance for employers, higher educational institutions and potential stu-

dents as how the MCP role would work and how the entry to the new profession might be managed [14]. The new programs are 24 months in length, and result in a post-graduate diploma with the option of "topping up" to a Master's degree either by full or part-time study [15]. Training is focused on General Medicine and Emergency Medicine. There is now preliminary evidence to suggest that the introduction of the MCP role, based on the proven North American PA model, may make a valuable contribution to clinical care in the NHS and represents an effective strategy for increasing medical capacity without jeopardising quality. However several fundamental issues remain to be resolved, including regulation, registration and prescribing. The realisation of this new profession for the UK now awaits the outcome of the national consultation process [16].

Australia

The government of Queensland recruited 2009 physician assistants from the US as part of a trial to assess their effect on the delivery of healthcare services. The year-long trial at five sites should assess team work, productivity, quality of care, as well as patient satisfaction [17]. Physician assistants should help to alleviate shortages in the workforce, particularly in rural, remote, and other areas with few doctors [18].

The Netherlands

Physician assistants were introduced in the Netherlands in 2000, using the extensive experiences from the United States. Formerly, doctor's assistants were working in the Netherlands, but these were variously qualified without a standardized national program [19]. At this moment there are about 400 PAs working in the Netherlands. PAs are active within almost all areas of the medical field. Many PAs are members of the Netherlands Association of Physician Assistants (NAPA). The Netherlands has educational programs at the Academie Gezondheidszorg in Utrecht, University of Arnhem/Nijmegen, the University of Groningen and the University of Leiden. Programs are 30 months in length. In order to be admitted to the Master Training Physician Assistant, the PA candidate must have proof of an advanced level of professional education (HBO) in healthcare (i.e. nursing or physiotherapy) and at least two years of relevant work experience.

Germany

In Germany the physician assistant is not jet clinically established, and there is no existing comparable academic education program as e.g. in the United States. In 2009 the private Sana-Kliniken started to train physician assistants at the Steinbeis-Hochschule, Berlin. The program is supported by the German Society of Orthopedics and Trauma Surgery and the German Heart Centre, Berlin. This program qualifies for a Bachelor of Science degree. Other PA programs are planned in Karlsruhe and Rheine. PAs are only allowed to practise under supervision of physicians. At the moment there are no existing laws defining the profession of German PAs and their role in the health care systems [20]. The German Society of Anaesthesiology and Intensive Care Medicine decided 2007 a resolution, which defines medical core competences and the possibility of delegation in anaesthesia and intensive care medicine. They emphasize that every patient must be treated by a board-certified or equivalently qualified anaesthesiologist [21, 22].

Operational area of physician extenders

Physician extenders are employed in diverse fields of the patient's care; the main operational areas are ambulatory care, operating room (OR), intensive care units (ICUs) and emergency departments (EDs).

Ambulatory care

Demand for primary care services has increased in many countries due to population aging, rising patient expectations, and reforms that shift care from hospitals to the community. At the same time, the supply of physicians is constrained [23] and there is increasing pressure to restrict costs. Shifting care from doctors to spe-

cial nurses is one possible response to these challenges. The expectation is that primary care nurses working in extended roles can:
- enhance the quality of services provided by doctors;
- safely substitute for doctors in an wide array of services, so reducing demand for doctors; and
- reduce the direct costs of services because nurses are less expensive to hire than physicians.

Several systematic reviews of doctor-nurse substitution in primary care have sought to identify whether nurses differ from doctors in terms of patient outcomes, process of care or resource utilisation [24]. Research into doctor-nurse substitution in primary care appears primarily to have been conducted in the USA, Canada and the UK, where physician extenders have been integrated into the health system for many years. The findings suggested that, as compared with doctor-led care, nurse-led care was associated with higher levels of patient compliance and satisfaction, longer consultations, and higher rates of laboratory testing. Health outcomes for patients were similar [25, 26].

Operating room (OR)

A registered nurse (RN) who assists with patient care in the operating room is also referred to as a perioperative nurse. Perioperative nursing includes activities in the preoperative, intraoperative and postoperative phases of surgery. They are organized in the Association of Perioperative Registered Nurses (AORN).

Perioperative nurses are RNs who work in hospital surgical departments, day-surgery units (also called ambulatory surgery), clinics and physician's offices. They work closely with the surgical patient, family members and other healthcare professionals to help plan, implement and evaluate treatment.

Historically, perioperative nursing practice has included the role of the registered professional nurse as an assistant during surgery. As early as 1977, documents issued by the American College of Surgeons supported the appropriateness of qualified RNs to first assist. The AORN position statement delineates the definition, scope of practice, and educational requirements for the perioperative registered nurse (RN) who practices as a registered nurse first assistant (RNFA) [27]. The RNFA works in collaboration with the surgeon and other health care team members to achieve optimal patient outcomes. Intraoperatively the RNFA practices at the direction of the surgeon and does not concurrently function as a scrub person. The minimum qualifications to practice as an RN first assistant include a certification in perioperative nursing (CNOR) and successful completion of an RNFA program that meets the "AORN standards for RN first assistant education programs".

Physician assistants play an important role in perioperative medicine. Starting in 1973 they were employed by the division of cardiothoracic surgery of the Emory University Hospital [28]. Additionally the Norwalk Hospital and the Yale University School of Medicine started in 1978 a PA residency program in surgery. The aim was to develop health professionals who could serve in a capacity similar to that of junior surgical residents. The PAs should deliver preoperative and postoperative care under the supervision of surgeons and assist in operations [29]. After the changes in the regulations of resident house staff duty hours in 2003 (80 hours per week limit), there has been resurgence in the need and demand of PAs. The PA has been able to relieve the residents of many time-consuming routine duties so that more of their time can be devoted to operating room and other more educational tasks. The exact role of PAs in surgery teams is determined by their clinical experience and the discretion of the attending cardiothoracic surgeon. In the division of cardiothoracic surgery of the Emory University Hospital the PAs play a vital role in

1. education of patients, families, nurses, PA students and residents in training;
2. They have administrative functions such as planning of admissions, scheduling of operation, maintaining records and clinical research;
3. PAs act as surgical first or second assistants during the performance of surgical procedures.

The cardiothoracic PA has a significant amount of autonomy in the operating room and performs the critical task of harvesting the saphenous veins or radial arteries for almost every coronary bypass procedure. Afterwards, PAs (either first or second) assist during the remainder of the case, including tasks of providing cardiac retraction, closure of the incisions in the lower extremity, and assist in cannulation and decannulation, as well as closure of the chest [30].

Several studies have examined the influence of physician extenders on surgical residents [31, 32]. Buch et al. performed a survey to determine how the integration of physician extenders into surgical teams has affected the surgical resident's perception of their education and overall residency experience in the department of surgery of the Mount Sinai School of Medicine, NY. They found out that residents and physician extenders agreed to work well together and that physician extenders contribute to resident education [33]. Additionally the implementation of PAs enabled an increase in the number of cases without employing more physicians [30].

Anaesthesia

Physician extenders play an important role in anaesthesia. Nurse anaesthetists have been providing anaesthesia care in the United States for nearly 150 years. The American Association of Nurse Anaesthetists (AANA) claims that nurse anaesthetists are the oldest nurse specialty group in the United States. Among the first American nurses to provide anaesthesia was Catherine S. Lawrence, who, probably along with other nurses, administered anaesthesia during the American Civil War (1861–1865) [34]. In the United States, a Certified Registered Nurse Anaesthetist (CRNA) is a registered nurse (RN) who has acquired graduate-level education in anaesthesia overseen by the American Association of Nurse Anesthetists's (AANA). Nurse anaesthetists must first complete a bachelor's degree, usually a Bachelor of Science in Nursing but it can be a Bachelor of Science in another science-related subject in some instances. They must be a licensed registered nurse. In addition, candidates are required to have a minimum of one year of full-time nursing experience in an acute care setting, such as medical intensive care unit or surgical intensive care unit. Following this year of experience, applicants apply to a Council on Accreditation (COA) accredited program of anaesthesia education and study for 24 to 36 months (http://www.aana.com/educuscrnas.aspx). Realistically, it takes a CRNA 8–10 years of education to achieve the complete CRNA training. Although all nurse anaesthetists currently graduate with a master's degree, one may continue their education to the terminal degree level, either earning a Ph.D. or similar research doctorate (DNS, DNSc), or a clinical/practice doctorate such as a DNAP (Doctor of Nurse Anaesthesia Practice), or DNP/DrNP (Doctor of Nursing Practice).

CRNAs practise in a wide variety of public and private settings including large academic medical centres, small community hospitals, outpatient surgery centres, pain clinics, or physician's offices, whether working together with anaesthesiologists, other CRNAs alone, or in solo practice. The licensed CRNA is authorized to deliver comprehensive anaesthesia care under the particular Nurse Practice Act of each state. Their anaesthesia practice consists of all accepted anaesthetic techniques (http://www.aana.com/scope.aspx). The degree of independence or supervision varies with state law; a specific supervision by an anaesthesiologist is not required in any state (http://www.aana.com/finalsupervisionfaqs.aspx, http://en.wikipedia.org/wiki/Nurse_anesthetist-cite_note-timeline-1#cite_note-timeline-1).

Discussions about extending the anaesthesia care team recently also took place in other countries. Many European countries have varying levels of assistant for anaesthesiologists. The UK provides operating department assistants or operating department practitioners who are relatively low-skilled. In continental Europe, assistants to anaesthesiologist are often called "anaesthetic nurses", and their scope of duties ranges from solely assisting anaesthesiologists (in Germany) to those of "nurse-anaesthetists" who have undergone an in-depth training programme and work relatively independently under the supervision of an anaesthesiologist (in Sweden and Switzerland). Current demographic and macroeconomic trends indicate that, in Europe, the demand for medical services will continue to increase. Employers will realize that they will not be able to recruit new anaesthesiologists in a sufficient number without offering flexibility of working practice and adequate compensation. Alternatively, more responsibilities and tasks

may be allocated to well-trained assisting personnel such as nurses. Some countries (Sweden, Switzerland) have shown the feasibility of such staffing for many years, whereas in other countries (Belgium, the UK), the introduction of anaesthesia nurses has only recently come under consideration [35].Many authors tried to answer the question if anaesthetic or surgical outcome is worse when medical anaesthetists delegate responsibility for all or part of the anaesthetic care to a nonmedical anaesthetist. To summarize, there is no good evidence of difference in outcome between medical and nonmedical anaesthetists. The circumstances of anaesthesia and surgery vary enormously between countries, and anaesthesia teams must be planned to accommodate the particular skills of the workforce, the working practices of surgeons and the physical arrangement of operating theatres. The whole system of anaesthesia care should be audited against criteria of outcome, patient satisfaction, cost and flexibility of working. Whoever administers anaesthesia and however their team is organized, it is most important to meet the standards that matter to the patient [36].

Emergency departments (EDs)

Emergency department overcrowding is a serious problem in the USA. Overcrowding is defined as a situation in which demand for emergency services exceeds the ability of a department to provide quality care within acceptable time frames. Emergency department overcrowding is a matter of patient safety when there is a delay in providing care as well as an issue with patient satisfaction [37]. The Joint Commission on Accreditation of Healthcare Organizations review of sentinel events has attributed patient deaths to delays in patient care. In hospital emergency departments, delay of treatment is the most common type of sentinel event [38]. The 2004 National Hospital Ambulatory Medical Care Survey (NHAMCS) reports an 18 % increase in the number of visits to emergency departments from 1994 to 2004 [39]. During the same period of time, there was a decrease of about 12 % in the number of hospital emergency departments in the United States. The 2004 NHAMCS also provides insight into the acuity of care being provided in emergency departments. Only 12.9 % of ED visits were classified as emergent with 37.8 % urgent, 21.8 % semi-urgent and 12.5 % non-urgent. This small percentage of ED visits classified as emergent suggests that nurse practitioners are suited ideally to providing care to the majority of ED patients. One national survey of hospitals, however, found that only 17 % of respondents employed nurse practitioners in the emergency department and only an additional 9 % were planning to hire new nurse practitioners. The emergency department is the only segment of the health care system in the USA that is mandated by federal law to screen and, if necessary, treat all patients who are presented to the emergency department for care. The emergency medical treatment ensures that the public has access to a medical screening exam in the emergency department regardless of the ability to pay. In the absence of a national universal health benefits program, hospital emergency departments are essentially the only place in the US health system where all patients are guaranteed medical care.

Several factors have created a need for alternatives to traditional physician staffing of emergency departments, including the shortage of board-certified emergency physicians, insufficient hospital funds to hire more physician providers, and difficulty with physician recruitment and retention in rural and other underserved areas. The emergency physician workforce supply has lagged behind the demand for emergency services, and with the forecasted growth in ED visits, the shortage is expected to continue for at least several decades [40].

In recent years, PAs and NPs have been used to augment physician staffing of EDs. Special programs for NP in the US have been established to train emergency nurse practitioners (ENPs). As there is no national certification for ENPs, graduates of these programs are also educated to qualify for national certification in other nurse practitioner areas. At Emory University, for example, graduates are eligible to become certified as family nurse practitioners. Although there are few programs educating emergency nurse practitioners, many primary care nurse practitioners are well suited to care for the majority of patients with non-emergent problems who present to the emergency department. The use of nurse practitioners in the emergency department, which

began in the 1970s, can complement the care of the emergency department physician and thereby improve ED efficiency. The responsibilities of the ED nurse practitioner should be consistent with her or his educational preparation, area of certification, and state scope of practice.

An analysis of ED visits from 1993 to 2005 documented in the NHAMCS shows that from 1993 to 2005 5.2 % of US ED visits were seen by PAs and 1.7 % by NPs. During the study period, PA visits rose from 2.9 % to 9.1 %, whereas NP visits rose from 1.1 % to 3.8 %. Compared to physician-only visits, those seen only by physician extenders arrived by ambulance less frequently (6.0 % vs. 15 %), had lower urgent acuity (37 % vs. 59 %), and were admitted less often (3.0 % vs. 13 %). An increasing use of physician extenders is particularly seen in non-profit hospitals and urban areas [41].

When assessing the potential benefits of a NP in the ED, primary outcome measures should include his or her impact on wait times, patient satisfaction, quality of care and cost-effectiveness [42]. Further, it is important to consider the study's country of origin when interpreting the results, because of missing international standards for the role of emergency nurse practitioners [43].

The cost-benefit ratio is another factor to consider. NPs appear to be more expensive than residents, on a per-patient-basis. Attending physicians are paid significantly more than are NPs, who in turn are better paid than residents and nurses. However, there are training costs to a residency program beyond the salary and it is unclear how much this was a factor in the analyses. The additional cost of having a nurse in the treatment area is offset in some of the systems by having the NP carry out the nursing treatment as well. Holistic care, or having the same health care provider during the entire ED visit, is advocated by some to improve the recognition of potential complications and a patient's knowledge of self-care or symptom management. However, it contributes to lower volumes of patients seen by the NP compared to a staff emergency physician (1–2 patients per hour versus 3–4 patients per hour) [42].

Quality of care is another important consideration. NPs did equally well at x-ray interpretation and were better at documentation and following protocols when compared with residents. The additional patient-contact time afforded by the NP encounter, along with improved communication and shorter length of stay, appear to translate into greater patient satisfaction [44, 45]. Patients receive more health information and better discharge instructions. Employing NPs in EDs is also very effective to archive new wait time benchmarks. Minor injury patients, representing a significant portion for ED visits, have waited the longest because of the use of a triage system. The addition of a NP to the ED did reduce wait times for the low acuity patients and was more cost effective than adding board-certified physicians to treat this category of patients [46]. The integration of physician extenders in a trauma service significantly reduced total hospital length of stay (LOS) and resident work hours without adversely effecting mortality [45].

Thus NPs represent a viable and effective option for the low acuity patients in overcrowded urban EDs and in the setting of rural EDs, allowing optimal use of limited physician resources and improving access to emergency care for the population. Several studies have been conducted to evaluate the quality of patients care as well as the cost effectiveness of physician extenders.

Intensive care units (ICUs)

ICUs vary significantly from hospital to hospital with respect to structure, services provided, personnel and their level of expertise, and organizational characteristics. In the United States most of the board-certified intensivists are of internal medicine background, with or without pulmonary subspecialty. But intensivists provide care only to a minority of ICU patients in the United States [9]. There are approximately 5,980 ICUs in the United States, caring for 55,000 patients daily [47]. Current staffing is heterogeneous with 26 % of ICUs having high-intensity and 73 % low-intensity intensivist coverage. In-house physician coverage is available in 20 % of the ICUs during weekend days, 12 % during weeknights, and 10 % during weekend nights [48]. A comparable situation exists in Canada. A survey of Canadian intensive care units for the Canadian Critical Care Trials Group showed that dedicated in-house physician coverage overnight was available in 60 % of the surveyed ICUs, but only in 15 % an ICU staff physician stayed in-house overnight. The

median level of postgraduate experience was 3 years, and 48 % had less than 3 months of ICU experience. Most of the shifts were more than 20 hours long [49]. A systematic review of observational studies comparing patients treated by an intensivist (dedicated ICU staff physician mostly with specialty training in internal medicine) and multidisciplinary teams was performed in 2002. The study showed lower mortality rates and shorter durations of ICU stay if patients were cared by an intensivist, than those associated with other models of care [50].

In order to improve patient safety and health care quality The Leapfrog Group called for an ICU physician staffing standard in 2001. Later in 2003 a Task Force of the American College of Critical Care Medicine (ACCM) established Guidelines of critical care services and personnel based on a system of categorization of three levels of care [51]. Due to a shortage of intensivists, implementation for the ACCM guidelines is not possible at this time. Despite some limitations, the Leapfrog standard is easier to implement and more likely to improve the care of the critically ill [52]. Faced with the limited availability of trained critical care physicians' and residents' work hour limits, an increasing number of physician extenders working in the ICU should help to provide appropriate care to the critically ill. Specially training programmes have been launched for physician extenders in intensive care medicine. The national certification for acute care nurse practitioner (ACNP) practice began in 1995 and currently, over 5,000 NPs have received certification as ACNPs, a role focused on providing care to acute and critically ill patients [53]. Also, physician assistants – traditionally oriented towards primary care – are currently working in critical care. Training for advanced responsibilities has traditionally been provided by the sponsoring physician. In addition several post-graduate programs in critical care medicine exist.

General roles and responsibilities of NPs and PAs include patient assessment, history and physical examinations, rounding with the multidisciplinary team and even performing invasive procedures if specially trained. Physician extenders can participate in several areas of patient care including consultations, discharges, admissions and routine care aspects, such as assessing patients at the bedside, ordering medications, reviewing and/or interpreting diagnostic and laboratory tests, nutrition, updating families and coordination of specialty consults.

Studies on the impact of physician extenders on patient care demonstrate that NP and PA-care has improved clinical and financial outcomes for mechanically ventilated patients including ventilator duration, LOS, mortality and cost savings. They also showed benefits for patients with chronic heart failure and vascular medicine patients. Physician extenders were proficient in skills such as intracranial pressure monitor placement, surgical assistants, invasive procedures and diagnostic cardiac catheterization. Physician extenders improved the implementation and compliance with clinical practice guidelines, including mechanical ventilation weaning, infection prevention measures and sepsis bundles [8].

In Europe, the situation of intensive care medicine (ICM) varies profoundly between countries [54]. The general model of ICU structure in Europe is the closed unit, where a specialised team of nurses and intensivists are responsible for the patients. There are differences in terms of structure as well as training and education in the different countries and hospitals. The situation of training and specialty status in Europe has been analysed in a survey by the European Society for Intensive Care Medicine (ESICM). Except in Spain, special competence in ICM is linked to a basic specialty (ICM as a subspecialty). In most European countries, access to postgraduate training in ICM is open to several disciplines, finishing with a specialist registration [55]. The structural organization of ICUs in Europe has not been analysed in a general, representative way. However, some important information can be extracted from the EPIC study (European Prevalence of Infection in Intensive Care). Vincent et al. analysed structural characteristics of 1417 Western European ICUs [56]. In 72% a committed 24-hour doctor was on duty. Italy and Spain had the highest number of ICUs with a full-time doctor, while The Netherlands and Finland had the lowest number. In a survey from the German Interdisciplinary Association of Critical Care Medicine (DIVI), Stiletto et al. evaluated 349 ICUs (25.5% of all ICUs in Germany), including a large spectrum of different hospitals [57]. An intensivist was present in 74% of the ICUs during working hours but in only 20% the ICUs during working hours but in only 20% at night. Outside working hours, non-specialist residents were present in the ICU in 56% of the hospitals. Obviously there are not enough intensivists available to provide 24-hour coverage for every ICU. The DIVI defined the requirements for certification of an ICU for training in ICM. Thus "patient care shall be provided continuously over a 24-hour period by physicians who are permanent staff members of the intensive care unit."

Although several European countries such as the UK, Ireland, the Netherlands, Belgium, Finland, Sweden and Switzerland launched education programmes at a graduate level for physician extenders in general, physician extenders play only a minor role in European intensive care medicine.

Summary

The role and education of physician extenders varies enormously in different countries. The benefit of physician assistants for the patients depends on the structural and educational conditions of the operational area. In intensive care medicine, physician extenders have been introduced mostly due to a shortage of trained intensivists to improve care giving. The benefit of physician assistants in intensive care giving has to be continuously assessed and may vary profoundly due to the differences in structure and organisation in different hospitals and countries.

The authors

Maria Wittmann, MD
Daniela Dewald, MD
Christian Putensen, Prof., MD
    Department of Anaesthesiology and
    Intensive Care Medicine | University
    Hospital Bonn | Bonn, Germany

Address for correspondence
    Maria Wittmann
    Department of Anaesthesiology and
    Intensive Care Medicine
    University Hospital Bonn
    Sigmund-Freud-Str. 25
    53105 Bonn, Germany
    E-mail: Maria.Wittmann@ukb.uni-bonn.de

References

1. Stead EA. Eugene A. Stead, Jr., MD Biography – PA History Center. In: 2010.
2. Braun JA, Howard DR and Pondy LR. The physician's associate-a task analysis. Am J Public Health 1973;63:1024–1028.
3. Glenn JK and Goldman J. Task delegation to physician extenders–some comparisons. Am J Public Health 1976;66:64–66.
4. Coye RD and Hansen MF. The "doctor's assistant". A survey of physicians' expectations. JAMA 1969;209:529–533.
5. Lawrence RS, DeFriese GH, Putnam SM, Pickard CG, Cyr AB and Whiteside SW. Physician receptivity to nurse practitioners: a study of the correlates of the delegation of clinical responsibility. Med Care 1977;15:298–310.
6. Fine LL and Silver HK. Comparative diagnostic abilities of child health associate interns and practicing pediatricians. J Pediatr 1973;83:332–335.
7. Mittman DE, Cawley JF and Fenn WH. Physician assistants in the United States. BMJ 2002;325:485–487.
8. Kleinpell RM, Ely EW and Grabenkort R. Nurse practitioners and physician assistants in the intensive care unit: an evidence-based review. Crit Care Med 2008;36:2888–2897.
9. Angus DC, Kelley MA, Schmitz RJ, White A and Popovich J, Jr. Caring for the critically ill patient. Current and projected workforce requirements for care of the critically ill and patients with pulmonary disease: can we meet the requirements of an aging population? JAMA 2000;284:2762–2770.
10. Hooker RS, MacDonald K, Patterson R. Physician assistants in the Canadian Forces. Mil Med. 2003;168(11):948–50.
11. Hutchinson L, Marks T and Pittilo M. The physician assistant: would the US model meet the needs of the NHS? BMJ 2001;323:1244–1247.
12. Stewart A and Catanzaro R. Can physician assistants be effective in the UK? Clin Med 2005;5:344–348.
13. Woodin J, McLeod H., McManus R and Jelphs K. Evaluation of US-trained Physician Assistants working in the NHS in England. In: Health Services Management Centre, University of Birmingham, 2005.
14. Abbott S, Stubbe K and Franklin GA. Local pilot, new profession: developing Medical Care Practitioners in primary care. In: 2006:188–193.
15. University of Hertfordshire. Physician Assistant Studies Medical Practice. In: 2010.
16. Parle JV, Ross NM and Doe WF. The medical care practitioner: developing a physician assistant equivalent for the United Kingdom. Med J Aust 2006;185:13–17.
17. Sweet M. Australia to try US-style physician assistants. BMJ 2008;337:a1407. doi: 10.1136/bmj.a1407.: a1407.
18. O'Connor TM and Hooker RS. Extending rural and remote medicine with a new type of health worker: physician assistants. Aust J Rural Health 2007;15:346–351.
19. Fischer I. Doctors' assistants and what they do in The Netherlands. World Health Forum 1994;15:269–270.
20. Ulsenheimer K. [Delegation of medical responsibilities to non-medical personnel. Options and limits from a legal viewpoint]. Unfallchirurg 2009;112:1004–1009.
21. Van AH and Landauer B. [Medical core competence and delegation in anaesthesia. Resolution of the German Society for Anaesthesiology and Intensive Care Medicine and the Professional Association of German Anaesthetists from 26.10.2007/08.11.2007]. Anaesthesist 2007;56:1273–4, 1276.
22. Van AH and Landauer B. [Medical core competence and delegation in intensive care medicine:resolution of the German Society of Anaesthesiology and Intensive Care Medicine and the Professional Association of German Anaesthetists from 11.12.2007]. Anaesthesist 2008;57:83–84.
23. Kane GC, Grever MR, Kennedy JI, et al. The anticipated physician shortage: meeting the nation's need for physician services. Am J Med 2009;122:1156–1162.
24. Laurant M, Reeves D, Hermens R, Braspenning J, Grol R and Sibbald B. Substitution of doctors by nurses in primary care. Cochrane Database Syst Rev 2005:CD001271.
25. Mundinger MO, Kane RL, Lenz ER, et al. Primary care outcomes in patients treated by nurse practitioners or physicians: a randomized trial. JAMA 2000;283:59–68.
26. Horrocks S, Anderson E and Salisbury C. Systematic review of whether nurse practitioners working in primary care can provide equivalent care to doctors. BMJ 2002;324:819–823.
27. AORN. AORN Standards for RN Assistant Education Programs. In: Perioperative Standards and Recommended Practices, 2009:692–694.
28. Miller JI and Hatcher CR. Physicians' assistants on a university cardiothoracic surgical service. A five-year update. J Thorac Cardiovasc Surg 1978;76:639–642.
29. Heinrich JJ, Fichandler BC, Beinfield M, Frazier W, Krizek TJ and Baue AE. The physician's assistant as resident on surgical service. An example of creative problem solving in surgical manpower. Arch Surg 1980;115:310–314.
30. Thourani VH and Miller JI, Jr. Physicians assistants in cardiothoracic surgery: a 30-year experience in a university center. Ann Thorac Surg 2006;81:195–199.
31. Resnick AS, Todd BA, Mullen JL and Morris JB. How do surgical residents and non-physician practitioners play together in the sandbox? Curr Surg 2006;63:155–1
32. Victorino GP and Organ CH, Jr. Physician assistant influence on surgery residents. Arch Surg 2003;138:971–975.
33. Buch KE, Genovese MY, Conigliaro JL, et al. Non-physician practitioners' overall enhancement to a surgical resident's experience. J Surg Educ 2008;65:50–53.

34. American Association of Nurse Anesthetists. AANA History: Hand in Hand with Nurse Anesthesia. In: 2007.

35. Egger Halbeis CB and Macario A. Factors affecting supply and demand of anesthesiologists in Western Europe. Curr Opin Anaesthesiol 2006;19:207–212.

36. Greaves JD and Eastland PJ. The role of nonmedical staff in the delivery of anaesthesia service. Curr Opin Anaesthesiol 2007;20:600–604.

37. Hoot NR and Aronsky D. Systematic review of emergency department crowding: causes, effects, and solutions. Ann Emerg Med 2008;52:126–136.

38. Bradley VM. Placing emergency department crowding on the decision agenda. J Emerg Nurs 2005;31:247–258.

39. McCaig LF and Nawar EW. National Hospital Ambulatory Medical Care Survey: 2004 emergency department summary. Adv Data 2006:1–29.

40. Moorhead JC, Gallery ME, Hirshkorn C, et al. A study of the workforce in emergency medicine: 1999. Ann Emerg Med 2002;40:3–15.

41. Ginde AA, Espinola JA, Sullivan AF, Blum FC and Camargo CA, Jr. Use of midlevel providers in US EDs, 1993 to 2005: implications for the workforce. Am J Emerg Med 2010;28:90–94.

42. Carter AJ and Chochinov AH. A systematic review of the impact of nurse practitioners on cost, quality of care, satisfaction and wait times in the emergency department. CJEM 2007;9:286–295.

43. Currie J, Edwards L, Colligan M and Crouch R. A time for international standards?: comparing the Emergency Nurse Practitioner role in the UK, Australia and New Zealand. Accid Emerg Nurs 2007;15:210–216.

44. Nyberg SM, Keuter KR, Berg GM, Helton AM and Johnston AD. Acceptance of physician assistants and nurse practitioners in trauma centers. JAAPA 2010;23:35–7, 41.

45. Christmas AB, Reynolds J, Hodges S, et al. Physician extenders impact trauma systems. J Trauma 2005;58:917–920.

46. Dowling D and Dudley WN. Nurse practitioners: meeting the ED's needs. Nurs Manage 1995;26:48C-E, 48J.

47. Angus DC, Shorr AF, White A, Dremsizov TT, Schmitz RJ and Kelley MA. Critical care delivery in the United States: distribution of services and compliance with Leapfrog recommendations. Crit Care Med 2006;34:1016–1024.

48. Gajic O and Afessa B. Physician staffing models and patient safety in the ICU. Chest 2009;135:1038–1044.

49. Parshuram CS, Kirpalani H, Mehta S, Granton J and Cook D. In-house, overnight physician staffing: a cross-sectional survey of Canadian adult and pediatric intensive care units. Crit Care Med 2006;34:1674–1678.

50. Pronovost P, Thompson DA, Holzmueller CG, Dorman T and Morlock LL. Impact of the Leapfrog Group's intensive care unit physician staffing standard. J Crit Care 2007;22:89–96.

51. Haupt MT, Bekes CE, Brilli RJ, et al. Guidelines on critical care services and personnel: Recommendations based on a system of categorization of three levels of care. Crit Care Med 2003;31:2677–2683.

52. Manthous CA. Leapfrog and critical care: evidence- and reality-based intensive care for the 21st century. Am J Med 2004;116:188–193.

53. American Assosiation of Critical Care Nurses. Standards for Acute and Critical Nursing. 2008.

54. Burchardi H and Moerer O. Twenty-four hour presence of physicians in the ICU. Crit Care 2001;5:131–137.

55. Bion JF, Ramsay G, Roussos C and Burchardi H. Intensive care training and specialty status in Europe: international comparisons. Task Force on Educational issues of the European Society of Intensive Care Medicine. Intensive Care Med 1998;24:372–377.

56. Vincent JL, Suter P, Bihari D and Bruining H. Organization of intensive care units in Europe: lessons from the EPIC study. Intensive Care Med 1997;23:1181–1184.

57. Stiletto R, Rothke M, Schafer E, Lefering R and Waydhas C. [Risk management–a new aspect of quality assessment in intensive care medicine: first results of an analysis of the DIVI's interdisciplinary quality assessment research group]. Zentralbl Chir 2006;131:388–392.

Hans U. Rothen

Organising the workflow in an ICU

Introduction

Caring for the critically ill is the key task of an ICU. To assure optimal patient care, a complex interplay between professionals of diverse occupational groups, using a wide range of medicines, treatments and procedures, is needed. In addition, many interventions are time-critical, and there are many external influences such as emergency admissions and guidelines or protocols developed by medical specialties other than intensive care medicine. Accordingly, the workflow in the ICU is complex and dynamic, with many shared tasks and overlapping activities. In addition, there is a constant need for knowledge acquisition, knowledge transfer, and knowledge documentation. Overall, integration of individual workflows into one single network of patient-centered activity is a challenge. Taking into account all these problems, it is surprising that the number of scientific papers covering this topic is still limited [1–5].

Before addressing specifically some key issues concerning workflow in the ICU, it may be appropriate to describe briefly the meaning of this term in a broader way. Workflow describes a sequence of specific tasks, performed by a single person or a team. In general, it is based on a set of procedural rules and aims at realisation of a 'business' objective. Process, on the other hand, is used as a more specific notion; it has a well-defined input, output and purpose. Both workflow and process are often described using flowcharts. Depending on the granularity (the amount of details included), such flowcharts can be easy to read or they can get very complicated. In healthcare, flowcharts may be used as basis to enhance pattern recognition, to identify opportunities of improved efficacy and efficiency in patient care, or to uncover situations with increased risk of medical error [3, 6].

In this chapter, we will discuss general principles that should be considered when analysing and improving workflow in the ICU. Many interventions that aim at an improvement of system performance are complex and consist of several components. The methods used come from the field of social sciences and quality management rather than from the well-established field of 'classic' experimental design familiar to clinicians [5, 7]. As the caring team in an ICU includes many professions such as nurses, physicians, physiotherapists, pharmacists, and as there are many medical specialities involved (intensive care medicine, cardiology and cardiac surgery, neurology and neurosurgery, to name just a few of them) communication and information transfer within the team and between teams is a key element that clearly deserves a few thoughts. In this respect, the handover needs special attention. Of course, an ICU cannot work if it does not fulfil minimal requirements of staffing. This topic will also be briefly mentioned here as it is closely related to the way teams communicate and interact. It is, however, discussed in more detail in other chapters of this book. In the last few paragraphs of the present chapter, standardisation in the process of care (and thus in workflow), the support of workflow by clinical information systems, and the use of performance measures to assess the actual state and changes in workflow will be addressed.

Overall, well-structured collaboration between physicians, nurses and all other professionals working in the ICU contributes to enhanced workflow and a better team climate. However, it is also associated with improved patient outcome [8–10], the ultimate goal of intensive care medicine and the 'raison d'être' of an ICU.

Analysing workflow

Nurses' and physicians' activities

For many years nursing activities and workload have been assessed and evaluated. Even though a universally accepted method does not exist [11], especially in intensive care medicine various scoring systems are used. Examples are the Therapeutic Intervention Scoring System, TISS [12, 13], Nine Equivalents of nursing Manpower use Score, NEMS [14], the Nursing Activity Score, NAS [15], and the Intensive Care Nursing Scoring System, ICNSS [16]. By contrast, few studies have been presented up to now evaluating physicians' activities and workload [17–19]. In addition, there is a lack of such research in the ICU. Physicians have a wide range of activities, some directly at the bedside, some not in the direct vicinity of the patient. Probably, indirect activities are often influenced by factors not related to the patient's status. Work sampling can be used to explore how time is used [20] and an analysis of workflow may help to redesign work allocation strategies and improve productivity [21, 22].

There are several methods to evaluate workflow and work activities [23]. They include subjective estimates of work activities, self-reporting of activities, time-motion analysis, and work sampling techniques. The self-reporting method is easy to administer and data are easy to obtain [24]. There is, however, a high risk of bias and reporting may be influenced by events other than the actual activity itself. Accordingly, this method is generally considered least reliable [25]. Time-

motion analysis is based on direct observation and measurement of the time spent on a specific activity [18, 19, 26–28]. The method is subject to observer and worker bias [19], and the measurement in itself influences the pattern of activities observed ('Hawthorne effect'). Also, the observer may misclassify activities. With the work sampling technique, data are collected at intervals of time. Such intervals are either fixed (e.g. every half-hour) or occur at random points (random work sampling). For random sampling, either pagers or personal digital assistants (PDA) can be used to notify the subject when it is time to record his or her activity.

An example of the results of random work sampling is shown in Figure 1. Data are based on a pilot study, performed recently in an ICU of a university-affiliated tertiary care hospital [29]. Note the relatively high proportion of indirect patient care (defined here as activity performed away from the patient's bed). Also, note that the amount of time used for learning and teaching was rather small.

Random work sampling has many advantages, such as ease of use and objectivity, and it avoids interaction between an observer and the subject being studied. Also, if a PDA is used, easy transfer of data to a main study database enhances timely analysis. Accordingly, this meth-

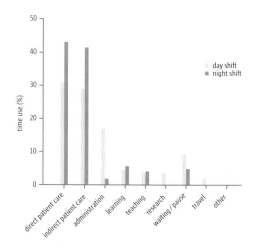

Fig. 1   Physicians' activities in the ICU. The relative distribution of physicians' activities is shown. [Data from 29.]

od has been used in various healthcare settings [15, 30]. It allows for easy calculation of the relative distribution of activities, but it does not result in an exact, absolute measurement of time per individual activity. To achieve acceptable accuracy, a rather high number of samples have to be collected [31]. In addition to the actual activity, other information can be collected and included for further evaluation. Examples are the level of physical effort, the perceived quality of the activity, an image of a key finding, etc.

Alternatively, data captured by radio frequency identification (RFID) can be used to visualise and analyse activities [6]. RFID tags can be used to capture the movements of medical staff, patients, or equipment. This technique is limited, however, by the difficulty of linking physical movement to actual activities.

In summary, various methods exist that allow analysing physicians' and nurses' or other healthcare professionals' activities. Yet up to now they have not been used extensively in intensive care medicine. Preliminary findings suggest that such tools might help to analyse, adjust, and ultimately improve workflow.

Workload

An accurate definition of workload is elusive. In general, the term 'workload' is used to characterise the task demands on an individual or a group of human operators. In principle, workload can be assessed based on the point of view of the operator carrying out a task, or it can be assessed using the point of view of the tasks to be carried out.

Using the point of view of the 'task operator' has been the focus of a number of studies on nursing workload. Overall, assessing workload in the ICU is not an easy task. Typically, many activities are related to each other, and a single person can accomplish several tasks in parallel (checking one patient's monitor while changing the dressing of another patient, talking to the patient's next of kin while washing the patient, inserting a central venous line while giving oral orders for setting another patient's ventilator, etc.). Also, the effective or the perceived amount of workload can differ, depending, among other things, on the level of education of the person

under observation and other, non-patient-related factors [32]. Furthermore, the quality of care delivered or the procedure carried out should be taken into account. Therefore it does not come as a surprise that it has been questioned whether workload can be reliably assessed at all [33, 34].

The 'tasks to be carried out' can serve as another starting point to assess workload. Employing this approach in the ICU, a number of measures can be used. Examples are: the number of procedures to be performed by a physician, the amount of time used for communication within the team or with patients and their next of kin, the number of teaching sessions, etc. The selection of the specific measure will depend on the question under scrutiny.

If, for instance, the workload of residents and fellows during their shift is to be analysed, the number of patients admitted and discharged from the ICU during a specific interval of the day can be calculated. Figures 2 and 3 show an example from a 30-bed ICU in a tertiary care hospital. In Figure 2, the relative hourly number of patients admitted and discharged from the ICU is presented. Note that 46 % of all patients were admitted between 08:00 and 15:59 (day shift), 42 % were admitted 16:00–23:59 (evening shift), and 12 % were admitted 00:00–07:59 (night shift). Thus, the average number of admissions in the evening shift is almost as great as the one during the day shift. On the other hand, if 'weighted patient moves' are used to assess workload, the relative distribution of day, evening and night shift is 65 %, 28 % and 7 % (see Fig. 3), which is markedly different from the first analysis. Based on these data, it can be concluded that between half and two-thirds of the workload of a full day has to be covered during the day shift. During the evening shift, workload is between one-third and almost half of the total 24-h workload. During the night shift, workload is about one-eighth to one-twelfth of the total 24-hour workload. Such time-dependent patterns of workload should be taken into account when planning schedules and staffing of shifts [35].

In summary, assessing workload in the ICU is difficult. Depending on the aim of an analysis, various approaches can be used, and even if the same database is explored, the results of analyses may differ markedly. An example has been presented in this chapter.

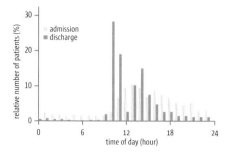

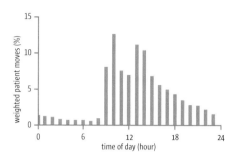

Fig. 2 Relative number of patients admitted to and discharged from an ICU vs. time of day. Relative number of patients admitted to (n = 2,419) or discharged (n = 2,395) from the ICU per hour Tuesday–Friday. Data from patients admitted/ discharged on other days of the week are not shown, as the pattern of distribution of these days differs. Unpublished data from the Department of Intensive Care Medicine, Bern University Hospital (Inselspital), Switzerland (32-bed multidisciplinary adult ICU). From January to December 2008, a total of 3,470 patients were admitted to the ICU.

Fig. 3 Weighted patient moves vs. time of day. The relative, weighted patient moves (admissions and discharges from an ICU) are shown. To calculate the weighted patient moves for a specific point in time, the sum of admissions during the previous two hours and the sum of discharges in the following two hours are added. Unpublished data from the Department of Intensive Care Medicine, Bern University Hospital (Inselspital), Switzerland (32-bed multidisciplinary adult ICU).

Keep an eye on patient safety

If the workload exceeds a certain amount, this can have negative effects on patient safety [36–39]. In addition, sleep deprivation can affect physician performance and consequently endanger patient safety [40]. Finally, extended work shifts may have adverse effects on health and safety among interns [41] and high workload may be associated with a high level of burnout in intensivists [42]. Such findings were, among others, the reason for an extensive change in working conditions in many parts of the Western world. Interestingly, some studies suggest that at least in the United States the resident duty hour reform did not result in a consistent and systematic improvement of patient safety indicators [43].

On the other hand, a positive relationship between patient volume and patient outcome has been shown in many studies [44–46]. In addition, ICUs may be able to cope with high workload [47]. In the latter study, consistent patient mortality outcomes were found even in periods of unusually high census (i.e. high workload), as measured by patient admissions per day. Whether this latter effect is due to a high level of quality of care in the ICUs included, a well-developed safety culture [48, 49], or some other causes, remains unclear. In any case, it is evident that workload *per se* is not the only determinant of patient safety. Accordingly, high workload does not necessarily result in decreased patient safety [50]. Finally, to cope with patient safety issues, approaches based on individual accountability today are considered to be far less effective than strategies that take into account patterns of workflow and the functioning of a system as a whole [51].

In summary, analysis and improvement of workflow clearly remain relevant issues also in respect to patient safety. Specifically, the complex nature of critical care work has to be taken into account, and strategies of improvement should use a patient- and not a silo-driven approach [52]. This includes a change in attitudes and behaviour of medical staff in respect to medical error [48] and a systematic review of all care delivered to a patient instead of concentrating only on workload [52].

The team – Interdisciplinary and interprofessional

Teamwork

Effective teamwork is considered to be crucial for providing optimal patient care in the ICU. For long, representatives of intensive care medicine have underscored the importance of effective interprofessional and interdisciplinary teamwork as the cornerstone for optimal delivery of care for the critically ill [53–55]. This contention is also confirmed by several studies showing as an example that daily multidisciplinary rounds are associated with lower mortality [56], or that the presence of interprofessional clinical rounds allows to separate "most efficient" from "least efficient" ICUs [10].

> Effective teamwork is associated with better patient care and better outcome.

Typically, a team in the ICU consists of nurses and physicians. In addition, depending on existing local or regional customs, national guidelines or regulations, other professionals such as pharmacists, respiratory therapists, or physiotherapists may be involved in care of the critically ill [55]. In any case, an adequate staffing level of the various groups is an important element to allow optimal teamwork.

Effective teamwork, related to improved outcome in the ICU, includes:

- Team communication
- Team leadership
- Team coordination (task management)
- Team decision-making [57]

Others have added to this list mutual performance monitoring and maintenance of standards and guidelines [58]. Several factors have been identified that may act as obstacles for team performance. Among others, they include physical environment (e.g. noise, amount of space), equipment (e.g. unavailability, misplacement), and relation to next of kin (e.g. lack of time spent with family) [59]. Developing the team process and thus optimising workflow should therefore take into consideration these various elements of teamwork.

Discussing all aspects of teamwork and of improving its performance is beyond the scope of this chapter. However, as communication is a key factor to maintain adequate functioning of a team [57], and as problems in communication are among the most often observed causes of medical errors and near mishaps [60], we will concentrate on this latter category in the next few paragraphs. The reader interested in other aspects of teamwork and in team training is referred to recently published reviews [57, 61–64].

Communicating within the team

Considering the sometimes complex workflow and high workload as described above, it is evident that open but structured and timely communication plays an important role in the ICU. As already noted, many errors in the ICU can be attributed to problems of communication [60, 65, 66]. Of note, medical professionals seem to be much less aware of such problems as compared to, for example, airline cockpit crews [48]. Accordingly, measures to improve communication play a crucial role in many respects [67].

> Problems in communication are the most common causes of medical errors.

Recently, five different categories have been described as relevant for communication and decision-making [68]. They include: pattern recognition, uncertainty management, strategic vs. tactical thinking, team coordination and maintenance of common ground, and creation and transfer of meaning through stories. Of note, these researchers conclude that junior house staff are struggling when required to move from the tactical level (task-oriented action) to a strategic level (thinking and acting at the level of a patient's overall treatment concept, or at the level of unit management) [68].

Typical elements of optimal communication in a team include [57, 58]:

- Use of direct verbal and nonverbal communication
- Accurate transfer of information during the written or verbal handoff
- Use of closed-loop communication (acknowledging information), in particular during patient emergencies
- Dissemination of information on newly admitted patients

- Distribution of information on patient treatment plans
- Abstaining from alterations of acute care (e.g. by a team leader) without verbal clarification of the performed therapy and without involving the team
- Appropriate requests of information during patient emergencies
- Avoidance of information overload from the team leader to team members during patient emergencies
- Speaking-up behaviour of junior team members

Until now, nurses, physicians and other members of a team in the ICU have generally been taught very different styles of communication. Whereas nurses tend to be broad and narrative in the description of a clinical situation, physicians are taught to be concise and to go quickly to the key points [66]. In addition, there are barriers such as hierarchy and the still prevailing belief that good and safe quality can be reached just by training and working hard. Even if appropriate knowledge and skills are a prerequisite to provide high standards of patient care, it should to be accepted that even skilled, experienced and motivated members of a team and the most respected expert can make mistakes and that there is always a "human factor" [69]. Effective communication can help to uncover and handle such errors in a timely manner [48, 66].

In summary, effective communication is a key element of teamwork and the basis of a well-functioning workflow. Failures in communication account for the majority of critical incidents and adverse events in an ICU. To change workflow and to improve patient safety, improving communication and changing the culture of teamwork is therefore a prerequisite.

The handover – A critical element

The ICU is a place of high turnover of patients, with a median length of stay around two days in many units [70, 71]. Within two days, the responsibility for care of a specific patient is thus transferred from the 'pre-ICU' team to the ICU team and thereafter to the 'post-ICU' team. Expanding the view gives an even more complex picture. As an example, a patient might pass through several interfaces, starting on the ward, with treatment in the operating room, the intensive care unit, and again returning to the ward. Counting in the shift changes of both physicians and nurses (and possibly other healthcare professionals) may add up to more than seven handovers even in this seemingly straightforward path of a patient [72]. Much higher numbers of handovers per patient are probably seen more often than expected! Nevertheless, the amount of published research on this topic is remarkably limited [73–76].

A handover can have multiple purposes [77], and health professionals from multiple professions (nurses, physicians, physiotherapists, etc.) and various medical specialties (emergency physician, anesthesiologist, intensivists, etc.) communicate with one another [78]. Even if oral communication is the preferred mode for most, there can also be communication via phone, or transfer of information via paper charts or electronic tools. If only verbal communication is used, very few facts are maintained correctly over several handover cycles. As an example, at the fifth handover, only 2.5 % of patient information was retained correctly if a verbal-only method was used, whereas the amount of correct information was markedly higher when notes were taken, and reached 99 % when a printed handout was used [79]. As a further example, in an pediatric acute care ward, residents indicated that they did not receive the adequate information for patient care during their night shift in one-fourth of all handovers [80]. In addition, physicians may overestimate the effectiveness of their communication [81].

The list of possible barriers to adequate transfer of information during handover is long [73, 82]. It includes communication barriers, lack of standardisation, lack of training, omitted (forgotten, missing) or wrong (distorted) information, physical barriers (noise, light, interruptions, and equipment), lack of time, difficulties due to high complexity or high number of patients, and human factors (stress, fatigue, etc.).

In recent years, tools to evaluate appropriateness of handover have been presented. The "handoff communication assessment" was developed to assess content and language form of handover communication between emergency physicians and hospitalists [83]. The "handover score" allows for measurement of the accuracy of information retained during handover [84]. However, further research still needs to be done.

In summary, transfer of information relevant to patient care is practiced almost continuously. In addition, medical responsibility is transferred several times per day from one caregiver to another. This process of handover is complex and up to now, only poorly analysed and understood. On the other hand, to improve workflow in the ICU, a well-designed process of handover with clearly defined aims and tasks of the various participants is needed.

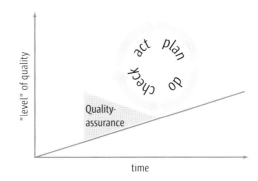

Fig. 4 A model for improvement [modified from Deming WE. Out of the Crisis. Massachusetts Institute of Technology, Cambridge, 1982, and from Müller HR. Qualitätsorientiertes Tourismus-Management. Haupt UTB, Bern, 2004, p. 44]

Changing workflow

General principles

To change and improve workflow, the same principles can be used as have been proposed for quality improvement. Key contributions to this field are based on the framework outlined by Deming and others [85]. The process of improvement requires timely identification of a problem, careful planning of interventions, reliable documentation, and open-minded analysis of results. An attempt to characterise this process in a simple way is shown in Figure 4. There are other models and methods that can be used in quality improvement such as Six Sigma, lean thinking, the Malcolm Baldrige model for performance excellence, or the EFQM model [86, 87]. Discussing all these models and methods is, however, beyond the scope of the present chapter.

The figure shows a simplified model, based on the assumption: quality management = quality assurance + PDCA cycle. PDCA: plan – do – check – act.

The plan-do-check-act (PDCA) cycle probably is the most often cited tool in quality management. It relies on repeated, often short sequences of learning by "trial and error" [88]. In many instances, PDCA probably is much more appropriate than a large-scale change, based on endless discussions and workshops, and never-ending trials to reach a common consensus on what is accepted as the best solution. The PDCA cycle is certainly also to be preferred to a 'quick and dirty' action aiming at a change in workflow without assessing its results.

Of course, the first step of PDCA will always be to identify a problem and to outline possible solutions. After all, without knowing whether a real problem exists and without any minimal agreement on the nature of the problem, any further action is meaningless. Thus, to use the PDCA cycle, one might start by answering the following four questions (modified from [85]):

- Is there a problem?
- What are we trying to achieve?
- How will we know that changes have occurred?
- What changes can we make that will result in improvement?

The following steps include: implementing a change, measuring its effect (i.e. compare expected with observed measures), and feedback (i.e. assess the results of a change, set up for a next cycle) [89]. Measurement in quality management uses specific tools that differ generally from those used in clinical research. They are briefly discussed below in a separate paragraph. Some further general principles of the "science of improvement" have been summarised recently [7].

In the following paragraphs, we will discuss only a few specific elements of workflow improvement. This does not mean, however, that those not included (staffing, modifying work shifts, etc.) are of less importance. Indeed, some of them are covered in other chapters of this book.

Improving the handover

As discussed previously, coordination of the caring team and establishing common grounds is an important element of workflow improvement. Accordingly, redesigning shift handovers and round procedures can be a key element to reorganising workflow [68]. Strategies to improve the handover can include [73]: Standardisation, enhancing communication skills, and improving the physical environment. In the following paragraph, a few examples of such approaches are presented.

> Improving handover includes: Standardisation, enhancement of communication skills, optimisation of the physical environment.

Among the strategies proposed, standardisation is the one most often cited. It was noted in 44 % of all strategies identified in a recently published review [73]. It is expected that standardisation increases accuracy and completeness of the handover [90, 91]. The use of mnemonics is an eye-catching subset of this category. An often cited mnemonic is SBAR (situation – background – assessment – recommendation) [92], and "Fast Hug" is another example (feeding, analgesia, sedation thromboembolic prophylaxis, head-of-bed elevation, stress ulcer prevention and glucose control) [93]. Whether the use of a mnemonic can improve handover has, however, not yet been studied extensively [92]. Appropriate teaching, especially of junior doctors, can help to improve the handover process [94]. Finally, it can be useful to compare the process of handover in the ICU with that of other settings and to take into account experiences from industry, aviation, etc. [95, 96].

Despite the relatively large number of proposed strategies, however, outcome studies are more or less lacking. Such studies should address effectiveness of handovers, determine which elements lead to improved patient outcome, and identify the best strategies to implement such elements in the handover process [73].

Using clinical guidelines and protocols

Using clinical guidelines and protocols can help to improve workflow, the overall process of pa-tient care and patient outcome. Eventually, this may also result in reduced costs. However, as described by many, there can be a large gap between ideal and actual care. Implementing new knowledge in clinical practice can sometimes take decades, as recently described for the use of -blockers in patients after acute myocardial infarction [86].

In general, effective strategies to implement clinical guidelines include multifaceted interventions, interactive education and reminders. On the other hand, strategies that use only one single intervention, or that are based on didactic education and passive dissemination, were found to be less effective [97, 98]. In addition, implementation is impeded if the guidelines are difficult to understand, if there is lack of support from peers or local opinion leaders, or if there are time restrictions or staff shortages [98–100].

In critical care medicine, additional barriers have been described. They include unwillingness of physicians to give up full control over therapy, or their disagreement with published evidence [101, 102], concerns over patient discomfort or unjustified adverse effects (oversedation, unplanned extubation, acidosis, hypercapnia, etc.) [101, 103], errors of omission [104], and unavailability of clinical protocols [105]. Furthermore, ICU leaders may overestimate their staff's adherence to protocols [106]. Overall, even if a large amount of evidence has accumulated in critical care medicine during the last few years, implementation in clinical practice is still rather slow [102]. Thus, inadequate transfer of existing knowledge is still a challenge. On the other hand, as stated recently, probably more lives can be saved by appropriate use of existing knowledge than by generating new knowledge [102].

In summary, standardising workflow helps to uncover deviations from the 'normal' and unnecessary variation in practice. Depending on the problem detected, this allows for intervention in a specific situation or modification of the existing guideline or protocol.

Using clinical information systems

A computerised provider order entry and electronic nursing documentation can markedly change the workflow of both nurses and physicians. Unexpectedly, a shift in physician time from interacting with nurses and patients toward retrieving information from the electronic patient record was observed in an emergency department [107]. However, a clinical information system may reduce the time needed by ICU nurses for documentation and increase the time used for direct patient care [108] and it may enhance implementation of treatment protocols [109]. Overall, the impact of a clinical information system on workflow remains unclear. There may be both increases and decreases in time spent charting and in direct patient care [110].

Using an appropriate display of physiological data is still a matter of research [111]. Probably, better integration of data from various sources, a search for new formats of displaying such data, including adaptation to a specific clinical context or a specific clinical task, may result in further improvement of workflow.

As many clinical information systems have been primarily initiated and driven by physicians, the workflow of nurses and other professionals may be less well supported by these systems. It even has been suggested recently that in respect to effective workflow of nursing care, the use of such systems may confuse nursing practice and result in poor quality of care [112].

Overall, clinical information systems and information technology probably play an important, although rather complementary role in the improvement of workflow in the ICU [113].

Is there improvement?

The ultimate goal of improving workflow is better care of the critically ill. This corresponds to the recently proposed general term of "value for patients = improvement in health outcome/money spent" [114]. In this equation, "improvement in health outcome" can be expressed as risk-adjusted outcome, and "money spent" refers to resources used. It can be assumed that good clinical performance is exactly what everyone working in healthcare (and specifically in the ICU) is aiming at anyway. On the other hand, wide variability in risk-adjusted outcome and resource use in intensive care medicine has been shown in a number of studies [10, 115–118], suggesting that there is still room for improvement in many aspects. Besides changes in workflow, other dimensions such as leadership and management process, impact on society, work satisfaction of staff, etc., deserve attention to achieve better value for patients.

"Although all improvement involves change, not all changes are improvement" [119]. Therefore, accurate and timely measurement is needed. There are two key questions for every ICU: 'Are we improving?' and 'How do we compare to others?' To deal with these issues, different approaches should be considered. Just applying the same methodology as used for clinical research may guide clinicians in the wrong direction. Table 1 shows typical characteristics of the various types of key variables used for performance measurement in clinical research, accountability, or improvement [120, 121]. Indeed, one type of measurement is not more correct than the other. Its appropriateness of use depends rather on the type of question that is addressed.

Some of the confusion and discussion around key performance measurement can be explained by the fact that there is overlap between the various approaches. In addition, clinicians probably still tend to interpret performance measures mostly from the point of view and with the background of their experience in clinical research [122]. It thus might be helpful to learn in more detail how to use and correctly interpret performance measures in improvement (statistical process control) such as run chart, Shewhart control chart, and cumulative sum control chart (cusum). Here, the reader is referred to some recently published papers explaining such tools [89, 123–125].

Many agencies and organisations, both from the private and the public sector, provide data which are open to the public. Still, whether public reporting contributes to improvement or to an increased speed of quality improvement remains unclear [126–129]. In this respect, the different characteristics as outlined in Table 1 have to be taken into account. In general, process indicators are more sensitive to differences in quality of care and workflow, whereas outcome indicators are of main interest to the general public but are very often influenced by many factors outside the control of providers [130]. Existing methods and tools have to be developed further and their effect on quality improvement has to be analysed [131].

In summary, to monitor the success of changes in workflow, process measures are the first

Tab. 1 Key aspects of performance measures. [Modified from 120, 121, 133]

Aim of measurement	Research	Comparison, accountability	Improvement of care and workflow
Key question	"What is the truth?"	"Are we better or worse than ...?"	"Are we getting better?"
Penalty for being wrong	Misdirection for the profession	Misdirected reward or punishment	Misdirection for an initiative
Measurement requirements and characteristics	Complete and accurate; controlled; glacial pace; expensive	Risk-adjusted; denominators attributable to individuals or organisations; validity	Real time; raw counts; consistent operational definitions; utility
Bias	Design study to eliminate bias	Adjust to reduce bias	Accept consistent bias
Determine if change occurred	Hypothesis testing using statistical methods	Not tested	Use process control methods such as run charts, Shewhart charts, etc.

choice. Their use and interpretation differs from that of process measures in clinical research and accountability. Instead, tools used in statistical process control should be used and developed further.

Conclusion

In the future, focusing on workflow and teamwork will be an integral part of ICU management [132]. Most healthcare professionals are hard workers, but what matter, is not how many patients a nurse cares for or how many procedures a physician performs, but rather the result of the team's work [122]. Achieving better health outcome while reducing cost will result in improved value for our patients. Accordingly, workflow has to be reorganised by eliminating unnecessary variation in practice, failures in communication, and specifically, by improving the handover. Indeed, probably more lives can be saved by appropriate use of already existing knowledge than by generating new knowledge. Tools to analyse workload and workflow should be further developed [5]. They will help to explore, adjust, and ultimately improve workflow in the ICU.

> Better workflow is an important basis for improving quality of care while limiting resource use.

The author

Hans U. Rothen, MD, PhD
Department of Intensive Care Medicine
Inselspital, Bern University Hospital,
and University of Bern
3010 Bern, Switzerland
E-mail: hrothen@insel.ch

References

1. Ali NA, Mekhjian HS, Kuehn PL, Bentley TD, Kumar R, Ferketich AK, et al. Specificity of computerized physician order entry has a significant effect on the efficiency of workflow for critically ill patients. Crit Care Med 2005;33:110–4.
2. Tang Z, Mazabob J, Weavind L, Thomas E, Johnson TR. A time-motion study of registered nurses' workflow in intensive care unit remote monitoring. AMIA Annu Symp Proc 2006:759–63.
3. Malhotra S, Jordan D, Shortliffe E, Patel VL. Workflow modeling in critical care: piecing together your own puzzle. J Biomed Inform 2007;40:81–92.
4. Shaw NT, Mador RL, Ho S, Mayes D, Westbrook JI, Creswick N, et al. Understanding the impact on intensive care staff workflow due to the introduction of a critical care information system: a mixed methods research methodology. Stud Health Technol Inform 2009;143:186–91.
5. Unertl KM, Novak LL, Johnson KB, Lorenzi NM. Traversing the many paths of workflow research:

developing a conceptual framework of workflow terminology through a systematic literature review. J Am Med Inform Assoc 2010;17:265–73.

6. Vankipuram M, Kahol K, Cohen T, Patel VL. Visualization and analysis of activities in critical care environments. AMIA Annu Symp Proc 2009;2009:662–6.

7. Berwick DM. The science of improvement. JAMA 2008;299:1182–4.

8. Knaus WA, Draper EA, Wagner DP, Zimmerman JE. An evaluation of outcome from intensive care in major medical centers. Ann Intern Med 1986;104:410–8.

9. Baggs JG, Schmitt MH, Mushlin AI, Mitchell PH, Eldredge DH, Oakes D, et al. Association between nurse-physician collaboration and patient outcomes in three intensive care units. Crit Care Med 1999;27:1991–8.

10. Rothen HU, Stricker K, Einfalt J, Bauer P, Metnitz PG, Moreno RP, et al. Variability in outcome and resource use in intensive care units. Intensive Care Med 2007;33:1329–36.

11. Twigg D, Duffield C. A review of workload measures: a context for a new staffing methodology in Western Australia. Int J Nurs Stud 2009;46:131–9.

12. Cullen DJ, Civetta JM, Briggs BA, Ferrara LC. Therapeutic intervention scoring system: a method for quantitative comparison of patient care. Crit Care Med 1974;2:57–60.

13. Miranda DR, de Rijk A, Schaufeli W. Simplified Therapeutic Intervention Scoring System: the TISS-28 items–results from a multicenter study. Crit Care Med 1996;24:64–73.

14. Iapichino G, Radrizzani D, Ferla L, Pezzi A, Porta F, Zanforlin G, et al. Description of trends in the course of illness of critically ill patients. Markers of intensive care organization and performance. Intensive Care Med 2002;28:985–9.

15. Miranda DR, Nap R, de Rijk A, Schaufeli W, Iapichino G. Nursing activities score. Crit Care Med 2003;31:374–82.

16. Pyykko AK, Ala-Kokko TI, Laurila JJ, Miettunen J, Finnberg M, Hentinen M. Validation of the new Intensive Care Nursing Scoring System (ICNSS). Intensive Care Med 2004;30:254–9.

17. Guarisco S, Oddone E, Simel D. Time analysis of a general medicine service: results from a random work sampling study. J Gen Intern Med 1994;9:272–7.

18. Melgar T, Schubiner H, Burack R, Aranha A, Musial J. A time-motion study of the activities of attending physicians in an internal medicine and internal medicine-pediatrics resident continuity clinic. Acad Med 2000;75:1138–43.

19. Blaivas M, Theodoro D. Comparison of perceived and actual times spent by residents performing ultrasound examinations on patients. Acad Emerg Med 2003;10:397–9.

20. Upenieks VV. Work sampling. Assessing nursing efficiency. Nurs Manage 1998;29:27–9.

21. Abrass CK, Ballweg R, Gilshannon M, Coombs JB. A process for reducing workload and enhancing residents'

education at an academic medical center. Acad Med 2001;76:798–805.

22. Bollschweiler E, Krings A, Fuchs KH, Pistorius G, Bein T, Otto U, et al. Alternative shift models and the quality of patient care. An empirical study in surgical intensive care units. Langenbecks Arch Surg 2001;386:104–9.

23. Sittig DF. Work-sampling: a statistical approach to evaluation of the effect of computers on work patterns in healthcare. Methods Inf Med 1993;32:167–74.

24. Burke TA, McKee JR, Wilson HC, Donahue RM, Batenhorst AS, Pathak DS. A comparison of time-and-motion and self-reporting methods of work measurement. J Nurs Adm 2000;30:118–25.

25. Oddone E, Guarisco S, Simel D. Comparison of housestaff's estimates of their workday activities with results of a random work-sampling study. Acad Med 1993;68:859–61.

26. Weinger MB, Herndon OW, Zornow MH, Paulus MP, Gaba DM, Dallen LT. An objective methodology for task analysis and workload assessment in anesthesia providers. Anesthesiology 1994;80:77–92.

27. Slagle J, Weinger MB, Dinh MT, Brumer VV, Williams K. Assessment of the intrarater and interrater reliability of an established clinical task analysis methodology. Anesthesiology 2002;96:1129–39.

28. Adomat R, Hicks C. Measuring nursing workload in intensive care: an observational study using closed circuit video cameras. J Adv Nurs 2003;42:402–12.

29. Siegemund M, Rothen HU, and Swiss ICU-network. Assessing physicians activities in the ICU using random sampling technique. Intensive Care Med 2006;32:S215.

30. Domenech MA, Payton O, Hill J, Shukla RK. Utilization of physical therapy personnel in one hospital. A work sampling study. Phys Ther 1983;63:1108–12.

31. Oddone E, Weinberger M, Hurder A, Henderson W, Simel D. Measuring activities in clinical trials using random work sampling: implications for cost-effectiveness analysis and measurement of the intervention. J Clin Epidemiol 1995;48:1011–8.

32. Rauhala A, Fagerstrom L. Are nurses' assessments of their workload affected by non-patient factors? An analysis of the RAFAELA system. J Nurs Manag 2007;15:490–9.

33. Taylor CJ, Bull F, Burdis C, Ferguson DG. Workload management in A&E: counting the uncountable and predicting the unpredictable. J Accid Emerg Med 1997;14:88–91.

34. Hughes M. Nursing workload: an unquantifiable entity. J Nurs Manag 1999;7:317–22.

35. Levin S, Aronsky D, Hemphill R, Han J, Slagle J, France DJ. Shifting toward balance: measuring the distribution of workload among emergency physician teams. Ann Emerg Med 2007;50:419–23.

36. Tarnow-Mordi WO, Hau C, Warden A, Shearer AJ. Hospital mortality in relation to staff workload: a 4-year

study in an adult intensive-care unit. Lancet 2000;356:185–9.

37. Aiken LH, Clarke SP, Sloane DM, Sochalski J, Silber JH. Hospital nurse staffing and patient mortality, nurse burnout, and job dissatisfaction. JAMA 2002;288:1987–93.

38. Landrigan CP, Rothschild JM, Cronin JW, Kaushal R, Burdick E, Katz JT, et al. Effect of reducing interns' work hours on serious medical errors in intensive care units. N Engl J Med 2004;351:1838–48.

39. Lockley SW, Cronin JW, Evans EE, Cade BE, Lee CJ, Landrigan CP, et al. Effect of reducing interns' weekly work hours on sleep and attentional failures. N Engl J Med 2004;351:1829–37.

40. Olson EJ, Drage LA, Auger RR. Sleep deprivation, physician performance, and patient safety. Chest 2009;136:1389–96.

41. Barger LK, Cade BE, Ayas NT, Cronin JW, Rosner B, Speizer FE, et al. Extended work shifts and the risk of motor vehicle crashes among interns. N Engl J Med 2005;352:125–34.

42. Embriaco N, Azoulay E, Barrau K, Kentish N, Pochard F, Loundou A, et al. High level of burnout in intensivists: prevalence and associated factors. Am J Respir Crit Care Med 2007;175:686–92.

43. Rosen AK, Loveland SA, Romano PS, Itani KM, Silber JH, Even-Shoshan OO, et al. Effects of resident duty hour reform on surgical and procedural patient safety indicators among hospitalized Veterans Health Administration and Medicare patients. Med Care 2009;47:723–31.

44. Kahn JM, Goss CH, Heagerty PJ, Kramer AA, O'Brien CR, Rubenfeld GD. Hospital volume and the outcomes of mechanical ventilation. N Engl J Med 2006;355:41–50.

45. Lin HC, Xirasagar S, Chen CH, Hwang YT. Physician's case volume of intensive care unit pneumonia admissions and in-hospital mortality. Am J Respir Crit Care Med 2008;177:989–94.

46. Ross JS, Normand SL, Wang Y, Ko DT, Chen J, Drye EE, et al. Hospital volume and 30-day mortality for three common medical conditions. N Engl J Med 2010;362:1110–8.

47. Iwashyna TJ, Kramer AA, Kahn JM. Intensive care unit occupancy and patient outcomes. Crit Care Med 2009;37:1545–57.

48. Sexton JB, Thomas EJ, Helmreich RL. Error, stress, and teamwork in medicine and aviation: cross sectional surveys. BMJ 2000;320:745–9.

49. Huang DT, Clermont G, Kong L, Weissfeld LA, Sexton JB, Rowan KM, et al. Intensive care unit safety culture and outcomes: a US multicenter study. Int J Qual Health Care 2010;22:151–61.

50. Mountain SA, Hameed SM, Ayas NT, Norena M, Chittock DR, Wong H, et al. Effect of ambient workload in the intensive care unit on mortality and time to discharge alive. Healthc Q 2009;12 Spec No Patient:8–14.

51. Patel VL, Cohen T. New perspectives on error in critical care. Curr Opin Crit Care 2008;14:456–9.

52. Amalberti R, Benhamou D, Auroy Y, Degos L. Adverse events in medicine: Easy to count, complicated to understand, and complex to prevent. J Biomed Inform 2009.

53. Critical care medicine. JAMA 1983;250:798–804.

54. Ferdinande P. Recommendations on minimal requirements for Intensive Care Departments. Members of the Task Force of the European Society of Intensive Care Medicine. Intensive Care Med 1997;23:226–32.

55. Durbin CG, Jr. Team model: advocating for the optimal method of care delivery in the intensive care unit. Crit Care Med 2006;34:S12–7.

56. Kim MM, Barnato AE, Angus DC, Fleisher LF, Kahn JM. The effect of multidisciplinary care teams on intensive care unit mortality. Arch Intern Med 2010;170:369–76.

57. Reader TW, Flin R, Mearns K, Cuthbertson BH. Developing a team performance framework for the intensive care unit. Crit Care Med 2009;37:1787–93.

58. Andersen PO, Jensen MK, Lippert A, Ostergaard D. Identifying non-technical skills and barriers for improvement of teamwork in cardiac arrest teams. Resuscitation 2010;81:695–702.

59. Gurses AP, Carayon P. Exploring performance obstacles of intensive care nurses. Appl Ergon 2009;40:509–18.

60. Williams M, Hevelone N, Alban RF, Hardy JP, Oxman DA, Garcia E, et al. Measuring communication in the surgical ICU: better communication equals better care. J Am Coll Surg 2010;210:17–22.

61. Salas E, DiazGranados D, Weaver SJ, King H. Does team training work? Principles for health care. Acad Emerg Med 2008;15:1002–9.

62. Lerner S, Magrane D, Friedman E. Teaching teamwork in medical education. Mt Sinai J Med 2009;76:318–29.

63. Manser T. Teamwork and patient safety in dynamic domains of healthcare: a review of the literature. Acta Anaesthesiol Scand 2009;53:143–51.

64. Buljac-Samardzic M, Dekker-van Doorn CM, van Wijngaarden JD, van Wijk KP. Interventions to improve team effectiveness: a systematic review. Health Policy 2010;94:183–95.

65. Donchin Y, Gopher D, Olin M, Badihi Y, Biesky M, Sprung CL, et al. A look into the nature and causes of human errors in the intensive care unit. 1995. Qual Saf Health Care 2003;12:143–7; discussion 47–8.

66. Leonard M, Graham S, Bonacum D. The human factor: the critical importance of effective teamwork and communication in providing safe care. Qual Saf Health Care 2004;13 Suppl 1:i85–90.

67. Pronovost P, Berenholtz S, Dorman T, Lipsett PA, Simmonds T, Haraden C. Improving communication in the ICU using daily goals. J Crit Care 2003;18:71–5.

68. Fackler JC, Watts C, Grome A, Miller T, Crandall B, Pronovost P. Critical care physician cognitive task analysis: an exploratory study. Crit Care 2009;13:R33.

69. Scanlon MC, Karsh B-T. Value of human factors to medication and patient safety i the intensive care unit. Crit Care Med 2010;38:S90-S96.

70. Metnitz PG, Moreno RP, Almeida E, Jordan B, Bauer P, Campos RA, et al. SAPS 3–From evaluation of the patient to evaluation of the intensive care unit. Part 1: Objectives, methods and cohort description. Intensive Care Med 2005;31:1336–44.

71. Moran JL, Bristow P, Solomon PJ, George C, Hart GK. Mortality and length-of-stay outcomes, 1993–2003, in the binational Australian and New Zealand intensive care adult patient database. Crit Care Med 2008;36:46–61.

72. Wurz J, Regli B. In one ear and out the other: communication barriers as a risk factor for critical incidents. Anesth Analg 2007;104:1319–21.

73. Riesenberg LA, Leitzsch J, Massucci JL, Jaeger J, Rosenfeld JC, Patow C, et al. Residents' and attending physicians' handoffs: a systematic review of the literature. Acad Med 2009;84:1775–87.

74. Riesenberg LA, Leisch J, Cunningham JM. Nursing handoffs: a systematic review of the literature. Am J Nurs 2010;110:24–34; quiz 35–6.

75. Gibson SC, Ham JJ, Apker J, Mallak LA, Johnson NA. Communication, communication, communication: the art of the handoff. Ann Emerg Med 2010;55:181–3.

76. Cohen MD, Hilligoss PB. The published literature on handoffs in hospitals: deficiencies identified in an extensive review. Qual Saf Health Care 2010.

77. Patterson ES, Wears RL. Patient handoffs: standardized and reliable measurement tools remain elusive. Jt Comm J Qual Patient Saf 2010;36:52–61.

78. Benham-Hutchins MM, Effken JA. Multi-professional patterns and methods of communication during patient handoffs. Int J Med Inform 2010;79:252–67.

79. Bhabra G, Mackeith S, Monteiro P, Pothier DD. An experimental comparison of handover methods. Ann R Coll Surg Engl 2007;89:298–300.

80. Borowitz SM, Waggoner-Fountain LA, Bass EJ, Sledd RM. Adequacy of information transferred at resident sign-out (in-hospital handover of care): a prospective survey. Qual Saf Health Care 2008;17:6–10.

81. Chang VY, Arora VM, Lev-Ari S, D'Arcy M, Keysar B. Interns overestimate the effectiveness of their hand-off communication. Pediatrics 2010;125:491–6.

82. Horwitz LI, Meredith T, Schuur JD, Shah NR, Kulkarni RG, Jenq GY. Dropping the baton: a qualitative analysis of failures during the transition from emergency department to inpatient care. Ann Emerg Med 2009;53:701–10 e4.

83. Apker J, Mallak LA, Applegate EB, 3rd, Gibson SC, Ham JJ, Johnson NA, et al. Exploring emergency physician-hospitalist handoff interactions: development of the Handoff Communication Assessment. Ann Emerg Med 2009;55:161–70.

84. Pickering BW, Hurley K, Marsh B. Identification of patient information corruption in the intensive care unit: using a scoring tool to direct quality improvements in handover. Crit Care Med 2009;37:2905–12.

85. Courtlandt CD, Noonan L, Feld LG. Model for improvement – Part 1: A framework for health care quality. Pediatr Clin North Am 2009;56:757–78.

86. Ting HH, Shojania KG, Montori VM, Bradley EH. Quality improvement: science and action. Circulation 2009;119:1962–74.

87. www.efqm.org. (accessed 20.05.2010)

88. Berwick DM. Developing and testing changes in delivery of care. Ann Intern Med 1998;128:651–6.

89. Randolph G, Esporas M, Provost L, Massie S, Bundy DG. Model for improvement – Part Two: Measurement and feedback for quality improvement efforts. Pediatr Clin North Am 2009;56:779–98.

90. McFetridge B, Gillespie M, Goode D, Melby V. An exploration of the handover process of critically ill patients between nursing staff from the emergency department and the intensive care unit. Nurs Crit Care 2007;12:261–9.

91. Wayne JD, Tyagi R, Reinhardt G, Rooney D, Makoul G, Chopra S, et al. Simple standardized patient handoff system that increases accuracy and completeness. J Surg Educ 2008;65:476–85.

92. Riesenberg LA, Leitzsch J, Little BW. Systematic review of handoff mnemonics literature. Am J Med Qual 2009;24:196–204.

93. Vincent JL. Give your patient a fast hug (at least) once a day. Crit Care Med 2005;33:1225–9.

94. Cleland JA, Ross S, Miller SC, Patey R. "There is a chain of Chinese whispers ...": empirical data support the call to formally teach handover to prequalification doctors. Qual Saf Health Care 2009;18:267–71.

95. Patterson ES, Roth EM, Woods DD, Chow R, Gomes JO. Handoff strategies in settings with high consequences for failure: lessons for health care operations. Int J Qual Health Care 2004;16:125–32.

96. Catchpole KR, de Leval MR, McEwan A, Pigott N, Elliott MJ, McQuillan A, et al. Patient handover from surgery to intensive care: using Formula 1 pit-stop and aviation models to improve safety and quality. Paediatr Anaesth 2007;17:470–8.

97. Prior M, Guerin M, Grimmer-Somers K. The effectiveness of clinical guideline implementation strategies – a synthesis of systematic review findings. J Eval Clin Pract 2008;14:888–97.

98. Francke AL, Smit MC, de Veer AJ, Mistiaen P. Factors influencing the implementation of clinical guidelines for health care professionals: a systematic meta-review. BMC Med Inform Decis Mak 2008;8:38.

99. Bero LA, Grilli R, Grimshaw JM, Harvey E, Oxman AD, Thomson MA. Closing the gap between research and practice: an overview of systematic reviews of interventions to promote the implementation of research findings. The Cochrane Effective Practice and Organization of Care Review Group. BMJ 1998;317:465–8.

100. Carlbom DJ, Rubenfeld GD. Barriers to implementing protocol-based sepsis resuscitation in the emergency department – results of a national survey. Crit Care Med 2007;35:2525–32.

101. Rubenfeld GD, Cooper C, Carter G, Thompson BT, Hudson LD. Barriers to providing lung-protective ventilation to patients with acute lung injury. Crit Care Med 2004;32:1289–93.

102. Kahn JM. Disseminating clinical trial results in critical care. Crit Care Med 2009;37:S147–53.

103. Tanios MA, de Wit M, Epstein SK, Devlin JW. Perceived barriers to the use of sedation protocols and daily sedation interruption: a multidisciplinary survey. J Crit Care 2009;24:66–73.

104. Byrnes MC, Schuerer DJ, Schallom ME, Sona CS, Mazuski JE, Taylor BE, et al. Implementation of a mandatory checklist of protocols and objectives improves compliance with a wide range of evidence-based intensive care unit practices. Crit Care Med 2009;37:2775–81.

105. Prasad M, Christie JD, Bellamy SL, Rubenfeld GD, Kahn JM. The availability of clinical protocols in US teaching intensive care units. J Crit Care.

106. Brunkhorst FM, Engel C, Ragaller M, Welte T, Rossaint R, Gerlach H, et al. Practice and perception–a nationwide survey of therapy habits in sepsis. Crit Care Med 2008;36:2719–25.

107. Asaro PV, Boxerman SB. Effects of computerized provider order entry and nursing documentation on workflow. Acad Emerg Med 2008;15:908–15.

108. Bosman RJ. Impact of computerized information systems on workload in operating room and intensive care unit. Best Pract Res Clin Anaesthesiol 2009;23:15–26.

109. Takala J, Dellinger RP, Koskinen K, St Andre A, Read M, Levy M, et al. Development and simultaneous application of multiple care protocols in critical care: a multicenter feasibility study. Intensive Care Med 2008;34:1401–10.

110. Mador RL, Shaw NT. The impact of a Critical Care Information System (CCIS) on time spent charting and in direct patient care by staff in the ICU: a review of the literature. Int J Med Inform 2009;78:435–45.

111. Effken JA, Loeb RG, Kang Y, Lin ZC. Clinical information displays to improve ICU outcomes. Int J Med Inform 2008;77:765–77.

112. Lee S, McElmurry B. Capturing nursing care workflow disruptions: comparison between nursing and physician workflows. Comput Inform Nurs 2010;28:151–9; quiz 60–1.

113. Reng M, The role of information technology in the ICU. 25 Years of Progress and Innovaton in Intensive Care Medicine, ed. R.M. Kuhlen, R. Ranieri, M. Rhodes, A. 2007; Berlin: Medizinisch Wissenschaftliche Verlagsgesellschaft. 375–82.

114. Porter ME, Teisberg EO. How physicians can change the future of health care. JAMA 2007;297:1103–11.

115. Keenan SP, Dodek P, Martin C, Priestap F, Norena M, Wong H. Variation in length of intensive care unit stay after cardiac arrest: where you are is as important as who you are. Crit Care Med 2007;35:836–41.

116. Niskanen M, Reinikainen M, Pettila V. Case-mix-adjusted length of stay and mortality in 23 Finnish ICUs. Intensive Care Med 2009;35:1060–7.

117. Straney L, Clements A, Alexander J, Slater A. Quantifying variation of paediatric length of stay among intensive care units in Australia and New Zealand. Qual Saf Health Care 2010.

118. Dodek PM, Keenan SP, Norena M, Martin C, Wong H. Review of a large clinical series: structure, process, and outcome of all intensive care units within the province of British Columbia, Canada. J Intensive Care Med 2010;25:149–55.

119. Batalden PB, Davidoff F. What is "quality improvement" and how can it transform healthcare? Qual Saf Health Care 2007;16:2–3.

120. Solberg LI, Mosser G, McDonald S. The three faces of performance measurement: improvement, accountability, and research. Jt Comm J Qual Improv 1997;23:135–47.

121. Lloyd RC. Helping leaders blink correctly. Split-scond decisions ahve patient safety implications. Healthcare Executive 2010:88–91.

122. Lee TH. Turning doctors into leaders. Harv Bus Rev 2010;88:50–8.

123. Henderson GR, Mead GE, van Dijke ML, Ramsay S, McDowall MA, Dennis M. Use of statistical process control charts in stroke medicine to determine if clinical evidence and changes in service delivery were associated with improvements in the quality of care. Qual Saf Health Care 2008;17:301–6.

124. Kao LS, Lally KP, Thomas EJ, Tyson JE. Improving quality improvement: a methodologic framework for evaluating effectiveness of surgical quality improvement. J Am Coll Surg 2009;208:621–6.

125. Lloyd RC. Navigating in the turbulent sea of data: the quality measurement journey. Clin Perinatol 2010;37:101–22.

126. Fung CH, Lim YW, Mattke S, Damberg C, Shekelle PG. Systematic review: the evidence that publishing patient care performance data improves quality of care. Ann Intern Med 2008;148:111–23.

127. Jarman B. In defence of the hospital standardized mortality ratio. Healthc Pap 2008;8:37–42; discussion 69–75.

128. Faber M, Bosch M, Wollersheim H, Leatherman S, Grol R. Public reporting in health care: how do consumers use quality-of-care information? A systematic review. Med Care 2009;47:1–8.

129. Lilford R, Pronovost P. Using hospital mortality rates to judge hospital performance: a bad idea that just won't go away. BMJ 2010;340:c2016.

130. Rothen HU, Takala J. Can outcome prediction data change patient outcomes and organizational outcomes? Curr Opin Crit Care 2008;14:513–9.

131. Nedza SM. Commentary: A call to leadership: the role of the academic medical center in driving sustainable health system improvement through performance measurement. Acad Med 2009;84:1645–7.

132. Amaral AC, Rubenfeld GD. The future of critical care. Curr Opin Crit Care 2009;15:308–13.

133. www.ihi.org. (accessed 20.05.2010)

Armand R.J. Girbes and Jan G. Zijlstra

Evaluating staff performance in the ICU

Introduction

Today, patients want to be informed about the hospital they go to, or the doctor or surgeon they go to, in terms of clinical performance. Lay journals such as Le Point in France, El Pais in Spain and Elsevier in the Netherlands publish ratings of hospitals and/or departments. Patients and the public at large are no longer satisfied with simply receiving the general message from a doctor or hospital board that everything is perfect in their hospital. Patients want figures on performance. Patients generally do not have the possibility of making a balanced choice for a given intensive care department. They are either admitted as an emergency, or the intensive care treatment is part of the course of their disease. Therefore, intensive care departments carry an even greater burden to make the quality of treatment of ICU patients the best possible quality of care.

In addition, there is a growing tendency toward accountability in patient care. Governments and administrators demand performance indicators. These indicators can be measured at the hospital or departmental level, albeit with a considerable degree of uncertainty [1]. To date only in a limited number of specialties, e.g. cardiac surgery, have attempts been made to measure at the level of individual doctors. Although no physician can function without infrastructure, the individual physician

is a key player with a great impact on performance. Excesses in patient care and scientific misconduct all over the world have taught us that assessment of performance is inadequate. And even if we diagnose substandard performance, it is not easy to take the correct measures because professionals are hard to coach and the legal framework of employment is complicated.

There exists in intensive care medicine a history of attention to the quality of treatment, especially in terms of patient outcome and complications. Performance of intensive care can be measured at several levels. The performance of an intensive care unit (ICU) as a whole, the performance of a group of healthcare workers within the ICU and the performance of individual healthcare workers, and therefore, of intensivists. Individuals are responsible, of course, for their own performance, but also for the accomplishment of the team and the ICU as a whole. On the other hand, ICU organisation and culture bear a certain responsibility for the performance of the individuals. The question arises how all these aspects can be measured in terms of performance, including that of individual physicians/intensivists. The quality control systems currently in use are not aimed at assessing individual healthcare workers. In the Netherlands, a nationwide initiative was introduced in 2005 to mandate individual performance interviews for medical specialists and consultants. The Royal Dutch Society of

Medicine stated in 2005 that individual performance interviews with each medical specialist or consultant must take place. There still is, however, a significant amount of hesitation and nervousness regarding the procedure. For decades it had been virtually unthinkable that physicians should be held accountable for their performance. The current procedure is therefore overcautious, and even the smallest reference to hierarchy in the procedure is omitted. However, the performance interviews are a new beginning for consultants working outside university hospitals, and may be the beginning of a straightforward accountability programme. In the university hospitals a regime of performance interviews with the department heads already existed. The primary goal is to improve performance and to identify and offer opportunities to help in this respect. In case of dysfunction, an appropriate procedure should be started and, if necessary, corrective measures must be taken. Intensivists, and physicians in general, have many responsibilities. Not only are they obliged to keep up with current knowledge and new developments in the medical professional field, but also the invidual's approach and basic attitude should be testable and verifiable, and the respective person prepared to take responsibility. Performance is not exclusively expressed in number of patients seen in the outpatient clinic, number of operations, number of anaesthetised patients per week or number of publications, but should also be measured in terms of good communication skills, drive for quality improvement, participation in quality networks, and a sound grasp of one's own performance in different situations. In this chapter we will discuss the possibilities and difficulties in assessing and improving the performance of individual doctors.

Staff and team performance

Intensivists are part of a complex process and work in teams. Therefore overall outcome parameters will not reflect the skills of a single intensivist. There are no standards for success rates for procedures such as central venous line access, intubation, etc. Even if there were, the small number of these interventions would not allow adequate statistics to compensate for chance and case mix. Although we could, as in aviation, standardise situations and measure performance in a simulator, we don't.

Measuring process parameters would be easier. As intensive care knows many guidelines and bundles, adherence to these protocols could be measured, but is not. We could ask patients, families, nursing staff, house staff, and colleagues about performance of individual physicians. Although they probably would give an indicative answer, it might be hard to get, and maybe therefore we don't ask. We could observe, check and control operating procedures. But they are colleagues, so we don't. There is another major obstacle. There is a large variation in practice. Best practice is hard to define and therefore deviations are difficult to detect. Not unimportantly, measuring individual performance focuses on underperformance. However, improving the mean has much more impact on healthcare than cutting out the excesses. Most excesses are detected long before they are really addressed. Excesses are therefore chiefly a handling problem and not a detection problem.

Intensive care medicine is teamwork, and thus it seems obvious that (mean) performance is measured in terms of outcome of the most important parameter the team produces: patient care. And indeed, in the past performance was synonymous with the standard mortality rate (SMR). The first studies on survival came from France [2]. Six years later Knaus and Le Gall compared the outcome data, in terms of adjusted mortality, for intensive care in France and the US [3]. Over the years the models for scoring patients were further refined, resulting in the development of better scoring systems such as APACHE IV, SAPS II, SOFA, TISS and MOD. However, it must be emphasised that all these scoring systems have their specific problems in terms of reliability in measuring performance. One of the important things to remember is that much can be measured, some is measured incorrectly, and much cannot be, or is not, measured [4, 5]. Meanwhile, repetitive measurements will beyond doubt help to improve performance and will enhance the incentive for the process of continuing improvement.

Other outcome indicators of team performance can be defined. The incidence of ventilator-associated pneumonia (VAP), incidence of central venous catheter-related infections, mean number of days on ventilation, admission duration in the ICU and in the hospital, or incidence of decubitus, are all examples of measurable performance indicators. It is, for example, not unreasonable to assume that in an ICU with a very low rate of VAP and CVC-related infection, generally speaking. good care is delivered. Next to outcome indicators, process indicators can be used. In this respect, one should think of length of stay in the ICU, duration of mechanical ventilation, occupancy rate (too high, i.e. > 85%, is undesirable, as is too low, < 70%), the occurence of complications and autopsy conferences. Finally, indicators on the structure of the department can be used: intensivist availability, patient-to-nurse ratio, policy to prevent medication errors, complication registration, absenteeism of both physicians and nurses, and registration of quality of life.

All these parameters will provide information on the performance of the team and thus of the individual members.

Additionally, in recent years more and more attention has been paid to other, so-called 'soft' issues, which can also be qualified as a measure of performance. Apart from long-term follow-up, and evaluating the patient's point of view, much interest has been shown in the experiences of families and family members of patients admitted to the intensive care unit (ICU). This has resulted in the publication of many studies on, among other things, family satisfaction, family involvement in end-of-life decisions and communication with the family. For sure, satisfaction on the part of the family members is associated with good communication skills of individual healthcare workers and the team. Treating patients and family members with respect and compassion is what should be seen all day in the ICU, although we do not have scoring systems for 're-spect' and 'compassion'. Neither is it expressed in yearly reports from departments. To create and enhance such a culture, leadership is very important. Not only should the leadership set the very best example at all times, but it should also address these issues and behaviour continuously and, importantly, talk to the healthcare workers about their conduct. As will be pointed out, the performance of the leader of the group is of the utmost importance.

Safety and error prevention in the ICU is also a subject appropriately receiving growing interest. Blame-free reporting, quality control cycles but also – and perhaps mostly – the attitude of individual professionals, combined with good leadership, are essential factors to lower the in-cidence of errors and create better structures to prevent previously made and potential errors. Involvement and willingness to participate in such a culture is an important factor that should be incorporated in measuring staff performance.

Staff performance is related to career, which is an important point of attention that should not be ignored. The task of good – servant – leadership is to help individual employees with their career and offer positive opportunities for self-development and self-improvement. In order to be able to assess the requirements, a proper evaluation of staff performance is necessary. Since the likelihood of developing burnout is significant in critical care clinicians and nurses, attention must be paid to associated factors in the evaluation of staff performance [6].

Audits

The way an intensive care unit/department is organised has a significant impact on the performance of the ICU, and therefore on the performance of the individual workers [7–10]. Consequently, even 'the very best intensivist in the world' will not perform very well on all aspects in a badly organised intensive care unit. Important aspects of ICU organisation are appropriate medical supervision by intensivists, continuity of medical and nursing care, a qualitatively and quantitatively sufficient presence of trained medical and nursing staff, the existence of quality improvement systems and regional networks. There is a large amount of evidence that intensivist-driven high-volume ICUs perform better in terms of patient outcome than small, open-format intensive cares. Unequivocal guidance of ICU nurses according to consistent approaches of medical care is a key factor in this respect.

Audits by peers, and preferably, external audits, are an excellent way to help to improve quality of care in the ICU. It is of utmost importance that audits should not aim to assign blame, but to provide a mirror to reveal challenges and possibilities for improvement. Avoidance of 'old boy networks' or 'Don Corleone politics' is essential. Audits can be done on a voluntary or obligatory basis, but it is our opinion that the voluntary approach, meaning that a drive to improve is present, is preferable. Probably, a voluntary basis is less likely to provoke a tendency to deceive. In the Netherlands, for more than 10 years now nationwide external audits have been performed by an ad-hoc audit committee consisting of multidisciplinary peers, i.e. ICU nurses and qualified intensivists. The audits are organised by and under the auspices of the National Audit for Intensive Care Quality Committee of the Dutch Intensive Care Society. All kinds of information, including prevailing protocols/guidelines and data on organisation and performance, are gathered before the actual one-day visit. During the one-day visit, the supplied information is verified by interviews with representatives of all sections and professionals involved in the intensive care department, and the ICU is inspected. The ad-hoc commission consists of two intensivists, two ICU nurses and a secretary. The audit commission then produces a report with conclusions and recommendations.

Lack of evaluation of individual performance

Over the past decades, little has been done regarding the evaluation of individual performance. In general, audits do not focus specifically on individual performance, and in our experience, being involved in audits for more than 10 years, one could even say that individual bad performances are kept secret. Recently, in one of the major non-university teaching hospitals in the Netherlands a formal external investigation endorsed by the Health Care Inspectorate was conducted after it had become public in January 2009 that a neurologist, J., had clearly dysfunctioned for many years [11]. He had been forced to leave the hospital six years earlier due to his dysfunctional professional behaviour. J. left the hospital in 2003 with a golden handshake, despite his professional misconduct. At the time it was accepted as true that he had erroneously prescribed hazardous medication to patients and made many wrong diagnoses. Because he moved on to work as a neurologist in Germany the story gained attention in the national media. And it became clear that this case had been covered up through some sort of hush-hush policy. The board of directors of the Dutch hospital as well as the neurologist's colleagues in 2003 were very well aware of the fact that he was incompetent.

After all the media attention, the current directorate of the hospital in January 2009 instituted an independent commission to investigate the facts regarding the actions of the expelled neurologist. The conclusions of the commission in September 2009 were devastating. It became clear that since 1992, J. had

- worked solitarily,
- hardly kept records on patients,
- made unfounded diagnoses,
- asked for unbridled and unfounded additional diagnostics,
- interpreted diagnostics his own way,
- frequently prescribed medication not indicated,
- falsified laboratory and neuropsychological results in order to be allowed to prescribe a specific drug (against Alzheimer's disease),
- done harm to his patients.

It remained unclear whether the neurologist informed patients about planned participation in medical research protocols, because the patient records were incomplete. The pivotal question was how it had been possible for this situation to persist for such a long time. It became clear that the cooperation between other members of the neurology department and the neurologist in question were characterised by numerous and severe conflicts. Neurologist J. did not comply with arrangements made within the department, he was not approachable and felt superior compared to his colleagues. At the time he was frequently interviewed on Dutch television about Alzheimer's disease and therefore seen as an expert in the field. The department made an appeal to the hospital's board of directors and staff leaders because of the conflicts – in vain. The department of neurology did not overtly express their concern about the medical incompetence of their colleague. In 1998 an interim deputy neurologist was confronted with the incomplete patient records and the wrong medication prescriptions of neurologist J. He informed the directorate of the hospital because he did not want to bear any responsibility for this. The board of directors, however, remained silent. The members of the neurological department apparently did not at any point in time wonder whether the incompetent behaviour of their colleague J. might harm his patients. Neither did they look for it. On the contrary, they gave ambivalent signals, and when an audit for qualification and license for training of (future) neurologists was carried out, they even concealed his shortcomings. A malpractice complaint by a patient in 1998 was settled by payment of compensation, and covered up. The patient even was, more or less, forced to remain silent. It was only when neurologist J. had stolen medication and falsified prescriptions, that action was taken by the board of directors and J. was sent on sick leave. He was not prosecuted, but was offered to be relieved from duty with pay until retirement. The Health Care Inspectorate had been aware of the conflicts within the department of neurology since the early 1990s. However, no investigation was undertaken and complaining patients were actually turned away. This case shows an incompetent, dysfunctioning consultant who being allowed to continue his work. The environment did not take appropriate action and more patients were harmed because nobody assumed responsibility. And no one asked: "What about the patients?" This case may seem exceptional but surely is not, although most departments and consultants do function well. Unfortunately, more serious cases of incompetent and unprofessional behaviour are known. Dysfunction of a single consultant or flaming rows within a department or between departments are not exceptionally rare. Several years ago, a university department of cardiothoracic surgery in the Netherlands had to be closed due to apparent incompetency and unprofessionalism and, consequently, high complication and mortality rates. This was related to the dysfunction of (only) a few players. The poor practice in the Bristol heart surgery, now more than a decade ago, is an example from the UK [12].

It is a great pity that signals are not picked up and appropriate actions for improvement stimulated in an earlier phase.

Performance interviews (see Tab. 1)

The appraisal of NHS consultants was started in the UK almost a decade ago [13]. In the Netherlands, as well as in many other countries, the healthcare authorities are quite reluctant to enforce implementation of appropriate individual performance interviews. Strangely, performance interviews for other staff in general, and especially in the public sector, are commonly obligatory. Performance interviews must be differentiated between assessment interviews, which contain a hierarchic appreciation of the performance, and evaluation interviews, i.e. appraisals. In the latter the interview and the preceding collection of information is mainly a process of facilitated self-reflection. It is meant to help the individual to review their professional activities comprehensively and to identify areas of real strength, and areas where there is a need for development and improvement. For most professionals in the public sector (but also in the non-public sector) both types of performance interviews are held with the executive manager, the boss. The evaluation interview, however, takes a horizontal and two-way approach. The evaluation interview is also meant to help the executive professional in terms of self-reflection and thus (self-)improvement. It is a time for 'boss' and 'professional' (in this case, the intensivist) to review the performance of the previous year, to give and receive feedback, clarify job duties, state expectations on both sides, and to set goals for the coming year. Ideally these evaluation interviews take place at least once a year. The key aspects of the performance interview (i.e. both assessment and evaluation interviews) are:

- Accomplishments – evaluation of success in performing identified duties/areas of responsibility. Issues such as good clinical care, maintaining good medical practice, relationships with patients and their families, working with colleagues, research and teaching/training should be discussed.
- Accountability & dependability – evaluation of success in contributing to the effectiveness of the department and the overall mission of the hospital
- Availability & flexibility – evaluation of success in dealing effectively with additional responsibilities, learning and applying new techniques/knowledge, and participation in training and educational opportunities
- Decision-making & problem-solving – evaluate success in making decisions, following safe work practices in compliance with hospital and legal policies. Additionally, evaluation of managerial abilities regarding human resources, i.e. colleagues, nurses, students, fellows, achieving success in line with the hospital's mission while setting appropriate

Tab. 1   Things to remember when introducing performance interviews

Ultimate goal is to improve performance, happiness and optimise career development	
Five-step model	■ Inform interviewee in time. Both participants of the interview can place (additional) points of discussion on the agenda. Timely setting of agenda with mutual agreement. ■ Settlement of agenda ■ Interview takes place, preferably with minutes secretary. ■ Reporting of performance interview. A clear report is made, clearly stating appointments made, action to be taken, conclusions and result of previous appointments. If both participants agree on the contents, both sign the report as "agreed". If one does not agree, it is signed as "seen". The latter may lead to an additional interview. ■ Both participants will make every effort to adequately carry out the appointments as they have been made. Both are accountable for that.
Sufficient time for the interview with sufficient comfort	■ The interview should be well planned in the agenda, allowing the interview to take place without disturbances ■ Comfortable chairs and good room temperature ■ Drinks present ■ Phone and beeper switched off ■ Atmosphere of trust
Underscore what went well, emphasise positive personal performances	
Performance interviews at least once a year	

examples for others to follow. This includes leadership performance.
- Career development and working hours
- Working conditions and non-attendance
- Specific personal situation, such as illness, special family circumstances, divorce, etc.
- Terms of employment and fringe benefits

Performance interviews should ideally be seen as a vibrant educational process, enhancing personal development. Plans can be made for the (near) future and individual education can be promoted and initiated, where appropriate. These interviews will thus contribute to the partnership between an individual and the employing organisation. In our opinion, such a process allows for timely measures to be taken to avoid burnout or post-traumatic stress in critical care physicians (and nurses), although studies to substantiate this are lacking. It is of note that the competence to perform good and effective performance interviews is not a given. Appropriate training is essential to make the process of performance interviews a success.

A special feature of the assessment interview is the added hierarchic element. This means that assessments can be translated into appropriate measures to be taken. Noticeably, at least in the Netherlands, it seems a difficult issue to incorporate any hierarchic issues in measuring the individual performance of consultants working outside university hospitals, where, naturally, a hierarchy exists with heads of departments in office. There is, however, no reason to believe that professional healthcare workers, such as intensivists, should be considered differently compared to other employees. Rather, the examples as given above should stimulate us to promote, initiate or continue performance interviews for staff physicians.

Conclusion

Evaluation of the performance of ICU staff comprises many aspects, from the performance as a team to individual performance. The 'very best individual intensivist' will not be able to deliver consistently excellent performance in a substandard ICU. The reverse situation is more accommodating to an individual, dysfunctioning intensivist, meaning that an incompetent intensivist will seemingly perform well in 'the world's very best intensive care unit', due to compensation and correction of the individual's bad performance by the ICU team and organisation. Repetitive measurement of different dimensions of an ICU's performance is required to adequately assess the accomplishments. This includes not only measuring patient outcome and patient complications, but also measuring individual performance. Measurement and discussion of individual performance will help to elicit appropriate self-reflection and induce a vibrant educational process. Performance interviews are an essential tool in this respect. The ultimate goal of all this is to help the individual staff and team member in his or her further professional development, and to detect, as soon as possible, any lapse and early signs of dysfunctioning and/or burnout. Needless to say that our patients deserve the very best medical team and individual staff members. That's what it is all about, for the good of the patients.

The authors

Armand R.J. Girbes, MD, PhD[1]
Jan G. Zijlstra, MD, PhD[2]

[1]Professor in Intensive Care Medicine | Department of Intensive Care | University Hospital VU Medical center | Amsterdam, The Netherlands

[2]Professor in Intensive Care Medicine | Department of Intensive Care | University Medical Center Groningen | Groningen, The Netherlands

Address for correspondence
Armand R.J. Girbes
Department of Intensive Care
University Hospital VU Medical Center
P.O. Box 7057
1007 MB Amsterdam, The Netherlands
E-mail: arj.girbes@vumc.nl

References

1. Lilford R, Pronovost P. Using hospital mortality rates to judge hospital performance: a bad idea that just won't go away. BMJ 2010;340:c2016.
2. Rapin M, Gomez Duque A, Le Gall JR et al. Les chances de survie des malades hospitalisés dans en service de réanimation. Nouv Presse Med 1976;6:1245-1248.
3. Knaus WA, Le Gall JR, Wagner DP et al. A comparison of intensive care in the USA and France. Lancet 1982;2:6420646.
4. Arends JJ, Vandenbroucke JP. What conclusions should be drawn between critical care physician management and patient mortality in the intensive care unit? Ann Intern Med. 2008 Nov 18;149(10):768-769. Comment on: Ann Intern Med. 2008 Jun 3;148(11):801-809.
5. Polderman KH, Jorna EM, Girbes AR. Inter-observer variability in APACHE II scoring: effect of strict guidelines and training. Intensive Care Med. 2001;27(8):1365-9.
6. Randall Curtis J, Puntillo K. Is there an epidemic of burnout and post-traumatic stress in critical care clinicians? Am J Resp and Crit Care Med 2007;175: 634-636.
7. Pronovost PJ, Angus DC, Dorman T, Robinson KA, Dremsizov, Young TL. Physician staffing patterns and nclinical outcome in critically ill patients. JAMA 2002;288:2151-2162.
8. Higgins TL, McGee WT, Steingrub JS, Rapoport J, Lemeshow SL, Teres D. Early indicators of prolonged intensive care unit stay: Impact of illness severity, physician staffing, and pre-intensive care unit length of stay. Crit Care Med 2003:31;45-51.
9. Dang D, Johantgen ME, Pronovost PJ, Jenckes MW, Bass EB. Postoperative complications: does intensive care unit staff nursing make a difference? Heart Lung 2002;31:219-228.
10. Amaravadi RK, Dimick JB, Pronovost PJ, Lipsett PA. ICU nurse-to-patient ratio is associated with complications and resource use after esophagectomy. Intensive Care Med 2000;26:1857-1862.
11. www.mst.nl/onderzoekscommissie/rapport/ samenvatting.pdf.
12. Treasure T. Lessons from the Bristol cae. More openness on risks and on individual surgeons' performance. BMJ 1998;316:1685-1686.
13. Conlon M. Appraisal: the catalyst of personal development. BMJ 2003;327:389-391.

C. Processes

The role of ergonomics in modern medicine _____ 251
Yoel Donchin

Creating the ideal ward round _____ 259
Martha M. Kennedy, Deborah J. Baker, Ayse P. Gurses and Peter J. Pronovost

Smoothing the way: Improving admission to and discharge from the ICU _____ 269
Hannah Wunsch, Yên-Lan Nguyen and Derek C. Angus

Surge management for critical care leaders _____ 277
Michael D. Christian, Bernard Lawless, Julie Trpkovski and Jeffrey R. Dichter

Evaluating and improving the effectiveness of our practices _____ 295
Stephen Streat

The contribution of technology assessment _____ 307
Carl Waldmann, Max Jonas, Liza Keating and Ian J. Rechner

Evaluating and improving organizational outcome _____ 317
Hans Flaatten

Education and training teamwork using simulation _____ 323
Guttorm Brattebø

Electronic prescribing: minimal requirements_____ 335
Kirsten Colpaert and Johan Decruyenaere

Should research be together with clinical practice?_____ 345
Sten Rubertsson

Yoel Donchin

The role of ergonomics in modern medicine

Between 1500 and 1812, bloodletting was used for treating patients with various complaints, and it most probably caused more harm than good. Though their knowledge was limited and they were unable to actually cure any disease, physicians nevertheless felt compelled to *do* something for their patients, so they used to administer "magic drugs", induce emesis or purge the lower intestine. However, they were aware of the potential dangers inherent in their practice – hence the basic rule of medicine, "First, do no harm" [1].

"Iatrogenic diseases" is the medical term for diseases caused by medical caregivers themselves, e.g. adverse effects of drug administration, wrong blood type transfusion, surgical complications, etc., to name just a few of the many problems created by modern medicine. The beginning of the 19th century, with the birth of microbiology, the discovery of the X ray, the development of ECG and blood banking as well as the general improvement in public health, saw medicine reach a new level of professionalism and adopt a new scientific approach to health issues. However, in the efforts to eradicate epidemics, to fight TB and to minimize the mortality rate of children from contagious diseases, the adverse effects of medi-

cine itself were ignored, like wounded soldiers left in the battlefield by soldiers marching on to a new battle. After 1940, medicine became an industry – gone was the physician making house calls on horseback; the emergency room (ER) became the place where patients came to get help (sometimes sent there by a primary physician).

The medical institution accumulated more and more technology (the OR needed a continuous supply of medical gases, radiology demanded high voltage electrical power), laboratories and other auxiliary services needed space and manpower, and this entire conglomerate of experts and technology evolved gradually into the modern medical centres, with thousands of beds and a multitude of services. The quality of a medical institute is measured by its ability to improve the medical state of patients who arrive at its gates in a critical condition by establishing an accurate diagnosis and providing them with a good therapy plan. For this purpose, the medical profession depends on teamwork. This is not an assembly line, and we do not have a routine repetitive task to perform – the patients who need our help and our care are each unique and full of surprises. And as it is impossible to limit the medical work according to a strict schedule of work hours, it is common for surgeons to operate for long hours without a break and simultaneously take care of 30 patient in a crowded ward, working 24 or 48 hour shifts; and it is common for nurses to work without a moment's rest in a semi-military regime. Little attention has been given to problems such as the ability of the surgeon to stay alert and make the right decisions after 24 hours with no sleep, or to the danger of drug labelling in small letters and inadequate colours.

Communication among the teams, sharing data and other "small" issues related to the human operator were overshadowed by the patient and his needs. And sure enough, mishaps and accidents that happened in the hospital began to be discussed even in the medical literature. (One of the first such public discussions, after the discovery of ether as an anaesthetic, was the case of Hannah Green, aged 15, who died following ingrown toenail surgery.) [2, 3] The number of "mishaps" increased with the technological advancements, but the issue still did not get the public's attention until the 1990s, when medical accidents, such as the wrong drug given to the wrong patient, "wrong side" surgery, and many other incidents, made it to the front pages of newspapers and TV programmes, alongside an increase in malpractice suits against physicians, nurses and hospitals. Obviously, these incidents did not go unnoticed by the medical community, and in fact quite a few medical publications claimed that there was even an epidemic! ("More patients died of errors than of AIDS and breast cancer.") [4] This was a real puzzle – how could it be, in spite of all the medical knowledge, the understanding of the way viruses enter the body, the biochemistry that processes control – how was it possible for a stupid, avoidable mistake (human error?) to ruin the medical efforts to save lives?

A very similar problem of technology not adapted to the human operator, though in a different realm, occurred at the end of WW1 and became crucial during WW2, as there was a desperate need for pilots to go into combat, without enough training and with war machines that were hostile to the operator, especially in situations where life or death decisions had to be made. That period saw the birth of a new profession, which started to look at the reasons why the best men are failing in their missions. The new professionals questioned why the display of gauges in the cockpit is designed the way it was, and attempted to figure out the effect of fatigue on performance.

A debate is still going on about whether it all started in Great Britain or whether it was actually the Americans were the first to coin the term 'ergonomics' for that new branch of science, a hybrid of cognitive psychology, anatomy and physiology, engineering, and design – a multidisciplinary approach which today is known by the name Human Factors Engineering (HF engineering). Even though it is a new domain, the basic ideas were expressed many years ago but went unnoticed. The monograph "De morbis artificum diatriba" (Diseases of Workers), a detailed description of work-related diseases by the Italian physician Bernardino Ramazzini (1633–1714), is considered the first book on occupational medicine. It deals with ailments which affected workers in very hot environments, such as the glass industry, or who were exposed to poisonous chemicals. He also described the carpal tunnel syndrome, long before the keyboard ever existed: "constant writing also considerably fatigues the hand and the whole arm, because of the perpetual tension of the muscles and tendons. I knew a man who used to write constantly and who began complaining of excessive weariness of his whole right arm, a weariness which no medicine could alleviate, and at last the pain went away after a complete rest of the whole arm."

More than 100 years later, the Polish biologist Wojciech Jastrzebowski (1799–1882) published his book "The Outline of Ergonomics, i.e. Science of Work, Based on the Truths Taken from the Natural Science" (1857), and the term Ergonomics came into being, to be used extensively only many years later. The word 'ergonomics' is derived from two ancient Greek roots: 'ergon' (work) and 'nomos' (law). Today the term is used for all aspects of human activity, in every domain that involves people, e.g. work, sports, leisure etc. The International Ergonomics Association (IEA), with 42 countries and approximately 18,000 ergonomists, is following in the steps of Ramazzii and Jastrzebowski. The US uses the term Human Factors Engineering, which emphasizes cognitive psychology, whereas the term Ergonomics has more to do with body measurements and the forces needed for operations such as turning on a faucet or deciding on the best height for the operator chair. Both terms are used to describe the man-machine interaction.

Human factors engineering and the medical environment

In 1816, the French physician René Laennec was facing a real problem: "I was consulted by a young woman presenting general symptoms of disease of the heart. The patient's age and sex did not permit me a close examination such as applying the ear directly to her chest. I then remembered a well-known acoustic phenomenon, whereby if you place your ear against one end of a wooden beam, the scratch of a pin on the other extremity is most distinctly audible ... I took a sheet of paper and rolled it into a very tight roll, one end of which I placed over the precordial region, whilst I put my ear to the other. I was both surprised and gratified at being able to hear the beating of the heart with much greater clearness and distinction than I had ever done by direct application [5]. This is possibly an application of technology in medicine for the purpose of improving the "man-machine" interaction.

Partly related to the term Ergonomics is the word 'surgery' (from ancient Greek *Khier* = hand, *Ourgos* = work). In the ruins of Pompeii, which was buried under volcanic ash in 79 AD, an arsenal of surgical instruments was found. Though their specific purpose and use are yet to be figured out, it is clear that they were designed to fit the human hand, for precision and maximum force [6].

Thus, surgical implements and machinery were invented and perfected to maximize their use and effect, but the working conditions in a strict regime, the patient bed and its surroundings, the daily battles to save lives and their emotional toll – all these were never an issue and were never addressed.

Anaesthesiologists, followed by intensive care physicians, whose work has the smallest degree of mistake tolerance, were the first to look into the causes of accidents and mishaps. The medical literature did not welcome papers on topics such as the detailed technical aspects of alarms and the hazards of 100 % nitrous oxide administration. Nonetheless, slowly but surely, the re-

search infiltrated into the main stream of medical publications.

The story of our first research project, completed more than 15 years ago, illustrates the way we tried, by using an HF approach, to figure out why errors occur in the intensive care unit (ICU) and what the extent of these errors would be [7]. The study began by motivating all participants' nursing staff, residents and senior doctors. We designed a form for reporting errors and mishaps that was simultaneously filled out by ICU team members and HF researchers, who – having been trained to understand the ICU environment – made their own observations so as to validate the medical team's reports. The HF observers brought a new and fresh look to our "work station" (we did not know we *had* a "work station" ... for us it was just the 6-bed ICU, where we worked). The HF observers noticed many gaps in the information transfer process and in the inter-personal communication of the staff, among themselves and with the families. We did not look at the adverse events in isolation; we measured all of the activities in the unit: the number of contacts a staff member (nurse or MD) had with a patient, the amount of time they spent around a patient's bed, etc. After three months of data gathering we had 601 incident reports, and we could demonstrate that nurses were doing most of the activities in the unit, but they were still less prone to err than the physicians! The numerical result was a surprise: 1.6 errors per bed per 24 hours, 1.6 potentially lethal incidents unless discovered and corrected in time. The reasons for this incidence were inherent in the unit, but could nonetheless be corrected in order to avoid further errors and mishaps.

It was not easy to publish such a paper in 1992, and several medical journals turned it down, noting that "it is of no interest to our readers". Finally, and after a lot of revisions, the Critical Care Medicine Journal accepted it for publication and in no time many others began quoting it; six years later the paper was already described as a classical paper and reappeared in another medical journal.

It was now clear to our colleagues in ICUs as well as to the hospitals' chief executive officers (CEOs) that HF engineers can be a part of the hospital's effort to overcome the epidemic of errors. Leading medical journals have published papers on medical human factors (e.g. British Medical Journal) and there are journals dealing with quality and safety in health care. A good introduction to the subject of Human Factors is to be found in the reference list at the end of this chapter.

For the purpose of illustrating the ability and power of HF in all aspects of medicine, let us now take a look at our main research projects at the Center for Safety at Work and Human Engineering at the Israel Institute of Technology (Technoin) in Haifa, in collaboration with the Hadassah Hebrew University Medical Center in Jerusalem, Israel. These examples are meant to demonstrate the wide spectrum of HF and its ability to change humans themselves more than its need to change the environment.

The examples cover the following topics:
- Process – operating room observations, drug administration
- Design of the work environment – drug cabinets, medical forms and checklists (hung on the walls rather than filed in the hospital records systems)
- Communication among medical teams (hand-over research)
- Accident simulation as a learning tool

Processing of an incision e.g. by surgery is just one step of many. Surgery is a multi-stage process which is susceptible to dire consequences if any one stage is not performed in the proper way. Wrong-side surgery should not happen, and is regarded as unacceptable. However, in order to figure out why it does in fact happen, it is not enough to investigate those rare cases when it happened, but it is vital to look at the chain of events leading to it, to inspect the system step by step, beginning with the decision to perform the surgery in the first place and ending with the patient's discharge. Close inspection of all the steps in the process can lead us to the weak points, namely those points of the highest probability for the wrong-side surgery to occur.

For the purpose of inspecting the system, trained observers from the Human Factors Department followed 417 patients scheduled for elective surgery. The observations began in the surgical ward, at the time when the nurse prepared the patients for transfer to the OR, and ended upon the patients' arrival to the recovery room after surgery. Even though nothing serious happened during the observation periods, we managed to identify "events" that – had they not been discovered on time – could have led to a mishap or would have delayed the procedure. We found that the potential for errors does exist, and that for each surgery there were 4.5 potential mishaps! The OR team rejected some of our findings as potential causes for errors, since a delay in the beginning of surgery or a missing laboratory value (not to mention patients that were not identified properly) were part of the daily routine in the OR. Nobody but external, non-biased observers could have identified these weaknesses and then suggest a way to overcome them [8].

Errors of drug administration are one of the major contributors to the epidemic of medical accidents. Instead of investigating an event, we propose observing and analysing the process, in the same way we observed the proceedings in the OR. Magnesium administration was chosen for this purpose because there were two fatal accidents due to overdosage of this drug. Instead of looking into the fatal cases themselves, we followed the whole process, beginning with the physician writing the order and ending with the nurse selecting the proper drip rate on the automatic syringe. Each step was documented and videotaped, to be analysed later by HF experts. A senior nurse volunteered to simulate the nurse's part in the process, namely she read the doctor's order, took the bottle off the shelf and performed the calculation. Analysis of the video recording, as well as the way the nurse struggled to calculate the right dosage, demonstrated the weak link in the chain of events. Furthermore, close inspection of the $MgSO_4$ bottle revealed misprints on the label. It was obvious that the complicated calculation imposed on the nurse, in the noisy demanding environment of the paediatric ward, is fertile ground for errors, as the mental workload of the nurse makes it hard for her to act properly. Therefore, a simple computer program was developed, which released the nurse from having to do the calculations herself; all she had to do was enter the patient's weight and the dosage the doctor ordered. The computer result was given in drops per minute with instructions how to dissolve the drug (see Fig. 1). Reducing workload and making the environment more friendly is

Drip-o-Mat for Pediatric Cardiac Surgery

(Developed by Dr. Yaacov Gozal and Dr. Alexander Avidan, Department of Anesthesiology/ CCM Hadassah Ein Karem)

Patient's weight 1.0 kg

Drug	mg/ml	µg/kg/min	3 mg/50 ml: 1 ml/h = 1 µg/kg/min	
Dopamine	40	2–10	0.075 ml	
Dobutamine	12.5	1–10	0.24 ml	
Phentolamine	10	1–2	0.3 ml	
Sodium Nitroprusside	10	0.5–8	0.3 ml	
Sodium Nitroprusside	6	0.5–8	0.5 ml	If diluted to 10 ml
Nitroglycerin	1	0.25–5	3 ml	

Drug	mg/ml	µg/kg/min	0.15 mg/50 ml: 1 ml/h = 0.05 µg/kg/min	
Adrenaline	1	0.05–1	0.15 ml	Bolus 1–10 µg
Noradrenaline	2	0.05–1	0.075 ml	
Isoprotenerol	0.2	0.05–0.5	0.75 ml	
Milrinone	1	0.25–0.75	0.15 ml	Loading 50 µg
Prostin	0.5	0.05–0.4	0.3 ml	
Phenylephrine	0.1	0.15–4	1.5 ml	Bolus 1–2 µg

Drug	mg/ml	µg/kg/min	60 mg/50 ml: 1 ml/h = 20 µg/kg/min	
Procainamide	100	20–80	0.6 ml	Loading 3–5 µg
Lidocaine	10	20–50	6 ml	Bolus 1–10 µg
Esmolol	10	50–300	6 ml	Bolus 0.5–1 mg
Esmolol	250	50–300	0.24 ml	Bolus 0.5–1 mg

Drug	mg/ml	Bolus mg	
Calcium	100	10–20	
Hydralazine	25	0.75	Divided in 4 doses
Verapamil (>1 year)	2.5	0.1–0.3	Repeatdose 0.1-0.2 mg
Adenosine	3	0.1–0.2	
Atropine	1	0.01–0.02	
Ephedrine	50	0.01–0.02	
Labetalol	5	0.25	

Defibrillation		
Defibrillation	2 W/kg	2 Watt

Coarctation	mg/ml	mg/kg	ml	mg
Dexamethasone	4	0.25	0.06	0.3
Mannitol 25 %	250	250	1.00	250
Heparin	50	1	0.02	1.0
Lidocaine 1 %	10	1	0.10	1.0

Fig. 1   The Drip-o-Mat – reduce workload of calculation

the domain of HF, and in this case we hopefully eliminated the potential for errors that might be fatal [9].

The design of forms used by the medical team is of the utmost importance, even when our communications are being handled by computers. The Oncology Institute of Hadassah, one of the largest medical centres in Israel, has had several near accidents related to an incorrect dosage of radiation. The Human Factors approach enabled us to locate the place where the data was supposed to be – the patient's radiation form. This form was used by many professionals who contributed to this complicated treatment: the surgeon, the oncologist, the physicist, the X-ray technician, nurses – each one contributes his own important input, some of them add a paper which is hidden in a side pocket of the form, others just write their orders, and this material is not very accessible, although it contains valuable information (e.g. patient's allergies, other drugs he or she is taking, etc.). In the spirit of the HF approach a new form was designed. In the designing stage each user was asked to specify his or her own needs and the relative importance of different data that were relevant to him/her in order to have a good picture of the patient's needs and situation.

A "war map" of the process needs to be created, so that the input of each member of the medical team is clear to the other team members. Based on HF principles we were able to create a form that is the official form now, and in a follow-up we found out that it reduces the possibilities of committing errors or the possibility of ignoring important physical values necessary for proper treatment.

Forms are one aspect, but the design of the nurses' station and drug labels is another. We managed to show that proper labelling of the intravenous (IV) drugs, not only on the containers but also on the IV tubing leading to the patient, can reduce the error rate and enable the nurse to quickly locate the path of an IV into the patient's vein within the tubing "macaroni" [10].

Information has to be communicated from one shift to the next, doctors' shifts and nurses' shifts; and patients transferred from internal medicine to a surgical ward have to carry with them the results of all clinical and laboratory tests. However, of no less importance is the need to communicate the deliberations that went on in the referring physician's mind. There is no structured way of communicating data – there are often simply habits and common practices. This area is a new subject of HF investigations. The HF engineer may look into the "hand-over" process either by field observations or by simulated setups in the laboratory. A preliminary study at the National University Hospital in Singapore has recorded the phone conversations between physicians of consecutive shifts who had to transfer information to the next shift and to look at the notes the previous shift physicians wrote to themselves. Another way to go about it is to ask the two groups involved in transferring their patients' data to "think aloud", record it and analyse the text.

A medical accident or an event that caused the death of a patient should be investigated like an air crash, namely by experts. Unfortunately, in medicine we do not have a specialty that is parallel to aerial accidents' investigations, and accidents are investigated by senior physicians (or lawyers) who are naturally biased. Human Factors experts, on the other hand, can investigate a medical mishap the same way the Three Mile Island accident or NASA failures are investigated. Rather than looking for someone to blame, investigations such as these aim to expose hidden chains of events, or gaps in the system that need to be corrected.

As mentioned above, one of the investigation methods is simulating incidents. This method was used for investigating the case of a patient who died in the ICU several hours after a cardiac catheterization, due to unnoticed bleeding from the femoral artery. A dummy served as the patient and the case was re-enacted by *all* those who were involved in the case, from the moment the patient was transferred to the gurney after angiography, then through the corridors to the exact ICU bed the patient had occupied. The setup of the ICU at the time of the event was reconstructed exactly, and the nursing staff was told to re-enact their every move, minute by minute, how they admitted the patient and how they discovered a disconnection in the flushing system left in the femoral artery. At the end of the simulation it was clear that the main reason for the death was not any "negligence" on the part of any nurse, but an engineering snag in the design of the ICU, which prevented the patient from being seen from the nurses' station. That incident and the hostile environment, in which one nurse had to deal with 7 patients – 2 of them hooked to ventilators, plus many other issues – given proper attention, could easily be fixed and help avoid another accident like this in the future.

Summary

Human Factors engineers are using many methods to look into the way we think and the way we interact with our work environment. However, the medical community is still very suspicious of research done by psychologists or anthropologists. It is crucial to cooperate with and learn from other disciplines. Medicine has for too many years ignored the fact that its doctors are also human beings, with limitations like any other people, e.g. their memory is limited and may fail especially when they need to sleep. Once medicine and HF engineering learn each other's language, our patients shall benefit from a new branch of medicine – Medical Ergonomics.

The author

Yoel Donchin, MD
    Head Patient Safety Unit
    Hadassah Hebrew University Medical center
    Jerusalem, Israel
    P.O. Box 12007, Jerusalem
    Israel 91120
    E-mail: yoel.donchin@gmail.com

References

1. Porter R. Blood & guts. A short history of medicine. Allen Lane – The Penguin Press. London 2002.
2. Knaus WA, Draper EA, Wagner DP, Zimmerman JE. An evaluation of outcome from intensive care in major medical centers. Ann Intern Med. 1986;104(3):410-418.
3. Beecher, HK. The first anesthesia death with some remarks suggested by it on the fields of the laboratory and the clinic in the appraisal of new anesthetic agents. Anesthesiology 1941;(2)443-449.
4. Leape LL, Brennan TA, Laird N, et al. The nature of adverse events in hospitalized patients. Results of the Harvard Medical Practice Study II. New England Journal of Medicine 1991;(6)324-384.
5. Bishop PJ. Evolution of The Stethoscope. J R Soc Med 1980;73(6)448-456.
6. Kirkup JR. The History and evolution of surgical instruments. Ann. R.S.C. of Surgeons of England 1981;63,279-285.
7. Donchin Y, Gopher D, Olin M, et al. A look into the nature and causes of human errors in the intensive care unit. Crit Care Med. 1995;23(2):294-300.
8. Einav Y, Gopher D, Kara I et al. Preoperative briefing in the operating room: shared cognition, teamwork, and patient safety. Chest. 2010;137(2):443-9.
9. Yariv Y, Kedmi E, Struachler Z et al. Analysis of MgSO4 administration (Hebrew) Publication of the center for safety at work and human factors engineering, Feb 2002.
10. Porat N, Bitan Y, Shefi D et al. Use of color-coded labels for intravenous high-risk medications and lines to improve patient safety. Qual Saf Health Care 2009;18(6):505-9.
11. Einav Y, Gopher D, Donchin Y. Taking action to reduce medical errors: don't put the cart before the horse. Crit Care Resusc 2005;7(2):128-30.

Martha M. Kennedy, Deborah J. Baker, Ayse P. Gurses and Peter J. Pronovost

Creating the ideal ward round

Introduction

Since the beginnings of western medical practice, care providers have walked amongst their hospitalised patients discussing issues related to diagnosis, treatment and prognoses, making a plan of care for the day – all with the goal of improving outcomes. This practice of "daily rounds" has evolved over time to become the foundation of clinical communication. The primary goal of any medical rounding process is communication of information within and between types of clinicians, assessment of patient's condition, setting strategic goals for both patient and provider, and assignment of tasks and responsibilities. In this discussion, we review the structure and process of rounds, expectations of teamwork and role fulfilment by participants, key components of ideal ward rounds, and the human and environmental barriers to achieving maximal performance.

Rounds – historical perspectives

Modern medical rounds grew from the vision and dedication of Dr. William Osler, who in the early 1890s developed the practice of bedside teaching at Johns Hopkins Hospital and Medical School. From the beginning, rounds had multiple goals, including teaching, patient care, and communication. Fundamental to his considerable reputation as both practitioner and educator was the belief that quality teaching and medical care begins and ends with the patient. His rounds were conducted at the bedside and included the patient in the discussion of disease, treatment, and outcome. He enforced the integration of clinical presentation and didactic instruction, and demonstrated the importance of the relationship between patient and practitioner.

Today, we find that there are many variations of rounds occurring in any given institution. They can be grouped into three main categories: work rounds, teaching rounds, and combined work and teaching rounds. *Work rounds* focus on evaluating patients, diagnosing problems, identifying tasks to be completed, and assigning the specific tasks to a team member. For example, the surgical team carries out a round on 20–35 service patients early in the morning, assessing intake and output, laboratory values, wounds and drains, and medications. Led by the senior resident, the team identifies tasks to be performed (e.g., pull back a drain, obtain blood cultures from a patient with a rising white count, evaluate a cinesophagram) and assigns a team member responsible for ensuring that the tasks are done that day. Work rounds are focused, spending a small amount of time per patient, enlisting various team members to play specific roles (examiner, scribe, order-writer). Communication to the patient, family and other caregivers is often deferred until after rounds.

Teaching rounds are focused on conveying information among team members, demonstrating and soliciting critical thinking, and case-based growth of knowledge by team members. Often led by the attending physician, registrar, or senior resident, the goal is education of team members utilising patient case information. For example, in the Intensive Care Unit (ICU), a patient with the acute respiratory distress syndrome may be discussed at length. Questions may be directed to any team member, most often to the more junior medical and nursing staff initially and then to more senior practitioners as the discussion becomes more complex. The focus is often on the physiology of the disease process, comparing treatments and their effectiveness, complications of both disease and interventions, and the influence of the particular patient's presentation on therapeutic choices. Teaching rounds are often lengthy, focus on a single patient or type of problem, integrate many different physiologic and therapeutic principles, and foster growth in critical thinking and knowledge.

A combination of the two previous categories, *work-teaching rounds* combine the patient-care focus of work rounds (i.e. what needs to be done, and who needs to do it) with the education component of teaching rounds. Rounds meet the functional work requirements of order-writing, goal setting, and establishing team communication. Work-teaching rounds may have more diverse case discussions than the more in-depth teaching-only rounds because of the number and type of patients seen while rounding. The structure of these work-teach rounds vary widely among hospitals, especially between academic and community hospitals. Nevertheless, most ICU rounds today fall into this category. The discussion, usually led by an intensivist, details for each patient the critical events of the past 24 hours, current problems, possible solutions, prioritisation of interventions, and back-up plans should the patient not respond as anticipated. Team members fulfil specific roles – identifying current concerns, presenting the patient summary, assessment, and plan for the day; writing orders; and documenting patient and team goals. Others review and critique the presentation and plan, reinforcing key management concepts, and facilitating focused discussions. Common discussion topics include ventilator management, fluid resuscitation, and sepsis management. Team organisation is determined by – and roles/responsibilities are assigned by – the intensivist and take into account the knowledge-base and mix of staff. The intensivist, based on work load and time constraints, determines the amount of time that will be devoted to teaching or tasks.

Rounds may be formal or informal, independent or collaborative, and have regimented or free-flowing discussions. The "rules" of the rounding process are set by the intensivist/team leader. Some prefer a formal organisation with delineated roles for each participant. For example, the leader may organise rounds so the overnight/primary provider presents the patient and proposes a management plan, the registrar amends the assessment and plan, and the final plan of care is determined by the leader. With this model, participants know what is expected of them, when it is appropriate to participate, and who is in charge. Less formal rounding achieves the same (or an even enhanced) level of decision-making but is more collaborative and flowing in style, may allow for more input from additional staff members who would otherwise be too intimidated to participate, and may have more open discussions than in the more formal setting. Both versions can achieve the same outcome regarding care decisions and education, and lead to the development of an improved teamwork and safety climate.

Creating the ideal ward round

The ideal ward round starts with an effective multidisciplinary team, working towards a common goal of providing excellent and comprehensive care, having well-defined roles, supporting and cross monitoring each other. The ideal ward round is one in which patients receive critical review, care is reviewed and critiqued, ongoing patient needs are recognised and addressed, and daily patient goals are established and shared among care providers. Nursing, medical, and ancillary providers work together to identify clinical issues and solutions, and monitor practice related to patient care delivery. Team members gain knowledge in clinical practice issues through patient-related discussions. Completing all of these tasks in a timely manner is the challenge of the modern-day work-teaching rounds.

The process of achieving ideal ward rounds starts first with the development of a cohesive team, as teamwork is the means by which the goals of rounding are obtained. This team-based approach to the care of critically ill patients has been a cornerstone of the Society of Critical Care Medicine since its inception. In today's healthcare system, we count on our team members to partner with us to ensure that our patients receive necessary and timely care. The shared expertise and efforts of a team dedicated to the care of critically ill patients is far reaching, with greater coverage than can be provided by even the most seasoned intensivist. As the shared skill and expertise of the team is developed by the intensivist, so does the application of that expertise across a group of patients, effectively extending the expert reach and influence of the more learned provider.

Creating that cohesive team of providers is the challenge faced by ICU leadership. While the housestaff in academic institutions is a constant source of team members, they are usually not able to fill all the necessary team roles. The team is comprised of unit-based staff (bedside nurses, charge nurse, midlevel providers, clinical nurse specialist, nurse manager), ancillary staff (respiratory therapist, pharmacists, social workers, physical and occupational therapists), and rotating staff (medical students, interns, residents, registrars). The ICU leadership is challenged to determine which positions or roles are required on a given team and who will underwrite their cost. Some roles, such as bedside nurse and charge nurse, are necessary and in place independent of the needs of the rounding team. Others, such as the respiratory therapist, pharmacist, and midlevel providers are not an "absolute need" within the unit or on the team unless deemed necessary by leadership or hospital standards. While the ward cannot run without nurses at the bedside, it can be argued that it can

run without the unit-based presence of a pharmacist or respiratory therapist. We will, however, in this discussion, counter that argument as we propose that the "ideal ward round" team starts with having the proper team members, and that certain roles are required, and not simply suggested (see Fig. 1).

Intensivist: We start first with the head of any team – the leader. All teams need a leader, and in the ICU setting the intensivist is usually the team leader. The intensivist is an expert in critical care, has no competing interests when attending in the ICU, is dedicated to the patient and support team, and can respond to emergencies in person or by phone within five minutes. The deployment of intensivists in ICU settings, and the resulting frequent and timely oversight of patients, has decreased ICU mortality, shortened ICU stays, and increased throughput. Rounds are the means by which the intensivist achieves these significant goals. We believe that the responsibility of the intensivist team leader is not only to direct care management but also to foster a collaborative teaching and team environment.

As leader, the intensivist chooses how rounds are implemented, who participates, and the manner in which learning will proceed. The intensivist sets the tone for interactions, determining if the rounds will be "open" and invite participation from non-provider staff, or "closed" to other than selected staff. He/she determines if it is "safe or

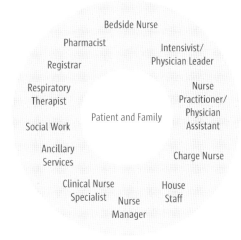

Fig. 1   The ideal team for ICU ward rounds

dangerous" to be uncertain or ask a question, and what role senior staff or trainees will have in directing patient care or leading teaching sessions. Creation of a collaborative and mutually respectful rounding atmosphere fosters multidisciplinary involvement in the care process and increases the likelihood that important observations or concerns are brought forth, accurate diagnoses are made and effective therapies identified and implemented.

To accomplish this, the intensivist should clearly identify the roles and responsibilities of individual team members, the manner in which he/she wants patient information provided, when discussion should take place, and the role of the senior trainees in the rounding process. Comments from ancillary staff members should be invited and appreciated, not as an add-on but as an integral component of rounds, especially when the patient issue falls within their expertise. Short and long-term goals should be articulated for each patient. Information should be summarised before moving on, and it should be validated that essential team members understand the goals for the day. Excellent teaching opportunities arise or can be manufactured during case discussions. The intensivist should follow the example set forth by Osler, whose "criticisms of students and their work were incisive and unforgettable, but never harsh or unkindly; they inspired respect and affection, never fear" [1]. When possible, these teaching moments provide an opportunity for the leader to support the senior residents or registrars in developing their own teaching skills. In the end, the intensivist is training all team members to think and perform above their current level, and in doing so increases the expertise within the ward at any given time.

Supporting any leader should be a team of qualified and invested individuals. In the ICU, those members range from the bedside nurse to the senior medical staff, and include specialty providers such as respiratory therapists, nutritionists, physical therapists, and pharmacists. At any given time, those team members should be able to articulate the goals for the patient, the steps planned or undertaken to achieve those goals, and deviations from the expected course. This level of attention and responsibility requires that individuals be educated in the care of their patients, feel valued as a team member,

and that they have the right to speak up within the group. The team leader sets the tone for team interactions.

Nursing: Nursing staff are the constant member in a team made of primarily transient staff. Nurses are the eyes and ears of any medical team, as well as the primary communicator with patients and families. They spend more time with the patient than any other provider, yet medical staff often discredit their experiential wisdom, believing that book knowledge is the only important domain of knowledge, and forgetting that time with the patient is equally important. Their awareness and analysis of changes in patient parameters and clinical presentation are critical to timely and appropriate interventions. They are essential to the quality care of ICU patients. Studies have demonstrated that increased nurse-patient ratios and any relative inexperience of nurses increase the risk of adverse events and length of stay [2–4].

The bedside nurse should be an active participant in rounds, be able to contribute to rounds, articulate the goal of care at the completion of rounds, thereby reducing the risk of a communication error. We count on them to communicate patient changes, identify problems, ensure that those problems are addressed, and be an active partner to the provider team. The charge nurse and clinical nurse specialist serve an equally important role, both supporting the bedside nurse in his/her patient role, and also in representing the entire unit in discussion of staffing levels and complex acuity/manpower issues. The charge nurse has global knowledge of the unit and staff that influence decisions made every day by the team leader. Nursing staff's critical thinking and evaluative skills develop with exposure to and participation in teaching sessions provided at the bedside or in more formal teaching sessions.

One effective method to improve communication between unit leadership each day is the use of "morning huddle" rounds between the charge nurse and intensivist. This is a brief meeting before rounds during which they discuss issues that arose overnight, review planned admissions and discharges, and try to plan out the unit workflow as much as possible. This review can be repeated in the afternoon/evening as the intensivist plans for the hand-off of overnight care.

Nurse educators and other nurse specialists play a critical role in ensuring quality of care. These nurses help to create protocols and policies, ensure that nurses know and comply with the protocols, problem solve practice issues, and offer coaching and mentoring. Yet in many hospitals, these "non patient care staff" are being eliminated. This will likely result in decreased quality and increased costs of care.

The nurse manager is a partner to the intensivist, and without his/her support the provider team may be severely handicapped. Nursing staff members look to the nurse manager for validation of practice, for support when taking on significant challenges, and to be their representative in meetings where their role and efforts are discussed. As such, the quality of partnership between the intensivist and nurse manager reflects the level of respect and collaboration between the two leaders, and is often mirrored by the nursing staff. The two leaders should have an open relationship where it is possible for each to identify and respond to problematic issues in a timely manner.

Housestaff and midlevel practitioners: Housestaff rotating through the ICU are often responsible for providing care to critically ill patients despite a relative lack of knowledge in the principles of critical care management. Their role on the team is to be both provider and student, directing care as they are gathering the skills required to critically review and analyse patient presentations. Should they rotate through one or more ICUs during their residency, the learning curve shifts and most become proficient in the management of acutely and critically ill patients. Their role on rounds varies according to their ability and experience. In many settings, the intern or resident managing the patient for the last 16–30 hours is responsible for gathering patient data, assessing the patient, synthesising the events of the last 24 hours, and proposing a management plan. This plan is then amended or supported by the senior residents or registrar, and finalised with the input of the intensivist.

An important issue for housestaff is how to balance the service and student roles, where they are expected to both provide care and also need to learn from more experienced staff and the intensivist. This education can be cased-based and take place during or after rounds, but without it the housestaff will not gain the skills necessary to be a safe ICU practitioner. It is up to the intensivist to recognise the knowledge and skill level of the individuals who make up the rounding team, and provide structure and content accordingly. This can be a tall order in a busy unit where housestaff vary widely in their knowledge and experience, members of the care team vary in the relative importance they place on the work and education goals of rounds, and teaching is often delegated to registrar staff or other well-trained ICU providers.

Midlevel practitioners play a vital and ever increasing role in ICU care. Needs for the role have been increased by the reduction in resident work hours and concerns with the balance between housestaff service versus student roles. Midlevel practitioners are nurse practitioners or physician assistants who have chosen to specialise in the care of acutely and critically ill patients. They are usually attached to a single unit or type of patient (for example medical or surgical, cardiac or neurosurgical ICU patients), and are valued members of the team. Midlevel providers are the constant presence among ICU providers, are generally respected for their clinical and organizational knowledge, and for their willingness to help others grow and learn. Because they usually work in one clinical area, they gain substantial patient or unit-specific experience, knowledge of ICU protocols and evidence-based practice, and knowledge of attending physicians preferences.

Midlevel providers generally participate in the education of housestaff, registrars, and nursing staff. As others rotate through the unit, the midlevel provider remains and retains practice and patient history across providers, an especially beneficial role with long-staying patients. The midlevel providers look to the intensivist for mentoring and coaching, for validation and critiquing of their knowledge base and decision-making, as well as for the push to continuously improve their practice level. On rounds, the midlevel provider can fulfil the role of support player or leader, depending upon the needs at that moment and the desire of the intensivist. In addition, midlevels play an important role in communicating with patients, their families and other clinicians, communication that is often time-consuming and important, but sometimes neglected.

Registrars: The ICU registrar or fellow is an intensivist-in-training. As such, they are a leader in the ICU, and expected to be able to mentor and train those less knowledgeable in the art of caring for critically ill patients. Throughout the year they should gain clinical acumen, leadership, and teaching skills. Registrars are expected to oversee all the patients, support the junior medical and midlevel staff, while at the same time challenge them to develop their own critical thinking and decision-making skills. On rounds, the registrar should be ready to give an opinion regarding management options and goals for any patient and the supporting rationale. They are expected to lead discussions based on a current case or a subject chosen by the intensivist.

Ancillary services: Ancillary services include respiratory therapists, nutritionists, pharmacists, physical and occupational therapists, social workers and discharge coordinators. Although ICU rounds can occur in their absence, there is ever growing evidence that their expertise is valuable and adds to the quality of rounds and patient care. Respiratory therapists may identify subtleties of patient-ventilator interaction missed by others determine that different settings would benefit the patient. Respiratory therapist-driven protocols have proven to be capable of decreasing the length of time on ventilators. The presence of pharmacist on rounds has proven to decrease adverse events, while being an excellent resource for team discussions of drug choice and dosing options. Physical therapists and other ancillary services provide additional "eyes on the patient" and in doing so, they increase the likelihood that pertinent issues will be identified and addressed in a timely manner.

Family: Family members should be invited to join rounds, and in doing so can provide insight into the patient, their history, beliefs, and desires. Unfortunately, few ICUs routinely invite families to participate, and this shortcoming needs to change. While many worry that the family will slow rounds or that providers will be uncomfortable discussing concerns and prognosis in front of a family, we and others have found that with practice, this is not the case [5, 6]. The addition of family members to rounds is usually beneficial, increasing patient and family satisfaction, clarifying questions, and in the long run saving provider time. These discussions facilitate providing care that is more consistent with the patient's wishes, especially in the care of chronically ill patients. Some families are a constant monitor of team processing over time, maintaining a detailed history, and recognizing subtle changes that might be missed by intermittent observation from providers. Other families are less detailed in their oversight, but feel they are part of the team working to help their loved one and appreciate the efforts being made on their behalf. This familiarity can lead to more frank discussions of outcome and prognosis. Providers benefit from interacting with the family and learning how to discuss difficult issues in their presence. It is important that when teaching occurs during rounds, the family understands that not all issues addressed are related to their family member, and that the scholarly questioning is a time-honoured learning process. Occasionally, it is necessary to move on with rounds even if all questions and concerns have not been addressed, but if this is indeed the case, it should proceed with the understanding that a team member will in fact return after rounds have been completed in order to continue the discussion.

Barriers to the ideal ward round

While the ideal rounds outlined above may be difficult to achieve, they still are possible. Rounds vary widely among ICUs and within an ICU over time, often defined by the intensivist style. Yet when they occur, ideal rounds are magical, improving patient outcomes, reducing length of stay, improving patient and family satisfaction, and restoring satisfaction to clinicians daily work. As such, we need to explore the barriers providing these rounds. To create such an ideal team and build the ideal ward rounds, there are human, environmental, and organizational factors that must be addressed.

Personnel: The intensivist/team leader role is fundamental to the ideal ward rounds – he or she must be ready to not only oversee the care of complex patients but also recognise and respond to the educational needs of the staff, employing various teaching techniques as warranted. They will need to provide positive and negative feedback in an appropriate manner, and provide end of rotation feedback to mentors and supervisors. This must be accomplished despite administrative and documentation/billing pressures. Hospital or university promotion and financial systems may not recognise or reimburse the effort put into teaching outside the classroom. The cognitive burden is substantial, and it is a special person who is both willing and qualified to take on this role.

Housestaff and registrars are subject to oversight by governing bodies that control their work hours. The rounds as described are often time consuming and require significant preparation. The extent to which the staff in training is able to fully participate in the rounds and related teaching will depend upon the balance between work hours and practice requirements. Midlevel providers can help fulfil the staffing needs in this and similar situations, but will require institutional support for role development, salary, and oversight.

Nurse-patient ratios, staffing and experience will influence the nurses' abilities to be active and consistent participants in rounds. The more patients that are assigned or less experience the nurse has in caring for such patients, the less likely he or she will be able to balance patient care needs with attention to rounds. This leads to diminished familiarity with the rationale behind decisions and less communication between the nurse and provider team.

Staff members also vary widely in the relative importance they assign to the work and education roles of rounds. This variation poses challenges to conducting rounds that meet all participants needs.

Institutional support is required for the allocation of ancillary staff to the ICU. Dedicated unit-based staffing of pharmacists, respiratory therapists, and other ancillary staff is not without cost. Without support of the integrated model, these roles will not be consistently represented on the team and the proven benefit will be lost.

Time constraints: As mentioned above, the ideal ward round may be time consuming. Preparing for such detailed rounds is also time consuming. Housestaff and/or midlevel providers must be able to collect and record the necessary information and synthesize it before rounds. This can be difficult if the patient load is extensive, filled with high acuity patients, or the provider is "stuck" at the bedside with a sick patient when they "should" be preparing for rounds.

Patient acuity and unit throughput needs may not always support extensive ward rounding. As patients are sicker, or bed availability decreases, there is increased pressure to have faster and more work-oriented rounds. In this case, the educational aspect of rounds may need to be deferred altogether or until after work rounds are completed.

Physical environment/tools: The ICU is often a noisy and busy environment, filled with staff members, multiple loud alarms and consulting or primary teams needing to see patients. It is not conducive to quiet thought and contemplation, and can be a source of sensory overload. Additionally, staff may be interrupted for phone calls related to bell allocation and pulled from rounds for patient problems. Even the most able provider can lose focus. To minimize these effects, the ward may need to enforce some "rules". To decrease noise, phones and pagers held by team members must be put on vibrate mode. The ward can put notices at the entrances that "rounds are in process" as a visual reminder to visitors that work is in process and quietness is appreciated. Nursing will be asked to not interrupt participants for requests that are not urgent, and in turn, providers will work to ensure that orders are entered completely and in a timely manner.

In some ICUs, the very size of the team may be a problem. For best communication and equality of discussion, team members should be in a circle and able to view each other during the presentation and discussions. This was easier when the team fit around a mobile rounding table and orders and notes were written in a single chart. The size of the team in an older, smaller unit can be daunting, especially with the addition of mobile computers to meet data entry and chart review needs. With the advent of computer-based order-writing systems, electronic patient records, and digital radiology, we have added considerable machinery to the rounding team. Not every team member needs their own access, however, and wards can organize their computer resources so that many may share or view a single console. This is an issue that can be resolved by the intensivist's organization of rounds, for example, mandating that there will be two computers in use during rounds – one for order input and one for data review.

More and more ICUs are utilizing computer-based technology for data collection.

Unfortunately, not all institutions have technology and process or team-based tools structured to allow retrieval and synthesis of data for rounds, especially by the inexperienced provider. Too much time is spent retrieving and sifting through data, and not enough on the synthesis and application. This will undoubtedly improve as informatics platforms develop and hospitals adopt more process-oriented tools that pull information from data sets compiled in the clinical setting.

Facilitating the ideal ward rounds

We have also identified several specific factors that facilitate rounds. First, the ICU should have sufficient staff to provide care for patients in the ICU, and all members of the care team must have sufficient resources to be able to provide care safely. To obtain and maintain these resources, hospital leaders must be made aware of the evidence supporting the benefits of intensivist staffing, good nurse-patient ratios, and dedicated pharmacist and respiratory therapy staffing. Hospital leadership should be encouraged to take a systematic rather than myopic view of ICU staffing costs, with reminders that better staffing reduces patient complications and length of stay, and cost of care. In the long run, better patient care and shorter ICU stays increases unit throughput and frees up beds for new admissions.

Secondly, the ICU physician leader must create a culture that supports ideal rounds. The leader can create and role model policies stating that patients/families must be invited to participate in rounds, and require that rounds do not start on a particular patient if the bedside nurse is not available. It is a very powerful statement in support of nurse-provider teamwork if the team agrees to round on a different patient until the nurse is available. Consistently requesting and encouraging participation by respiratory therapists, pharmacists, and other specialty staff sends the message that non-physician expertise is appreciated and respected. The leadership can support unit staffing with midlevel providers, not only as a means of reducing workload but also for the less tangible benefit of continuity and consistency of care, and education of team members.

Thirdly, there are tools that can be used to foster communications. These tools include the morning briefing ("huddle rounds") and use of a daily goal sheet. The daily goal sheet is a structured tool that clarifies goals of care for each patient and ensures that all members of the care team are able to articulate those goals. The use of the daily goal sheet reduces communication and medication errors, decreases length of stay, and saves nursing and provider time as goals and expectations are clearly stated. If the bedside provider knows what the goal is meant to be, then they are more likely to notify the provider if the patient or system are not going to meet that goal – problems are addressed and corrective action is initiated more quickly.

Lastly, the team needs feedback regarding how effective rounds are. One practical way to accomplish this is to ask one member of the care team (nurse, house officer, midlevel, etc) to observe the effectiveness of teamwork and communication during rounds on a single patient each day or week. The staff member then reports back these results to team members, helping all to recognise what is going well or needs improvement. This requires that staff members understand the attributes of effective teamwork and feel safe to give difficult feedback. Most importantly, the team must be humble enough to accept feedback – it is often best if the attending sets the tone by asking for the direct feedback. Leaders who routinely do this find it to be a positive and rewarding experience, improving the teamwork skills for all. This can be especially beneficial for new attendings'/registrars' working to develop their leadership skills.

Research opportunities

As more institutions strive to attain best practice standards for rounding, research opportunities present themselves. There are opportunities to measure the quality of the teamwork climate and its impact on length of stay, error reporting, patient bounce-backs, staff satisfaction and turnover, and patient/family satisfaction. Other areas to be researched include determining the optimum number of participants, testing rounding structure, format and duration for clinical and educational effectiveness across provider type, and the effect of integration of new technology platforms into rounds.

Conclusion

The ideal ward round is one that facilitates team members working together to accomplish a common goal-providing comprehensive, expert, and humanistic care. The patient and family are well cared for, the staff is respected and respectful, and the team ends the day with more of the knowledge and skills required to take care of patients than they had at the start of the day. The team is led by a clinical expert, with well-developed collaborative and teaching skills, who is responsible for guiding the expert care of a group of patients, and in doing so challenges the staff to improve their interpersonal and professional skills. Communication of patient information, clinical assessment, provider interventions, and patient response are the constant conversation of an intensive care unit. The rounding process is the structured sharing of that conversation, and is fundamental to providing excellent patient care.

The authors

Martha M. Kennedy, PhD RN CRNP[1]
Deborah J. Baker, MS RN CRNP[2]
Ayse P. Gurses, PhD[3]
Peter J. Pronovost, MD, PhD[4]
[1]Nurse Practitioner | Surgical Intensive Care Department of Surgery | Baltimore, Maryland
[2]Director of Nursing, Surgery | Department of Surgery | Baltimore, Maryland
[3]Assistant Professor | Department of Anesthesiology and Critical Care | Quality and Safety Research Group | Baltimore, Maryland
[4]Professor | Department of Anesthesiology and Critical Care Medicine | Baltimore, Maryland

Address for correspondence
Martha M. Kennedy
Nurse Practitioner, Surgical Intensive Care
600 North Wolfe Street
Halsted 600
Baltimore, Maryland 21287, USA
E-mail: Mkenned2@jhmi.edu

References

1. Golden RL. William Osler at 150: an overview of a life. JAMA 1999;282:2252–2258.
2. Morrison AL, Beckmann U, Durie M, Carless R, Gillies DM. The effects of nursing staff inexperience (NSI) on the occurrence of adverse patient experiences in ICUs. Aust Crit Care 2001;14:116–21.
3. Penoyer DA. Nurse staffing and patient outcomes in critical care: a concise review. Crit Care Med 2010;38:1521–1528.
4. Thorens JB, Kaelin RM, Jolliet P, Chevrolet JC. Influence of the quality of nursing on the duration of weaning from mechanical ventilation in patients with chronic obstructive pulmonary disease. Crit Care Med 1995;23:1807–1815.
5. Davidson JE, Powers K, Hedavat KM, Tiesczen M, Kon AA, Shepard E, et al. Clinical practice Guidelines for support of the family in the patient-centered intensive care unit: American College of Critical Care Medicine Task Force 2004–2005. Crit Care Med 2007 Feb;35:605–22.
6. Muething SE, Kotagal UR, Schoettker PJ, del Rey JG, DeWitt, TG. Family-Centered Bedside Rounds: A New Approach to Patient Care and Teaching. Pediatrics 2007;119:829–832.

Hannah Wunsch, Yên-Lan Nguyen and Derek C. Angus

Smoothing the way: Improving admission to and discharge from the ICU

Some of the hardest decisions for clinicians and most fraught times for patients are during the potential transitions in and out of an intensive care unit (ICU). The decisions to admit or discharge a patient are complicated by the challenges of identifying the current appropriate level of care for a patient, as well as understanding the trajectory of that individual's health status. A poor decision at any point can result in complications or even death. Moreover, the actual processes of transfer may be complex, leading to the recognition that the periods surrounding admission and discharge can be particularly dangerous for critically ill patients. Few guidelines exist that provide clear direction regarding admission and discharge decisions or practice. This dearth of guidance is primarily due to the fact that we have little data to support precisely when and what type of patient will gain benefit from transfer into or out of the ICU. Yet, targeting aspects of admission and discharge as areas for improvement remains essential for the well-being of critically ill patients. This chapter explores the specific issues surrounding admission to and discharge from the ICU, and emphasises the data available to help guide decision-making and potentially improve these processes of care.

Admissions

Assessing a patient's need for intensive care remains a challenge. A lack of studies in the area of admission practice, and also the difficulty of interpreting data that may come from different healthcare systems limits the ability to provide broad guidance in this area. For example, ward care may differ with regard to nurse-to-patient ratios or the ability to deliver specific interventions; intermediate care rooms may or may not exist, and in fact, even the definition of an ICU remains variable [1]. For a few situations, such as after coronary artery bypass grafting, there is general agreement regarding the decision to admit a patient to the ICU. But for the majority of patients who receive intensive care, the admission decision remains subjective and often emergent. However, there is a consistent set of decisions that need to be made for each patient that ultimately leads to the decision to admit a patient or to care for him or her elsewhere. All of these decisions can contribute to delivery of best care, sub-optimal care without any complications, or detrimental care (see Fig. 1).

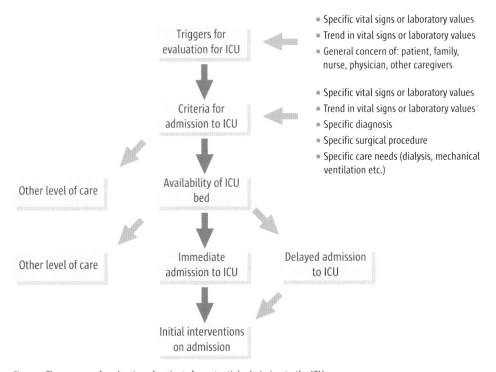

Fig. 1 The process of evaluation of patients for potential admission to the ICU

Identifying patients at risk

Over the past ten years, many hospitals across different countries have introduced Rapid Response, also called "Outreach", "Track and Trigger", or "Medical Emergency", teams in an effort to identify earlier the patients who require intensive care, and to decrease the need for intensive care through earlier intervention [2–4]. The large variation both in the staffing patterns and specific triggers for such teams demonstrates the inherent uncertainty in this new area. For example, some teams may include physicians and others may be staffed by nurses and respiratory therapists. Clinicians also struggle to decide whether specific vital signs alone, trends over time, aggregate scores, computers, nurses, physicians, or families should flag the need for evaluation and potential intervention. Such teams also show mixed results when studied, with some single-centre data suggesting that the rates of cardiopulmonary resuscitation decrease, and admission to ICU at night decreases [5, 6], but with

large multicentre studies yet to demonstrate any substantial impact on outcomes [3, 7].

Criteria for admission

Once evaluated, the decision of whether or not to admit a patient to the ICU is fraught with difficulties, combining evaluation of the severity of illness of a patient, the probable benefit to be gained from receiving ICU-specific care, and (potentially) limited bed availability, which may necessitate rationing decisions. The Society of Critical Care Medicine provides "Guidelines for ICU Admission, Discharge, and Triage" [8]. These guidelines acknowledge the difficulty of deciding whom to admit, stating that "unfortunately, few studies have examined the indications for and the outcomes of ICU care". In a review of observational studies that followed all patients who were evaluated to receive intensive care, refusal of ICU admission was associated with older age, higher severity of illness, and having a medical diagnosis (versus having had surgery) [9]. No studies have systematically examined practice across hospitals, or identified areas of consensus or disagreement regarding ICU admission practice. Consequently, decisions regarding what constitute appropriate interventions and levels of care can differ dramatically. For example, a simulation study at a single centre demonstrated that, even within one institution, the decision to admit a patient to the ICU, or provide mechanical ventilation, varied dramatically depending on the caregiver making the choice. With the given scenario 30 % of physicians admitting the patient to the ICU, 4 % intubated the patient, and 48 % initiated palliative care outside of the ICU [10].

National data from the United Kingdom identified 12 % of surgical patients who incurred 84 % of the hospital mortality [11], and subsequent work in a single centre identified lack of admission to ICU as a potential cause of the high mortality [12]. Another single study, in a cross-national comparison, examined post-surgical outcomes for high-risk surgical patients in a hospital in New York City versus a hospital in London and found a higher hospital mortality associated with surgery in London [13]. The authors speculated that the difference could be due to the lower ICU admission rate in the hospital in London, arguing in favour of more aggressive use of intensive care. Potential harm from denial of intensive care is backed up by data from a systematic review by Sinuff et al. looking at rationing of intensive care beds. The review found that refusal of ICU was associated overall with an increased risk of hospital death [9]. However, these were observational studies where patients who did not receive intensive care were refused admission for a variety of reasons (including expected futility of care). Therefore, it is difficult to determine whether these were appropriate decisions and whether admission to an ICU might have provided benefit for some or all of these patients.

Deciding not to admit a patient

It is also important to emphasise that intensive care is not always necessary or appropriate. Reasons for deciding not to admit a patient to the ICU (besides bed availability) include that the patient may not choose to escalate care, that the patient does not actually require intensive care, (with quality care appropriately delivered elsewhere in the hospital), or that a decision is made regarding the futility of higher-level care, with initiation of a change of goals and end-of-life planning [14]. Many people, including physicians caring for a patient and family members, often view the ICU as "safe" and are reluctant to hear that a patient should (appropriately) receive care elsewhere. Based on this perception, aggressive admission to ICU and extended ICU stays would be considered the best care at all times. However, one cannot forget the potential harm from intensive care and the fact that these risks must be balanced against the benefit. A few studies in the surgical literature have addressed the question of intensive care after carotid endarterectomy and suggest that intensive care is not always necessary; choosing to *not* admit a patient to the ICU could substantially decrease the hospital length of stay without any change in patient outcomes [15, 16]. Risks associated with unnecessary intensive care include an increased number of hand-offs of care between teams, exposure to infections, iatrogenic complications from invasive monitoring, debilitation due to decreased mobility or restrictions on movement, excessive noise and interruptions with potential for sleep deprivation, delirium, and (often) more restrictive visiting hours for families. Delayed transfers out of the ICU may also unnecessarily prolong a patient's overall hospital stay. From a systems perspective, unnecessary care in the ICU can increase costs, and also has the potential to cause delayed admission or refusal for another patient who may gain benefit.

Bed availability and timing of admission

In discussing the decision of whether or not to admit a patient to the ICU, there is an assumption that an ICU bed is available if required. However, this assumption is not always valid. For example, different countries have different availability of ICU beds for a given population which must, by necessity, change the frequency and timing of admissions to ICU [1]. Delays in providing the appropriate level of care, or refusal of admission, may occur. Queuing theory demonstrates that the ability to admit patients to an ICU without substantial delay is a combination of the ICU occupancy and also the size of the ICU [17]. Moreover, relatively small increases in occupancy level can exponentially increase delays. Thus, larger ICUs can operate at higher occupancy than smaller ICUs without substantially affecting admission timing. A few studies have looked specifically at the effect of delayed ICU admission on patient outcomes, concluding that prompt transfer is associated with improved mortality [18]. For sepsis, time to antibiotic therapy has been shown to be associated with hospital mortality [19]. The movement towards early goal-directed therapy [20], and a focus on the first six hours of care as the time window for the "resuscitation bundle" emphasised by the Surviving Sepsis Campaign, are examples of some of the ways in which prompt care may constitute best care, and delays may result in worse care, with significant consequences for patients [21].

The related question of the time of day of admission (independent of any delay) has also been raised. The concern is that patients who deteriorate at night and on weekends are cared for by fewer staff both in the ICU and/or on the wards, which could inadvertently lead to harm when a patient requires immediate stabilisation. But these concerns are not consistently borne out by the literature, with some studies finding improved outcomes with admission during the day, and others finding no differences [22–24]. Moreover, a recent study examining whether the ICU occupancy affects outcomes for patients who *do* gain admission to the ICU demonstrated no differences on high versus low census days, concluding that ICUs already demonstrate a remarkable ability to scale up operating conditions as needed [25].

Changes to admission practice

Recent efforts to improve the quality of care have focused on the need to affect patient care prior to the possibility of an admission to the ICU. Whether or not rapid response teams impact outcomes, they are being implemented worldwide. Such teams are changing the time at which the evaluation process for critically ill patients begins, as well as potentially affecting who is admitted, by allowing for a less emergent evaluation of a patient's needs. Moreover, there is greater understanding of the need to address the appropriateness of care, and to enhance palliative care services so that patients who will not benefit from ICU care are re-routed appropriately to receive other services [26]. And studies into early goal-directed therapy and the Surviving Sepsis Campaign have raised awareness of the potential need to recognise critical illness early and to intervene in a timely fashion by initiating therapies and speeding up the time to transfer to the ICU. We do not yet fully understand the impact of all of these initiatives, and un-bundling the effect of one versus the other remains a challenge [27], but it is clear that there is a heightened awareness of the urgency for more research and greater focus on this "front end" of critical care.

Discharges

Perhaps even more fraught than the problem of when and how to initiate admission to the ICU is determining whether or not a patient is appropriate for discharge from the ICU and facilitating safe transfer of care. Mistakes in this decision and the breakdown of care that can occur are measured by readmissions to the ICU, unexpected deaths on hospital wards, and also unnecessary time spent in the ICU.

Predicting outcomes at discharge

Many studies have sought to predict outcomes for patients on discharge from the ICU in an attempt to identify patients who are at high risk of either readmission or death. But no study has been able to satisfactorily identify individual patients. The Acute Physiology Score has been calculated for patients at ICU discharge, as have many other severity of illness measures [28, 29]. A recent analysis concluded that they could "identify risk factors associated with death and readmission to intensive care [but] it was not possible to produce a definitive model based on these risk factors for predicting death or readmission in an individual patient" [30]. What is relatively consistent across countries is readmission rates and the percentage of deaths for ICU patients that occur outside of the ICU [28], suggesting that these problems remain universal.

While patient factors may not easily predict individual outcome, one systems factor has clearly been shown to be associated with worse outcomes: premature discharge [31]. Goldfrad and Rowan demonstrated an increased odds of death of 1.2 for patients discharged at night, which they used as a proxy for premature discharge, and other studies in different countries have come to the same conclusion [22, 32]. Encouragingly, recent "modernisation" efforts in the UK, including an increase in the number of ICU beds, additional funding, and various ICU-associated programmes and protocols were shown to decrease the percentage of patients who experienced premature discharge from the ICU, suggesting that systems changes can impact the discharge process in positive, quantifiable ways [33].

Location

One unknown in the ICU literature is the role of step-down (also called intermediate care or high-dependency) beds in the transition of patients out of the ICU, versus direct transfer to a normal hospital ward. The first problem with studying this issue is the potential for enormous variation in what constitutes care in either a step-down unit or a general ward. For example, "Level 2" intensive care in the United Kingdom is defined as the need for support of a single organ (excluding mechanical ventilation), such as dialysis or inotropic support [34], generally staffed with one nurse for two patients, and described as "high-dependency" care. However, this same nursing ratio may be found in many ICUs in the United States, and potentially in other countries, with step-down care involving more patients for each nurse. Since different nurse-to-patient ratios have been implicated in differences in complication rates for patients and mortality, these variations in staffing models may have large implications for discharge practices [35]. Even if there was a standard definition for ICU, step-down, and ward, many questions remain unanswered, such as whether patients do better if there is a step-down bed, or whether an intermediate step just represents yet another hand-off of care with the potential for lost information, changes in nursing, and geographic movement within the hospital. Finally, a model of discharge from the

ICU that, while not unique to the United States, is certainly more common than in other countries, is the practice of direct discharge of patients from the ICU to either long-term acute care facilities or other skilled care facilities, including ventilator weaning facilities. There are few data examining these different models of post-ICU care, although continued high mortality in these settings remains a concern [36].

Hand-offs

The actual process of a transfer out of an ICU can also put patients at risk, irrespective of the appropriateness of the discharge. Transfer of knowledge, transfer of care teams, and the physical transfer of patients are all areas of risk (see Fig. 2). One study by Horwitz et al. studied "sign-out" of clinical information among internal medicine house-staff teams, examining hand-offs for 184 patients [37]. The authors found that five patients had delays in diagnosis, one required transfer to the ICU and four patients had near misses due to sign-out omissions. The study identified missing information that included the clinical condition of the patient, recent or scheduled events, and tasks to complete. Given the complexity of ICU patients these problems seem likely to be exacerbated during transfer of care. The period of transfer of patients out of the ICU is one way in which "closed" ICUs, with care by intensivists, may not facilitate improved care, since primary teams may struggle to resume the day-to-day management on these extremely complex patients, even when appropriately stable for transfer. Medicine reconciliation, in particular, remains a problem on transfer. In a study of the discontinuity of chronic medications in patients discharged from the ICU, 33 % had one or more chronic medications omitted at hospital discharge [38].

Changes to practice

Some aspects of admitting and discharging, such as bed availability, may require large systems changes for improvement. But hand-offs and in particular, medicine reconciliation, are areas where relatively small changes in practice may improve patient safety. For example, Patterson et al. used examples from other setting "with high consequences for failure", such as space shuttle mission control, nuclear power plants, and railroad discharges, to determine ways in which hand-offs can be made safer [39]. The authors identify 21 hand-off coordination and communication strategies, including making hand-offs face-to-face verbal updates with interactive questioning, and deliberate delay of transfer of responsibility during critical activities.

Finally, one relatively new concept that has emerged from operations research, and spread from areas such as obstetrics is the concept of "universal rooms", combined with "variable-acuity nursing" which allows the system to flex up or down to accommodate the changing needs of a patient within the same space. Such a design

1. mitigates the need to identify a defining moment when a patient can "step down" to a lower level of care,
2. removes concerns regarding physical transfer of patients, and
3. potentially minimises hand-offs among staff (see Fig. 2) [40–42].

A modified version of this model is to maintain the ICU as a separate space, but then to have all other levels of care in a single room, which may be a more feasible model in many hospitals and for many types of patients [41]. While a few hospitals have been able to redesign spaces as universal rooms, primarily for cardiac patients, for most this model remains conceptual rather than implementable [42]. Moreover, there are few data to support whether this model of care does result in improvements. At the moment there is still no "best system", and further work is clearly needed in this area if we are to improve readmission and death rates after ICU discharge.

Conclusion

The periods of admission to and discharge from the ICU are critical times for patients. With the recognition that intensive care begins and ends outside of the ICU for many patients [43, 44], we are poised to address many of the fundamental, and still unanswered questions regarding how to improve the care of patients during these transitions. Most important to the process is the recognition that these periods require extra vigilance. Perhaps the biggest challenge going forward is in interpreting the data that do exist as results may be heavily influenced by different models of care with regard to staffing, availability of beds, and the physical constraints of an individual hospital. However, it is this very variability that may allow us to compare systems and ultimately determine what constitutes best practice.

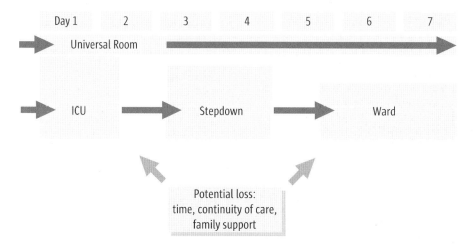

Fig. 2   Models of care transfer for patients admitted to and discharged from the ICU [modified from 41]

The authors

Hannah Wunsch, MD, MSc[1]
Yên-Lan Nguyen, MD, MPH[2]
Derek C. Angus, MD, MPH[3]

[1]Department of Anaesthesiology | Columbia
University | New York, NY USA
[2]Service de Réanimation Médicale | Centre
Hospitalier de Saint-Antoine | Assistance
Publique des Hôpitaux de Paris | Paris,
France
[3]The CRISMA Laboratory (Clinical Research,
Investigation, and Systems Modeling of
Acute Illness) | Department of Critical
Care Medicine | University of Pittsburgh |
Pittsburgh, PA USA

Address for correspondence
Hannah Wunsch
Division of Critical Care
Department of Anaesthesiology
Columbia University
622 West 168th St, PH5-527D
New York, NY 10032
E-mail: hw2125@columbia.edu

References

1. Wunsch H, Angus DC, Harrison DA, Collange O, Fowler R, Hoste EA et al. Variation in critical care services across North America and Western Europe. Crit Care Med 2008, 36:2787–2789.
2. Gao H, Harrison DA, Parry GJ, Daly K, Subbe CP, Rowan K. The impact of the introduction of critical care outreach services in England: a multicentre interrupted time-series analysis. Crit Care 2007, 11:R113.
3. Cuthbertson B. The impact of critical care outreach: is there one? Critical Care 2007, 11:179.
4. Gao H, McDonnell A, Harrison DA, Moore T, Adam S, Daly K et al. Systematic review and evaluation of physiological track and trigger warning systems for identifying at-risk patients on the ward. Intensive Care Med 2007, 33:667–679.
5. Bellomo R, Goldsmith D, Uchino S, Buckmaster J, Hart GK, Opdam H et al. A prospective before-and-after trial of a medical emergency team. Med J Aust 2003, 179:283–287.
6. Buist MD, Moore GE, Bernard SA, Waxman BP, Anderson JN, Nguyen TV. Effects of a medical emergency team on reduction of incidence of and mortality from unexpected cardiac arrests in hospital: preliminary study. BMJ 2002, 324:387–390.

7. Merit Study Investigators. Introduction of the medical emergency team (MET) system: a cluster-randomised controlled trial. Lancet 2005, 365:2091–2097.
8. Guidelines for intensive care unit admission, discharge, and triage. Crit Care Med 1999, 27:633–638.
9. Sinuff T, Kahnamoui K, Cook DJ, Luce JM, Levy MM. Rationing critical care beds: a systematic review. Crit Care Med 2004, 32:1588–1597.
10. Barnato AE, Hsu HE, Bryce CL, Lave JR, Emlet LL, Angus DC et al. Using simulation to isolate physician variation in intensive care unit admission decision making for critically ill elders with end-stage cancer: a pilot feasibility study. Crit Care Med 2008, 36:3156–3163.
11. Pearse RM, Harrison DA, James P, Watson D, Hinds C, Rhodes A et al. Identification and characterisation of the high-risk surgical population in the United Kingdom. Crit Care 2006, 10:R81.
12. Jhanji S, Thomas B, Ely A, Watson D, Hinds CJ, Pearse RM. Mortality and utilisation of critical care resources amongst high-risk surgical patients in a large NHS trust. Anaesthesia 2008, 63:695–700.
13. Bennett-Guerrero E, Hyam JA, Shaefi S, Prytherch DR, Sutton GL, Weaver PC et al. Comparison of P-POSSUM risk-adjusted mortality rates after surgery between patients in the USA and the UK. Br J Surg 2003, 90:1593–1598.
14. Joynt GM, Gomersall CD, Tan P, Lee A, Cheng CA, Wong EL. Prospective evaluation of patients refused admission to an intensive care unit: triage, futility and outcome. Intensive Care Med 2001, 27:1459–1465.
15. Kraiss LW, Kilberg L, Critch S, Johansen KJ. Short-stay carotid endarterectomy is safe and cost-effective. Am J Surg 1995, 169:512–515.
16. Rigdon EE, Monajjem N, Rhodes RS. Criteria for Selective Utilization of the Intensive Care Unit following Carotid Endarterectomy. Annals of Vascular Surgery 1997, 11:20–27.
17. Green LV. How many hospital beds? Inquiry 2002, 39:400–412.
18. Simchen E, Sprung CL, Galai N, Zitser-Gurevich Y, Bar-Lavi Y, Gurman G et al. Survival of critically ill patients hospitalized in and out of intensive care units under paucity of intensive care unit beds. Crit Care Med 2004, 32:1654–1661.
19. Kumar A, Roberts D, Wood KE, Light B, Parrillo JE, Sharma S et al. Duration of hypotension before initiation of effective antimicrobial therapy is the critical determinant of survival in human septic shock. Crit Care Med 2006, 34:1589–1596.
20. Rivers E, Nguyen B, Havstad S, Ressler J, Muzzin A, Knoblich B et al. Early goal-directed therapy in the treatment of severe sepsis and septic shock. N Engl J Med 2001, 345:1368–1377.
21. Dellinger RP, Carlet JM, Masur H, Gerlach H, Calandra T, Cohen J et al. Surviving Sepsis Campaign guidelines for

management of severe sepsis and septic shock. Crit Care Med 2004, 32:858–873.

22. Laupland KB, Shahpori R, Kirkpatrick AW, Stelfox HT. Hospital mortality among adults admitted to and discharged from intensive care on weekends and evenings. J Crit Care 2008, 23:317–324.

23. Luyt CE, Combes A, Aegerter P, Guidet B, Trouillet JL, Gibert C et al. Mortality among patients admitted to intensive care units during weekday day shifts compared with "off" hours. Crit Care Med 2007, 35:3–11.

24. Wunsch H, Mapstone J, Brady T, Hanks R, Rowan K. Hospital mortality associated with day and time of admission to intensive care units. Intensive Care Med 2004, 30:895–901.

25. Iwashyna TJ, Kramer AA, Kahn JM. Intensive care unit occupancy and patient outcomes. Crit Care Med 2009, 37:1545–1557.

26. Gade G, Venohr I, Conner D, McGrady K, Beane J, Richardson RH et al. Impact of an inpatient palliative care team: a randomized control trial. J Palliat Med 2008, 11:180–190.

27. Chiche JD, Angus DC. Testing protocols in the intensive care unit: complex trials of complex interventions for complex patients. JAMA 2008, 299:693–695.

28. Rosenberg AL, Watts C. Patients readmitted to ICUs: a systematic review of risk factors and outcomes. Chest 2000, 118:492–502.

29. Rosenberg AL, Hofer TP, Hayward RA, Strachan C, Watts CM. Who bounces back? Physiologic and other predictors of intensive care unit readmission. Crit Care Med 2001, 29:511–518.

30. Campbell AJ, Cook JA, Adey G, Cuthbertson BH. Predicting death and readmission after intensive care discharge. Br J Anaesth 2008, 100:656–662.

31. Goldfrad C, Rowan K. Consequences of discharges from intensive care at night. Lancet 2000, 355:1138–1142.

32. Priestap FA, Martin CM. Impact of intensive care unit discharge time on patient outcome. Crit Care Med 2006, 34:2946–2951.

33. Hutchings A, Durand MA, Grieve R, Harrison D, Rowan K,

Green J et al. Evaluation of modernisation of adult critical care services in England: time series and cost effectiveness analysis. BMJ 2009, 339:b4353.

34. Audit Commission National Report. Critical to Success. The place of efficient and effective critical care services within the acute hospital. London; 1999.

35. Needleman J, Buerhaus P. Nurse staffing and patient safety: current knowledge and implications for action. Int J Qual Health Care 2003, 15:275–277.

36. Wunsch H, Guerra C, Barnato AE, Angus DC, Li G, Linde-Zwirble WT. Three-year outcomes for Medicare beneficiaries who survive intensive care. JAMA 2010, 303:849–856.

37. Horwitz LI, Moin T, Krumholz HM, Wang L, Bradley EH. Consequences of inadequate sign-out for patient care. Arch Intern Med 2008, 168:1755–1760.

38. Bell CM, Rahimi-Darabad P, Orner AI. Discontinuity of chronic medications in patients discharged from the intensive care unit. J Gen Intern Med 2006, 21:937–941.

39. Patterson ES, Roth EM, Woods DD, Chow R, Gomes JO. Handoff strategies in settings with high consequences for failure: lessons for health care operations. Int J Qual Health Care 2004, 16:125–132.

40. Pati D, Harvey T, Cason C. Inpatient Unit Flexibility; Design Characteristics of a Successful Flexible Unit. Environment and Behavior 2008, 40:205–232.

41. Gallant D, Lanning K. Streamlining patient care processes through flexible room and equipment design. Crit Care Nurs Q 2001, 24:59–76.

42. Brown KK, Gallant D. Impacting patient outcomes through design: acuity adaptable care/universal room design. Crit Care Nurs Q 2006, 29:326–341.

43. Angus DC, Carlet J. Surviving intensive care: a report from the 2002 Brussels Roundtable. Intensive Care Med 2003, 29:368–377.

44. Hillman K. Critical care without walls. Curr Opin Crit Care 2002, 8:594–599.

Michael D. Christian, Bernard Lawless, Julie Trpkovski and Jeffrey R. Dichter

Surge management for critical care leaders

Introduction

As a very busy clinician and/or administrator reading this text on organisational management, one of the very first questions you should ask yourself, and you likely already have, is 'why should I read this chapter, disasters are rare and I already have enough issues to worry about in my ICU every day?'. There are actually two truths in this statement, both of which provide very strong reasons as to why, as a critical care leader, it is essential that you read this chapter and take away a comprehensive, practical understanding of surge capacity management.

Let us consider the second part of the statement first, that you have enough worries in your ICU every day. Given that in many countries around the world ICUs operate at near 100 % capacity on a daily basis due to a variety of issues including shortages of health human resources (staff), financial constraints and patient flow issues. This situation, combined with the very nature of acute care in which demand for services fluctuates, occasionally unexpectedly, results in a common scenario where demand outstrips supply. This, by definition, is a surge. The main point is that surges occur every day and include everything from the unexpected extra two OR admissions due to intra-operative complications right through to the mass casualty disaster. Surge manage-

ment provides a framework and strategies to allow continued provinsion of safe care in all of these situations.

The second truth in the statement is that disasters are rare. However, because they are rare, many critical care leaders, along with many hospital administrators, live under the false assumption that when disasters do occur it is really only the emergency department that is impacted. Hence this is the reason why most hospital disaster plans often focus exclusively on emergency department planning. In fact, following a major surge event, in-patient services such as critical care and the operating rooms/surgical services often face a much greater impact on services than the emergency department. The London transit bombings of 2005 provide an excellent insight into this issue [1, 2]. During this incident the Royal London Hospital received 195 casualties, 7 of whom were critically ill. Their 16-bed ICU operated at near 100 % capacity. In response to the incident they opened 8 new ICU beds using their post-anaesthetic care unit and a stepdown unit. The emergency department declared a major incident at 09:26 that day, at 12:40 they stood down and at 13:30 the emergency department was open for business as usual. Meanwhile, for those critically ill the length of stay ranged from 6 to 22 days (average 12.4 days) with many extra sessions in the operating theatres required for weeks to follow. Similar experiences are described following the Rhode

Island night club fire [3] and Madrid train bombings [4].

This chapter will provide a high-level overview of surge management including key actions that critical care leaders should undertake and initiatives they should advocate in their hospitals. We will begin by discussing concepts in surge management as well as useful response strategies, this will be followed by highlighting key concepts related to surge management including coordination, communication, triggers for altering standards of care, allocating scarce resources and financial implications of surge management. To illustrate how these principles can be combined and effectively implemented, a case study of the development and implementation of a comprehensive surge capacity management programme in Ontario, Canada, following SARS will be presented. After reading this chapter you as a critical care leader should have a firm grasp of the main concepts in surge management. However, to truly master these concepts one must translate the knowledge into action by applying the concepts within your institution. Further, training is also available through courses such as the Fundamentals of Disaster Management run by the Society of Critical Care Medicine (http://www.sccm.org/FCCS_and_Training_Courses/FDM/Pages/FDM_Resources.aspx).

Surge capacity & response strategies

Definitions and conceptual frameworks

Surge capacity is a broad term which is applicable to a continuum of daily fluctuations in demand for services through to extraordinary circumstances and from technical through to clinical settings in healthcare [5–9]. Given this great span for the concept of operations of surge capacity, it is not surprising that there is great variability in the definitions offered for surge capacity as well as a fairly heterogeneous collection of research and academic publications on this topic [10]. Although many tend to focus on moderate to major surge in the context of disasters or pandemics, it is essential that the concept of a continuum of surge is not lost as the systems and processes used to address moderate and major surge should build upon the same systems and processes used daily to address minor surge.

The size of the surge, in terms of magnitude of increase in demand, is only one factor that in-

fluences the impact of the surge event. The time course over which the surge occurs is the second important determinant of the impact. Large numbers of patients presenting over a short period of time present a greater challenge for managing than would the same number of patients over a longer period of time. Further, slower-onset surges with some degree of forewarning allow for efforts at preparation and mitigation as opposed to sudden-impact disasters. Finally, although much less common, it is important to remember that surge situations are not only the result of an increase in demand. Given that surge situations result from a disequilibrium of the supply/demand equation, significant decreases in the supply of resources can also cause a relative surge situation. Sudden loss of resources may result from events such as systems failures, failures of the supply chain, or outbreaks causing the closure of beds or wards, i.e. nosocomial infections or SARS [11].

The defining works most relevant to conceptualising surge management has been done by Joseph Barbera and his colleagues [12, 13]. They highlight the critical distinction between two important concepts, "surge capacity" and "surge capability".

- **Surge capacity:** The ability to respond to a markedly increased number of patients
- **Surge capability:** The ability to address unusual or very specialised medical needs

These definitions focus on the objectives or aims of the actions; however, they do not identify the specific process through which these are achieved. In its most simplified construct, mechanisms to mitigate surges address either the demand for healthcare services or the supply of healthcare services. Healthcare services are dependent upon the availability of necessary inputs of staff, stuff and space. In almost all cases, the true rate-limiting factor is either staff or stuff [14].

Approaches to decrease demand entail two components:

- Decreasing existing demands upon the system there by freeing capacity for surge response
- Diverting new demands for services away from the system, thus preventing the consumption of resources

When resources become scarce decisions about allocation including prioritisation and rationing are required which constitute the process of triage. Triage and resource allocation will be addressed separately in a subsequent section of this chapter.

In a minor surge event interventions involving demand typically involve achieving operational efficiencies. This process begins with understanding the various sources of demand through process mapping the journey of critically ill patients within your institution. Management of minor surge typically does not require or involve actions to alter the demand side of the equation. In moderate and major surges however, efforts to decrease demand, at least temporarily, are important components of an effective response strategy.

Barbera states, "the controlled (planned and monitored) degradation of services when maximum capacity is exceeded is engineered failure" [12]. This orderly de-escalation of services serves two purposes, the first is to protect the ability to provide essential services by preventing catastrophic failure of the system and secondly, to free up resources for the response. The most commonly cited example of this is to 'cancel elective surgery'. This is often a knee-jerk response that is easier to operationalise in a sudden isolated large surge event but much more complex in a prolonged surge situation such as a pandemic [6]. When considering what services to de-escalate, considerations should include the potential impact on patients, the potential of critical resources being made available by cancelling the service, which services may be provided at potential partner hospitals or hospitals remote from the event, and finally, the ability to provide the service at all when significantly altered standards of care are in practice. For example, cancelling all elective surgeries that are day surgeries, performed primarily with local or regional anaesthetics would do little to increase the availability of ventilators or critical care capability. However, stopping all but emergent cardiac surgeries would make available a large number of ventilators and critical care resources. Certain procedures, such as heart-lung transplants, may be emergent and life-saving, but if the situation is such that the alterations in the standards of care only allow for 1:4 post-op ICU nursing and

limited availability of a single vasopressor, this level of care could not support such resource-intensive procedures.

The key to diverting non-essential demands for service and relieving pressure on the healthcare institution is to identify earlier points of contact in the overall system and institute appropriate diversionary tactics at those points of contact. This requires healthcare institutions to think and engage partners beyond their own walls.

On the supply side, response efforts focus on increasing the amount of resources that are available or maximising the output that can be obtained from existing resources. Increasing the amount of resources available often involves increasing acquisitions or stockpiling. However, there are significant financial and logistical constraints which make stockpiling impractical as the sole solution for managing surges in demand, thus the discussion that follows will also address maximising the output from existing resources. Further, many resources, in particular staff, simply cannot be stockpiled or acquired rapidly [14]. Despite these limitations institutions and authorities must work, within the financial and logistical constraints they face, to stockpile critical resources in their requirement to exercise due diligence. Unfortunately, due diligence regarding emergency preparedness is often overlooked by hospital boards [15]. Several excellent papers provide recommendations regarding critical care supplies and equipment (stuff) that should be stockpiled to prepare for major surges [16–19].

To manage a surge, a critical care leader must know what resources he or she has available to them and how to access them at any time of day or night. Key to identifying what 'stuff' is available is understanding the supply-chain system for your institution. In efforts to achieve financial savings many hospitals have moved to 'just-in-time' supply chain management systems. By design such systems minimise any excess within the system. While these systems work well in routine, stable operations they present significant vulnerabilities and limitations in managing surges situations [6]. Stockpiles of critical resources are necessary to compensate for sudden variations in demand for services. The next step in establishing a plan to extend the capacity of staff, stuff or space is to develop and maintain accurate inventories documenting what resources are available. These inventories should be skills- or functional criteria-based, not 'role'-based. For example, the staff inventory should identify nurses anywhere in the hospital who possess key skills and experience required to care for critically ill patients, not simply those who are or have served in the role of a critical care nurse [18, 20]. Similarly, when considering space, develop an inventory of locations in the hospital which posses the key functional requirements for providing critical care: oxygen, suction, medical gas, electrical outlets, and space for equipment. Finally, when preparing inventories, particularly of equipment, it is important to identify not only equipment currently in use for patient care but also equipment that may be in storage or used for training that could be mobilised for patient care during a surge.

Response efforts to maximise the potential output from existing resources forms the core of what has come to be referred to as 'altered standards of care'. The works of Rubinson [21–25] and Hicks [26, 27] have significantly advanced the understanding of mechanisms through which the standard of care may be altered to maximise healthcare services during a surge. They advocate the considerations of various strategies to substitute, adapt, conserve, and re-use stuff, space and staff to extend their capacity. As discussed below, the degree of deviation from normal practices depends upon the magnitude of the surge and should be proportional to discrepancy between the demand and supply of resources. In a minor surge small modifications to usual practice would be required, whereas in a major surge event mass critical care would be required [21]. Mass critical care is both a different model and standard of critical care from what is practiced under normal circumstances. Simply stated, the goal of mass critical care is to provide a few key interventions (those with the highest impact and potential to save lives) to many people rather than providing very resource-intensive interventions to only a few. Efforts to substitute, adapt, conserve and re-use aim to decrease this supply/demand gap. It is only if this gap cannot be overcome with such strategies that triage should be undertaken.

A particular challenge faced when implementing response strategies that address either demand or supply issues is how to scale the responses and implement triggers for their deployment. Scaling on the supply and demand side occur in opposite directions but should be based upon common information sources and integrated triggers. The requirement for scaling the response is derived from the ethical principle of proportionality, which dictates that actions to mitigate resource shortfalls should be proportionate to the degree of the shortfall expected or experienced [28, 29]. Implicit in any discussion of scaling and triggers is the need for situational awareness and an effective communication network as detailed earlier. Two common approaches to scaling are found within the published literature. The first is that of Hicks who divides responses into "conventional", "contingent", and "crisis" [27]. This scaling approach is largely descriptive and does not provide specific data inputs or thresholds upon which the scales are based. A more widely used approach is to construct triggers based upon the 6-tier system (see Fig. 1) propagated by Barbera and colleagues [13]. Triggers based upon the tier system typically set thresholds based upon resources in geopolitical regions becoming overwhelmed. There are two primary limitations of this approach. The first is that in order to recognise that a threshold has been reached and subsequently to trigger a response, data collection, data analysis and communications capabilities must already be in place. This can be particularly challenging during the initial phases of an event. The second limitation is that this tends to set up a reactive rather then proactive response. Once established in a reactive mode it can be challenging to 'get ahead of the curve' in responding to the crisis.

Key actions & initiatives

1. All initiatives should recognise the nature of surge as a continuum from common minor daily events through to rare overwhelming events. Thus, critical care leaders should develop systems for moderate and major surges which build upon the process and systems used to address minor surge. Stand-alone systems should be avoided.

2. Critical care leaders should participate in regional healthcare coalitions or structures

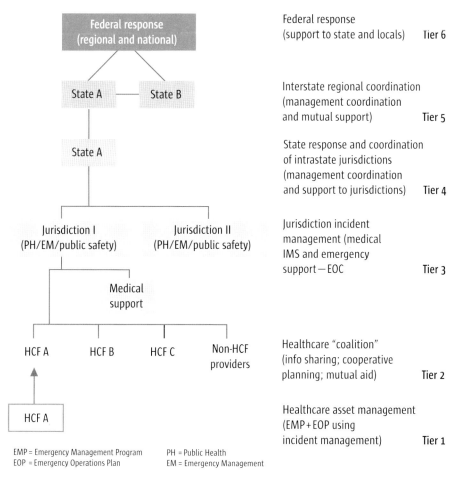

Federal response
(support to state and locals)   Tier 6

Interstate regional coordination
(management coordination
and mutual support)   Tier 5

State response and coordination
of intrastate jurisdictions
(management coordination
and support to jurisdictions)   Tier 4

Jurisdiction incident
management (medical
IMS and emergency
support – EOC   Tier 3

Healthcare "coalition"
(info sharing; cooperative
planning; mutual aid)   Tier 2

Healthcare asset management
(EMP + EOP using
incident management)   Tier 1

EMP = Emergency Management Program   PH = Public Health
EOP = Emergency Operations Plan   EM = Emergency Management

Fig. 1   This six-tier construct depicts the various levels of health and medical asset management during response to mass casualty or complex incidents. The tiers range from the individual HCF and its integration into a local healthcare coalition, to the coordination of Federal assistance. Each tier must be effectively managed internally in order to coordinate and integrate externally with other tiers. [From Medical Surge Capacity and Capability Handbook, 2nd edition, published September 2007. Copyright © 2007 The CNA Corporation, www.cna.org. Prepared for the U.S. Department of Health and Human Services by the CNA Corporation under Contract Number 233-03-0028. Authors: J. A. Barbera, A. G. Macintyre. Editors: A. Knebel, E. Trabert]

which have a central committee, imbued with adequate situational awareness to coordinate moderate and major surge responses.

3. Should decisions regarding the de-escalation of services be required, the decision about which services can/will be provided and which cannot/will not be provided should be based upon a consideration of:

   ▪ The consequence to patients of suspending or delaying the service,

   ▪ the resource requirements of that service and

   ▪ which services may be provided at potential partner hospitals or hospitals remote from the event, and

   ▪ the ability to provide the resources in the context of altered standards of care. These activities should be supported at a national level by professional societies developing classifications for prioritising patients.

When possible these should be based upon existing schemes.

4. Critical care leaders should work cooperatively within their healthcare coalitions to ensure that within a geographic region or between regions, capacity to provide non-deferrable essential services is maintained.

5. Critical care leaders should ensure their healthcare institution has prepared plans which detail options for substituting, adapting, conserving and where appropriate re-using critical supplies which may face shortfalls during a surge. This activity should be supported by scientific guidance from organisations such as the CDC and FDA. Hospitals should specifically consider planning for substituting, adapting, conserving and re-using the following:

- Ventilators and components (i.e. circuits, endotracheal tubes)
- Antibiotics
- Sedatives and analgesics
- Vasopressors/inotropes
- Oxygen
- Vascular access devices (i.e. central lines, PICC lines and peripheral i.v.s)

6. Critical care leaders should prepare plans within their institution to alter the standard of care to extend staff and space resources, drawing upon the advice from the Task Force on Mass Critical Care which recommends:

- Critical care should occur in hospitals or similarly designed and equipped structures (e.g. mobile medical facility designed for critical care delivery, veterinary hospital, or outpatient surgical procedure center). After ICUs, post-anaesthesia care units and emergency departments reach capacity, hospital locations for EMCC should be prioritised in the following order: (1) intermediate care units, step-down units, and large procedure suites; (2) telemetry units; (3) hospital wards.
- Non-medical facilities should be repurposed for critical care only if disasters damage regional hospital infrastructure by making hospitals unusable, and if immediate evacuation to alternate hospitals is not available. Principles for staffing models should include the following: (1) Patient care assignments for caregivers

should be managed by the most experienced clinician available; (2) assignments should be based on staff abilities and experience; (3) delegation of duties that usually lie within the scope of some workers' practice to different healthcare workers may be necessary and appropriate under surge conditions; (4) systematic efforts to reduce care variability, procedure complications, and errors must be used when possible. Plans to implement these recommendations should be established for all categories of healthcare workers including physicians, nurses and other allied healthcare workers.

Communication and coordination during a pandemic, and development of healthcare coalitions

Situational awareness based on accurate, timely and complete information is essential for responding to any surge events [30]. Hospitals and their local healthcare partners must share information with each other effectively, and then use it to coordinate resources in providing the best and safest possible patient care across their region. Communication and coordination (command and control) are therefore the foundations for situational awareness, and effective implementation of altered standards of care during a pandemic.

Clear lines of command are critical to mounting an effective response. However, traditional organisational structures used in healthcare are very horizontal and lack the hierarchy required for effectively managing moderate or major surge events. The incident management system (IMS) is rapidly being adopted by healthcare systems [31] and is ideal for structuring a response to surge events. IMS is a scalable, objective-driven tool, based upon a consistent structure and common terminology, for organising an institution's response to an event. Most commonly it has been used by a wide variety of organisations, public- and private-sector, for managing crisis events. However, it can be used for managing any event, not just emergencies. When used properly, IMS facilitates effective communication and coordination between other organisations and agencies also responding to the surge using IMS.

In some areas healthcare institutions are organised within a formal structure (usually governmental), such as a regional health authority, which allows for an organised response to a surge event. However, in large parts of North America and Europe hospitals are autonomous institutions without any formal linkages. In such areas healthcare coalitions can be used to structure responses to moderate or major surge events. Healthcare coalitions may be defined as a formal collaboration among hospitals and health systems, public health departments, emergency management and response organisations, and other organisations that provide support during a surge event [32]. Coalitions serve to facilitate planning and interaction between individual hospitals, local coalitions, or jurisdictional response agencies [32]. Mature healthcare coalitions have developed to a level of sophistication that is capable of providing effective and coordinated surge responses to their communities, and have been recommended as being the foundation of a national disaster health system [33].

The key deliverables required of healthcare coalitions during a moderate or major surge all revolve around situational awareness (see Box 1). Perhaps the most important functions in the event of a moderate or major surge range from developing effective two-way communication processes between coalition partners to providing accurate, up-to-date information on the number and severity of cases and the resource supply and demand ("staff, space, and stuff"). This information is crucial in determining if and when altered standards of care need to be implemented.

Box 1: Key deliverables needed from healthcare coalitions

Effective 2-way communication protocols and processes between coalition partners and member organisations, and with other coalitions through regional authority
- Communication processes may be as simple as conference call capability, web-based tools, telephones, or even ham radios as a back-up system

Effective information exchange between coalition partners
- Accurate and updated information on the number and severity of cases that are being seen
- Accurate and updated information on internal resources already utilised and remaining capacity still available
- Tracking patients and beds, assets and resources, staff and volunteers, and other resources

Develop the means to establish a database of key information, and analysis capability

Utilising available information to develop situational awareness in knowing when to implement altered standards of care, and awareness for how far to go, including implementation of scarce resource and allocation protocols

Support for each other
- 'Share' local academic experts or specialists available to all partners
- Peer support during very stressful periods in a crisis
- Working together in coordinating public relations

Once a healthcare coalition is formed, Boxes 2 and 3 describe the organisational and functional characteristics for success [32]. Organisational success is determined by the commitment of member organisations to the coalition, defined through written agreements, strong leadership and governance. Inclusion of local health departments in the planning is important, and the significance of this will be discussed further below in relation to triggers. Functional success is ultimately determined by the level of trust and teamwork that is built within the coalition. The ability of organisations in the coalition to work together as a team will be foundational in the planning process and subsequently operationalising the plan's response to a real surge event. Further, coalitions are far stronger if they have a well-respected local leader or organisation to coordinate and direct the coalition. Successful coalitions likely demonstrate iterations of these characteristics of success over months to years.

Box 2: Organizational characteristics that contribute to coalition success
Cooperation between coalition partners, which is strengthened through formal compacts or mutual aid agreements, and the establishment of defined governance
- This provides the basis for information exchange, cooperation with resource sharing, and coordination/redistribution of patient movement

A high level of coalition leadership and involvement, and members' commitment to the organisation
- Often built on pre-existing relationships and structures, or by having a 'dominant' health system organise the group

Having the public health department involved in the coalition, with other members contributing as a resource for policy- and decision-making, and to provide support
- Facilitates the state/local government's ability to exercise legal authority to support local healthcare organisations if a pandemic occurs

Geographically flexible, and inclusive of most, if not all, local organisations

Box 3: Functional characteristics that contribute to coalition success
Plan together, and then train together

Develop communication plans together
- Develop common communication protocols and tools
- Jointly determine back-up communication strategies: ham radios, etc.
- Work on public relations together
- Others

Develop hazard vulnerability analyses together

Provide each other with real-time data and information, to optimise situational awareness

Key actions & initiatives

1. Critical care leaders should support, promote, and facilitate healthcare coalition development in their communities, if a formal regional health authority structure does not exist.
2. Promote formation and definition of healthcare coalition official organisational agreements, governance, and leadership, if they do not already exist. These may need to be informal initially but efforts should be made over the longer term to formalise these relationships through memorandum of understanding or mutual aid agreements.
3. Promote and facilitate healthcare coalition (continued) development of defined communication standards and protocols, utilising tools that include internet-based programmes, conference calls, phone contact, and any other available means.
4. Develop a database of common elements, including accurate and up-to-date information on the number and severity of cases, utilisation and capacity ('staff, space, and stuff'), and other information crucial for situational awareness. The variables collected should be consistent from the regional level up to the national level and will contribute to the development of a common information picture.
5. Continue to promote and facilitate healthcare coalition familiarity and trust. Activities that may further this mission include:
   - Coalition partners meeting in person and sharing direct and reliable contact information. Experience has demonstrated that informal contacts are remarkably effective for developing communication links in the midst of a crisis.
   - Organise committees and/or working groups composed of representatives from member organisations, with particular focus on hazard vulnerability analysis (HAV) for surge events.
   - Having local experts available for consultation, by defined communication vehicle(s), to other healthcare professionals in the coalition, and having regularly scheduled conference calls to update all involved. These were both recommended strategies learned from experience during the SARS epidemic [11, 34, 35].

Consider developing support groups, or other support mechanisms, for healthcare professionals within the coalition when responding to a moderate or major surge event. Again, previous experience with the SARS epidemic demonstrated that a crisis creates circumstances that lead to damaged healthcare provider morale [11, 34, 35].

6. At the individual hospital level, continue to promote hospital based preparedness but also encourage the integration of effective communication and planning with coalition partners.

The challenges and potential problems in developing successful coalitions are noted in Box 4. Of these, financing the cost of coalition involvement may be the most significant, and is discussed separately in a later section.

> **Box 4: Challenges to coalition success**
> **Organisational sensitivities**
> - Insufficient trust between member organisations, which must be developed through relationship-building over time
> - Sharing proprietary information
> - Insufficient funding and/or staff shortages
>
> May need public health department/legal authority to support and expect equal and fair participation
>
> Financing of the surge response – The financial cost of a disaster may be great to both healthcare organisations and providers
> - Without a means to help underwrite disaster services, the potential cost serves as a disincentive for involvement

Triggers and supports for altered standards of care during a moderate or major surge

Triggers to initiate altered standards of care (ASCs) should be based on the volume of patients that are actually being hospitalised, or at risk for being admitted, (the demand) compared to available resources (the supply). Though this data is focused at the individual hospital level, a broader perspective of this information, at a minimum

at the regional coalition level, is essential in order to determine when to implement ASCs. As discussed above, regional healthcare coalitions are a good vehicle for obtaining supply and demand data and then transmitting decisions back to individual hospitals.

The formal authority to make a decision to implement altered standards of care is held by regional, state, or federal government agencies. The reasons for this are their likelihood of having sufficient information available through coalition involvement to make best decisions, and because they possess the legal authority to implement them. This authority is crucial for mobilising resources, and in providing support for healthcare professionals who will be providing care in an altered environment.

The data assessed regarding triggers for implementing altered standards of care comes from four states that have formally developed ASC protocols or studied them (Colorado, Minnesota, Utah and New York), the Veteran Administration, from the work done in Ontario, Canada, and documents published in CHEST [14, 21, 23, 24, 28, 36–38]. The common theme from these documents emphasises the urgency in implementing altered standards of care when either

1. the demand for hospital services exceeds any given hospital's capacity, and/or
2. the rate of increasing cases is so rapid that there is risk that a regional coalition's capacity may be overwhelmed.

The most specific identified triggers are either an increasing number of hospitals declaring "internal disasters" (elective procedures delayed, staff recalled, etc.) or an increasing number of hospitals "going on ER divert" [21, 24]. All four state protocols would be activated in a major surge, a pandemic in these examples, with an emergency declaration by the governor, often in conjunction with the state Department of Health. The triggers for terminating ASCs are equally nonspecific, and highlighted that the need for altered standards of care would end when capacity came back into balance with the needs.

Another important consideration is the legal protection for workers that should coincide with the altered standards of care. Without such provisions, healthcare provider liability concerns regarding legal or professional reprisals for practicing altered standards of care and/or triage would serve as a further disincentive for coming to work in a potential surge event, particularly bio-event disasters.

The timing of when to implement ASCs is a balance between the risk of early activation prior to a clear need, versus late activation and potentially not being fully prepared if the surge event escalates. Given the potential lag time required for surge capacity response, the earliest appropriate trigger should be used [33].

Key actions & initiatives

1. In order to facilitate the greatest beneficial impact of altered standards of care ASCs should be initiated at the earliest point where there is evidence of the healthcare system potentially becoming overwhelmed, and likely (hopefully) before any hospital is yet overwhelmed. Each local community may be affected differently, and initiation of altered standards of care may be implemented by region, as/when/if needed.
2. A 'hard' ASC regional activation trigger during a surge event would be when one hospital either declares an 'internal disaster' (as described above) or otherwise determines that it has insufficient resources to provide routine care without moving to an altered standards of care status. When even one hospital is overwhelmed with cases to this point, all regional coalition hospitals are presumed to be at imminent risk.
   - Hospitals should be authorised to implement altered standards of care internally for a limited time of no more than 24 hours, unless further authorisation is received from a jurisdictional government.
3. When either of the above conditions is met, government leadership at the federal, state, and local levels should declare a public health emergency, in order to facilitate and support the healthcare systems' efforts to provide the most amount of care to the greatest number of patients.
4. Healthcare providers should be protected from professional or legal consequences when providing care in good faith during a declared state of public health emergency.

5. The trigger for terminating altered standards of care should be when all hospitals in a regional coalition are able to provide normal, safe care to patients with usual resources. This return to normal services can also be implemented in a step-wise fashion. Similar to initiation of altered standards of care, a specific termination trigger is difficult to define, and no specific best practices can be cited.

Allocation of scarce resources

Overview

If shortages of vital resources occur during a disaster despite efforts to substitute, adapt, conserve and reuse, then reallocation strategies must be employed. Triage should be used to direct the allocation of those resources in order to optimise efficiency, maintain ethical tenets, and help the greatest number of people possible [1, 11]. Triaging of scarce resources entails two elements:
- Prioritising patients for treatment
- Rationing of resources.

Such decisions must be made within a sound ethical framework. A variety of ethical perspectives may inform the triage process, but a utilitarian perspective is most commonly applied.

In order to maintain ethical distribution, it is important that both horizontal and vertical equity are achieved. This means, similar patients are treated equally and unlike patients are treated differently. Achieving such ethical standards requires appropriate structures and systems to be in place.

Types of triage protocols can be categorised based upon the where they are intended to be applied. Primary triage protocols are used in the pre-hospital phase, secondary triage protocols in the ER and tertiary triage protocols are used within hospitals to allocate patients to definitive care areas. The primary and secondary triage protocols which have been used over the past centuries were developed in response to mass casualty incidents caused by warfare, natural disasters and man-made disasters, for example, bombings or plane crashes [12, 13]. These types of events rarely produce large volumes of patients requiring critical care [14]. Further, since World War

II on only a few occasions in Western societies has triage been conducted in civilian healthcare systems where there was the need to make decisions which required that life-supportive therapies would be denied to some patients. In most cases, given the isolated nature of the event, additional resources can be deployed to the affected area or patients transferred to unaffected areas.

Specific types of events, such as pandemics (e.g. H1N1) and CBRN incidents, do, however, have the potential to create surges in demand for critical care resources impacting broad geographic regions. The remainder of the discussion will focus on triage considerations is these types of events.

Comparisons & contrasts of proposed triage protocols

Although much of the attention with regard to allocation of scarce resources during a major surge event has focused on decisions around critical care (tertiary triage), primary and secondary triage will also play a vital role in the response to a major sure. As discussed in the earlier section on surge, there is a need to divert non-essential demands for service prior to presentation to the hospital, and if resources in the pre-hospital and emergency department become scarce, decisions as to how to allocate these resources will also be required. Primary, secondary and tertiary triage are intrinsically connected and must build upon each other for effective resource management to occur. Given the focus of this text on critical care, we will briefly compare the existing tertiary triage protocols.

The first draft of a comprehensive tertiary triage protocol was published in 2006 by a working group of the Ontario pandemic planning committee [15]. The Ontario protocol is composed of detailed inclusion criteria, exclusion criteria, minimum qualifications for survival (MQS) and a prioritisation tool using the SOFA score. The exclusion criteria and MQS are aimed at identifying patients with a low (< 50%) 1- or 2-year survival rate even if they were to receive critical care, particularly in the face of altered standards of care. This protocol has formed the basis for the majority of pandemic protocols that have been developed internationally and nation-

ally including in New York, Colorado, Utah, and Alaska, to name only a few.

The Ontario protocol also provided the foundation for the triage protocol developed by the Task Force on Mass Critical Care which elaborated upon the Ontario protocol by providing details regarding the infrastructure required to support a triage system and suggested triggers for initiating triage [16].

A group in Minnesota led by Hicks has also provided guidance regarding the allocation of ventilators during a pandemic [17]. This group also suggested using the SOFA score; however, they recommend that every time a new patient is being considered for critical care, that patient should be triaged against all patients currently in the ICU. This presents both logistical challenges in addition to applying information from the SOFA in a fashion that is significantly different than the manner in which the SOFA score was validated. The Ontario protocol attempts to match the application of the SOFA score with the manner in which it was derived. The most significant contribution of the Minnesota approach is the use of a tiered application of exclusion criteria as resources become increasingly scarce. This tiered approach provides a concrete method through which the restrictions can be balanced to match the degree of the resource shortfall. This is consistent with the philosophy recommended in the Ontario protocol and several of the more recent triage protocols developed by states have incorporated this approach into their adaptations of the Ontario protocol.

Despite these recent advances in developing draft protocols, the ability to conduct triage, especially tertiary triage, in a major surge faces a number of significant and potentially insurmountable obstacles. Firstly, while many of the tertiary triage protocols were developed by extrapolating from research evidence where it existed, overall, like most primary triage [12] protocols, tertiary triage protocols are not strictly evidence-based and are only in the earliest stages of testing. Early results of a small pilot study (currently under review for publication in Critical Care) shows promising results of the Ontario triage protocol's ability to identify patients that are most likely to benefit from ICU care and to mobilise resources. However, the study also reveals that further modifications of the protocol are required to improve its sensitivity and specificity. The second major obstacle is the lack of infrastructure necessary to support an ethical and effective triage process in civilian healthcare systems [18]. This includes the need to have systems or processes to train triage officers, achieve situational awareness, modify protocols as needed, communicate changes and monitor triage outcomes [16]. Thirdly, a legal process to create this infrastructure and provide appropriate legal (civil and criminal) protection for triage officers is required. No jurisdictions have fully addressed these legal issues yet.

Regardless of whether a formal triage process is in place, if resource shortfalls occur, allocation decisions will be made. However, without a standardised process these decisions are unlikely to result in an ethical or efficient use of resources. The inequities that result from these decisions have the risk of undermining public confidence in the healthcare system and could lead to collapse of the healthcare system during the time it is most required [18].

Key actions & initiatives

1. Should triage be necessary, critical care leaders should ensure that coordination of the triage process occurs at the state level. Healthcare coalitions cannot posses a sufficiently broad level of situational awareness to make independent decisions regarding the initiation or coordination of triage.
2. Critical care leaders should work with their state (or national) governments to develop plans for triage utilising the protocol developed through the Task Force on Mass Critical Care's collaborative process, and their existing state legislation, to implement the protocol. These plans should include mechanisms to address triage infrastructure and triage officer liability issues. The infrastructure should include a process to systematically review the decisions of the triage officers by a review committee to ensure that inequities are not occurring and assess patient outcomes to modify the triage protocol if required.
3. The allocation committee established by healthcare coalitions to oversee resource allocation should liaise with the state level central

triage committee to provide information on resource supply and demand status to the state triage committee and communicate triage directives from the state to coalition members.
4. Critical care should be rationed only after all efforts at augmentation have been exceeded or a tier level 6 (see Fig. 1) has been attained or exceeded.
5. Critical care leaders should ensure their healthcare institution develops a surge management plan that includes a senior intensivist acting as a triage officer and a team to support the triage officer. Prior to resource shortfalls occurring, the role of this senior intensivist should be to coordinate resource utilisation (ICU admissions & discharges) across the expanded critical care units within an institution established as part of the EMCC response. This individual should remain free of direct clinical responsibilities so that he/she can maintain a level of objectivity and be available to liaise when required with the hospital's emergency management group in the emergency operations center.

Financing healthcare costs during surge events

Healthcare financing of a disaster has profound implications for all of the recommendations herein contained. The cost of disaster care during a major surge, particularly a prolonged event such as a pandemic, would likely be huge for hospitals, healthcare organisations, and healthcare professionals, and is often the 'elephant in the room' when discussing disasters. The costs include providing care for a much larger population, many likely to be uninsured, and expending far greater resources in the process. It also includes the cost of likely foregoing many of the services that are revenue-generating, such as elective surgeries [39]. In addition, usual documentation of services during an emergency might necessarily be drastically decreased, in order to focus on the delivery of care. Although healthcare organisations and providers are driven by their passion and love of caring for their patients, it is unfair to ask them to shoulder the entire financial responsibility, too. Furthermore, failing to address this most important issue essentially penalises those who are ethically most compelled to act and participate, and an incentive for others who might look for opportunities to participate less, or not at all. This issue is well addressed by the Agency for Healthcare Research and Quality [1].

Key actions & initiatives

Critical care leaders should work with their appropriate level of government to develop plans to compensate hospitals, healthcare organisations and healthcare providers during the time that a formally declared healthcare emergency is in effect. A possible approach may be as follows:

- A daily rate that is equal to the average daily income of physicians for the previous 365 days immediately before the emergency declaration is calculated.
- This daily rate will begin the day of the emergency declaration, and will continue through the day the declaration is discontinued. If hospitals, healthcare organisations or healthcare providers continue to bill and collect for services rendered, these services would be subject to all usual and standard documentation and regulatory requirements.

Conclusion

This chapter has emphasised the key considerations in surge management: stuff, staff and space. In order to manage a surge, one must manage episodes of disequilibrium in the supply-demand balance. Key components to any response are command and control, communication and utilising a scalable approach to manage minor through to major surges. The final section of this chapter presents a case study to illustrate how these concepts have been applied in one jurisdiction.

Case study:
Surge capacity management in Ontario

Background

To date, planning for a sudden influx of patients requiring urgent or emergent care has largely focused on pandemic planning or preparing for large-scale disasters. The impact of widespread infectious disease processes such as severe acute respiratory syndrome (SARS) and H1N1 had highlighted the potential weakness in the overall healthcare system caused by lack of coordination of critical care services within hospitals and across regions. The inability of individual hospitals and the healthcare system to respond appropriately to surge events, or sudden demands for services, compromises access to care in a patient population for whom timely access can affect outcomes. Moreover, the breach in what should be a seamless continuum of care between the community, emergency department, critical care units and hospital wards becomes glaringly apparent.

The *Final Report of the Ontario Critical Care Steering Committee* [40] recognised a need to develop a system to accommodate these surges in critical care. This committee was formed and the report created in response to lessons learned from the local outbreak of SARS. The report outlines a number of key recommendations for making improvements in the overall system. During SARS, it became apparent that there were challenges in handling the acute rise of critically ill patients, some of whom required specialised care and isolation, and the impact this subsequently had on other patient services [34, 35]. It was clear that there existed a lack of a principled approach, not only between critical care units, but even within hospitals, to surge capacity planning. This held true despite the fact that most hospitals have in place protocols for disaster or pandemic planning. SARS also highlighted a lack of standardisation in processes, language and communication when dealing with this type of increase in patient volumes. It was realised that there had to be a better way to deal with the increased demand for critical care services and develop plans that would help minimise the impact on other patient services.

Core to addressing the issue of surge capacity planning is having an understanding and agreement on the definition of surge. In the *Final Report of the Ontario Critical Care Steering Committee* the definitions for surge capacity management are categorised into minor surge, moderate surge and major surge. A minor surge is defined as an acute increase in demand for services within an individual hospital up to 15% beyond normal operating capacity. The event could be managed within the resources of the individual hospital for a short period of time. If the event precipitating the surge lasts longer than 48 hours, or the ability to safely care for patients is compromised, a moderate surge response would be declared. In a moderate surge the increase in demand for critical care services impacts beyond an index hospital response and requires a regional response from a group of hospitals. A major surge is an unusually high increase in demand. The resources at a regional level are overwhelmed and a provincial level response is required.

Key surge capacity management elements in the Ontario plan

The following elements make up the key platform in surge capacity planning and their consistent application is required for success across all levels of responding to a surge event (see Fig. 2).

- **Management**: This identifies the person or delegates in a management level position who have accountability for oversight of the surge event. They are able to coordinate activity and ensure that the pre-established processes are put into effect for a system level response to be carried out.
- **Human resources**: It is important to catalogue not only how many staff members are available to work, but also to maintain a list of their skill sets. During a surge event this becomes

useful to inform staffing models, ensure efficient and maximum use of the entire skills available.

- **Alternative physical space**: To be able to flex above normal operating capacity it is key to identify what physical space is available and appropriate to house patients.
- **Equipment and technology**: Once physical space is identified it is then imperative to know what equipment is available to safely monitor and care for the patient.
- **Surge processes**: When all the planning, inventory taking, flow mapping and decision-making algorithms are in place, it is important that the correct processes are created to ensure that the plan can actually be operationalised when needed.

Key surge response principles in the Ontario plan

Regardless of the magnitude of the surge event, there are key principles that should be intricately woven into the planning that is done in preparation for responding to the needs of a surge event as outlined above. Without incorporating these principles the success of properly responding to the needs of patients, and supporting the needs of those who will be on the front line, will be in jeopardy.

- **Central authority**: Regardless of the level of event precipitating a surge response, be it within a single hospital, or requiring coordinated efforts across multiple hospitals and jurisdictions, it is important to be able to identify someone who is in charge. This person should be able to make decisions that may be necessary regarding changes to staffing models and deploying other resources. It is also important that someone with executive level authority be aware that a surge is occurring and could impact on other services in the hospital.
- **Readiness to act for all categories of surge**: Hospitals are responsible for ensuring that the plans for responding to surges in patient volumes focus on the key elements described above are in place. This involves more than having the plans on paper and sitting on a shelf. It is important that all staff is aware, educated, and supported to play the role expected during a surge response.

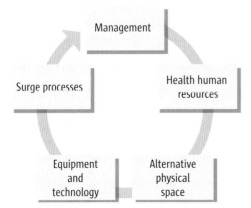

Fig. 2   Key elements of the Ontario Surge Management Plan [from Critical Care Secretariat, Ontario Ministry of Health and Long-Term Care]

- **Response built on partnerships**: Maximising the use of existing staff and resources requires that strong partnerships are established across departments and care areas in the hospital. Successful sharing of space, equipment, or staff requires these partnerships to be in place and awareness by the people who may potentially be impacted. In the event that what initially may be a minor surge event escalates or is sustained to require a moderate surge response, strong partnerships and accountability will be necessary between local partner hospitals and relevant stakeholders such as Local Health Integration Networks, patient transport emergency medical services, municipalities and their agencies and the Ministry of Health and Long-Term Care.

- **Tiered escalation response**: Regardless of whether the surge event is minor, moderate, or major, the response to each event is predicated on the same key elements and principles. Hospitals are expected to use the standardised approach outlined in their planning for identifying physical space, additional equipment, staffing models and surge processes. In this way, the response framework remains the same; hospitals do not need to develop, implement and rehearse separate plans for the different categories of surge.

- **Operational capabilities will be scalable, flexible and adaptable**: As surge events may vary in size and complexity, hospitals are accountable for being able to ensure the ability to carry out appropriate response for minor surges through to a major surge. This will include the need to make decisions *a priori* on the potential impact on other services otherwise routinely carried out by the hospital (outpatient services, elective surgical procedures) that may need to be scaled down in order to focus resources and priorities on responding to the surge.

A large-scale implementation for surge capacity management

Surge capacity planning is one of the 7 core key initiatives being implemented under the Ontario Critical Care Strategy (OCCS). This work is supported by the Ministry of Health and Long-Term Care through a dedicated Critical Care Secretar-

iat. The key goals of the strategy are to improve patients' access to care, to improve the quality of care being provided and to promote system-wide integration so that individual critical care units and hospitals are breaking away from an operational 'silo' way of functioning.

In 2006, as part of the Performance Improvement Initiative of the OCCS, hospitals could apply to receive a coaching team for assistance in developing performance improvement plans for issues identified by the hospital as areas needing improvement. The coaching teams were comprised of clinical and administrative peers who received training in the use of coaching techniques to guide the development of action plans for performance improvement. In the first iteration of this programme, several hospitals identified surge capacity planning as an area in which their organisations could benefit if they could develop better plans to deal with the regular spikes in demand for critical care services. The increasing number of hospitals requesting a coaching team for surge capacity planning was a clear indication that this type of planning should be undertaken more broadly across the province.

A pilot programme for surge capacity planning involving 18 hospitals was developed and implemented. Based on the 5 key elements for surge capacity planning and incorporating the 5 key principles outlined above, the 18 acute care hospitals, each with critical care units of varying capacity and capability, used a standardised framework and algorithms to develop plans for responding to minor surge events. Each hospital undertook daily data collection and patient flow mapping exercises to better understand the 'business' of critical care in their own organisations. This exercise promoted an understanding of concepts such as knowing from where patients were admitted to the ICU, barriers to timely discharge of ICU patients, trends in when the ICU was operating at or near full occupancy, what the staffing complements were during these trends, and identifying processes that would improve handling the unexpected surges that may occur on a day-to-day basis. This level of detail in the planning fostered improved partnerships between critical care units and other care areas of the hospital such as the wards, the emergency department, the OR office, and post-anaesthetic care units. As part of the planning, the hospitals participated together in regular teleconferences and webinars to report on milestones in executing their action plans as well as to share successes or make inquiries about how to troubleshoot regarding specific issues. This concept of a group of hospitals planning together fostered a better mutual understanding about the realistic capacity and capabilities of each of the critical care units in the geographic area. It is the essence of this understanding which promoted and fostered stronger communication and partnerships between the hospitals; all of which would be key to forming strong critical care networks and laying the foundation of preparing the critical care units and hospitals to respond together to larger levels of surge.

Based on the successful implementation of the initial Surge Capacity Management Pilot programme, approval was given to expand the project on a province-wide basis. Over a time period of one year and with ongoing oversight and support by the Critical Care Secretariat, 124 hospitals representing close to 200 critical care units implemented a standardised plan for responding to minor surge events in their hospitals. With this level of planning completed, the hospitals are now prepared to move forward, building on key partnerships and using a common response framework, to undertake planning for moderate surges. A key philosophy in all of the planning is that when it comes to larger-scale disasters or pandemics, the hospitals will be able to deploy the same activities that they use for responding to minor surges; something that happens on a far more regular basis than a large-scale disaster.

Critical success factors and challenges faced in the role of the Ontario surge plan

Challenges

One of the key challenges in having hospitals participate was the firmly held belief that they had already done this level of planning for surge events. "We already have a Code Orange plan or a disaster plan. Do we really need to carry out this detailed level of planning?" For some hospitals, some of the planning they had already undertaken was aligned with the elements and principles described above. However, it required clear consistent messaging to promote the understanding that this level of surge planning was targeted toward preparing for the more common day-to-day surges in demand for resources and that the framework and tools used would also be the basis for responding to larger-scale events. Another key challenge identified by the hospitals was being able to commit time and resources to carry out the action plan items, especially in the face of other key priorities or implementation of other government-sponsored programmes. Many of the people on the individual hospital surge team are front-line healthcare providers, managers or senior administrators who took on the activities of implementing surge plans in addition to their usual job activities. The greatest factor in helping to overcome these challenges was the eventual realisation that it was necessary to do this level of planning – to build the confidence that any of the hospitals would be able to successfully handle a minor surge event. The onset of the second wave of H1N1 during the implementation phase of the programme provided a very real scenario that stressed the importance of having a standardised response framework to be used by the hospitals.

Success factors

A number of factors are related to the success of one of the largest implementations of a standardised framework for surge capacity planning. The first of these would be the development, coordination and support of the programme at a centralised level, in this case the Critical Care Secretariat. This ensured consistency of communication and standards for implementation. Another success factor, related to the first, is that this programme was not implemented in isolation, but rather intimately linked with other initiatives of the OCCS anchored on the goal of improving access, quality of care and system integration. As part of the OCCS, each of the 14 Local Health Integration Networks (LHIN) across the province has a dedicated critical care physician in the role of Critical Care LHIN Lead. These physicians worked closely with the hospitals to support the implementation of the programme and foster the development of local critical care networks.

The authors

Michael D. Christian, MD, MSc, FRCPC[1]
Bernard Lawless, MD, MHSc, CHE, FRCSC[2]
Julie Trpkovski, RN[3]
Jeffrey R. Dichter, MD, SFHM, FACP[4]
[1]Major | 1 Canadian Field Hospital (Canadian
Forces) | Attending Physician, Infectious
Diseases & Critical Care | Mount Sinai
Hospital & University Health Network | University of
Toronto | Department of Medicine | Toronto, Canada
[2]Provincial Lead | Critical Care and Trauma
Secretariat | Ministry of Health and Long Term Care
Trauma Surgery, General Surgery, Critical Care |
St. Michael's Hospital | Toronto, Ontario, Canada
[3]Director | Critical Care Secretariat | Ministry of
Health and Long Term Care | St. Michael's Hospital |
Toronto, Ontario, Canada
[4]Medical Director | Cardiovascular Intensive Care |
Regions Hospital | Saint Paul, Minnesota, USA

Address for correspondence
Michael D. Christian
Department of Medicine
University of Toronto
600 University Ave
Rm 18-232-1
Toronto, ON M5G 1X5, Canada
E-mail: michael.christian@utoronto.ca

References

1. Aylwin CJ, Konig TC, Brennan NW, Shirley PJ, Davies G, Walsh MS, Brohi K. Reduction in critical mortality in urban mass casualty incidents: analysis of triage, surge, and resource use after the London bombings on July 7, 2005. Lancet 2007;368:2219–2225.
2. Shirley PJ. Critical care delivery: the experience of a civilian terrorist attack. J R Army Med Corps 2006;152:17–21.
3. Mahoney EJ, Harrington DT, Biffl WL, Metzger J, Oka T, Cioffi WG. Lessons learned from a nightclub fire: institutional disaster preparedness. J Trauma 2005;58:487–491.
4. Gutierrez de Ceballos JP, Fuentes FT, Diaz DP, Sanchez MS, Llorente CM, Guerrero Sanz JE. Casualties treated at the closest hospital in the Madrid, March 11, terrorist bombings. Crit Care Med 2005;33:S107-S112.
5. Asplin BR, Flottemesch TJ, Gordon BD. Developing models for patient flow and daily surge capacity research. Acad Emerg Med 2006;13:1109–1113.
6. Barbisch DF, Koenig KL. Understanding surge capacity: essential elements. Acad Emerg Med 2006;13:1098–1102.
7. Jenkins JL, O'Connor RE, Cone DC. Differentiating large-scale surge versus daily surge. Acad Emerg Med 2006;13:1169–1172.
8. Kaji A, Koenig KL, Bey T. Surge capacity for healthcare systems: a conceptual framework. Acad Emerg Med 2006;13:1157–1159.
9. Stratton SJ, Tyler RD. Characteristics of medical surge capacity demand for sudden-impact disasters. Acad Emerg Med 2006;13:1193–1197.
10. Phillips S. Current status of surge research. Acad Emerg Med 2006;13:1103–1108.
11. Booth CM, Stewart TE. Severe acute respiratory syndrome and critical care medicine: the Toronto experience. Crit Care Med 2005;33:S53-S60.
12. Barbera JA, Macintyre AG. Medical and Health Incident Management (MaHIM) System: A Comprehensive Functional System Description for Mass Casualty Medical and Health Incident Management. Washington, D.C.: Institute for Crisis, Disaster, and Risk Management, The George Washington University, 2002.
13. The CNA Corporation. Medical Surge Capacity and Capability: A management system for integrating medical and health resources during large-scale emergencies. Department of Health and Human Services, 2004.
14. Christian MD, Devereaux AV, Dichter JR, Geiling JA, Rubinson L. Definitive care for the critically ill during a disaster: current capabilities and limitations: from a Task Force for Mass Critical Care summit meeting, January 26–27, 2007, Chicago, IL. Chest 2008;133:8S-17S.
15. Seeman N, Baker GR, Brown AD. Emergency Planning in Ontario's Acute Care Hospitals: A Survey of Board Chairs. Healthc Policy 2008;3:64–74.
16. Hota S, Fried E, Burry L, Stewart TE, Christian MD. Preparing your intensive care unit for the second wave of H1N1 and future surges. Crit Care Med 2010;38:e110-e119.
17. Rubinson L, Branson RD, Pesik N, Talmor D. Positive-pressure ventilation equipment for mass casualty respiratory failure. Biosecur Bioterror 2006;4:183–194.
18. Rubinson L, Hick JL, Curtis JR, Branson RD, Burns S, Christian MD, Devereaux AV, Dichter JR, Talmor D, Erstad B, Medina J, Geiling JA. Definitive care for the critically ill during a disaster: medical resources for surge capacity: from a Task Force for Mass Critical Care summit meeting, January 26–27, 2007, Chicago, IL. Chest 2008;133:32S-50S.
19. Sprung CL, Kesecioglu J. Chapter 5. Essential equipment, pharmaceuticals and supplies. Recommendations and standard operating procedures for intensive care unit and hospital preparations for an influenza epidemic or mass disaster. Intensive Care Med 2010;36 Suppl 1:S38–S44.

20. Sandrock C. Chapter 4. Manpower. Recommendations and standard operating procedures for intensive care unit and hospital preparations for an influenza epidemic or mass disaster. Intensive Care Med 2010;36 Suppl 1:S32-S37.

21. Devereaux A, Christian MD, Dichter JR, Geiling JA, Rubinson L. Summary of suggestions from the Task Force for Mass Critical Care summit, January 26–27, 2007. Chest 2008;133:1S-7S.

22. Rubinson L, Nuzzo JB, Talmor DS, O'Toole T, Kramer BR, Inglesby TV. Augmentation of hospital critical care capacity after bioterrorist attacks or epidemics: recommendations of the Working Group on Emergency Mass Critical Care. Crit Care Med 2005;33:2393-2403.

23. Rubinson L, Hick JL, Curtis JR, Branson RD, Burns S, Christian MD, Devereaux AV, Dichter JR, Talmor D, Erstad B, Medina J, Geiling JA. Definitive care for the critically ill during a disaster: medical resources for surge capacity: from a Task Force for Mass Critical Care summit meeting, January 26–27, 2007, Chicago, IL. Chest 2008;133:32S-50S.

24. Rubinson L, Hick JL, Hanfling DG, Devereaux AV, Dichter JR, Christian MD, Talmor D, Medina J, Curtis JR, Geiling JA. Definitive care for the critically ill during a disaster: a framework for optimizing critical care surge capacity: from a Task Force for Mass Critical Care summit meeting, January 26–27, 2007, Chicago, IL. Chest 2008;133:18S-31S.

25. Rubinson L, O'Toole T. Critical care during epidemics. Critical Care 2005;9:311-313.

26. Hick JL, Hanfling D, Burstein JL, DeAtley C, Barbisch D, Bogdan GM, Cantrill S. Health care facility and community strategies for patient care surge capacity. Ann Emerg Med 2004;44:253-261.

27. Hick JL, Barbera JA, Kelen GD. Refining surge capacity: conventional, contingency, and crisis capacity. Disaster Med Public Health Prep 2009;3:S59-S67.

28. Devereaux AV, Dichter JR, Christian MD, Dubler NN, Sandrock CE, Hick JL, Powell T, Geiling JA, Amundson DE, Baudendistel TE, Braner DA, Klein MA, Berkowitz KA, Curtis JR, Rubinson L. Definitive care for the critically ill during a disaster: a framework for allocation of scarce resources in mass critical care: from a Task Force for Mass Critical Care summit meeting, January 26–27, 2007, Chicago, IL. Chest 2008;133:51S-66S.

29. University of Toronto Joint Centre for Bioethics Pandemic Influenza Working Group. Stand On Guard For Thee: Ethical considerations in preparedness planning for pandemic influenza. 2005.

30. Burkle FM, Jr., Hsu EB, Loehr M, Christian MD, Markenson D, Rubinson L, Archer FL. Definition and functions of health unified command and emergency operations centers for large-scale bioevent disasters within the existing ICS. Disaster Med Public Health Prep 2007;1:135-141.

31. Christian MD, Kollek D, Schwartz B. Emergency preparedness: What every healthcare worker needs to know. Canadian Journal of Emergency Medicine 2005;7:330-337.

32. Courtney B, Toner E, Waldhorn R, Franco C, Rambhia K, Norwood A, Inglesby TV, O'Toole T. Healthcare coalitions: the new foundation for national healthcare preparedness and response for catastrophic health emergencies. Biosecur Bioterror 2009;7:153-163.

33. Courtney B, Toner E, Waldhorn R. Preparing the Healthcare System for Catastrophic Emergencies. Biodefense Strategy, Practice, and Science 2009;7:33-34.

34. Booth CM, Stewart TE. Communication in the Toronto critical care community: important lessons learned during SARS. Crit Care 2003;7:405-406.

35. Hawryluck L, Lapinsky S, Stewart T. Clinical review: SARS – lessons in disaster management. Critical Care 2005;9:384-389.

36. Christian MD, Hawryluck L, Wax RS, Cook T, Lazar NM, Herridge MS, Muller MP, Gowans DR, Fortier W, Burkle FM. Development of a triage protocol for critical care during an influenza pandemic. CMAJ 2006;175:1377-1381.

37. Minnesota Department of Health OoEP. Minnesota Healthcare System Preparedness Program: Pandemic recommended cctions for healthcare facilities. 2008.

38. Powell T, Christ KC, Birkhead GS. Allocation of ventilators in a public health disaster. Disaster Med Public Health Prep 2008;2:20-26.

39. Achonu C, Laporte A, Gardam MA. The financial impact of controlling a respiratory virus outbreak in a teaching hospital: lessons learned from SARS. Can J Public Health 2005;96:52-54.

40. Ministry of Health and Long-Term Care. Final Report of the Onatrio Critical Care Steering Commitee. 2005.

Stephen Streat

Evaluating and improving the effectiveness of our practices

Introduction

Before we can evaluate and improve the effectiveness of our practices in intensive care medicine, we must know what the objectives of our practices are and must have reliable ways to measure the extent to which we meet those objectives.

As we confront the daunting health implications of the demographic and economic challenges of the early 21st century we should learn from our history when seeking to define what should be the objectives of intensive care services. We must elucidate and define the roles that we should fulfil in both the care of patients and the overall functioning of the modern hospital. In doing so, we would do well to consider the comments made by the late English moral theologian Gordon Dunstan [1] – "The success of intensive care is not, therefore, to be measured only by the statistics of survival, as though each death were a medical failure. It is to be measured by the quality of lives preserved or restored; and by the quality of the dying of those in whose interest it is to die; and by the quality of human relationships involved in each death" [2].

Performance is more than effectiveness

Although this chapter focuses on *effectiveness*, we should also seek to evaluate and improve other do-

mains of our performance including the *efficiency* of our practices, and their *cost-effectiveness*, both within the scope of intensive care medicine and in comparison to other health interventions. Performance may be constrained by external factors which may not be obvious to us or over which we may exercise little or no control (e.g. reimbursement practices, financial and other incentives, institutional policies, professional codes of practice and legal decisions). If we are to improve *performance* in general, we must have effective ways of measuring what we seek to improve and of changing clinical practice in ways that do in fact achieve that goal. Unfortunately, after nearly 60 years of modern intensive care medicine, we lack much of the clinical, economic and behavioural information that we need and are only now beginning to systematically address these fundamental questions [3].

Effectiveness

Historically intensive care medicine and nursing was simplistically viewed as a specialised healthcare activity, taking place in a separate area of the hospital with its own important structural and organisational features [4, 5]. Intensive care had as its (sole) objective the 'rescue from imminent death' of a patient with an acute life-threatening illness and accordingly, we focussed almost exclusively on ICU survival as our measure of effectiveness [5]. We treated patients in a dynamic and individualised way, substantially guided by changes in physiology [4] and used a variety of often complex and expensive medical and surgical therapies to do this. At the time, the survival benefit of simple intensive therapies (e.g. intubation, ventilation and circulatory support) was often immediately obvious in an individual patient [6, 7] and there was very little randomised trial evidence to guide any treatment decisions.

Intensive care evolved rapidly in complexity, particularly during the late 1970s, when more patients with high-lethality multiple organ failure [8] began to recover after the addition of enteral and parenteral nutrition, cimetidine and haemodialysis [9] to prolonged cardio-respiratory support. Treatment practices, including various modes of physiological support and the use of investigations, pharmaceuticals and monitoring modalities, became established by tradition and via extrapolation from first principles, again without randomised trial evidence of benefit. Most of the very few randomised controlled trials that were conducted were small and had surrogate outcomes, often only short-term changes in physiological values. A few years after the burgeoning of technology in the ICU in the late 1970s, methods were developed to describe and quantify the severity of chronic comorbidity, acute illness and treatment intensity [10–14]. These measures were used to classify, at least roughly and phenomenologically, specific intensive care syndromes and to predict the risk of death, at least of cohorts of patients, in the ICU. They allowed for comparisons to be made between large cohorts of patients treated in various ways and in differing healthcare settings [15, 16]. This 'case mix- and severity-adjusted outcome' methodology is still in widespread use, although the considerable limitations of this approach are recognised, particularly in terms of defining the 'quality of performance' of an ICU [17–19]. Although comparing outcomes of patients treated in different intensive care settings is possible, while attempting to control for confounding factors, such as lead-time bias or illness severity, such comparisons are necessarily imprecise – even large cohorts of patients (>1000 in each group) may fail to demonstrate significant differences in apparent effectiveness.

Evidence of effectiveness

However, the tools for risk adjustment have proven useful in randomised trials in intensive care medicine, which began to increase rapidly in number only in the late 1980s. In recent years, evidence about the comparative effectiveness (or lack of effectiveness) of various clinical practices has begun to emerge. A few trials have shown increased mortality from 'innovative' treatments (e.g. L-NMMA [20], growth hormone [21] or intensive insulin therapy [22]) and such treatments should be avoided, at least outside of further randomised controlled trials with appropriate safeguards designed to avoid such harm. Most trials have reported similar mortality outcomes between 'innovative' and 'standard' treatments (many of which themselves had become established practice in the absence of high-level evidence of their effectiveness compared to 'no treatment'). In some of these trials, secondary outcomes or other features (e.g. morbidity [23], cost [24, 25] or treatment simplicity [26]) may lead clinicians to prefer one treatment over the other. Very few trials have shown convincing or durable evidence of reduced mortality, e.g. induced hypothermia for hypoxic-ischaemic encephalopathy after cardiac arrest [27, 28]. Perhaps uniquely for interventions with apparently strong evidence of mortality benefit [29] antibiotic prophylaxis (as part of selective decontamination) remains poorly taken up and is subject to considerable ongoing research. There are a number of ongoing studies in areas of continued dubiety, e.g. drotrecogin alfa recombinant in sepsis [30, 31] and goal-directed therapy in sepsis [32, 33]. There is more evidence of benefit for strategies or therapies that reduce *morbidity* rather than *mortality* – e.g. use of a checklist of five strategies to reduce central line-associated bloodstream infections [34], noradrenaline rather than dopamine to reduce dysrhythmia in shock [23], or early enteral feeding to reduce infectious complications [35].

Guidelines and bundles

Although some clinicians were quick to adopt some treatments that were apparently beneficial in single RCTs, others retained equipoise and participated in subsequent studies which showed no difference [24] or even harm [22]. Notably, some apparently beneficial strategies were rapidly and perhaps prematurely incorporated into 'care bundles' – weakening professional support for some of these endeavours [36, 37].

These experiences highlight the risks of making premature practice changes and assuming that patient outcomes will necessarily improve. Nevertheless, consensus statements and even 'care bundles' containing some recommendations based on early data were developed with the implication that compliance with these should inevitably and consequently improve patient outcomes, in line with an overall strategy of 'improving quality by implementing proven measures' [38].

An association between 'guideline compliance' and 'improved patient outcome' has indeed been shown in some settings. Most notably perhaps, central line-associated blood stream infection (CLABSI) can be seen as the prototype of a specific complication which is amenable to implementation of a 'checklist' approach [39, 40] and in which compliance with that process has been shown to be associated with lower CLABSI rates [34]. Eighteen months after that publication, despite widespread acceptance of the feasibility and desirability of reducing CLABSI rates, only 22 % of US states reported CLABSI rates and only 12 % had an active prevention programme [41]. Encouragingly, however, reduced CLABSI rates in ICUs in Michigan which undertook the prevention strategy have remained low for 3 years afterward, suggesting that effective implementation of strategic approaches can lead to durable 'culture change' within the ICU [42].

Despite the apparent robustness of the CLABSI experience, an association between 'bundle compliance' and outcome does not necessarily provide evidence of efficacy of specific components of a 'care bundle'. In sepsis, for example, improvement may be due to earlier attention to likely time-critical aspects of treatment (e.g. time to effective antibiotic administration). More generally, ICU mortality overall, and for a number of common clinical syndromes encountered in the ICU (e.g. sepsis, trauma, subarachnoid haemorrhage) has been falling over time, even in the absence of apparently novel treatments [43, 44]. The relative contributions of different factors to this underlying trend are poorly understood or quantified. Auditing of compliance with 'bundles' or processes of care as a measure of effectiveness

should not therefore be assumed to have equivalent value as evaluating and monitoring patient outcomes directly [45].

Intensive care unit organisation

It does seem very likely that different organisational and administrative aspects of intensive care service delivery contribute both to differences in outcomes amongst various regions of the world and different intensive care units, and perhaps to changes in underlying mortality with time within intensive care units. Aspects that are amenable to systematic change include in particular the intensity of intensivist staffing and a culture of safety. Although high-intensity physician staffing [46–48] and the presence of a strong safety culture [49, 50] are associated with improved clinical outcomes, it is not possible to define precisely what organisational changes, alone or in combination, will reliably improve patient outcomes and to what extent.

There are many other aspects of clinical practice which impact on ICU performance, particularly on the efficiency and cost-effectiveness of the ICU, but also to some extent on its effectiveness. These include admission and discharge policies and practices, patient assessment practices, ward round and handover practices, infection control practices, interdisciplinary teamwork and communication, documentation and record-keeping, data management and processes for audit, quality improvement and research.

It is clear that the cost-effectiveness of the ICU is greatest when the patient is most likely to benefit – i.e. where the likelihood of death is neither very low, nor almost certain, but within a range where intensive treatments can be reasonably expected to change an unfavourable outcome into a favourable one. An ICU which admits a large number of patients who could do equally well in a lower-intensity treatment setting is contributing to overall healthcare costs, without commensurate additional benefit. Similarly, admission of large numbers of patients with high-lethality conditions may be justifiable if only those with favourable responses to therapy continue to receive those therapies, and those with unfavourable responses have them limited and withdrawn. These difficult scenarios continue to vex all intensivists worldwide, despite widely different access to intensive care services in different countries. Although thresholds for decisions about beginning, limiting and withdrawing intensive treatments will vary according to the locally available resources, there is surely a duty on all intensivists to exercise moral leadership and engagement in these matters.

The initial consideration by the intensivist of the appropriateness of ICU admission and the application of intensive therapies is often undertaken on the basis of a telephone conversation with another, usually junior, physician who has assessed the patient, sometimes in a remote hospital. Within this conversation there are opportunities for misunderstanding and error, with important clinical consequences. A systematic approach to this situation has the potential to reduce these risks and a number of checklist initiatives have been developed over the last five years, prototypically the SBAR (situation, background, assessment, recommendation) model [51]. An adaptation of SBAR (isobar – identify, situation, observations, background, agreed plan, read back) was developed in 2007 as a standardised clinical handover process and checklist in rural Western Australia [52], has been accepted and is widely used by clinical staff in both pre-

hospital and in-hospital settings, including shift handovers. We developed a similar 'shared mental model' for ICU medical staff, modelled after our earlier ward round and handover process (see Tab. 2), and supported this with a pocket-sized laminated card in 2003 (see Tab. 1).

Similar systematic handover processes, including one developed in consultation with experts in motor racing and aviation [53], have indeed been shown to reduce handover errors in intensive care settings [54]. Multidisciplinary collaboration in healthcare is associated with higher performance [55–57], and collaboration may be jeopardised as a side-effect of the physical configuration of electronic patient records during ward rounds and handovers [58].

We developed a formal structured ward round and handover process in 1986 which systematically reviews all aspects of clinical care, including family issues, which is explicitly taught to new medical staff and summarised in Table 2. Although similar mnemonics which encourage review of *some* aspects of clinical care have been promulgated by advocates of 'bundles' (e.g. FASTHUG [59] – feeding, analgesia, sedation, thromboembolic prophylaxis, elevation of the head of the bed, ulcer prophylaxis, and glucose control), we believe that a systematic review of

Tab. 1   Template for communicating information about patients

1. **Circumstances**: Comment on the circumstances of your encounter with the patient you are describing, e.g. "I am in the ED with a trauma team call to a young man who climbed into the tiger's cage at the zoo …"

2. **Premorbid state**: Describe the patient giving as much information as is available and relevant about the patient's prior health and functional level, i.e. what he/she was like before this acute illness. This includes age and sex, relevant past history, social history, family history, all comorbidities, and what he/she can do, i.e. functional level; use the term "fit and well" only if there are no comorbidities at all, e.g. "This is a 78-year-old retired psychiatrist with a long complicated past history including …"

3. **Acute illness**: Describe the sequence of events from the start of the present illness until now; include relevant blood, x-ray and other investigations and therapies; mention what other people or teams are involved so far in the patient's care.

4. **Your assessment**: Describe the current status of the vital signs and organ systems, including ABC, conscious level and neurologic deficit, renal function, liver function etc. Be as objective as possible and give specific values, e.g. "urine output is over 200 ml in last 2 hours and serum creatinine is 90 µmol/l".

5. **Therapy:** Describe the current or recent treatment, e.g. O_2, ventilation, fluid therapy, inotropes, antibiotics, etc.

6. **Plan:** Describe the intended plan of action by other staff and yourself. Don't be afraid to advance your own opinion on what the problem is and what should be done, especially "Does this patient require intensive therapies and ICU admission and is that appropriate?"

Tab. 2   Morning ward round

The morning ward round is a disciplined activity which follows a set format. Side conversations should be avoided. All issues relevant to a patient should be discussed before the ward round leaves each bed space. The format is:

a) **Case presentation** by the handover registrar or intensivist;

either **Succinct case summary** (for a new admission or a previous admission to new staff) using the Admission Note as a crib sheet: Prior health status, Sequence of events, Assessment of vital systems, Diagnosis, Injury List (for trauma patients), Treatment already undertaken, Treatment and Investigations being planned, Who the family are, who has spoken with them and what they have been told;

or **Brief progress report** (for other patients): Changes and Events of the last 24 hours, Problems and Plans for the next 24 hours

b) **Information from the patient's nurse**

c) **Systematic review** of all aspects of patient care. The systematic review is led by the intensivist of the day. The responsibility for charting and recording all decisions on the 24-hour chart lies with the Long Day registrar. The review follows a sequence designed to cover all aspects of care of the critically ill patient:

   a) **Airway**: type, patency, tracheobronchial secretions, cough

   b) **Breathing**: type, blood gases, ventilator settings, turns, physiotherapy, x-ray changes

   c) **Circulation and Fluids**: fluid input and output from all sites, haemodynamic status, biochemistry, nutrition, cardiovascular medications, renal function

   d) **Infection and Antibiotics**: signs of infection, bacteriology results, antibiotics and levels, specimens required

   e) **Neurologic**: signs of consciousness (eye opening, motor responses, vocal responses), lateralising signs, sedative and relaxant medications, ICP, EVD, CT scan, SEPs, EEG

   f) **Miscellaneous**: lab results, special procedures, dressings, medications, etc.

   g) **Instrumentation**: tubes, lines, catheters, etc.

   h) **Documentation**: review of charting; the previous day's duty intensivist will update the Document Form.

   i) **Communication**: make sure that the Special Nurse and the Long Day registrar have no unanswered questions

   j) **Family issues** as above

all aspects of clinical care, for all patients, preserves appropriate scepticism about some of the evidence base for the mnemonic (e.g. sedation [60], elevation of the head of the bed [61] and glucose control [22]) and has greater potential to reduce harm from issues being overlooked which were not included in acronyms.

Many ICUs contribute patient data to large clinical databases maintained by research groups often affiliated to professional societies (e.g. the [UK] ICS, ANZICS, and SCCM). Such databases now contain very large amounts of patient data and can show significant outcome changes over time. They have also been used by clinical trials groups to help to define areas of fruitful research activity. However, the usefulness of the pooled data to the self-understanding of the performance of an individual ICU is less obvious. Be-

cause changes in patient and ICU characteristics within an individual ICU are likely to be gradual – with similar case mix, treatments and administrative structures from year to year, it is possible to monitor various aspects of performance over time by collecting a simple dataset containing standardised elements of patient, treatment, resource-use and outcome data.

We began such an endeavour in 1984 and now have data on more than 28,000 patients, including linked data on bereaved family outcomes. Comprehensive financial systems enable us to monitor expenditure not only on pharmaceuticals and disposables but also staff costs, capital equipment, depreciation, laboratory and other investigations, blood products and use of other hospital services. Using financial data along with data from the clinical database enables us to monitor crude trends in cost-effectiveness at least. Within a few years, this database provided evidence of continued reductions in ICU mortality for various clinical conditions, reductions in length of ICU stay and marked changes in the use of various treatments and investigations [62, 63].

Effectiveness in interpersonal processes

Effectiveness is often defined in business as how well the output of a process meets the requirements of the end user or customer. From the perspective of the intensive care unit, there are a number of 'end-users' of intensive care services – including, of course, the patient, but also including the patient's family, other health professionals involved in the care of the patient during the period of illness and even the healthcare facility itself.

In thinking about effectiveness, we traditionally focussed most closely on the need of the patients. We considered how well treatment maximises their opportunity not only to survive, but to recover well, while minimising the burden of treatment (including morbidity and other costs). However, in so doing we often overlooked the importance of providing the patient with an appropriate balance between curative and comfort objectives, of ensuring that suffering (including iatrogenic suffering) is anticipated and ameliorated, and of allowing the patient to achieve their own goals, within the limits of their capability. Nowhere more is this deficiency seen than in patients with unpredictable and treacherous disease conditions (e.g. pancreatitis, multiple organ failure, subarachnoid haemorrhage) where too much attention can be paid to a curative objective, and too little to achieving comfort and spiritual and emotional needs, until death is both inevitable and proximate [64].

Patient-centredness as an attribute of healthcare delivery has a strong tradition in some other areas of clinical practice, notably in palliative care and general practice. The concept of patient-centredness is linked to another concept in the care of critically ill patients – that is 'family-focussed' care. These two concepts recognise that the care of critically ill patients should focus on the needs (and preferences) of the patient, while recognising and also attending to the needs of the patient's family. This does not imply that intensive care practitioners should simply provide any and all specific treatments simply because the patient or the family desire them. However, it should cause all practitioners to pay attention to establishing the needs and preferences of the patient and the degree to which intensive therapies could meet those needs and preferences. It should not be assumed that all patients would chose similar health outcomes as being desirable to them, nor that they would be prepared to endure a similar extent of 'iatrogenic suffering' in order to achieve those outcomes.

It is, unfortunately, not common to have the opportunity to discuss these matters with critically ill patients, in a situation remote from the immediate, life-threatening crisis. The exceptional circumstance is where patients are contemplating non-emergency surgery with significant risk to life or functional recovery. In these situations it is possible to discuss risks (and benefits) of various courses of action, including non-operative treatment, and perhaps more importantly, to define with the patient what should (and should not) be done if serious complications develop. It is salutary to note that, at least in a realistic simulation scenario, doctors are often reluctant to discuss non-operative options or the risks of unfavourable outcomes (other than early death), and are reluctant to offer advice – even when requested by the patient to do so [65], a finding recently replicated in a US setting [66].

In a study with a related theme, elderly patients expressed a strong preference not to undergo intensive treatment in circumstances that might rescue them from an acute crisis occurring on the background of a progressive loss of functional independence [67]. Notably, however, the great majority of the (adult) children of these elderly persons, despite agreeing that such a preference was 'the right thing' for their parent, would demand that intensive treatment be given. Family members may commonly reflect their own wishes for incompetent critically ill patients and it should not be assumed that they accurately reflect the preferences of the patients themselves [68, 69]. Whilst the concept of a single 'designated surrogate decision-maker' may provide a legally robust decision-making framework for patients lacking decision-making capacity, it does not provide confidence that such decision-making would closely accord with patient preferences and has less resonance outside of the US.

In legal systems which do not recognise the equivalence of the decisions made by a substituted decision-maker on behalf of another person to informed consent by that person, a more nuanced and explicitly consensual approach to decision-making is usual [70, 71], which accords closely with recent (US) consensus recommendations for end-of-life care in the ICU [72]. These recommendations acknowledge the importance of the social (including family) structure surrounding the patient and highlight the importance of good communication between health professionals and families to improving both patient care and family outcomes.

Defining and evaluating measures of effectiveness for intensive care practices that appropriately address these interpersonal issues has proved even more difficult than monitoring definable medical complications such as CLABSI, or ICU readmission rates. Seven domains of end-of-life care which were identified by literature review and a consensus process have been suggested as areas where quality could be measured [73]. These domains are patient- and family-centred decision-making, communication, continuity of care, emotional and practical support, symptom management and comfort care, spiritual support and emotional and organisational support for intensive care unit clinicians. A large number of quality indicators within these seven domains were also proposed. More recently, ten selected indicators were pilot-tested in several ICUs, found to be feasible and to reveal opportunities for practice improvement [74]. For example, the provision of a family information leaflet, a quality indicator within the communication domain, which has itself been shown to improve some measures of family members' comprehension and satisfaction [75] occurred in only 43% of occasions.

Measurements of patient and family satisfaction can provide some useful information, particularly when collected systematically and used as part of a quality improvement cycle. As an example, we have provided a follow-up service for bereaved family members for 15 years [76] and use systematically collected information from that service to alter clinical practice (in particular about the frequency, timeliness and conduct of family meetings). Interviews with patients and their families about what they consider the most important aspects of 'palliative' care echo previously well-described themes of "communication by clinicians about the patient's condition, treatment, and prognosis; patient-focused medical decision-making; clinical care of the patient to maintain comfort, dignity, personhood, and privacy; and care of the family" [77]. Reports of disappointing performance in these areas continue [78], despite the existence of a large number of potentially helpful simple strategies [75, 79–82] including ethics consultations, palliative care consultations, routine family meetings, provision of information leaflets, the use of non-medical language by doctors and providing more time and opportunity for family members to speak (and for staff to listen) in family meetings.

Effectiveness outside the walls of the ICU

The practice of intensive care medicine is not confined to the care of patients within the intensive care unit. Intensivists have been involved in the design and implementation of processes which help to identify at an early stage patients who might benefit from intensive therapies and ensure that such treatments are given. Some of these involvements have been in pre-hospital emergency care as well as in-hospital systems within the emergency department and other hospital wards and departments. Many such systems have evolved, including most recently the Medical Emergency Team (MET) system, in which intensivists play vital roles alongside other health professionals. The effectiveness of such 'early warning systems' and 'emergency treatment systems' in reducing mortality has proved difficult to demonstrate [83–85] reflecting in part the difficulties inherent in a cluster randomised trial design of a complex intervention [86]. Nevertheless, there is a strong suggestion of a 'dose-effect' relationship between the frequency of activation of 'emergency calls' within a MET system and improvement in some patient outcomes [87, 88] and this in part has led to considerable uptake of such systems.

A further significant effect of such systems is to allow for a more considered appraisal of the appropriateness of intensive therapies in patients with catastrophic illness, before the tyranny of immediate threat to life or even cardiac arrest lead inexorably to provision of such treatments 'without due consideration' [89]. This feature alone may justify the establishment of a MET on the grounds of improvement in the quality of care for dying patients and is likely to be cost-effective over ICU admission.

Similarly, post-ICU follow-up systems, usually nurse-based but sometimes multidisciplinary, have also evolved which facilitate the earlier transfer of patients from an ICU to a ward setting by providing support and expertise to ward staff to look after such patients effectively. Some post-ICU follow-up systems have also included long-term follow-up of hospital survivors, and follow-up of the bereaved family members. These systems have often highlighted the fact that health related-quality of life is often considerably reduced in ICU survivors and that functional impairment can persist long-term. Follow-up of bereaved family members [76] has identified areas in which better intensive care practice [90] might reduce at least dissatisfaction, if not psychological morbidity [91] in members of the deceased's family.

The effectiveness and cost-effectiveness of such varied follow-up systems is still unclear. A recent randomised evaluation of long-term nurse-based follow-up of hospital survivors of intensive care admission failed to show effectiveness, and consequently was not cost-effective [92]. However, the outcomes assessed (health-related quality of life, psychological well-being, costs and 1-year mortality) although fundamentally important, did not include the issue of in-hospital post-ICU secondary deterioration and subsequent ICU readmission, which itself is a risk factor for in-hospital mortality [93]. Risk factors for ICU readmission are being defined – and include prolonged ICU stay (7 days or more), non-elective initial ICU admission, acute renal failure and ICU admission from general wards, the emergency department or other hospitals rather than immediately postoperatively [94]. Whether post-ICU follow-up or even shared ward care between intensivists and others for patients recognised as high risk for ICU readmission can prevent readmission (and also reduce mortality) is not yet clear [84, 95].

Conclusion

Intensive care medicine is entering a mature phase of development characterised by relative stability of ICU technology, treatment processes, and clinical outcomes, an increasing evidence base and a focus on achieving, maintaining and improving high levels of quality and safety in patient care. The suggestion that increasing the implementation of proven measures should improve both quality and safety [38] has intuitive appeal and has been widely taken up. Human factors involved in such endeavours are beginning to receive appropriate attention and simple, yet time- and resource-intensive, strategies which recognise these factors and work with them are being recommended [96, 97], including the creation of the appropriate team, identification, prioritising and scoping the area of problem, creation of systems for data collection and reporting, introducing appropriate strategies for behaviour change, measuring the effects of the intervention and further refining the intervention in an iterative process. The success of such endeavours will crucially depend on both clinical and institutional leadership and support.

The author

Stephen Streat, BSc, MB, ChB, FRACP
Intensivist | Department of Critical Care Medicine | Auckland City Hospital | Auckland, New Zealand
Clinical Director | Organ Donation New Zealand
Honorary Clinical Associate Professor | Department of Surgery | University of Auckland, New Zealand

Address for correspondence
Stephen Streat
Department of Critical Care Medicine
Auckland City Hospital
2 Park Road
Grafton
Auckland 1023, New Zealand
E-mail: stephens@adhb.govt.nz

References

1. Shotter E. Obituary: Professor the Reverend Canon G R Dunstan. J Med Ethics 2004;30:233–234

2. Dunstan GR. Hard questions in intensive care. Anaesthesia 1985; 40:479–482

3. Weinert CR, Mann HJ. The science of implementation: changing the practice of critical care. Curr Opin Crit Care 2008; 14:460–465

4. Spence M. The emergency treatment of acute respiratory failure. Anesthesiology. 1962 Jul–Aug; 23: 524–537

5. Spence M. An organization for intensive care. Med J Aust. 1967 Apr 22;1(16): 795–801

6. Trubuhovich RV. August 26th 1952 at Copenhagen: 'Bjørn Ibsen's Day'; a significant event for Anaesthesia. Acta Anaesthesiol Scand. 2004 Mar;48(3):272–7

7. Trubuhovich RV. From respiratory support to critical care: my early days in intensive care medicine. Crit Care Resusc. 2007 June;9(2):123–126

8. Eiseman B, Beart R, Norton L. Multiple organ failure. Surg Gynecol Obstet. 1977 Mar;144(3):323–6

9. Routh GS, Briggs JD, Mone JG, Ledingham IM. Survival from acute renal failure with and without multiple organ dysfunction. Postgrad Med J. 1980 Apr;56(654):244–7

10. Knaus WA, Zimmerman JE, Wagner DP, Draper EA, Lawrence DE. APACHE-acute physiology and chronic health evaluation: a physiologically based classification system. Crit Care Med. 1981 Aug;9(8):591–7

11. Teres D, Brown RB, Lemeshow S. Predicting mortality of intensive care unit patients. The importance of coma. Crit Care Med. 1982 Feb;10(2):86–95

12. Wagner DP, Knaus WA, Draper EA. Statistical validation of a severity of illness measure. Am J Public Health. 1983 Aug;73(8):878–84

13. Le Gall JR, Loirat P, Alperovitch A, Glaser P, Granthil C, Mathieu D, Mercier P, Thomas R, Villers D. A simplified acute physiology score for ICU patients. Crit Care Med. 1984 Nov;12(11):975–7

14. Keene AR, Cullen DJ. Therapeutic Intervention Scoring System: update 1983. Crit Care Med. 1983 Jan;11(1):1–3

15. Knaus WA, Draper EA, Wagner DP, Zimmerman JE. An evaluation of outcome from intensive care in major medical centers. Ann Intern Med. 1986 Mar;104(3):410–8

16. Zimmerman JE, Knaus WA, Judson JA, Havill JH, Trubuhovich RV, Draper EA, Wagner DP. Patient selection for intensive care: a comparison of New Zealand and United States hospitals. Crit Care Med. 1988 Apr;16(4):318–26

17. Berenholtz SM, Dorman T, Ngo K, Pronovost PJ. Qualitative review of intensive care unit quality indicators. J Crit Care. 2002 Mar;17(1):1–12

18. Khanduja K, Scales DC, Adhikari NK. Pay for performance in the intensive care unit–opportunity or threat? Crit Care Med. 2009 Mar;37(3):852–8

19. Kahn JM, Scales DC, Au DH, Carson SS, Curtis JR, Dudley RA, Iwashyna TJ, Krishnan JA, Maurer JR, Mularski R, Popovich J Jr, Rubenfeld GD, Heffner JE; American Thoracic Society Pay-for-Performance Working Group. An official American Thoracic Society policy statement: pay-for-performance in pulmonary, critical care, and sleep medicine. Am J Respir Crit Care Med. 2010 Apr 1;181(7):752–761

20. López A, Lorente JA, Steingrub J, Bakker J, McLuckie A, Willatts S, Brockway M, Anzueto A, Holzapfel L, Breen D, Silverman MS, Takala J, Donaldson J, Arneson C, Grove G, Grossman S, Grover R. Multiple-center, randomized, placebo-controlled, double-blind study of the nitric oxide synthase inhibitor 546C88: effect on survival in patients with septic shock. Crit Care Med. 2004 Jan;32(1):21–30

21. Takala J, Ruokonen E, Webster NR, Nielsen MS, Zandstra DF, Vundelinckx G, Hinds CJ. Increased mortality associated with growth hormone treatment in critically ill adults. N Engl J Med. 1999 Sep 9;341(11):785–92

22. NICE-SUGAR Study Investigators, Finfer S, Chittock DR, Su SY, Blair D, Foster D, Dhingra V, Bellomo R, Cook D, Dodek P, Henderson WR, Hébert PC, Heritier S, Heyland DK, McArthur C, McDonald E, Mitchell I, Myburgh JA, Norton R, Potter J, Robinson BG, Ronco JJ. Intensive versus conventional glucose control in critically ill patients. N Engl J Med. 2009 Mar 26;360(13):1283–97

23. De Backer D, Biston P, Devriendt J, Madl C, Chochrad D, Aldecoa C, Brasseur A, Defrance P, Gottignies P, Vincent JL; SOAP II Investigators. Comparison of dopamine and norepinephrine in the treatment of shock. N Engl J Med. 2010 Mar 4;362(9):779–89

24. RENAL Replacement Therapy Study Investigators, Bellomo R, Cass A, Cole L, Finfer S, Gallagher M, Lo S, McArthur C, McGuinness S, Myburgh J, Norton R, Scheinkestel C, Su S. Intensity of continuous renal-replacement therapy in critically ill patients. N Engl J Med. 2009 Oct 22;361(17):1627–38

25. Finfer S, Bellomo R, Boyce N, French J, Myburgh J, Norton R; SAFE Study Investigators. A comparison of albumin and saline for fluid resuscitation in the intensive care unit. N Engl J Med. 2004 May 27;350(22):2247–56

26. Australian and New Zealand Intensive Care Society (ANZICS) Clinical Trials Group. Bellomo R, Chapman M, Finfer S, Hickling K, Myburgh J. Low-dose dopamine in patients with early renal dysfunction: a placebo-controlled randomised trial. Lancet. 2000 Dec 23–30;356(9248):2139–43

27. Bernard SA, Gray TW, Buist MD, Jones BM, Silvester W, Gutteridge G, Smith K. Treatment of comatose survivors of out-of-hospital cardiac arrest with induced hypothermia. N Engl J Med. 2002 Feb 21;346(8):557–63

28. Hypothermia after Cardiac Arrest Study Group. Mild therapeutic hypothermia to improve the neurologic outcome after cardiac arrest. N Engl J Med. 2002 Feb 21;346(8):549–56

29. Liberati A, D'Amico R, Pifferi S, Torri V, Brazzi L, Parmelli E. Antibiotic prophylaxis to reduce respiratory tract infections and mortality in adults receiving intensive care. Cochrane Database Syst Rev. 2009 Oct 7;(4):CD000022

30. Efficacy and Safety of Drotrecogin Alfa (Activated) in Adult Patients With Septic Shock, NCT00604214, available via http://clinicaltrials.gov

31. Activated Protein C and Corticosteroids for Human Septic Shock (APROCCHS), NCT00625209, available via http://clinicaltrials.gov

32. Australasian Resuscitation In Sepsis Evaluation Randomised Controlled Trial (ARISE), NCT00975793, available via http://clinicaltrials.gov

33. Protocolized Care for Early Septic Shock (ProCESS), NCT00510835, available via http://clinicaltrials.gov

34. Pronovost P, Needham D, Berenholtz S, Sinopoli D, Chu H, Cosgrove S, Sexton B, Hyzy R, Welsh R, Roth G, Bander J, Kepros J, Goeschel C. An intervention to decrease catheter-related bloodstream infections in the ICU. N Engl J Med. 2006 Dec 28;355(26):2725–32

35. Marik PE, Zaloga GP. Early enteral nutrition in acutely ill patients: a systematic review. Crit Care Med. 2001 Dec;29(12):2264–70

36. Hicks P, Cooper DJ, Webb S, Myburgh J, Seppelt I, Peake S, Joyce C, Stephens D, Turner A, French C, Hart G, Jenkins I, Burrell A. The Surviving Sepsis Campaign: International guidelines for management of severe sepsis and septic shock: 2008. An assessment by the Australian and New Zealand intensive care society. Anaesth Intensive Care. 2008 Mar;36(2):149–51

37. Dellinger RP, Levy MM, Carlet JM, Bion J, Parker MM, Jaeschke R, Reinhart K, Angus DC, Brun-Buisson C, Beale R, Calandra T, Dhainaut JF, Gerlach H, Harvey M, Marini JJ, Marshall J, Ranieri M, Ramsay G, Sevransky J, Thompson BT, Townsend S, Vender JS, Zimmerman JL, Vincent JL; International Surviving Sepsis Campaign Guidelines Committee; American Association of Critical-Care Nurses; American College of Chest Physicians; American College of Emergency Physicians; Canadian Critical Care Society; European Society of Clinical Microbiology and Infectious Diseases; European Society of Intensive Care Medicine; European Respiratory Society; International Sepsis Forum; Japanese Association for Acute Medicine; Japanese Society of Intensive Care Medicine; Society of Critical Care Medicine; Society of Hospital Medicine; Surgical Infection Society; World Federation of Societies of Intensive and Critical Care Medicine. Surviving Sepsis Campaign: international guidelines for management of severe sepsis and septic shock: 2008. Crit Care Med. 2008 Jan;36(1):296–327

38. Krimsky WS, Mroz IB, McIlwaine JK, Surgenor SD, Christian D, Corwin HL, Houston D, Robison C, Malayaman N. A model for increasing patient safety in the intensive care unit: increasing the implementation rates of proven safety measures. Qual Saf Health Care. 2009 Feb;18(1):74–80

39. Gawande A. The Checklist Manifesto: How to Get Things Right. New York, Metropolitan Books, 2009.

40. Winters BD, Gurses AP, Lehmann H, Sexton JB, Rampersad CJ, Pronovost PJ. Clinical review: checklists – translating evidence into practice. Crit Care. 2009;13(6):210

41. Murphy DJ, Needham DM, Goeschel C, Fan E, Cosgrove SE, Pronovost PJ. Monitoring and Reducing Central Line-Associated Bloodstream Infections: A National Survey of State Hospital Associations. Am J Med Qual. 2010 Jun 4. Epub ahead of print. DOI: 10.1177/1062860610364653

42. Pronovost PJ, Goeschel CA, Colantuoni E, Watson S, Lubomski LH, Berenholtz SM, Thompson DA, Sinopoli DJ, Cosgrove S, Sexton JB, Marsteller JA, Hyzy RC, Welsh R, Posa P, Schumacher K, Needham D. Sustaining reductions in catheter related bloodstream infections in Michigan intensive care units: observational study. BMJ. 2010 Feb 4;340:c309

43. Moran JL, Bristow P, Solomon PJ, George C, Hart GK; Australian and New Zealand Intensive Care Society Database Management Committee (ADMC). Mortality and length-of-stay outcomes, 1993–2003, in the binational Australian and New Zealand intensive care adult patient database. Crit Care Med. 2008 Jan;36(1):46–61

44. Higgins TL, Teres D, Copes WS, Nathanson BH, Stark M, Kramer AA. Assessing contemporary intensive care unit outcome: an updated Mortality Probability Admission Model (MPM0-III). Crit Care Med. 2007 Mar;35(3):827–35

45. Kastrup M, von Dossow V, Seeling M, Ahlborn R, Tamarkin A, Conroy P, Boemke W, Wernecke KD, Spies C. Key performance indicators in intensive care medicine. A retrospective matched cohort study. J Int Med Res. 2009 Sep-Oct;37(5):1267–84

46. Pronovost PJ, Angus DC, Dorman T, Robinson KA, Dremsizov TT, Young TL. Physician staffing patterns and clinical outcomes in critically ill patients: a systematic review. JAMA. 2002 Nov 6;288(17):2151–62

47. Kim MM, Barnato AE, Angus DC, Fleisher LF, Kahn JM. The effect of multidisciplinary care teams on intensive care unit mortality. Arch Intern Med. 2010 Feb 22; 170(4):369–76

48. Hawari FI, Al Najjar TI, Zaru L, Al Fayoumee W, Salah SH, Mukhaimar MZ. The effect of implementing high-intensity intensive care unit staffing model on outcome of critically ill oncology patients. Crit Care Med. 2009 Jun;37(6):1967–71

49. Huang DT, Clermont G, Kong L, Weissfeld LA, Sexton JB, Rowan KM, Angus DC. Intensive care unit safety culture and outcomes: a US multicenter study. Int J Qual Health Care. 2010 Jun;22(3):151–61

50. Sexton JB, Helmreich RL, Neilands TB, Rowan K, Vella K, Boyden J, Roberts PR, Thomas EJ. The Safety Attitudes Questionnaire: psychometric properties, benchmarking data, and emerging research. BMC Health Serv Res. 2006 Apr 3;6:44

51. Haig KM, Sutton S, Whittington J. SBAR: a shared mental model for improving communication between clinicians. Jt Comm J Qual Patient Saf 2006; 32: 167–175

52. Porteous JM, Stewart-Wynne EG, Connolly M, Crommelin PF. iSoBAR–a concept and handover checklist: the National Clinical Handover Initiative. Med J Ausl. 2009 Jun 1;190 (11 Suppl):S152–6

53. Catchpole KR, de Leval MR, McEwan A, Pigott N, Elliott MJ, McQuillan A, MacDonald C, Goldman AJ. Patient handover from surgery to intensive care: using Formula 1 pit-stop and aviation models to improve safety and quality. Paediatr Anaesth. 2007 May;17(5):470–8

54. Pickering BW, Hurley K, Marsh B. Identification of patient information corruption in the intensive care unit: using a scoring tool to direct quality improvements in handover. Crit Care Med. 2009 Nov;37(11):2905–12

55. Zwarenstein M, Goldman J, Reeves S. Interprofessional collaboration: effects of practice-based interventions on professional practice and healthcare outcomes. Cochrane Database Syst Rev. 2009 Jul 8;(3):CD000072

56. Wheelan SA, Burchill CN, Tilin F. The link between teamwork and patients' outcomes in intensive care units. Am J Crit Care. 2003 Nov;12(6):527–34

57. Reader TW, Flin R, Mearns K, Cuthbertson BH. Developing a team performance framework for the intensive care unit. Crit Care Med. 2009 May;37(5):1787–93

58. Morrison C, Jones M, Blackwell A, Vuylsteke A. Electronic patient record use during ward rounds: a qualitative study of interaction between medical staff. Crit Care. 2008;12(6):R148

59. Papadimos TJ, Hensley SJ, Duggan JM, Khuder SA, Borst MJ, Fath JJ, Oakes LR, Buchman D. Implementation of the 'FASTHUG' concept decreases the incidence of ventilator-associated pneumonia in a surgical intensive care unit. Patient Saf Surg. 2008 Feb 12;2:3

60. Strøm T, Martinussen T, Toft P. A protocol of no sedation for critically ill patients receiving mechanical ventilation: a randomised trial. Lancet. 2010 Feb 6;375(9713):475–80

61. Drakulovic MB, Torres A, Bauer TT, Nicolas JM, Nogué S, Ferrer M. Supine body position as a risk factor for nosocomial pneumonia in mechanically ventilated patients: a randomised trial. Lancet. 1999 Nov 27;354(9193):1851–8

62. Streat S, Judson JA. Cost containment: the Pacific. New Zealand. New Horiz 1994 2(3):392–403

63. Streat SJ, Plank LD, Hill GL. An overview of modern management of patients with critical injury and severe sepsis. World J Surg 2000 Jun;24(6):655–663

64. Streat SJ. Illness trajectories are also valuable in critical care (letter). BMJ. 2005 May 28;330(7502):1272

65. Corke CF, Stow PJ, Green DT, Agar JW, Henry MJ. How doctors discuss major interventions with high risk patients: an observational study. BMJ. 2005 Jan 22;330(7484):182

66. White DB, Malvar G, Karr J, Lo B, Curtis JR. Expanding the paradigm of the physician's role in surrogate decision-making: an empirically derived framework. Crit Care Med. 2010 Mar;38(3):743–50

67. Corke CF, Lavery JF, Gibson AM. Choosing life support for suddenly severely ill elderly relatives. Crit Care Resusc. 2005 Jun;7(2):81–6

68. Marks MA, Arkes HR. Patient and surrogate disagreement in end-of-life decisions: can surrogates accurately predict patients' preferences? Med Decis Making. 2008 Jul-Aug;28(4):524–31

69. Shalowitz DI, Garrett-Mayer E, Wendler D. The accuracy of surrogate decision makers: a systematic review. Arch Intern Med. 2006 Mar 13;166(5):493–7

70. Streat S. When do we stop? Crit Care Resusc. 2005; 7:227–232

71. Zib M, Saul P. A pilot audit of the process of end-of-life decision-making in the intensive care unit. Crit Care Resusc. 2007 Jun;9(2):213–8

72. Truog RD, Campbell ML, Curtis JR, Haas CE, Luce JM, Rubenfeld GD, Rushton CH, Kaufman DC; American Academy of Critical Care Medicine. Recommendations for end-of-life care in the intensive care unit: a consensus statement by the American College of Critical Care Medicine. Crit Care Med. 2008 Mar;36(3):953–63

73. Clarke EB, Curtis JR, Luce JM, Levy M, Danis M, Nelson J, Solomon MZ; Robert Wood Johnson Foundation Critical Care End-Of-Life Peer Workgroup Members. Quality indicators for end-of-life care in the intensive care unit. Crit Care Med. 2003 Sep;31(9):2255–62

74. Nelson JE, Mulkerin CM, Adams LL, Pronovost PJ. Improving comfort and communication in the ICU: a practical new tool for palliative care performance measurement and feedback. Qual Saf Health Care. 2006 Aug;15(4):264–71

75. Azoulay E, Pochard F, Chevret S, Jourdain M, Bornstain C, Wernet A, Cattaneo I, Annane D, Brun F, Bollaert PE, Zahar JR, Goldgran-Toledano D, Adrie C, Joly LM, Tayoro J, Desmettre T, Pigne E, Parrot A, Sanchez O, Poisson C, Le Gall JR, Schlemmer B, Lemaire F. Impact of a family information leaflet on effectiveness of information provided to family members of intensive care unit patients: a multicenter, prospective, randomized, controlled trial. Am J Respir Crit Care Med. 2002 Feb 15;165(4):438–42

76. Cuthbertson SJ, Margetts MA, Streat SJ. Bereavement follow-up after critical illness. Crit Care Med. 2000 Apr;28(4):1196–201

77. Nelson JE, Puntillo KA, Pronovost PJ, Walker AS, McAdam JL, Ilaoa D, Penrod J. In their own words:

patients and families define high-quality palliative care in the intensive care unit. Crit Care Med. 2010 Mar;38(3):808–18

78. Curtis JR, Engelberg RA, Wenrich MD, Shannon SE, Treece PD, Rubenfeld GD. Missed opportunities during family conferences about end-of-life care in the intensive care unit. Am J Respir Crit Care Med. 2005 Apr 15;171(8):844–9

79. Schaefer KG, Block SD. Physician communication with families in the ICU: evidence-based strategies for improvement. Curr Opin Crit Care. 2009 Dec;15(6):569–77

80. Gries CJ, Curtis JR, Wall RJ, Engelberg RA. Family member satisfaction with end-of-life decision making in the ICU. Chest. 2008 Mar;133(3):704–12

81. Curtis JR, Engelberg RA, Wenrich MD, Nielsen EL, Shannon SE, Treece PD, Tonelli MR, Patrick DL, Robins LS, McGrath BB, Rubenfeld GD. Studying communication about end-of-life care during the ICU family conference: development of a framework. J Crit Care. 2002 Sep;17(3):147–60

82. McDonagh JR, Elliott TB, Engelberg RA, Treece PD, Shannon SE, Rubenfeld GD, Patrick DL, Curtis JR. Family satisfaction with family conferences about end-of-life care in the intensive care unit: increased proportion of family speech is associated with increased satisfaction. Crit Care Med. 2004 Jul;32(7):1484–8

83. Hillman K, Chen J, Cretikos M, Bellomo R, Brown D, Doig G, Finfer S, Flabouris A; MERIT study investigators. Introduction of the medical emergency team (MET) system: a cluster-randomised controlled trial. Lancet. 2005 Jun 18–24;365(9477):2091–7

84. McGaughey J, Alderdice F, Fowler R, Kapila A, Mayhew A, Moutray M. Outreach and Early Warning Systems (EWS) for the prevention of intensive care admission and death of critically ill adult patients on general hospital wards. Cochrane Database Syst Rev. 2007 Jul 18;(3):CD005529

85. Chan PS, Jain R, Nallmothu BK, Berg RA, Sasson C. Rapid Response Teams: A Systematic Review and Meta-analysis. Arch Intern Med. 2010 Jan 11;170(1):18–26

86. Hillman K, Chen J, May E. Complex intensive care unit interventions. Crit Care Med. 2009 Jan;37(1 Suppl):S102–6

87. Chen J, Bellomo R, Flabouris A, Hillman K, Finfer S; MERIT Study Investigators for the Simpson Centre; ANZICS Clinical Trials Group. The relationship between early emergency team calls and serious adverse events. Crit Care Med. 2009 Jan;37(1):148–53

88. Santamaria J, Tobin A, Holmes J. Changing cardiac arrest and hospital mortality rates through a medical emergency team takes time and constant review. Crit Care Med. 2010 Feb;38(2):445–50

89. Chen J, Flabouris A, Bellomo R, Hillman K, Finfer S; MERIT Study Investigators for the Simpson Centre and the ANZICS Clinical Trials Group.. The Medical Emergency Team System and not-for-resuscitation orders: results from the MERIT study. Resuscitation. 2008 Dec;79(3):391–7

90. Kross EK, Curtis JR. Burden of psychological symptoms and illness in family of critically ill patients: what is the relevance for critical care clinicians? Crit Care Med. 2008 Jun;36(6):1955–6

91. Siegel MD, Hayes E, Vanderwerker LC, Loseth DB, Prigerson HG. Psychiatric illness in the next of kin of patients who die in the intensive care unit. Crit Care Med. 2008 Jun;36(6):1722–8

92. Cuthbertson BH, Rattray J, Campbell MK, Gager M, Roughton S, Smith A, Hull A, Breeman S, Norrie J, Jenkinson D, Hernández R, Johnston M, Wilson E, Waldmann C; PRaCTICaL study group. The PRaCTICaL study of nurse led, intensive care follow-up programmes for improving long term outcomes from critical illness: a pragmatic randomised controlled trial. BMJ. 2009 Oct 16;339:b3723. doi: 10.1136/bmj.b3723

93. Cooper GS, Sirio CA, Rotondi AJ, Shepardson LB, Rosenthal GE. Are readmissions to the intensive care unit a useful measure of hospital performance? Med Care. 1999 Apr;37(4):399–408

94. Frost SA, Tam V, Alexandrou E, Hunt L, Salamonson Y, Davidson PM, Parr MJ, Hillman KM. Readmission to intensive care: development of a nomogram for individualising risk. Crit Care Resusc. 2010 Jun;12(2):83–9

95. Pirret AM. The role and effectiveness of a nurse practitioner led critical care outreach service. Intensive Crit Care Nurs. 2008 Dec;24(6):375–82

96. Bion JF, Abrusci T, Hibbert P. Human factors in the management of the critically ill patient. Br J Anaesth. 2010 Jul;105(1):26–33

97. Curtis JR, Cook DJ, Wall RJ, Angus DC, Bion J, Kacmarek R, Kane-Gill SL, Kirchhoff KT, Levy M, Mitchell PH, Moreno R, Pronovost P, Puntillo K. Intensive care unit quality improvement: a "how-to" guide for the interdisciplinary team. Crit Care Med. 2006 Jan;34(1):211–8

Carl Waldmann, Max Jonas, Liza Keating and Ian J. Rechner

The contribution of technology assessment

Introduction

> *"No system has sufficient funds to provide the best possible treatment for all patients in all situations" [1]*

Healthcare budgets cannot be infinite and the costs of healthcare have increased in parallel with population demographics. Increasing age, combined with the public's expectation that the healthcare system will be able to cope with an increasing array of diseases has led to a significant increase in healthcare spending in relation to GDP. In summary there has to be some rational use of these funds.

Critical care consumes a disproportionate amount of resource for relatively few patients. Financial analysis, especially with current fiscal pressures, may make it difficult to justify delivering prolonged intensive care for patients with a poor prognosis or who are discharged into rehabilitation requiring continuing access to the healthcare system [2]. It is therefore manifestly important, following recognition of a finite budget, that preventing inappropriate prolonged treatment in patients who do not ultimately survive, and improving the processes for other patients must be regarded as essential. Rationing of healthcare is a difficult area and quickly focuses the mind particularly in critical care [3]. This issue confuses non medical per-

sonnel particularly as there is a wide variation in patient care processes. This may happen on many levels: between countries, between intensive care units (ICU) in neighbouring hospitals as well as in the same ICUs when consultants do not agree on management protocols [4].

In 1811 the Luddite movement began in Nottingham under the fictitious character Captain Ludd. The Luddites set about destroying stocking frames, – the new technology of the time, which they considered would threaten their livelihood. They managed to cause a considerable amount of damage before the rebellion was squashed. Today 'Luddite' is used to refer to the individuals who oppose technological change. One of the challenges of introducing changes in process particularly where there is a use of new technology is the reluctant healthcare professional.

New technology presents the opportunity to reshape the way in which we deliver healthcare, and in particular critical care. Whilst the adoption of new technology is critical to progress, its objective assessment is critical to the development of a service. The costs associated with the adoption of newer technologies must be balanced by the inevitable need for resource allocation and hence a decrease in resources available to other areas of health [5].

As the technologies available to critical care have continued to expand, the need for more precise evaluation of new technologies has arisen. The current economic climate has crystallised the need for accurate assessments. The situation is likely to become increasingly more acute and relevant as healthcare systems are working under increasingly tight financial restraints. However it remains clear that economic evaluation of any new technology must be driven by valid and relevant clinical outcomes that remain patient centred.

One recent example of the adoption of a new healthcare technology is that of the introduction of analgo-sedation using remifentanil for cardiac surgery in Leipzig [6]. In this study for the cost of purchasing what was considered an expensive drug remifentanil (16,500 Euros) the estimated savings made as a result of improved patient flow through the unit calculated was 315,000 Euros.

Analysis of this study clearly implied that it was not just the drug that made the difference but the whole process. The objective of the study was to speed up recovery times while maintaining safety and improving costs. A total of 421 patients given remifentanil were treated in a fast track area and were compared retrospectively with patients who had been treated by a standard protocol. The primary outcomes were time to extubation, length of stay in the ICU and treatment costs. The results showed that the times to extubation were significantly shorter with 75 min (range 45–110 min) compared to 900 min (range 600–1140 min) in the standard group. Intensive care unit stay and hospital length of stay were also significantly shorter (p < 0.01). The reduction of treatment costs of intensive care for patients was 53.5 % corresponding to savings of 738 Euros per patient. As a conclusion, the protocol for cardio-anaesthesia including the central elements of switching opiate therapy to remifentanil and switching patient recovery to a special post-anaesthesia recovery and care unit, shortened therapy times and showed itself to be safe and economically effective.

As a result many intensive care units have reconsidered their policies and process of sedation. Merely changing the drug has not been the recipe for success.

The need for analgesia and converting from a hypnotic based sedative regime to analgosedation (with newer drugs such as remifentanil and importantly the involvement of the hospital pain team) has been the crucial combination in improving patient throughput. The processes involved and patient pathways have had to be revisited with the use of sedation holding, sedation scoring, delirium scoring and the initiation of rehabilitation programmes as early as possible for an improved outcome for patients. For this process to be successful it is important that the process is introduced

carefully with a carefully planned educational programme for all levels of staff. Furthermore this educational programme needs to be assessed by monitoring compliance with the process of sedation and that the education programme is repeated appropriately so that the staff are kept up-to-date.

What is health technology assessment (HTA)

'Health technologies' are broadly defined to include all interventions used to promote health, prevent and treat disease, improve rehabilitation and long-term care. This may include drugs, devices, procedures (surgical techniques, screening and counselling) and even the settings of care such as general practice, hospitals and care homes.

The NHS Technology Assessment Programme was set up in 1993 and the findings and output from this Programme directly influence key decision-making bodies such as the National Institute for Clinical Excellence (NICE). Although the definition of HTA presents a wide spectrum of interventions, with the exception of drug based technologies, most of the principles involved can be considered with reference to medical devices.

"Health technology assessment is a multidisciplinary process that summarises information about the medical, social, economic and ethical issues related to the use of health technology in a systematic, transparent, unbiased, robust manner. Its aim is to inform the formulation of safe, effective, health policies that are patient focused, and seek to achieve best value" [7].

Health technology assessment is one facet of healthcare research. Interestingly, whilst the hierarchy of levels of evidence categorically states that for the evaluation of drugs and therapeutics the randomised controlled trial remains the gold standard, the accepted level of evidence for the evaluation of new medical devices is lower down the pyramid and is often based on case control studies.

The current system in the United Kingdom is the National Institute for Clinical Excellence (NICE). Although government-funded it remains an independent authority. Its main purpose is to deliver guidance in several areas. It concentrates on public health guidance and health promotion: the areas of relevance to critical care are clinical practice guidelines and health technology assessment [8]. Thus it has the ability to direct the new direction of travel of health and at the same time offer guidance on the tools required.

The aim of the process of technology assessment is to standardise access to healthcare across the United Kingdom. Indeed following a HTA by NICE the NHS is then legally obliged to fund and resource the medicine and treatments recommended. The technological assessments undertaken by NICE represent an objective reproducible technique upon which evaluations are undertaken.

The recommendations from NICE are based on both clinical and economic evidence. The process of HTA through NICE is essentially based on three stages:

- The initial phase is the scoping stage. This consists of the call for proposals. The proposals can be received from individuals, industry and organisations. An advisory committee on topic selection coordinates the process and clarifies the timeline. A scoping document is drafted and a decision is made by the health minister as to whether or not this is an appropriate topic for review. This decision is made within the context of health benefit that maybe derived, the potential impact to health, resources involved and what this may add to health guidance [8].

- If accepted, the process of assessment is then started. The appraisals committee invites all stakeholders thought to be associated with the topic. The stakeholders represent a comprehensive group from a wide background: patient/carer groups, representation from industry – both pharmaceutical and medical devices, relevant medical disciplines and from academia. An extensive assessment is drawn up and this forms the basis of the assessment report.

- This is then passed onto the appraisal committee which considers all available evidence in a transparent and reproducible fashion. The evidence is summarised and preliminary recommendations are made and published in the form of an appraisal consultation document. This is an extensive process which adheres to a tight pre-specified schedule. Inherent to this process is a cost-effectiveness analysis in the form of an incremental cost-effec-

tiveness ratio. A relevant example of this process to critical care is technology appraisal 84: drotrecogon alfa (activated) for sepsis (severe). A consistent approach is adopted for all appraisals [9].

Inevitably the economic aspects have predominated: the ethical aspects of health technology assessment are also relevant. Although the process of health technology assessment incorporates many aspects of the problem, the integration of the ethical aspects to the problem are at times neglected [10, 11].

Whilst large scale application of HTA is integral to the day to day running of any healthcare system, local application is also important.

The drug-based technologies and pharmaceutical industry are tightly legislated and require assessments ranging from animal studies to large interventional clinical trials. In contrast, medical devices have relatively little legislature surrounding clinical introduction and there frequently may not be a consensus as to what constitutes adequate assessment. There is as a result a need for further developments of the science relating to HTA. This is especially pertinent when considering the escalating numbers of devices for which manufacturers make claims relating to patient care. The ensuing HTA exercises stipulate study design and assessment of these new technologies in an attempt to judge and evaluate short and long-term benefits.

In effect there are two questions to answer: does the device have a positive clinical impact, and are the resultant economics affordable in the context of local/national healthcare funding? The requirement for a balanced approach of science versus economics ensures that the assessment design will draw on expertise from clinicians, engineers, statisticians, economists, ethicists and of course lawyers.

The ASSESSMENT Process

The HTA process has 3 core areas:
- device safety,
- device performance,
- device cost.

Device safety

This is a complex area where there may be safety aspects related to the using a device as well as the clinical process and context in which the device is used. Safety also encompasses accuracy of the device as inappropriate clinical decisions can result from inaccurate measurements. Frequently overlooked, it is the obverse component of the assessment process which should scrutinise the impact of not using the device.

Assessing the safety of the device or box itself is a statutory requirement and includes elements of electrical safety, detailed multilingual instructions, packaging, conformation to environmental specifications and disposal instructions. All of these issues are dealt with using a European Standard, referred to as the CE mark (La Conformité Européenne), which certifies that technical manufacturing standards have been met. It is not a functional guarantee that the device or process will be of benefit or be safe in clinical use. In the US, the Food and Drug Administration (FDA) fulfils a similar role but in addition, before granting approval for sale in the US, has a remit beyond the technical qualifications of the CE mark and mandates some assessment of clinical operation. The FDA uses clinical experts to review investigational studies relating to the device to ascertain whether the product does what is claimed by the manufacturer and/or presents unreasonable risks to the patient. The FDA classify devices into three classes according to the risk of potential harm to the user, ranging from Class 1 devices that present minimal risk to the user e.g. home blood pressure kits, to Class 3 e.g. Dialysis machines or ICU ventilators.

Device performance

Efficacy and effectiveness are used to assess device performance. The efficacy relates to the device performance under ideal conditions and the effectiveness is the performance under normal clinical working conditions. This is an important distinction as efficacy ratings may indicate the necessity for 'experts' to operate the device, whereas effectiveness relates to the performance limitations under average clinical conditions. Overall, when reviewing technology, the new approach should offer improvement over current technologies. This may be because the device can obtain measurements with less risk to the patient i.e. is less invasive, or has some other aspect which is advantageous.

Efficacy

Assessing efficacy usually means comparison of the device against a known 'gold' standard. When the measurement is well defined e.g. cardiac output, the efficacy becomes the mathematical correlates of accuracy.

Accuracy is the closeness of the device measurement to the actual value and can be described by:

- Correlation (degree of association between readings),
- Precision (the closeness of repeated measurements),
- Bias (the difference between the means of the measurements)

The repeatability and inaccuracy of the gold standard is important as if it has a varying accuracy then the limits of agreement between it and the technology under scrutiny become wider, less meaningful and makes definitive comparisons difficult. e.g. thermodilution cardiac output vs. other technologies.

Where a gold standard reference does not exist then it is necessary to show that the technology has a clinical utility, usually in relationship to patient outcomes.

Effectiveness

Assessment of effectiveness requires clinical trials in which the technology is used as it would be under average conditions. Standard rules of engagement for conduct of comparative studies are important to produce valid results and it must be appreciated that there may be issues related to study design.

The two obvious trials are a technology versus a control, or the technology with its measurement guiding subsequent therapeutic management. For the former type of trial, the data are usually comparative, whereas for the latter the results tend to be clinical outcome based. For outcome data the ideal measurement is considered to be mortality, but because of the resource implications of numbers needed to power studies for mortality, the use of surrogates such as length of hospital stay or number of complications is common. If using a device to guide therapy it is important to consider the relative contributions of the device being assessed as opposed to the therapeutic interventions of the protocol which may be the important determinant of the results.

Device cost

The economics related to health technologies is a key driver for technology assessment. These principles provide a safeguard for a finite and shrinking health budget and represent an attempt to ensure that resources and benefits are spread and do not favour one particular group. The area of cost containment is complex as in many situations the only costs considered are 'direct' costs relating to the technology and disposables. Frequently the indirect costs such as training and storage are ignored and these may represent a considerable financial load. e.g. a clinical information system may have a monetary cost per bed but staff training, education and maintenance personnel may generate considerable additional on-costs.

Procurement

In the hospital arena the principles of HTA are used to enable decisions for device procurement. When purchasing a device the functionality i.e. safety and performance, has to be considered in relation to the cost. The selection criteria for the purchase and replacement of medical devices depends on cost and numbers being purchased. The selection process should also include an evaluation of the manufacturer/supplier in terms of track record, profile in the local and national healthcare market, company financial stability/survival and service capability and response times.

Technologies have to understandably undergo rigorous safety checks before they can be used on patients. Once a CE mark has been given to the technology, then the process of procurement to

the healthcare industry occurs. When these barriers are overcome and the technology arrives within the Intensive Care environment, how does it fit into the processes which are involved in the care of the acutely ill patient? Factors such as staff confidence, availability and "user friendliness" of equipment, along with being able to withstand the rough environment and perceived benefit of the end user, all play a role in successful implementation of technology. Technological advancement is moving at such a pace that once the technology is being used at the "coal face", there may be another more modern version available.

Examples of technology assessment and processes

Beds

Beds are probably the most frequently used medical device for individual patient care. The majority of beds for standard ward care are not suitable for critical care. Frequently thought of as passive devices offering little more than support and a surface on which a patient is placed, there has been a failure to recognise that beds have therapeutic potential and enable the delivery of a wide variety of therapies, hence the term 'therapeutic bed'. These therapies include thermoregulation, pressure related wound therapy, position therapy such as proning and lateral rotational therapy. The procurement of beds however may not involve the clinical staff which may result in a suboptimal solution. One should warn against the lack of clinical involvement; with beds in ICU the ability to reach the airway is important and may be compromised with certain beds: Figure 1 demonstrates difficulty of access to the head to manage airway on a critical care bed.

Clinical information systems (CIS)

Clinical benefit of health technology – the ideal scenario!

In any walk of life, if a device is robust, easy to use, inexpensive, looks "sexy", saves money through improved processes, and makes the life of the user easier – then it will be a sure winner.

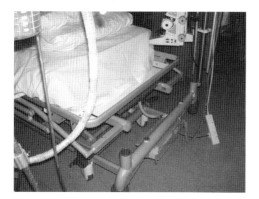

Fig. 1   Demonstration of difficulty of access to the head to manage airway on a critical care bed

Looking at the mobile phone industry and how the media have advertised mobile phones along with how many health care professionals use them, shows that we are living in an era where information technology is part of our everyday life. Imagine a life without television, a laptop (on which we write this!) and the internet. It is in this environment that technology within healthcare will thrive.

There are many types of technology found within the intensive care providing clinical data. One of the ways this is all coordinated is through the clinical information system (CIS), or in the Leyton Orient football parlance 'the central midfield controller'. This records all the observations that are made on the patients, the blood results and investigations along with the clinical history. The CIS in addition has reporting functionality to assess the costs, quality and outcomes of the intensive care unit. The necessity or mandate for developing the CIS comes from the reports of the Institute of Medicine (IOM) – part of the National Academy of Sciences. The report from the IOM 'To err is human' suggested that up to 98,000 people die in hospitals in the USA annually due to preventable medical mistakes, more than are killed from road traffic accidents, breast cancer and AIDS [12].

One of the commonest errors is medication mistakes [13].

The IOM strategy for improvement in this form of error is by implementing the computerised order entry, standardising processes for medication doses, dose timing and dose scales in a given patient unit and ensuring reporting of errors. Only once the errors and error rates are known can these errors be managed.

Medical informatics provides an answer to ensuring patient safety by ensuring standardisation of patient care and processes, allowing physician order entry systems with online clinical decision support. The electronic patient record should be seen as the 'enabler' of the process of patient management before during and after critical care. It will be of particular importance to ensure that the process of rehabilitation starts and is documented on the ICU and is continued throughout the post intensive care period. Rehabilitation for the critically ill patient has been mandated by NICE [14].

Procurement of CIS technology

A project initiation document is probably the most crucial part of the project in the procurement and development of a CIS. This is the link between what the end user wants and what the technology is able to provide. Within the intensive care there are many healthcare professional who work together to deliver patient care. It is important to ensure the end user has what they want and time must be spent developing a project initiation document and the formation from this of a *scope document* which will help the end user to understand exactly what to expect during the course of the project.

Project initiation document

This process should involve all members of the healthcare team (medical, nursing, technicians, physiotherapists, dieticians and pharmacist), the information technology department and support services (radiology, pathology and microbiology). The final and probably most important member is a previous ICU patient. The group then need to sit down and plot the patient's journey through the ICU and what information is required from investigations, clinical information and monitoring data. Pharmacy data and prescribing along with order communications such as radiology and pathology need recording. Various different clinic scenarios need to be thought about to ensure the different clinical scenarios are all accounted for in the CIS. This includes factors such as paediatric patients, surgical and medical and ICU compared to HDU patients. Once this *statement of need* is finalised this has to be placed in the project initiation document which is then sent out to tender to the different companies that can provide a CIS for a critical care unit.

Statement of need (SON)

Determining which company is granted the contract will depend on which company can match the statement of need. This will relate to cost, matching of the statement of need and the time scale over which the project can be delivered.

The statement of need and the project initiation document are then merged to form a "project scope", which will help the end user to understand exactly what to expect during the course of the project.

Potential pitfalls of the project scope

Like any binding contract between two individuals, it is only with time and what the user sees as the end product that potential problems arise. Those of us who have been involved in house or hospital building projects provide good experience of such a scenario. As a project develops there might be new technologies or treatments available. Project development might be delayed so that the money originally put aside by the contractor does not cover the task that it was originally set aside for. You may argue that this is the contractor's problem, but if the vendor has caused delays by for example not giving the contractor access to the clinical area, problems might occur.

Project development

Once the contract has been tendered and awarded, the project is moved from the sales team of the company to the development side. Most companies are set up so that these two departments are separate and as long as there is not too much

deviation from the scope, a good relationship starts to develop between the company developers and the ICU project administrator team. A CIS project takes approximately 6 to 12 months to set up. The hardware for the servers needs to be set up first and then the software is loaded onto these, which have to be mirrored and backed up in a fire and flood proof place. Training for configuration of the system them starts. The configuration is based on the original meeting of all the hospital employees who developed the project initiation document.

Testing of data quality

All configurations and interfacing of devices such as blood gas results and monitoring data which come across automatically to the CIS have to be tested. A parallel testing CIS system which mirrors the CIS which is ultimately used to enter patient data on must exist.

To ensure the data quality data, you must have minimum and maximum bound for parameters. This means that for example the range for something like central venous pressure should be -5 to 30 mmHg. If a value such as 250 mmHg is entered it will be rejected. In addition, normal reference ranges can be entered and if these are exceeded then the data item can appear in a different colour. Mandatory data fields can be entered to ensure data fields get populated. By doing this data which is used to calculate scores or predictive tools becomes valid. These can then be used in alerts to the clinical user that there is a potential adverse clinical situation developing with the patient which needs to be addressed sooner rather than later.

Test data must include all interfaced devices (monitoring, laboratory, ventilator and infusion pump information), prescribed drugs, fluid balance calculations and audit data such as APACHE and SAPS scores. This involves entering actual patient data into the test CIS and then getting a third party to check that these data are correct.

Staff training

Once the system has been developed and tested then the end users have to have training in the use of the system. If the processes of care are not very different from those used before, then essentially the training is mainly getting the staff used to a new CIS. Processes of care can be altered with the use of information technology to benefit the patient and staff. Data can automatically be acquired from the bedside monitors and ventilators. These data have to be verified by the user but will in addition come under the scrutiny of the data parameters which were set in the original system development.

Advisories and calculations

Information systems have the ability to carry out calculations on data which is entered into the system. An example would be if the patient's blood sugar is greater than 10 mmol/l then an advisory message appears in the bedside computer screen. This message then has to be acknowledged and this leaves an audit trail. Calculations can be configured to ensure for example that if the cerebral perfusion pressure is below a certain value then an advisory is triggered.

Audit and reporting systems

Once the system "goes live" following system testing and staff training then live patient data can start being collected. This is one of the paradoxical issues with report and audit writing, which is that only when you have data can these reports be looked at.

Quality of care reports

Technology within the CIS ensures that data are entered in mandatory fields and the quality is good by putting bounds on these data. In addition with the use of advisories and calculations data quality can be further enhanced and known clinical care which benefits patients such as keeping the blood sugar below 10 mmol/l is achieved. With data it is hugely important to ensure it is entered correctly in the first place, rather than having to correct it at a later date. After 48 hours it is sensible to ensure that certain data types such as vitals and ventilator parameters cannot be altered. This stops the data from being corrupted by unscrupulous investigators. In addition, most individuals are not likely to remember data figures after 48 hours.

Reports can be automatically generated at monthly intervals to ensure that the ICU is practising to a certain standard. Examples of this include factors such as care bundle adherents for sepsis, veno thromboembolic prophylaxis and safe ventilation with low tidal volumes. In addition – as ICU is best described as a complex interaction of a multitude of factors in a process of care which is delivered to the patient – performance of this system can be evaluated using tools such as cumulative summation of mortality (CSUM) and standardised mortality ratios (SMR) against known outcomes.

Using technology to alert processes of care

Technology with the CIS ensures that data have to be entered; otherwise the user cannot progress to the next screen or entry. Similarly advisories can appear which instruct staff to carry out certain tasks. Provided the clinical user sees these advisories as aid memoirs rather than dictatorial instructions, processes of care can be altered. Then with the use of the tools such as the CSUM and SMR mentioned early performance of the ICU can be monitored.

Summary

1. Health care is expensive and budgets are not limitless.
2. Traditional processes of care may need to be challenged because they are not cost-effective.
3. Introducing a new process will only be effective if introduced carefully and constantly evaluated.
4. New processes of care are often associated with new technologies that would have undergone a rigorous period of evaluation to ensure they do the job they are designed to do.
5. New technologies such as a CIS may have an important role to play in improving patient safety but often require patient processes to be re-thought.

The authors

Carl Waldmann, MD, MA, MB, Bchir, FRCA, EDIC[1]
Max Jonas, MB, BCh, FRCA[2]
Liza Keating, MB, ChB, MSc, MRCP, FCEM, DICM[1]
Ian James Rechner, MD, BSc MB, BS, FRCA[1]
  [1]ICU | Royal Berkshire Hospital, Reading, UK
  [2]ICU | Southampton University Hospital, UK

Address for correspondence

Carl Waldmann
Intensive Care Unit
Royal Berkshire
NHS Foundation Trust
London Road
Reading
RG5 4EU, United Kindom
E-mail: cswald@aol.com

References

1. Hope T, Savulescu J and Hendrick J. Medical Ethics and Law. The Core Curriculum. Oxford: Churchill Livingston Elsevier 2008.
2. Stricker K, Rothen HU and Takala J. Resource use in the ICU: short- vs. long-term patients. Acta Anaesthesiol Scand 2003;47:508–15.
3. Terblanche M, Adhikari NK. The evolution of intensive care unit performance. J Crit Care 2006;21:19–22.
4. Suter, P. Some ICUs save more lives than others: we need to know why! Intensive Care Med 2005;31:301–302.
5. Sachdeva R. Measuring the impact of new technology: An outcomes-based approach. Crit Care Med 2001;29:N190–N195.
6. Hantschel D, Fassl J, Scholz M, Sommer M, Funkat A, Wittmann M and Ender J. Leipzig fast-track protocol for cardio-anesthesia. Effective, safe and economical. Anaesthesist, 2009;58:379–86.
7. EUnetHTA. HTA definition, 2010. Accessed 26/6/2010. http://www.eunethta.net/Public/HTA/
8. Ridley S. NICE regulation in the UK. Care of the Critically Ill 2007 (April);23(2):49–52.
9. NICE. Drotrecogin alpha (activated) for severe sepsis. Technology Appraisal TA84, 2004.
10. Goetghebeur M, Wagner M, Khoury H, Rindress D, Gregoire J and Deal C. Combining multicriteria decision analysis, ethics and health technology assessment: applying the EVIDEM decisionmaking framework to growth hormone for Turner syndrome patients. Cost Eff Resour Alloc. 2010; 8, 2010.
11. Sacchini D, Virdis A, Refolo P, Pennacchini M and de Paula IC. Health technology assessment (HTA): ethical aspects. Med Health Care Philos 2009;12:453–7.
12. Karlsson G. Cost effectiveness analysis and capital costs. Soc Sci Med 1998; 46:1183–1191.
13. Leape LL, Bates DW, Cullen DJ, Cooper J, Demonaco HJ, Gallivan T, Hallisey R, Ives J, Laird N, Laffel G et al. Systems analysis of adverse drug events. ADE Prevention Study Group. JAMA 1995;274:35–43.
14. NICE. Critical illness rehabilitation. Clinical Guideline CG83, 2009.

Further Reading

Jonas M, Waldmann C and Imhoff M. Technology Assessment and Procurement In Monitoring the monitor. ESICM, 2008.
Waldmann C, Imhoff M and Martich D. Patient safety and health informatics. In Patient Safety and Quality of Care in Intensive Care Medicine, eds. Chiche, Moreno, Putensen & Rhodes. ESICM, 2009.
PACT module on Technology Assessment in press.

Hans Flaatten

Evaluating and improving organizational outcome

If you don't know where you are going,
every road will get you nowhere.

Henry A Kissinger

Anyone using a map needs to know two basic pieces of information: Where you are and where you plan to go. Then you can plan the journey. The similarities to outcome evaluation and improvements are striking. You first have to know the present status of your intensive care unit (ICU), and then set up a goal for what you want to achieve. The first step could be called an organizational evaluation, and the second step is the "goal", hopefully an improvement, and the passage from your present place to the goal is the improvement process.

A simple example may illustrate this:

In your ICU there is a growing concern about the increasing time ICU patients spend "on the ventilator". You know that ventilator time is a major determinant of ICU length of stay (LOS), and that reducing ventilator time may decrease ICU LOS and hence make your ICU able to care for more patients. The first step is then to collect information about the ventilator time in your unit. Most ICUs will count the hours and then convert the number of

hours to days. To define the start is usually easy (intubation, start of mask ventilation), the end of a ventilator session may be more difficult to define. A fixed time (usually a year) is often used to collect data. Now you can do simple calculations and run descriptive statistics to find the median and mean ventilator time. Data show your median ventilator time to be 2.8 days, and the mean is 6.2 days. You decide that your goal is to decrease this by 25 %. Now you know where you are and where you want to go. The work you plan to do in order to achieve this goal is what we often refer to as quality improvement and that is the content of this chapter.

What is meant by outcome-based evaluation?

In this context we define the organization at the ICU level (it could however also be at the hospital level or national level).

Outcome's evaluation analyses the impacts/benefits/changes to ICU patients (as a result of your treatment and care) during and/or after their ICU stay.

Furthermore, outcome evaluation can examine these changes in the short-term, intermediate term and long-term.

An outcome evaluation can be described by its basic components. One way to do this is to think of the ICU stay in terms of inputs, activities/ processes, outputs and outcomes (see Fig. 1 and Tab. 1). Such systematic view can be useful to examine any program! Be aware that in this description, output data do not necessarily have anything to do with outcome.

Planning the evaluation

Many people tend to think that an evaluation process is a complex activity not readily available for the "common" intensive care doctor or nurse. On the contrary, the principles are quite simple and can be used in any ICU. To start plan evaluation of your ICU you need to answer some basic questions (taken from http://managementhelp.org/ evaluatn/outcomes.htm):

- Who are the primary audiences (recipients) for the results?
- What kind of information would be required?
- When is information needed?
- Where can one get information and how is it to be retrieved?
- What resources are available for me to get necessary information?
- How does one analyse and report results in a timely way?
- What decisions do you want to make as a result of the evaluation?

In the example above, this could mean:
- The main recipients are the ICU personnel and hospital administrators
- We need information about the time "on" the ventilator
- We need this information by the end of the year
- We must retrieve the ventilator times from individual patients records (charts) and store them
- The main resources are the ICU chart (manual or electronic) and the ICU nurses
- We want to use SPSS for an analysis of these data
- Pending the results, we must create a goal for the mean ventilator time in the coming year, and the ways to achieve this goal

Methods to improve outcome at the ICU level

A number of methods have been used in order to implement changes in the ICU; these introduce new treatments/equipment, making/changing written procedures or discussions with ICU physicians and nurses. There are several pitfalls in most methods, and very often attitudes of the involved ICU personal tend not to change for more than a short period of time. This is particularly true if changes are implemented using a top-down process.

In order to achieve changes that will be retained in the ICU it is important to create some kind of "ownership" in the process for all stakeholders. The following are some important steps in this regard:
- All involved ICU personnel must agree on "where we are"; this means that they must all accept the present situation, and that the numbers and results must be known and acknowledged by the whole ICU staff and on all levels.
- There must be a common understanding and acceptance of the goal, or "where we want to be next year". This is especially true when any requirement for changes comes from the ICU physicians and involves other personnel groups like those of the ICU nurses
- You should try to be as specific as possible (if relevant) to the changes you want to achieve (for example like the choice of a 25% reduction in ventilator time mentioned above). A description of goals merely consisting of terms such as: "reducing", "increase", or "including" etc. is to be avoided.
- It is recommended to communicate the process to all personnel (remembering that some of the staff may only work night-shift or are only infrequently present in the ICU), and to use different methods: verbal communication (staff meetings), electronic communication (sms, e-mail, home page announcement etc) and poster/whiteboard information at strategic places in the ICU.
- Choose a process strategy for change that is easy to track and enable feedback to the ICU personnel as the process continues.
- Discuss after the implementation period how one can achieve sustained improvement (after the implementation phase).

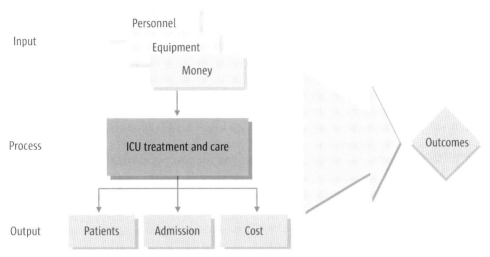

Fig. 1   The ICU seen as a chain of input, process, and output. Different combinations make up the outcome.

Tab. 1   Outcome evaluation in the ICU (modified from http://managementhelp.org/evaluatn/outcomes.htm)

Components	Description
Input	These are materials and resources that the ICU uses in its activities, or processes, to serve patients, e. g., equipment, staff, facilities, money, etc. These are often easy to identify and many of the inputs seem common to many organizations and programs.
Activities	These are the activities, or processes, that the ICU undertakes with the patient in order to meet their needs, for example, observation, monitoring, specific treatment, care, etc. Note that when identifying the activities in a program, the focus is still on the ICU or program itself, and still is not very much on actual changes in the patients.
Output	These are the units of service regarding your program, for example, the number of people treated in the ICU, the number of ICU days, the resources used (usually in term of costs), etc. Such numbers often mean nothing at all about the actual impacts/benefits/changes in your ICU patients.
Outcomes	These are the actual impacts/benefits/changes for patients during or after their ICU stay. For example the number of patients surviving ICU/hospital stays, the number of patients able to get back to their home, the number able to take up work etc. Notice that this outcome is quite different from outputs such as the number of ICU patients and admissions. These changes, or outcomes, are usually expressed in terms of:
	▪ Knowledge and skills (these are often considered to be rather short-term outcomes)
	▪ Behaviours (these are often considered to be rather intermediate-term outcomes)
	▪ Values, conditions, and status (these are often considered to be rather long-term outcomes)
Outcome targets	These are the number and percent of ICU patients which you want to achieve the outcome, for example, an outcome goal of a reduction of ICU stay to a mean of 6 days, to reduce the standardized mortality rate to 0.75 % or to get at least 90 % of survivors to return to their homes and an independent life-style.
Outcome indicators	These are observable and measurable "milestones" toward an outcome target. These are those things that you'd see, hear, and read, etc., that would indicate to you whether you're making any progress toward your outcome target, or not.

The quality circle and Plan-Do-Study-Act

Very often this concept is applied for implementing changes, and the method can be found under different names. Most often it is known as the "quality circle", indicating that improving quality is a continuous process. This way to implement changes was developed in Japan under its industrial "revolution" after the Second World War. The concept was called "Kaizen", which literally means improvement, and the Kaizen strategy calls for continuous efforts for improvement involving everyone in the organization – managers and workers alike. The concept was gradually also introduced in the western world, soon also to be adopted by their health care [1]. A number of studies have been published using this concept, also within intensive care [2, 3]. An outline of the concept is shown in Figure 2.

The process starts by planning the process (PLAN), which includes the method of retrieving data from your own ICU (see the above discussion) and the developing a plan of how to change or alter processes. For the latter part, most often a local protocol is used specifically for the project. This protocol often describes important steps in the process of patient care.

The next step is to launch the project (DO) and get the information out to all stakeholders. The third phase (STUDY) is both an ongoing process feeding information back to the ICU personnel during the study, and the formal procedure of working with the results after study completion. The last phase (ACT) is to permanently change processes of care on basis of the study. Did the process lead to the changes you planned, and, if yes, what was the success factor; if no, how can you approach the problem using an alternative method/protocol.

Implementation of new knowledge

A growing problem is the gap between best practice (best evidence) and common practice (the care actually given to patients). This is also true for intensive care, and was recently well documented in a study from Germany [4]. In that study, perceived versus practice adherence regarding the surviving sepsis guidelines was studied in 366 patients with septic shock in 214 ICUs. The following results were found:

- A low tidal volume < 6 ml/kg/predicted bw was documented in only 2.6% of a subgroup of patients with ARDS. At the same time, the mean tidal volume was 10 ml/kg/bw! The perceived adherence was close to 80%.
- Blood glucose levels of 4.4–6.1 mmol/l were documented in 6.2% of their patients, while the perceived adherence was 66%
- Actual practice was influenced only to a small degree by hospital size or university affiliation (although this was not significant)

The authors called for implementation strategies involving all staff in the ICU both at local and at national levels in order to fill this gap.

The Institute for Health Care Improvement (IHI) (www.ihi.org) has for more than a decade now advocated what they call a "framework" for a good spread of knowledge transfer [5]. In that paper, the message from different publications in organizational and health care literature on the spread of innovations is reviewed. The authors have gone further and interviewed organizations about their success stories. In short, an organization must:

- Be prepared for spread
- Establish an aim for spread
- Develop, execute, and refine a spread plan

Such a framework could easily be implemented using the method described above. Other meth-

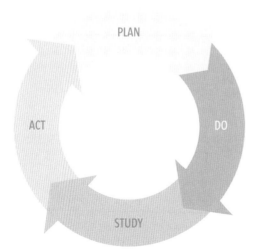

Fig. 2   The quality improvement cycle (plan-do-study-act)

ods such as using checklists are valuable, and can be used as a "stand-alone" solution or as a part of the STUDY phase as described above. The use of checklists can allow a change in the behaviour of individuals and teams in order to achieve a better outcome. In the Keystone ICU project, Pronovost reported a dramatic reduction of catheter-related bloodstream infections after introducing simple evidence-based interventions and development of a "team checkup tool" (Check-list) [6].

Conclusion

Evaluating and improving outcome should be given high priority in the ICU. A number of effective methods are available, and their usefulness has been well documented, also within intensive care.

The author

Hans Flaatten, MD, PhD
Haukeland University Hospital
Department of Anaesthesia and Intensive Care
Jonas Liesvei 65
5021 Bergen, Norway
E-mail: hans.flaatten@kir.uib.no

References

1. Plsek PE. Quality improvement methods in clinical medicine. Pediatrics, 1999. 103(1 Suppl E): p. 203–14.
2. Brattebo G, et al. Effect of a scoring system and protocol for sedation on duration of patients' need for ventilator support in a surgical intensive care unit. Bmj, 2002. 324(7350): p. 1386–9.
3. Robinson BR, et al. An analgesia-delirium-sedation protocol for critically ill trauma patients reduces ventilator days and hospital length of stay. J Trauma, 2008. 65(3): p. 517–26.
4. Brunkhorst FM, et al. Practice and perception–a nationwide survey of therapy habits in sepsis. Crit Care Med, 2008. 36(10): p. 2719–25.
5. Massoud MR, et al. A Framework for Spread: From Local Improvements to System-Wide Change., in IHI Innovation Series white paper. 2006, Institute for Healthcare Improvement: Cambrigde MA.
6. Pronovost P. Interventions to decrease catheter-related bloodstream infections in the ICU: the Keystone Intensive Care Unit Project. Am J Inf Control, 2008. 36: p. S171.el-5.

Guttorm Brattebø

Education and training teamwork using simulation

It has been said that while medicine used to be simple, ineffective but relatively safe, it's now highly effective, extremely complex and potentially dangerous. The well-being of patients in the intensive care unit depends heavily on the health care workers that are involved in their treatment. This may especially apply to modern intensive care medicine with its interwoven system of technical equipment, highly potent medications and sophisticated techniques, making it possible to treat or mitigate failures in most of the body's organ systems. There is little disagreement about the value of most treatment protocols or approaches to treating the many diseases or organ failures that acutely ill or injured patients may develop. However, as the complexity of intensive care has increased, we've also realised the need for focusing on how such complex systems sometimes fail, resulting in adverse events and harm to patients. This is a painful realisation, but also a requirement for achieving safer care. Much emphasise has been placed on safeguarding technical equipment and hardware, and redundancy when it comes to infrastructure. Guidelines and protocols based on consensus and current scientific knowledge has also become more accepted, reducing unnecessary variation in the way care is delivered. Such unwanted variation is mainly due to the health professionals' own personal preferences or local cultural differences. In this context, the importance of how the teams working in modern intensive care unit interact must not be underestimated. Analyses of adverse events have shown that human factors are the most prevalent contributing factor to patient harm. This should come as no surprise since there are so many people involved in the health care system and the extreme complexity of a modern hospital. Health professionals are nearly always educated and trained in "silos" with their peers, seldom training practical skills with the other professional groups they are required to work with in a clinical situation. Given the need for being able to act quickly and with precision when emergencies occur, such situations often result in suboptimal care and adverse events. Based on the growing body of literature as well as the author's experience in trauma simulation, this chapter will discuss some possibilities for increasing safety margins in the intensive care unit by training non-technical team skills, in addition to the success factors for such training.

Modern medicine is very complex and the intensive care unit (ICU) with its sophisticated technical equipment and advanced treatment options is among the most challenging clinical environments in a hospital. While this gives hope for effectively treating very severe conditions, it also increases the possibilities for unwanted harm to patients. Such events have been labelled adverse events (AE), and may occur in as much as 5–10 % of all hospital admissions [1–3]. Based on thorough investigations of AE there are reasons to believe that a significant proportion of them could have been prevented at least theoretically, since the root causes often are human factors and suboptimal team cooperation [4–7]. While only a small proportion of AE results in death, significant morbidity, suffering and costs are caused by AE. In Table 1 some of the common examples of management care problems are given. On the other hand, it is important to recognise that medical errors are nearly never the result of negligence, sloppiness, poor motivation or incompetence [10]. Rather, health care can be regarded as one of the most complex social systems [11]. There is scientific support for the relation between teamwork and patient safety in highly dynamic domains such as intensive care units (ICU), surgical theatres, and trauma rooms [12–14]. During recent years the importance of well functioning teams has been acknowledged as a crucial factor in both the causation and prevention of AE [12, 14]. Investigations have also shown that human factors like suboptimal team cooperation, lack of leadership and clear communication lead to disasters [7, 15, 16]. On the other hand, team training and simulator use is often mentioned as one important way of reducing the risk for patient

harm [1, 17, 18]. To mitigate the problems of failing team work, the aviation industry developed the concept of team training, called crew resource management training (CRM) [19]. The main goal of this training is to address the challenges of situational awareness, leadership, communication, and cooperation. The same causes of errors and lack of quality have been identified in medicine, and CRM training using simulations has been applied to the operation room environment as in full-scale anaesthesia simulators, in the delivery room, and the trauma room. Hence, the use of simulation to improve teamwork seems to be a sound strategy for improving health care [10, 11, 20]. This situation can and must be changed, but unfortunately health care is rather behind other high-risk industries in its attention to ensuring basic safety for our patients. Focus must shift from blaming the individual person treating the patient, to trying to prevent harm by improved system understanding and design. In the ICU environment special attention should be spent on communication and safe drug use, e.g. using proven medication safety practices [1, 21, 22].

Simulation training is especially useful for training the non-technical skills mentioned, but complicated or new procedures can also be trained in this way. Such training requires actually no fancy or expensive technical equipment, but some hospitals have advanced computer-based simulation mannequins available. On the other hand, simulation is just an educational method, with strengths but also certain limitations.

Team training and simulator use is regarded as one very important way of reducing the risk for patient harm [1, 17, 18]. It is human nature to err, but as important as our tendency for e.g. forgetting important details, is our ability to spot abnormalities and to create immediate solutions and better alternatives to meet the challenges ahead. We are normally well trained in the science of medicine for evaluating and caring for the individual patient, but we are less capable to understand the systemic safety issues involved in the complex interaction between team members [10]. However, when regarding human's fallibilities it is important to acknowledge our special ability for pattern recognition and mental simulation, which is far better than what computers can perform. These abilities have also been pointed out as the fundamental basis for expert

Tab. 1   Some examples of care management problems [modified from www.sikkerpatient.dk and 8, 9]

Not following agreed protocols without clinical justification, or applying incorrect protocols

Inadequate supervision of junior staff, or not seeking help when needed

Wrong treatment given, or treatment given to incorrect patient or body site

Failure to identify correct patient

Failure to monitor, observe, or act

Incorrect risk assessment (e.g. risk of suicide or self harm)

Inadequate handover and low quality communication

Failure to discover faulty equipment

Failure to carry out preoperative checks or misunderstanding / lack of tests behaviour, a capacity that can be trained in a simulator environment [23–25]. Cook and colleagues have studied and described how trained clinicians are able to anticipate and foresee possible safety threats and discontinuities in patient care. Then they will "bridge" those gaps, offsetting some of the expected consequences or limiting the impact of the gaps. By doing this, they create safety instead of threatening the safety of patients as depicted in Figure 1. This has the paradoxical effect of making gaps seem less significant, because they don't always have as detrimental effects as they would have had without experienced clinicians in the system [26]. Accordingly, this is a primary source of the robustness of health care. Asking experienced clinicians about possible gaps in the care of patients can therefore be used as a first step for choosing relevant topics and constructing simulator training sessions. The aim for simulation in this context can be viewed as a way of making health care more failure-proof or resilient towards the possible harmful effects of errors. On the other hand, the opportunity for "learning by doing" rarely occurs in modern medicine when one considers the handling of seldom occurring crises, and it would hardly be acceptable from a patient safety perspective either [17]. For example, trauma teams are expected to function efficiently and smoothly when treating major trauma cases, even though the teams are often without previous training [27]. The team members are usually sufficiently trained professionals individually, but with limited experience in team work [28].

In obstetrics, another dynamic domain of medicine, the British confidential enquiries into maternal and child health (CEMACH) in December 2007 concluded that "... the assessors were struck by the number of health care professionals who appeared to fail to be able to identify and manage common medical conditions or potential emergencies outside their own immediate area of expertise. Resuscitation skills were also considered to be poor in an unacceptably high number of cases." Furthermore: "In many cases the care provided was hampered by a lack of cross disciplinary or cross agency working and problems with communication. These included: poor or non-existent team working, inappropriate delegation to junior staff, inappropriate or inadequate consultations by phone, the lack of sharing of relevant information between health professionals, including between general practitioners (GPs) and the maternity team, poor interpersonal skills" [9].

Studies indicate that as many as one fourth of trauma related deaths are preventable, and that most treatment errors and protocol devia-

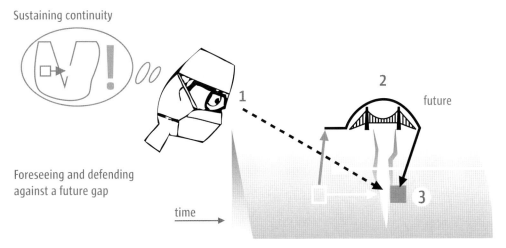

Sustaining continuity

Foreseeing and defending against a future gap

time

1

2

future

3

Fig. 1   How experienced clinicians can foresee and defend ("bridging") against a future gap in the continuity of care. [Reproduced with permission from Cook RI. A brief look at gaps in the continuity of care and how practitioners compensate for them. www.ctlab.org]

tions occur in the admission phase. It has also been shown that improving the systems for treating severely injured patients can significantly reduce the proportion of preventable deaths [29]. Regarding teamwork, the most difficult task to improve seems to be communication, but situational awareness, leadership, and co-operation is also very important [7, 16, 18, 30]. Based on an extensive literature review, Manser identified and described safety aspects of teamwork [12]. Table 2 lists aspects of teamwork based on recent studies and reports. The nature of many medical emergency teams and the conditions they are supposed to function under, pose specific challenges to optimal team function because conditions change (dynamism), teams may be assembled ad hoc, work together only for a brief period, consist of many professions, and therefore must integrate various professional cultures [12, 33]. The obvious answer to these issues is to give such teams the opportunity to train together as a team. The military has a slogan: "Train as you fight!" This is very suitable for ICU teams as well.

Communication as the most important key element in teamwork has been studied extensively, and several ideas have been put forward trying to describe a format for optimal communication in clinical settings. The so-called SBAR (situation, background, assessment and recommendations) is one simple but effective way of structuring communication [31]. Various models of the relationship between specific communication practices and patient safety have been proposed [34, 35]. The practices brought forward here are in good agreement with anaesthetists' non-technical skills (ANTS) [25, 30].

In their review of contributory factors underlying critical incidents, Reader and colleagues found an overlap between the non-technical skills requirements for the ICU and anaesthesia, with both domains having a need for good teamwork, situation awareness, task management and decision-making skills [24]. Furthermore they recommend that non-technical skill training programmes should be integrated into the technical aspects of a domain, when professionals have an adequate level of technical competence. Then the cognitive load of having to learn both technical and non-technical skills will be reduced simultaneously. It is further argued that the framework of non-technical skill categories identified in the ANTS taxonomy also applies to the ICU environment [24, 31]. The need for training these skills is important for both experienced and novice personnel,

Tab. 2 Aspects of teamwork relevant to patient safety [modified from 12, 23, 25, 31, 32]

Aspects	Characteristics
Situational awareness	Actively seeking information, recognising and understanding data and information (e.g. pattern recognition)
	Anticipation
Communication	Openness of communication and exchange of information
	Quality of communication (e.g. shared frames of reference)
	Specific communication practices (e.g. team briefing, closed-loop, SBAR)
Shared mental models	Shared perception of a situation, and understanding of team structure, tasks, and team roles
Quality of collaboration	Mutual respect and trust between team members
Leadership	Leadership style (value contributions from staff, encourage participation in decision-making)
	Adaptive leadership behaviour (e.g. increased explicit behaviour in critical situations)
Coordination	Adaptive coordination (e.g. shift between explicit and implicit coordination; increased information exchange and planning in critical situations)
Decision making	Identifying options
	Balancing risks and mental simulation
	Re-evaluation and change of solution/decision

since none so far have been extensively trained in team skills. It is then reasonable to agree that there is good scientific evidence for using simulation to improve quality of teamwork in the ICU.

The next issue is then to decide how to develop a simulation programme in order to achieve better performing teams. Fernandez and colleagues have described a very useful model for defining teamwork in emergency medicine, including some key recommendations to guide the implementation of their proposed taxonomy into routine simulation based training [36, 37]. Salas and colleagues also provide evidence-based principles for the planning, implementation and evaluation of team training programmes based on extensive reviews of the literature [18]. The relevant questions to be considered before a simulator-training programme is implemented are listed in Figure 2.

The most basic stage is the assessment of the educational needs: What are the problems? Which safety threats or emergency procedures ought to be addressed in the training? Simulation is a method that can be used in many different ways, and hence it is important to decide on the explicit educational goals (e.g. changes in behaviour) that must be demonstrated. Then one has to build the actual cases and scenarios to be simulated. One useful starting point for this can be to use selected AE reports [38]. It is also strongly recommended to construct scenarios based on real patients with those clinical problems which the participants can readily identify from their own experience, so that they "believe" the case and problems presented. When constructing a training scenario one can "pick and choose" from several real cases. The best challenges are the ones where there is not always a definite "correct answer"; e.g. to intubate or not. The scenario must include certain events that should trigger the specific wanted behaviours. These triggers should preferably be independent on each other, so that the entire scenario progress doesn't rely solely on only one single item. It is fascinating to observe how similar teams can choose quite different approaches to the same challenge. On the other hand, one must avoid too complicated scenarios, because they will be difficult to facilitate. The facilitator must be able to decide on the patient's clinical development right away, without having to consult the manuscript too often. This will obstruct the flow of simulation, and make the session less natural. Therefore, it's best to rely on common and relevant clinical problems that are easy to remember and then to follow during the simulation. It is also recommended to run a pilot before starting, just to "try out" the scenario. Table 3 shows a sample of scenarios and clinical challenges that can be trained.

Then there is need for a checklist or scale for evaluating the actual performance of the teams. This is very important for the feedback. The list

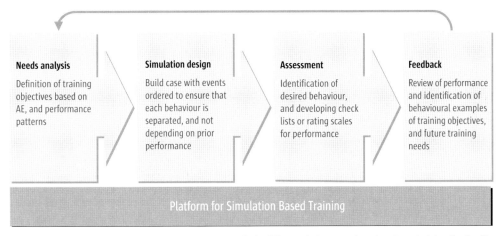

Needs analysis

Definition of training objectives based on AE, and performance patterns

Simulation design

Build case with events ordered to ensure that each behaviour is separated, and not depending on prior performance

Assessment

Identification of desired behaviour, and developing check lists or rating scales for performance

Feedback

Review of performance and identification of behavioural examples of training objectives, and future training needs

Platform for Simulation Based Training

Fig. 2   Description of taxonomy in simulation training, with the different design steps from 'needs analysis' to 'feedback' and identification of future training needs [modified from 36 and 37]

Tab. 3   Clinical situations and topics suitable for simulator training in the ICU environment

Advanced cardiopulmonary life support in cardiac arrest

Admittance of a new patient with threatened vital signs

Emergency endotracheal intubation, especially with a difficult airway

Accidental patient self-extubation or loss of airway

Treatment of acute tension pneumothorax, with chest tube insertion

Telling families that the patient is dying or dead

Communicating with families in relation to possible organ donation

Sudden technical failures in vital equipment or disruption of infra-structure (e.g. loss of electricity or piped gas supply)

Handling of serious adverse events (incl. patient, family, involved health personnel)

Handling of emotional upset families, including language problems

Prioritising resources when several patients are admitted at same time

Fast hand-over of complicated patients to /from e.g. the operation theatre

Testing of new treatment protocols or technical equipment

must describe which specific behaviours one wished to observe, e.g. was the identity of the patient checked, did the patient receive a high flow of oxygen, or was the blood pressure recorded? One must also decide on whether or not the patient should be "allowed to die" during the simulation. The author warns against this, because it is possible to make the patient deteriorate to indicate that the team must reassess, identify life-threatening issues, and offer correct treatment. Perhaps there are more effective ways of making the team realise that they have not performed to standards, other than letting them completely "fail" by loosing the patient.

The most important part of the simulation is the debriefing and the feedback session immediately after the simulation. In the Better & Systematic Trauma Care (BEST)-programme we usually seat the participants in a horseshoe formation, so that everybody can see each other's faces when reflecting and discussing the simulation. Be sure to have enough time for debriefing and keep all participants together. The main purpose is to give the participants the possibility for reflection and discussion on their performance. This is also the reason for running two simulations after each other, so that the teams will have the opportunity to demonstrate improvement based on the feedback and discussions. Regarding the important aspects of clinical feedback in medicine, Jack Ende's classic discussion of this is in my opinion still valid [39]. Especially, it is important to use a non-evaluating language, dealing with the specific and observed behaviours, and aiming at decisions and actions and not assumed intentions. Some tips for clinical feedback are listed in Table 4.

When building a simulation-based training programme, it must also be decided on which technological level the simulator or simulation should be placed: high-fidelity or low-fidelity simulation. There are a number of highly sophisticated simulators on the market, with a vast possibility for complicated responses to various inputs, e.g. medications [40]. These simulators are relying on computer programmes, where different algorithms are constructed based on physiological models. The strengths of these sophisticated simulators are that they are more real and can be subjected to more clinical procedures. On the other hand, they are expensive, must be programmed and often there is need for a second person just to take care of these technical issues [41]. In our experience it is possible to have effective team training using just regular resuscitation

Tab. 4   Guidelines for feedback in medical education [modified from 39]

Facilitator and trainee should be working as allies, with common goals

Feedback must be based on first-hand data and come as no surprise

It must be limited to behaviours that can be changed

Use descriptive and non-evaluative wording

Deal with specific performances, not generalisations

Focus on decisions and actions, not assumed intentions or interpretations mannequins. Experienced teams will not need a very expensive mannequin to train inter-personal skills, because they can easily relate the current situation to previous real life experiences. Moreover, regardless of the possibility of even more realistic simulators in the future, one must realise that simulation training is and will always remain an artificial situation; not real life. This is also the experience gained from a US-based programme that has been running local team training in obstetric units at rural hospitals in Oregon [42]. They started out with a very sophisticated simulation set-up, but ended up using simple mannequins.

Critical success factors for team training

It is easy to believe that when there is so much literature in favour of simulator training than the effects should be clearly demonstrated. This is not the case. However, recently there have been published some interesting papers analysing costs of adverse drug events and effect of team training to reduce medication errors [43, 44]. Salas and colleagues have also nicely pointed out the success factors for team training as listed in Table 5 [45]. The first thing is to make sure that the training objectives are in line with the goals for your organisation. With this in place it is also easier to provide support for the initiative, which is the second prerequisite. The next goal is to get the frontline care leaders on board. If they don't believe in and support the initiative, failure is likely to ensue. Then one must prepare the environment and

Tab. 5   Critical success factors for team training
in health care [45]

Align team training objectives
and safety aims with the organisational goals

Provide organisational support
for the team training initiative

Get frontline care leaders on board

Prepare the environment and trainees for team training

Determine required resources
and time commitment and ensure their availability

Facilitate application of trained teamwork skills on the job

Measure the effectiveness of the team training programme

trainees for the training, and also determine the required resources and time needed for the training. The persons responsible for manpower must also be committed and ensure that the needed resources are available for the training session. Application of the trained team skills in the job situation is also needed and important. And last but not least, one must measure the effectiveness of the team training programme itself [45]. Other researchers have also tried to identify reasons why team training initiatives are successful or not [46].

Some pitfalls in simulation sessions

It is easy mainly to focus on medical procedures or specific clinical issues in the debriefing sessions. Then the physicians in the team could certainly go on arguing by citing publications and sources of (contradictive) information for hours. However, the medical content is *per se* not the most important issue in a simulation exercise. The crucial point is to be able to pose some challenges that will demand demonstration of good situational awareness and adequate skills in communication, cooperation and leadership. Therefore, the dicussion must be focused explicitly on these team behaviours. On the other hand, a case that can be identified as relevant, and a team composition that reflects what is normally the situation when a team like this works together, will help the team to behave as if the simulation was in fact a real situation. Often, some team members are reluctant to act, because they find the training situation artificial or even embarrassing. If other team members (especially physicians) act in, this usually makes the team exercise develop well and to a larger degree resemble a real case. The debriefing can be started by shortly stating what the key clinical issues in the scenario was, and what the correct treatment would be. Then one can proceed to discussing the relevant team issues.

In the following, an example of the briefing and case for a team simulation is given. This set-up uses a low-fidelity "dead" mannequin or a live model, where clinical information and parameters are given verbally by the facilitator on demand [39 and www.bestnet.no]. One obvious advantage to this solution is the facilitator's ability for adjusting the patient's response and case progression to the specific team's decisions and actual performance.

Examples of briefing for an ICU team prior to a simulation session

Let's say that you are a member of the ICU team, about to take part in a simulated admission of a new acute patient with suspected sepsis. The patient is a simple resuscitation mannequin, but a facilitator will give all relevant information when prompted during the session. Clinical data will be given after the relevant procedure has been performed. You will have to simulate any invasive procedures and clinical examinations, and say aloud what you are doing e.g. "I am auscultating the chest, what do I hear?" Everything that you would do in a real situation like this should be carried out as normal, e.g. connecting monitoring devices and performing relevant XRs. Intravenous drugs or fluids should be prepared as normal but not delivered into the venous cannulas. Please note that the main purpose of the simulation is to train team communication, cooperation and leadership during the initial resuscitation and stabilisation of the patient. After the training, there will be a discussion and feedback session, before a second simulator run. The simulations will be video recorded, intended for possible help during the debriefing.

Clinical scenario

The patient is a 24 year-old male who was admitted to the hospital approximately 20 minutes ago with signs of severe sepsis. He has been ill for 4 days, with fever and malaise. He has open airways, is breathing spontaneously at a rate of 34 breaths a minute, reacting to painful stimuli by eye opening, swearing, and localising pain. He is very pale, and the skin is cold and damp. He has pale-blue extremities. Please, go ahead and perform an initial assessment and resuscitation.

The structure for team debriefing and reflection as used in the BEST-programme is described here:

1. Participants' own opinions on the simulation in general

Take a short session where all the participants have the possibility for "tension release".

Let them comment briefly on questions like: "How did the simulation affect you?" and ask the participants to focus especially on the posi-

tive aspects of the simulation. The team leader is the last person to comment on the performance, so that the team is not "silenced" by the leader before they are able to make their own remarks.

2. Short feedback from the instructor focusing on the successful aspects

Explain to the participants that feedback related to the professional content will be given in connection with review of the videotape.

3. The professional content in the simulation

These include order of actions, important decisions to be made, efforts to initiate, and equipment needed. Give all the participants a chance to suggest improvements. The instructor then sums up by writing all the suggestions e.g. on a whiteboard. This is an important part of the feedback session as the participants by proposing improvements themselves will be responsible for improving issue in the ICU environment. Normally this is a good time for the instructor to give a short feedback on the professional content.

4. Show some of the video footage

Everyone wants to see themselves on the video at the same time as they are a bit scared or embarrassed by the idea. It might be a good idea to show the first five minutes of the video only commenting in general terms. Further on, the feedback session should focus on the previously stated objectives for the simulation. The main objectives are demonstration of improved cooperation, communication, and leadership behaviour. It might be a good idea to start every round with a brief definition of successful objectives.

5. Summing up and closing remarks

It seems important that every participant leave the room with a feeling that they all had a chance to comment on the simulation. Remember that it is the whole team which should be the main focus, not individuals. Closing up the session should therefore include questions like "Are there any other issues, aspects etc. that haven't been asked for and that you would like to comment on?" It might also be a good idea to ask if there is need for any subsequent theoretical sessions that can be part of the unit's regular educational programme in the ICU. It is also recommended to tell the team that the video will be destroyed and not stored or used for any reprimanding of individuals.

Use of video

Video recording of the simulation can be useful for highlighting certain aspects of the team's performance [47]. However, there is no need for sophisticated audio-visual equipment. A simple video camera will do, preferable fitted with a wide-angle lens, since many treatment rooms are rather small. On the other hand, a wireless microphone is nice to have, since it will enhance the sound quality of the communication, if it is placed over the "patient". We also recommend placing the camera high in the room, with the "patient" centred, and maintaining a steady view throughout the session. Trying to follow e.g. the team leader or specific procedures will often result in a busy "music video" recording that will be difficult to follow during the viewing. Likewise, it is highly recommended to test the equipment for sound, light, recording quality, battery capacity, and replay on the actual projector or TV-set to be used. Your ability to fix technical problems should not be the main part of the debriefing session.

Example of the BEST trauma team training course

The one-day multi-professional course with simulated trauma patients is organised locally at each hospital, and the training takes place in each hospital's own trauma room [48]. The one-day course consists of three hours of lectures and case discussions, followed by four hours of practical training. All personnel involved in trauma treatment participate on the lectures, which are followed by the simulation where two of the hospitals' own trauma teams participate in two simulation sessions each. The course focuses on the need for optimal team function and a strict and hierarchical progression in the patient assessment and treatment. The theory is based on current best practice principles, but the course elab-

orates significantly more on communication, co-operation and leadership. Case stories and instructors are from identifiable hospital levels. Discussions and didactic exchange of ideas and experience is encouraged throughout the course. Training takes place in the trauma room using a standard resuscitation mannequin as the simulated patient. After a brief review of the emergency call to the medical dispatch centre, the team is given a few minutes to plan and prepare for admitting the simulated patient.

The teams use their own familiar team set-up and procedures, and all necessary disposable equipment. Each team member plays his/her own professional role. A short report from the ambulance crew is also given to the participants before the simulated patient arrives, to encourage preparations. The preparation and treatment of the simulated victim is video-recorded. During the simulation the instructor will give the physiological data after each monitoring or diagnostic procedure has been performed properly.

After approximately 20–30 minutes, or when the patient and team are ready to leave the emergency room for e.g. the OP theatre or XR-lab, the instructor stops the simulation. After the simulation, the complete team is debriefed in a separate room (without observers), reviewing the video using a structured format focusing on what went in a good manner and what can be improved. This session normally takes 30–40 minutes. A second simulation is then done with the same team, but with a new case. Debriefing is done again, and finally the team is encouraged to summarise areas of potential improvement discovered during the simulation and discussions. If possible, the staff that not participating in the simulation discusses case stories in a theoretical format during the simulations. The simulation case histories are based on real cases, with appropriate XR films and lab results. After the course, all educational material (CD-ROM) is left at the hospital, and the hospital is encouraged to copy and edit this material, in order to arrange for further local training.

Conclusion

There are many situations in the ICU that can be trained in a simulator setting. Especially emergency situations should be trained this way. Speed and correct completion of life-saving procedures is important for patient outcome. This normally relies heavily on so many local circumstances that there is always room for improvement. For more than 14 years the BEST Foundation has used interdisciplinary team training based on AE reports, and we firmly believe that such training increases the emergency teams' robustness to AE and ability to handle critical incidents. Building team resilience against safety threats is perhaps the most effective strategy in our search towards safer health care. Simulator team training in the ICU must be explored and refined further to meet the needs for cost-effectiveness.

The author

Guttorm Brattebø, MD
> Consulting Anaesthetist | Department of Anaesthesia and Intensive Care | Haukeland University Hospital | Bergen, Norway
> Board Chairman | The BEST Foundation: Better & Systematic Trauma Care

Address for correspondence
> Guttorm Brattebø
> Haukeland University Hospital
> 5021 Bergen, Norway
> E-mail: guttorm.brattebo@helse-bergen.no

References

1. Kohn LT, Corrigan JM, Donaldson MS. To err is human: building a safer health system. Washington, DC: National Academy Press, 1999.
2. Baker GR, Norton PG, Flintoft V, Blais R, Brown A, Cox J, et al. The Canadian adverse events study: the incidence of adverse events among hospital patients in Canada. CMAJ 2004;170:1678–86.
3. Schioler T, Lipczak H, Pedersen BL, Mogensen TS, Bech KB, Stockmarr A, et al. Danish adverse event study. [Incidence of adverse events in hospitals. A retrospective study of medical records]. Ugeskr Laeger 2001;163:5370–8.
4. The joint commission. Root causes of sentinel events. http://www.jointcommission.org/NR/rdonlyres/FA465646-5F5F-4543-AC8FE8AF6571E372/0/root_cause_se.jpg.
5. Stein-Parbury J, Liaschenko J. Understanding collaboration between nurses and physicians as knowledge at work. Am J Crit Care 2007;16:470–7.
6. Pronovost PJ, Thompson DA, Holzmueller CG, Lubomski

LH, Dorman T, Dickman F, et al. Toward learning from patient safety reporting systems. J Crit Care 2006;21:305–15.
7. Williams R, Silverman R, Schwind C, Fortune JB, Sutyak J, Horvath KD, et al. Surgeon information transfer and communication: factors affecting quality and efficiency of inpatient care. Ann Surg 2007;245:159–71.
8. Vincent C, Taylor-Adams S, Chapman EJ, Hewett D, Prior S, Strange P, et al. BMJ 2000;320:320:777–81.
9. Lewis G (ed). Executive summary and key recommendations. The confidential enquiry into maternal and child health (CEMACH). The seventh report on confidential enquiries into maternity deaths in the UK: 2003-CEMACH: London, 2007. www.cemach.org.uk.
10. Brindley PG. Patient safety and acute care medicine: lessons for the future, insights from the past. Critical Care 2010;14:217.
11. Aron D, Headrick L. Educating physicians prepared to improve care and safety is no accident: It requires a systematic approach. Qual Saf Health Care 2002;11:168–73.
12. Manser T. Teamwork and patient safety in dynamic domains of healthcare: a review of the literature. Acta Anaesthesiol Scand 2009;53:143–51.
13. Reader TW, Flin R, Cuthbertson BH. Communication skills and error in the intensive care unit. Curr Opin Crit Care 2007;13:732–6.
14. Jain M, Miller L, Belt D, King D, Berwick DM. Decline in ICU adverse events, nosocomial infections and cost through a quality improvement initiative focusing on teamwork and culture change. Qual Saf Healthcare 2006;15:235–9.
15. Christian CK, Gustafson ML, Roth EM, Sheridan TB, Gandhi TK, Dwyer K, et al. A prospective study of patient safety in the operating room. Surgery 2006;139:159–73.
16. Greenberg C, Regenbogen S, Studdert D, Lipsitz SR, Rogers SO, Zinner MJ, et al. Patterns of communication breakdown resulting in injury to surgical patients. J Am Coll Surg 2007;204:533–40.
17. Perkins GD. Simulation in resuscitation training. Resuscitation 2007;73:202–11.
18. Salas E, DiazGranados D, Weaver SJ, King H. Does team training work? Principles for health care. Acad Emerg Med 2008;15:1002–9.
19. Helmreich RL, Merritt AC. Culture at work in aviation and medicine. National, Organizational and Professional Influences. Aldershot, UK: Ashgate, 1998.
20. Dunn W, Murphy JG. Simulation: About safety, not fantasy. Chest 2008;133:6–9
21. Pronovost P, Weast B, Schwarz M, Wyskiel RM, Prow D, Milanovich SN, et al. Medication reconciliation: a practical tool to reduce the risk of medication errors. J Crit Care 2003;18:201–5.
22. Kozer E, Seto W, Verjee Z, Parshuram C, Khattak S, Koren G, et al. Prospective observational study on the

incidence of medication errors during simulated resuscitation in a paediatric emergency department. BMJ 2004;329;1321–5.

23. Klein G. The sources of power: how people make decisions. Massachusetts: MIT Press, 1998.

24. Reader T, Flin R, Lauche K, Cuthbertson BH. Nontechnical skills in the intensive care unit. Br J Anaesth 2006;96:551–9.

25. Fletcher G, Flin R, McGeorge P, Glavin R, Maran N, Patey R. Anaesthetists' Non-Technical Skills (ANTS): evaluation of a behavioural marker system. Br J Anaesth 2003;90:580–8.

26. Cook RI. A brief look at gaps in the continuity of care and how practitioners compensate for them. www.ctlab.org.

27. Wisborg T, Rønning TH, Beck VB, Brattebø G. Preparing teams for low-frequency emergencies in Norwegian hospitals. Acta Anaesthesiol Scand 2003: 47:1248–50.

28. Sexton JB, Thomas EJ, Helmreich RL. Error, stress, and teamwork in medicine and aviation: cross sectional surveys. BMJ 2000;320:745–9.

29. Esposito TJ, Sanddal TL, Reynolds SA, Sanddal ND. Effect of a voluntary trauma system on preventable death and inappropriate care in a rural state. J Trauma 2003;54:663–70.

30. Fletcher GCL, McGeorge P, Flin RH, Glavin RJ, Maran NJ. The role of non-technical skills in anaesthesia: a review of current literature. Br J Anaesth 2002;88:418–29.

31. Haig KM, Sutton S, Whittington J. SBAR: Ashared mental model for improving communication between clinicians. Jt Comm J Qual Patient Saf 2006;32:167–75.

32. Jeffcott SA, Mackenzie CF. Measuring team performance in healthcare: review of research and implications for patient safety. J Crit Care 2008;23:188–96.

33. Malhotra S, Jordan D, Shortliffe E, Patel VL. Workflow modelling in critical care: piecing together your own puzzle. J Biomed Inform 2007;40:81–92.

34. Lingard L, Whyte S, Espin S, Baker GR, Orser B, Doran D. Towards safer interprofessional communication: constructing a model of "utility" from preoperative team briefings. J Interprof Care 2006;20:471–83.

35. Pronovost PJ, Berenholtz SM, Dorman T, et al. Improving communications in the ICU using daily goals. J Crit Care 2003;18:71–5.

36. Fernandez R, Kozlowski SWJ, Shapiro MJ, Salas E. Toward a definition of teamwork in emergency medicine. Acad Emerg Med 2008;15:1104–12.

37. Fernandez R, Vozenilek JA, Hegarty CB, Motola I, Reznek M, Phrampus PE, et al. Developing expert medical teams: toward an evidence-based approach. Acad Emerg Med 2008;15:1025–36.

38. Kyrkjebø JM, Brattebø G, Smith-Strøm H. Improving patient safety by using interprofessional simulation training in health professional education. J Interprof Care 2006;20:1–10.

39. Ende J. Feedback in clinical medical education. JAMA 1983.250.777–81.

40. Cooper JB, Taqueti VR. A brief history of the development of mannequin simulators for clinical education and training. Postgrad Med J 2008;84:563–70.

41. Kyle RR, Murray WB (eds). Clinical simulation: operations, engineering and management. Burlington, MA: Academic Press, 2008.

42. Guise JM, Segel S. Teamwork in obstetric critical care. Best Pract Res Clin Obstet Gynaecol 2008;22:937–51.

43. Nuckols TK, Paddock SM, Bower AG, Rothschild JM, Fairbanks RJ, Carlson B, Panzer RJ, Hilborne LH. Costs of intravenous adverse drug events in academic and non-academic intensive care units. Med Care 2008;46:17–24.

44. Ford DG, Seybert AL, Smithburger PL, Kobulinsky LR, Samosky JT, Kane-Gill SL. Impact of simulation-based learning on medication error rates in critically ill patients. Intensive Care Med 2010 Mar 19. [Epub ahead of print].

45. Salas E, Almeida SA, Salisbury M, King H, Lazzara EH, Lyons R, et al. What are the critical success factors for team training in health care? Joint Commission J Quality Patient Safety 2009;35:398–405.

46. Wisborg T, Brattebø G. Keeping the spirit high: why trauma team training is (sometimes) implemented. Acta Anaesthesiol Scand 2008;52:437–41.

47. Mackenzie CF, Xiao Y, Hu FM, Seagull FJ, Fitzgerald M. Video as a tool for improving tracheal intubation tasks for emergency medical and trauma care. Ann Emerg Med 2007;50:436–42.

48. Wisborg T, Brattebø G, Brinchmann-Hansen Å, Uggen PE, Hansen KS. Effects of nationwide training of multi-professional trauma teams in Norwegian hospitals. J Trauma 2008;64:1613–8.

Kirsten Colpaert and Johan Decruyenaere

Electronic prescribing: minimal requirements

Introduction

The prescribing and administrating of medication represents a substantial part of today's medicine. Therefore, it is particularly cumbersome to note that an extensive number of reports have revealed large scales of error within these processes [1–8]. Already more than a decade ago, the IOM declared that at least 44,000 to 88,000 medical defects occur annually as a result of medication errors in the United States [9]. The cost associated with preventable adverse drug events is estimated to be as high as 17 to 29 billion dollars [9]. Based on these data, electronic prescribing has been advocated as a means of reducing medication errors, in order to deliver higher quality care while at the same time decreasing costs [10–13]. However, many hospitals still refrain from such information technology (IT), because of the high cost, the technical implementation, the unclear cost-effectiveness and the reluctance of physicians to accept and use new IT systems. This is clearly demonstrated by the persistently low adoption rates, which, according to the most recent surveys, vary between 5 and 17 % [14–17]. The recent survey by Aarts et al. shows that the adoption rate of electronic prescribing is apparently more pronounced in high-tech hospital environments such as intensive care units (ICU) [18]. But even in ICUs, implementation rates are low, and vary between 5 % to 22 % [19–22].

Furthermore, it is important to realize that IT implementation projects in general are often not successful, with figures varying between 40 % and 70 % [23–26], and that even up to 19 % may fail outright [26]. Unfortunately, only a small number of data is available on IT implementation failures in the health care domain, because most are covered up, ignored or rationalized [27]. Examples of failures are implementations which are suspended or only partially developed because of protests by physicians, extreme overspending, errors and delays [27]. Recently, the US's Joint Commission on Accreditation of Healthcare Organizations pointed out the problem of medical errors' emergence through poor design and implementation of health IT [28–30], and even issued a sentinel alert recommending good management practices [31].

What is electronic prescribing?

Depending on the country, the electronic prescription of medication may be referred to under various names. In the UK, it is called "electronic prescribing", which refers to "the utilization of electronic systems to facilitate and enhance the communication of a prescription or medicine order, aiding in the choice, administration and supply of a medicine through knowledge and decision support ..." [32].

In the USA on the other hand, the most commonly used term is CPOE, which originally stood for "Computerized Physician Order Entry". However, since the prescribing author has shifted from physician to other groups of staff (e.g. nursing staff, etc.) this term is referred to nowadays as "Computerized Provider Order Entry". CPOE sometimes also encompasses medical orders other than drug prescriptions, as laboratory tests, imaging and many other activities may be involved.

In this review we focus exclusively on electronic medication prescribing, and will use the term "Electronic Prescribing" (EP).

Level of Electronic Prescribing

Most studies evaluating electronic prescribing in ICU used home grown systems [33–42]. Currently however, the development of home grown systems has become virtually unachievable, as a result of the complexity of the software needed and the necessity of interfacing the system with other software systems, e.g. electronic patient record (EPR), syringe pumps, etc.. Today, ICUs have the choice between implementing:

1. an electronic prescription tool which is part of the hospital's health information system (HIS);
2. a standalone electronic prescription system, which preferentially has a linkage to the HIS (especially EPR, pharmacy and billing department);
3. an intensive care information system (ICIS), which always comes with CPOE built-in, and usually has at least some basic form of clinical decision support (CDS) incorporated.

A wide variety of EP systems is available on the market, all having different functionalities and lay-outs. A basic EP system already has some inherent and important benefits over paper-based prescribing: it avoids handwriting errors and the need for rewriting daily paper charts, thereby diminishing transcription errors; it allows for the use of order sets and assists for the preferential use of local formulary drugs. Depending on the linkage with the hospital information system, it

improves turnaround times of drugs and improves prescription handling by linking with the pharmacy department, and creates potential for automated billing.

Nowadays, increasingly complex EP systems with incorporated CDS are available on the market (see Tab. 1). These are especially useful in the ICU, as it is a highly sophisticated environment with a large number of monitors and other high-tech devices. CDS tools can steer physicians in making appropriate decisions based on medical evidence. It uses information both actively and passively in order to prevent errors of omission or commission and, as such, interacts with the workflow of the nurse and/or physician and intervenes at opportune moments to inform and advise. Errors of commission are more readily available, for example, during the prescription of an incorrect dose of a drug, a notification will appear prompting that corrective measures should be taken. However, errors of omission are far more difficult to implement and configure, as this warrants the detection of an error that has not yet occurred. There are

Tab. 1   Clinical decision support functionalities (in order of level of complexity)

Drug-allergy screening

Drug-drug interactions

Drug dosage screening according to:
- renal function
- age
- laboratory results (e.g. drug levels)

Drug choice screening according to:
- documented co-morbidities
- laboratory results (e.g. diuretics in case of hypokalaemia, antibiotics related to available microbiology)
- patients' status (e.g. if enteral feeding works switch to an enteral formula instead of an intravenous administration)

Access to decision support tools and/or alerting devices
- integration with local/standard guidelines
- suggestion of more cost-effective alternatives
- suggestion of appropriate duration of drug therapy
- prevention of error of commission/omission

two levels at which such errors of omission occur: synchronous errors of omission (i.e. on prescribing or entering the system, for instance the detection of not entering allergy data at the time of prescribing antibiotics), or asynchronous errors (i.e. detection of failure of prescription of antibiotics for a patient with a high temperature and increasing evidence of a new infection; the failure of administration of antibiotics within 2 hours after dialysis). To date, however, only a few commercial systems are capable of delivering built-in rule engines capable of generating this kind of alerts.

Key factors for successful implementation

The adoption of health IT requires a substantial increase in investment by hospitals, so that logically, it is of utmost importance that the probability of implementation failures is kept to an absolute minimum. Although many organizations are reluctant to publish anything on these problems, the available literature shows that frequently reported causes of implementation failures stem from poor project planning, poor communication, and lack of end-user involvement.

We will discuss five important issues which are crucial for successful implementation:

- management,
- hardware,
- software,
- the implementation process itself, and
- end-user acceptance.

Management

Although there is currently widespread agreement about the importance of health IT investment [43], the lack of clear financial benefits continuously feeds the recurrent question as to whether these investments are justified. Unfortunately, the economic impact of health IT investment is difficult to evaluate, and computers are unlikely to impact standard markers of outcomes such as mortality, length of ICU or hospital stay, drug expenditure and quality of life after ICU/hospital discharge. On the other hand, it is rather difficult to evaluate the "Total Cost of Ownership (TCO)" of an IT system beforehand, as this is defined as the total cost of acquiring, installing, using, maintaining, changing and upgrading this system over its predicted useful lifespan. Moreover, the normal tools used by managers, such as cost-benefit analyses or other return on investment methods, are not very helpful [44]. Typically, cost-benefit analyses [45–48] focus mainly on indirect earnings (e.g. quality and continuity of care, users' satisfaction, and process optimization) transformed into the monetary value of implementing a particular clinical information system component (e.g. CPOE, clinical decision support (CDS) or picture archiving and communications systems (PACS)) [44, 49–54]. Another frequently underestimated problem is the typical delay between technology implementation and its perceived benefits [55]. For instance, all the cost-benefit analyses of implementing an EHR system recently as described in the taskforce document by Shekelle et al. predicted that the financial benefits would significantly outweigh the costs in a timeframe that varied from three to thirteen years [45]. Yet another report stated that cost reductions in EHR could be made in the same year, but generally would take 2–5 years to break even [55]. Unfortunately, the overall ROI of a single project, such as the implementation of EP, is more difficult to determine, since related studies are mostly limited to the impact on medication errors, adverse drug events or workflow, thereby neglecting the overall added project value at a strategic level [56].

The Chief Information Officer (CIO) is crucial to the process of implementing health IT, as his/her job is to focus resources in implementing the right systems in the right sequence at the right time, thereby allowing information to flow actively from those who know to those who need to know [57]. Unfortunately, it will always be an imbalance between what the CIO wants, and what the CEO provides. It is, however, important that a shared vision is clearly stated, and careful integrated planning is made. This requires multidisciplinary teams at all levels of management (clinical, administrative) who all know what goals have to be met. The Japanese saying: "Vision without action is a daydream; action without vision is a nightmare", applies perfectly well here.

Hardware

It is obvious that specific computer hardware forms an essential part of electronic prescribing. However, this depends greatly on each particular hospital situation and the network and hardware already available. There are several key elements for EP implementation, which are listed below:

1. **Central and/or bedside workstations:** crucial for user acceptance is the availability of a sufficient number of personal computers (PCs). According to a Canadian survey by Lapinsky et al., the threshold for the perception of an adequate number of workstations in the ICU is 0.44 computers per bed [19]. Also Holden et al. found in a very recent questionnaire that a lack of computer stations precludes volitional EP use [58]. Mobile PCs include laptops, tablet PCs or personal digital assistants (PDAs). Laptops allow for more functionalities but require a trolley to be put on. Furthermore, even laptops usually do not have large enough screens to allow two or more health care workers to work with them simultaneously, and this can impede normal workflow, for instance during ward rounds [59].

2. **Network infrastructure:** this is essential for the server-client software architecture and for linkage to the different hospital information systems, as well as the billing and stock department.

3. **Server and back-up server systems:** the EP software runs on the server. In case of a server breakdown (which one can never rule out), there needs to be an immediately available thorough backup plan together with a backup server.

4. **Paper:** in case of a system breakdown, one needs to guarantee high quality patient care. Particularly in the ICU, it is advocated to always have backup files of the medication and fluids administered, as well as the most crucial monitoring data from the previous 24 hours. In that way, one is able to print out these recent files, and continue patient care while avoiding serious problems related to drug therapy. Furthermore, as is mentioned in the study by Morrison [59], the paper printouts containing basic information on every admitted patient in the ICU for each member of the medical staff helped them orient themselves towards interaction during daily ward rounds. This is a common finding across the various sectors [60].

Software

Is there a potential benefit of an advanced EP system with sophisticated CDS, and does this outweigh the extra cost and more complex implementation process? Furthermore, is there a linear relationship between level of IT and benefit, or is there a threshold for a minimum level of CDS functionalities?

Unfortunately, although we expect that most benefit is to be gained from more sophisticated systems, the answer is not as straightforward as it seems.

From the literature, we know that not all CPOE systems show beneficial effect, and especially older systems tend to have problems arising from poor man-machine interfacing, where many screens are needed in order to make a medication prescription [30]. More recent technologies however have user interfaces that are far more intuitive and better designed to fit physician workflow.

Clinical decision support systems also come in many different forms [61] and can be implemented in many different ways, thereby making an evaluation of these systems a daunting task. By now, many studies have clearly shown beneficial effects of clinical decision support [62–66], while others were unable to show improved quality of care [62]. The question here arises as to whether the "failure" is due to poorly designed decision support technology, or to poor use of the technology by physicians. Furthermore, most of the reports of successful decision support systems come from sites that have self-developed rather than commercial systems [67]. Wright et al. [61] have reported that not all commercially available clinical information systems have the same decision support capabilities, and the best system in their review had only one missing feature from a total of 42 predefined clinical decision support contents [68], while the worst system missed out on 18. This marked variability should alert future CPOE purchasers to exercise careful perseverance to ensure that the preferred CPOE system will meet their needs. It is worth noting that the introduction of advanced CDS has potential pitfalls in itself, because frequent alerts and warnings can interrupt workflow thereby causing messages to be ignored or overridden. Generating alerts for everything will surely cause alert fatigue, which is known to be a cause of decreased beneficial effects.

Thus, it seems that there is no real answer to the question of "what is required minimally?" The answer seems to be "the more complex, the better", although special care should be taken finding a perfect balance between benefits and alert fatigue. And furthermore, complex systems require considerably more implementation knowledge and efforts than more simple electronic prescription tools.

The implementation process

Apparently, the potential benefits not only depend on the choice of a particular EP system but perhaps even more on the way the system is being configured and implemented. This is clearly illustrated in the following two studies evaluating the implementation of CPOE in paediatric hospitals. The first study by Han et al. [28] found an unexpected increase in mortality to be coincident with the implementation of CPOE in their paediatric ICU. However, a second investigation by Delbeccaro et al. [29], using the same CPOE system, was published one year later but could not confirm this, and even described a trend toward decreased mortality 5 months after implementation. The same commercial CPOE system was used in both hospitals, and both institutions configured and used real-time decision support in the form of allergy checking, dose checking, and custom rules. However, the major difference lay in the pre-configuration of order sets: In the study by Han, no ICU-specific order sets had been programmed at the time of CPOE implementation but instead these were developed over time after the implementation. On the other hand, the other study by Delbeccaro preconfigured 230 disease and/or departmental order sets, 2,500 order "sentences", and a high degree of filtering (code-set filtering) that was designed to provide the most frequently needed orders while minimizing the number of "clicks" required by a provider to enter an order. Further-

more, similar and frequently ordered medications and infusions, laboratory, radiology, and nursing care order sentences combined with order sets were built in before the implementation. These were all evaluated by multidisciplinary workgroups. The second important difference was the degree of training and support delivered: in the first centre, training was begun approximately 3 months before CPOE implementation, through a mandatory 3-hour computer tutorial and practice session. Designated CPOE experts were present to provide "hands-on" consultation support during the immediate post implementation period, after which support was reduced to telephone consultation. In the second centre, training also began several months before implementation, though the training was role specific and ranged between 2 and 4 hours at a minimum, and additional training help was provided if deemed necessary. Each discipline also designated certain individuals who received extra training and were dubbed "super users". These super users helped in training others and providing peer support in the clinical units during and after the implementation. Additional extensive go-live support was provided in house 24 hours a day for 2 weeks and then tapered over the next week. Thus, it seems that the well-prepared implementation strategy, together with the intense training and support of users, reported in the study of Delbeccaro et al. resulted in a beneficial CPOE implementation.

This example stresses once again that it is complex, labour-intensive and costly to set up EP systems properly. Furthermore, they will need to be updated continuously for configuration of new drugs, for fixing bugs and for installing updates. According to Leah Binder, Leapfrog's CEO, hospitals face the challenge of customizing the off-the-shelf software to meet their specific needs, as these are not plug-and-play systems [68].

End-user acceptance

One of the most important and prevalent barriers to successful CPOE implementation is resistance by physicians [70]. Health IT can only improve health care outcomes when it is accepted and used effectively by clinicians [70–71]. In order to accomplish this, the full engagement of physicians throughout planning and implementation of CPOE is essential. They must comprehend and share the vision of the organization. According to a Holden et al., numerous studies have shown that even the most motivated and safety oriented clinicians do not always use available IT [72–74]. They often override or work around it [76–77], or use only some of the available features [78–79]. Success stories from numerous hospitals restate the importance of "special people" [80], i.e. those high-level leaders and technical specialists who assist physicians in using EP.

Last but not least, there is the underestimated factor of speed regarding end-user acceptance. Speed is even the parameter that users value most [81], and is rated much higher than quality improvement aspects. At our centre, we recently had a problem with a dramatically slower ICIS after upgrading, which caused an immediate marked decline in user satisfaction, and a demand to return to the previous version (with less decision support). Fortunately, the problems could be solved after identifying and eliminating the bugs.

Conclusion

Electronic drug prescribing has been advocated as a means of reducing medication errors, in order to deliver a higher quality of care while at the same time decreasing costs. However, the realisation of these benefits is not obvious and therefore, a thorough software implementation strategy is essential in order to minimize the occurrence of new medication errors or adverse drug events. Electronic prescribing depends on an appropriate level of clinical decision support combined with a well-thought-out software configuration. Moreover, the speed of the system together with an intuitive user-interface are additional key elements for optimal end-user acceptance.

The authors

Kirsten Colpaert, MD[1]
Johan Decruyenaere, MD, PhD[2]
   [1]Intensivist | Department of Intensive Care
   Medicine | Ghent University Hospital |
   Ghent, Belgium

[2]Professor of Medicine, Head of
Department | Department of Intensive
Care Medicine | Ghent University Hospital |
Ghent, Belgium

Address for correspondence
   Kirsten Colpaert
   Department of Intensive Care Medicine
   Ghent University Hospital
   De Pintelaan 185
   9000 Ghent, Belgium
   E-mail: kirsten.colpaert@ugent.be

References

1. Donchin Y, Gopher D, Olin M. A look into the nature and causes of human errors in the intensive care unit. Crit Care Med 1995;23(2):294–300.
2. Bates DW, Cullen DJ, Laird N, Petersen LA, Small SD, Servi D et al. Incidence of adverse drug events and potential adverse drug events. Implications for prevention. ADE prevention Study Group. JAMA 1995;274(1):29–34.
3. Leape LL, Bates DW, Cullen DJ, Cooper J, Demonaco H, Gallivan T et al. Systems analysis of adverse drug events. ADE Prevention Study Group. JAMA 1995;274(1):35–43.
4. Colpaert K, Decruyenaere J. Computerized physician order entry in critical care. Best Pract Res Clin Anaesthesiol. 2009 Mar;23(1):27–38.
5. Moyen E, Camiré E, Stelfox HT. Clinical review: Medication errors in critical care. Crit Care 2008;12(2):208.
6. Colpaert K, Claus B, Somers A, Vandewoude K, Robays H, Decruyenaere J. Impact of computerized physician order entry on medication prescription errors in the intensive care unit: a controlled cross-sectional trial. Crit Care. 2006 Feb;10(1):R21.
7. Cullen DJ, Bates DW, Leape LL. Adverse Drug Event Prevention Study Group. Prevention of adverse drug events: a decade of progress in patient safety. J Clin Anesth 2000;12(8):600–14.
8. Herout PM, Erstad BL. Medication errors involving continuously infused medications in a surgical intensive care unit. Crit Care Med 2004;32(2):428–32.
9. Kohn LT, Corrigan J, Donaldson MS. Institute of Medicine. To Err Is Human: Building a Safer Health System. Washington, DC: National Academia Press;1999
10. Bates DW, Leape LL, Cullen DJ, Laird N, Peterson L, Teich J et al. Effect of computerized physician order entry and a team intervention on prevention of serious medication errors. JAMA: The Journal of the American Medical Association 1998; 280(15): 1311–1316.
11. Bates DW, Teich JM, Lee J et al. The impact of computerized physician order entry on medication

errorprevention. Journal of the American Medical Informatics Association 1999 Jul–Aug; 6(4): 313–321.

12. Evans RS, Pestotnik SL, Classen DC. Preventing adverse drug events in hospitalized patients. Ann Pharmacother 1994;28(4):523–7.

13. The leapfrog Group for Patient Safety: Rewarding Higher Standards. www.Leapfroggroup.org. Accessed 16–06–2008.

14. Kuperman GJ, Bobb A, Payne TH, Avery AJ, Gandhi TK, Burns G et al. Medication-related clinical decision support in computerized provider order entry systems: a review. Journal of the American Medical Informatics Association 2007; 14(1): 29–40.

15. Ash JS, Gorman PN, Seshadri V, Hersh WR. Computerized physician order entry in U.S. hospitals: results of a 2002 survey. J Am Med Inform Assoc. 2004;11(2):95–9.

16. Cutler DM, Feldman NE, Horwitz JR. U.S. adoption of computerized physician order entry systems. Health Aff. 2005;24(6):1654–63.

17. Jha AK, DesRoches CM, Campbell EG, Donelan K, Rao SR, Ferris TG et al. Use of electronic health records in U.S. hospitals. N Engl J Med. 2009;360(16):1628–38.

18. Aarts J, Koppel R. Implementation of computerized physician order entry in seven countries. Health Aff. 2009;28(2):404–14.

19. Lapinsky SE, Holt D, Hallett D et al. Survey of information technology in Intensive Care Units in Ontario, Canada. BMC Medical Informatics and Decision Making 2008;Jan 24:8:5.

20. Levy M. Computers in the ICU. Journal of Critical Care 2004;19(4):199–200.

21. Manjoney R. Clinical information systems market – an insider's view. J Crit Care. 2004 Dec;19(4):215–20.

22. Amarasingham R, Pronovost PJ, Diener-West M, Goeschel C, Dorman T, Thiemann DR, Powe NR. Measuring clinical information technology in the ICU setting: application in a quality improvement collaborative. J Am Med Inform Assoc. 2007;14(3):288–94.

23. ITCortex. Failure rate: Statistics over IT projects failure rate. Available at: http://www.it-cortex.com/Stat-Failure_Rate.htm. Accessed: April 16,2010.

24. Lewis B. The 70-percent failure. InfoWorld. Available at: http://infoworld.com/articles/op/xml/01/10/29/011029/opsurvival.xml. Accessed: April 16,2010.

25. McManus J, Wood-Harper T. Understanding the sources of information systems project failure. Manag Serv 2007 (Autumn): 38–43.

26. Rubinstein D Standish Group. Report: There's Less Development CHAOS Today. vol 1, March: SDTimes, 2007. Available at: http://www.sdtimes.com/content/article.aspx?ArticleID-30247. Accessed: April 16,2010.

27. Kaplan B, Harris-Salamone KD. Health IT success and failure: recommendations from literature and an AMIA workshop. J Am Med Inform Assoc. 2009;16(3):291–9.

28. Han Y, Carcillo J, Venkataraman S, et al. Unexpected increased mortality after implementation of a commercially sold computerized physician order entry system. Pediatrics 2005;116(6):1506–12.

29. Del Beccaro MA, Jeffries HE, Eisenberg MA, Harry ED. Computerized provider order entry implementation: no association with increased mortality rates in an intensive care unit. Pediatrics 2006;118(1):290–5.

30. Koppel R, Metlay JP, Cohen A, et al. Role of computerized physician order entry systems in facilitating medication errors. J Am Med Assoc 2005;293(10):1197–203.

31. Joint Commission on Accreditation of Healthcare Organizations (JCAHO). Safety implementing health information and converging technologies. Sentinel Event Alert 2008, December 11.

32. http://www.connectingforhealth.nhs.uk/. Accessed April 05, 2010

33. Chertow GM, Lee J, Kuperman GJ, Burdick E, Horsky J, Seger DL et al. Guided medication dosing for in-patients with renal insufficiency. JAMA 2001;286(22):2839–44.

34. Peterson JF, Kuperman GJ, Shek C, Patel M, Avorn J, Bates DW. Guided prescription of psychotropic medications for geriatric in-patients. Arch Intern Med 2005;165(7):802–7.

35. Maurer C, Lecointre K, Cachin N, Latawiec K, Ouadfel F, Lahmek P, Fauvelle F, Piquet J. Impact of medical prescription computerisation on the incidence of adverse drug effects. Rev Mal Respir 2003; 20:355–63.

36. Oliven A, Michalake I, Zalman D, Dorman E, Yeshurun D, Odeh M. Prevention of prescription errors by computerized, on-line surveillance of drug order entry. Int J Med Inform 2005;74(5):377–86.

37. Pestotnik SL, Classen DC, Evans RS, Burke JP. Implementing antibiotic practice guidelines through computer-assisted decision support: clinical and financial outcomes. Ann Intern Med 1996;124(10):884–90.

38. Teich JM, Merchia PR, Schmiz JL, Kuperman GJ, Spurr CD, Bates DW. Effects of computerized physician order entry on prescribing practices. Arch Intern Med 2000;160(18):2741–7.

39. Kirk RC, Li-Meng Goh D, Packia J, Min Kam H, Ong BK. Computer calculated dose in paediatric prescribing. Drug Saf 2005;28(9):817–24.

40. Evans R, Pestotnik S, Classen D, et al. A Computer-Assisted Management Programme for Antibiotics and Other Antiinfective Agents. N Engl J Med 1998;338(4):232–260.

41. Mullett CJ, Evans RS, Christenson JC, Dean JM. Development and impact of a computerized paediatric antiinfective decision support programme. Paediatrics 2001;108(4):E75.

42. Potts AL, Barr FE, Gregory DF, Wright L, Patel NR. Computerized physician order entry and medication errors in a paediatric critical care unit. Paediatrics 2004;113:59–63.

43. Blumenthal D. Stimulating the adoption of health information technology. N Engl J Med 2009;360(15):1047-1049.

44. Arlotto P,Oakes J. Return on Investment: Maximizing the Value of Healthcare Information Technology, HIMMS, Chicago, USA, 2003;3-57.

45. Shekelle PG, Morton SC, Keeler EB. Costs and Benefits of Health Information Technology. Evidence Report/ Technology Assessment No. 132. (Prepared by the Southern California Evidence-based Practice Center under Contract No. 290-02-0003.) AHRQ Publication No.06-E006. Rockville, MD: Agency for Healthcare Research and Quality. April 2006.

46. Pekka T, Hannu S. The Economic evaluation of Medical Information Systems. TUCS Center for Computer Science, September 1998; TUCS technical report 195.

47. Gardner RM, Hulse RK, Larsen KG. Assessing the effectiveness of a computerized pharmacy system. Symposium on Computer Applications in Medical Care 1990;14:668-672.

48. Grover V, Jeong SR, Segars AH. Information system effectiveness: the construct pace and patterns of application. Inform Manag 1996;31(4):117-191.

49. Stroetmann KA, Jones T, Dobrev A, Stroetmann VN. eHealth is Worth it: The Economic Benefits of Implemented eHealth Solutions at ten European Sites. Office for Official Publication of the European Communities, Luxembourg 2006;13-30.

50. Menachemi N, Saunders C, Chukmaitov, Brooks RG. Hospital quality of care: does information technology matter? The relationship between information technology adoption and quality of care. Health Care Manag Rev 2008;33(1):51-59.

51. Menachemi N, Brooks RG. Exploring the Return on Investment Associated With Health Information Technologies. Florida State University College of Medicine: Center for Patient Safety 2005;15-45.

52. Barlow S, Johnson J, Steck J. The economic effect of implementing an EMR in an outpatient clinical setting. J Healthc Inf Manag 2004;18(1):46-51.

53. Cooper J. Organization management, implementation and value of EHR implementation in a Solo pediatric practice. J Healthc Inf Manag 2004;18(3):51-55.

54. Wang SJ, Middleton B, Prosser LA, Bardon CG, Carchidi PJ,Kittler AF et al. A cost-benefit analysis of electronic medical records in primary care. Am J Med 2003;114(5):397-403.

55. Beard N, Elo K, Hitt L-M, Housman MG, Mansfield G. Information technology and hospital performance: an econometric analysis of costs and quality. (Accessed April 5, 2010, at http://www.pwc.com/healthcare).

56. Meyer R, Degoulet P. Choosing the right amount of healthcare information technologies investments. Int J Med Inform 2010;79(4):225-31.

57. Cotter CM. Computerized physician order entry from a chief information officer perspective. J Crit Care 2004;19(4):283-9.

58. Holden RJ. Physicians' beliefs about using EMR and CPOE: in pursuit of a contextualized understanding of health IT use behavior. Int J Med Inform 2010;79(2):71-80.

59. Morrison C, Jones M, Blackwell A, Vuylsteke A. Electronic patient record use during ward rounds: a qualitative study of interaction between medical staff. Crit Care 2008;12(6):R148.

60. Sellen AJ, Harper RH: The Myth of the Paperless Office Boston: MIT Press; 2001.

61. Wright A, Sittig DF, Ash JS, Sharma S, Pang JE, Middleton B. Clinical decisionsupport capabilities of commercially-available clinical information systems. J Am Med Inform Assoc 2009;16(5):637-44.

62. Garg AX, Adhikari NK, McDonald H, Rosas-Arellano MP, Devereaux PJ, Beyene J et al. Effects of computerized clinical decision support systems on practitioner performance and patient outcomes: a systematic review. JAMA 2005;293(10):1223-38.

63. Rothschild JM, McGurk S, Honour M, Lu L, McClendon AA, Srivastava P et al. Assessment of education and computerized decision support interventions for improving transfusion practice. Transfusion 2007;47(2):228-39.

64. Rana R, Afessa B, Keegan MT, Whalen FX, Nuttall GA, Evenson LK et al. Transfusion in the ICU Interest Group. Evidence-based red cell transfusion in the critically ill: quality improvement using computerized physician order entry. Crit Care Med 2006;34(7):1892-7.

65. Boord JB, Sharifi M, Greevy RA, Griffin MR, Lee VK, Webb TA et al. Computer-based insulin infusion protocol improves glycemia control over manual protocol. J Am Med Inform Assoc 2007;14(3):278-87.

66. Celi LA, Hinske LC, Alterovitz G, Szolovits P. An artificial intelligence tool to predict fluid requirement in the intensive care unit: a proof-of-concept study. Crit Care 2008;12(6):R151.

67. Chaudhry B, Wang J, Wu S, Maglione M, Mojica W, Roth E et al. Systematic review: impact of health information technology on quality, efficiency, and costs of medical care. Ann Intern Med 2006;144(10):742-52.

68. Wright A, Goldberg H, Hongsermeier T, Middleton B. A description and functional taxonomy of rule-based decision support content at a large integrated delivery network. J Am Med Inform Assoc 2007;14(4):489-96.

69. Anderson HJ. CPOE: it don't come easy. Health Data Manag Mag 2009; Jan 01. Accessed online April 20, 2010.

70. Poon EG, Blumenthal D, Jaggi T, Honour MM, Bates DW, Kaushal R. Overcoming the barriers to implementing computerized physician order entry systems in US hospitals: Perspectives from senior management. Health Aff 2004;23(4):184-90.

71. Blumenthal D, Glaser JP. Information technology comes to medicine. N Engl J Med 2007;356:2527–2534.

72. Holden RJ, Karsh B. A theoretical model of health information technology usage behaviour with implications for patient safety. Behav Inform Technol 2009;28:21–38.

73. Zheng K, Padman R, Johnson MP, Diamond HS. Understanding technology adoption in clinical care: clinician adoption behavior of a point-of-care reminder system. Int J Med Inform 2005;74:535–543.

74. Holden RJ, Karsh B. A review of medical error reporting system design considerations and a proposed cross-level system research framework. Hum Factors 2007;49:257–276.

75. Lapointe L, Rivard S. Getting physicians to accept new information technology: insights from case studies. CMAJ 2006;174:1573–1578.

76. Weingart SN, Toth M, Sands DZ, Aronson MD, Davis RB, Phillips RS. Physicians' decisions to override computerized drug alerts in primary care. Arch Intern Med 2003;163:2625–2631.

77. Vogelsmeier AA, Halbesleben JR, Scott-Cawiezzel JR. Technology implementation and workarounds in the nursing home. J Am Med Inform Assoc 2008;15:114–119.

78. Sequist TD, Cullen T, Hays H, Taualii MM, Simon SR, Bates DW. Implementation and use of an electronic health record within the Indian Health Service. J Am Med Inform Assoc 2007;14:191–197.

79. Simon SR, Kaushal R, Cleary PD, Jenter CA, Volk LA, Orav EJ, et al. Physicians and electronic health records: a statewide survey, Arch. Intern. Med. 167 (2007) 507–512.

80. Ash JS, Stavri PZ, Dykstra R, Fournier L. Implementing computerized physician order entry: the importance of special people. Int J Med Inform 2003 Mar;69(2–3):235–50.

81. McDonald CJ, Overhage JM, Mamlin BW, Dexter PD, Tierney WM. Physicians, information technology, and health care systems: a journey, not a destination. J Am Med Inform Assoc. 2004 Mar-Apr;11(2):121–4.

Sten Rubertsson

Should research be together with clinical practice?

Intensive care medicine evolved as a branch of medicine due to the recognition that patients with acute, life-threatening illness or injury could be better treated if they were placed in special units within the hospital. These units became more organized and defined at the beginning of the polio epidemic in 1947–1948 and with the development of mechanical ventilation, during the 1950s. Borås in Sweden, and Copenhagen in Denmark were the first cities to organize these units. The demand for postoperative care due to more and more advanced surgery, and the possibility to treat more sick patients further sped up the development of intensive care units (ICUs).

Most of us believe that science is the foundation for our medical profession and how we practise and treat our patients. This is combined with accumulated experience and knowledge both in the medical community and the individual doctor treating these patients. Even if evidence-based medicine have been acknowledged as a demand for the practice of medicine, intensive care medicine still has a long way to go to be able to fulfil this. This was clearly illustrated in a literature search recently performed and published by Ospina et al. that found rela-

tively few randomized multicentre trials of an intervention in intensive care medicine in order to show a positive or a negative effect on outcome when mortality was used as a primary endpoint [1]. Most of the studies came out with neutral results between interventions. It is a difficult task to design a study dealing with sick ICU patients who display a great heterogeneity in age, underlying diseases, genetic composition etc. Patients cared for in the ICU also have a relatively high mortality compared to other patient categories. Primary outcome measures other than mortality clearly need to be discussed and used. Even if mortality is viewed as the most important outcome, other measures such as a consideration of the number of days cared for in the ICU and morbidity after the ICU treatment are interesting not only for the patient but also in a discussion of resources and finances.

Furthermore, future challenges are already here today with a demand of cost effective health care and patients asking for the best treatment available. Even if the patients cared for in the ICU are most of the time unable to ask for or demand a special treatment, their relatives will increasingly do so in the future. Information regarding available treatment is today more readily available especially due to the fact that the internet is making this possible. To meet this demand we need to have active research and quality assurance of the delivered treatment. Regarding costs we have to remember that the costs per patient day cared for in the ICU is one of the most expensive in health care. We therefore need to motivate this cost for the hospital leaders and also for the politicians. This will not be easy to motivate in the future if we cannot show that treatment with intensive care medicine makes a difference. The only way to get this financial support is to motivate costs documented from an active research community within our ICUs and thereby present reliable data. Therefore leaders within intensive care medicine actively have to include costs for research in their budget presented to hospital leaders. Unfortunately, today the message in most countries from politicians to hospital administrators is that more care has to be provided with less money. To counteract this, both national and international societies in intensive care medicine have to play a more active role by an ongoing dialogue with politicians pointing out the importance of funding active research besides medical care within our ICUs.

Even if today university hospitals are also under more pressure to produce more, usually for less money, it is absolutely vital that research in these institutions is maintained and defended. From these institutions any collaboration with non-university hospitals should not only involve clinical practice but also research. Today there are several networks that have been doing so, the *Australian and New Zealand Intensive Care Society (ANZICS)* and the Canadian Critical Care Trials group (CCCTG) are two of the most successful in this regard. By using networks within research in intensive care medicine, intensivists outside the university hospitals will get more involved and feel that they too can substantially contribute to the progressive development within our medical field.

One key component to achieve this goal is to implement the importance of research together with clinical practice already from the start of the education made available to doctors, nurses and other medical professionals working in the ICUs. This implementation needs to be included not only during their basic education but also during their special training to become intensive care doctors and nurses. If this is accomplished, research projects could be better defended and at the same time be a natural part of the clinical practice. To better understand science and research also makes it easier to evaluate what kind of treatments should be implemented in the ICU care. This is vital for our speciality in justifying our practice.

Intensive care medicine is in most countries a subspecialty or a branch of anaesthesiology or different specialities within internal medicine or surgery. In some countries in Europe, but also in North America, intensive care medicine has gained an individual status and has become an independent specialty. Irrespective of how treatment is organized, intensive care medicine is a multidisciplinary interest. To defend its status within the medical community, collaboration needs to be defended with mutual respect based upon a sound scientific foundation. This is an additional reason why research has to be implemented together with clinical practice within intensive care medicine. We can only gain respect from collaborating colleagues by showing that our treatment of patients in the ICU is based on skills together with a high level of scientific knowledge of our medical field. It could also be expressed as "defeat par excellence" (Åke Grenvik, Professor emeritus, Division of Critical Care Medicine, University of Pittsburgh).

To clearly strengthen our speciality we therefore need to further integrate science within our clinical practice. It has to start by asking appropriate clinical questions and, where appropriate, by addressing them to researchers within basic sciences. The link to basic science need to be emphasized as a vital link for clinical research. Hopefully we then can design studies which will have a better chance to have an impact on treatment and care of our intensive care patients.

One way to do this is to integrate PhD programs into clinical practice. This has been done for many decades in Scandinavian countries. Many of these PhD programs include collaboration with researchers of basic science. Most of the PhD students are recruited already during their training to become a specialist. The program is integrated within their period of clinical training with some time allocated simply for research alone. The PhD program in most places also involves several courses in statistics, epidemiology, scientific design of studies, and evidence-based medicine etc. as granted by the university. Being in possession of a PhD degree is in many university clinics a prerequisite to obtain a position as a senior consultant and at the same time allows a better choice of the future specialist – at least one already having ambitions to stay within an academic institution. Far from all doctors with a PhD degree will stay at the university hospitals but will move to a non-university hospital and thereby bring an academic view to these institutions.

The European Society of Intensive Care Medicine (ESICM) has developed several tools for better support of the education to become an intensive care doctor. The ESICM also took the initiative to develop *CoBaTrICE* which is an international "*Competency Based Training programme in Intensive Care Medicine for Europe and other world regions*" [2]. The *CoBaTrICE* was created to better harmonise training in intensive care medicine worldwide and the project was funded by the European Commission Leonardo da Vinci programme. There are 12 clinical competencies describing the knowledge, skills, attitudes and behaviours required in performing a particular task and what standard that is required in its performance. In addition to these 12 competencies there is a syllabus called basic science including a brief description of research methods. To enforce the importance of a stronger link between research and clinical practice, a thirteenth competency could be created with an expansion of basic science. Another option would be to include in each of the 12 competencies appropriate sections of basic science. Missing knowledge gaps could also be mentioned stimulating an active search for further evidence to clinical practice.

Since 1998, the Scandinavian Society of Anaesthesiology and Intensive Care Medicine (SSAI) has co-ordinated an advanced training program in Intensive Care Medicine [3]. Until today more than 300 fellows have completed the training program in Scandinavia. The training period is 2 years and during the training period, the SSAI organises 6 courses. The trainee is expected to attend the examination for the European Diploma in Intensive Care Medicine and acquire the European Diploma in Intensive Care (EDIC) awarded by the ESICM. Since the

previous program which started in 2009, the fellows will also have to complete a "minor project" during their two-year training. This project could be part of an on-going or recently passed PhD research but could also be a small research project or a quality assurance/development project. This project could take place within their own department or collaboration within the network created by the participants of the program. The aim of this project is to train fellows in science and research to be more able to independently evaluate the literature in regard to how much support for treatments practiced in intensive care medicine is already available. Hopefully, this project will also further stimulate the implementation for research in their clinical practice.

Another threat to the link between research and clinical practice is the fact that the structure for leadership of the departments is changing. This is at least an experience we have in Scandinavia with chairmen of clinical departments having less scientific education. This has even become a reality for leadership in our university hospitals. With this structure there is a potential risk that the link between research and clinical practice could be weakened. For the future we must find a solution to this.

In summary, research should be together with clinical practice, as there is no other option to this.

The author

Sten Rubertsson, MD, PhD, EDIC, FCCM
Professor
Dept. of Surgical Sciences/Anaesthesiology & Intensive Care Medicine, Uppsala University
Uppsala University Hospital
SE-751 85 Uppsala, Sweden
E-mail: sten.rubertsson@akademiska.se

References

1. Ospina-Tascón GA, Büchele GL, Vincent JL. Multicenter, randomized, controlled trials evaluating mortality in intensive care: doomed to fail? Crit Care Med 2008;36:1311–22.
2. http://www.cobatrice.org/en/index.asp3.
3. http://www.ssai.info/Education/ intensive_care_training_program.html.

D. Outcomes

Patient safety – An essential paradigm in intensive care medicine _____ 351
Andreas Valentin

Evaluating and reporting nosocomial infections _____ 359
Stijn I. Blot, Sonia O. Labeau and Jordi Rello

Self-reporting of errors and adverse events in the intensive care unit (ICU) _____ 369
Hans Flaatten

Benchmarking the intensive care unit _____ 375
Rui P. Moreno, Ana Cristina Diogo, Susana Afonso de Carvalho and Andrew Rhodes

Nosocomial infection: outcome indicator? _____ 383
Mercedes Palomar Martínez

The role of risk profile management in the evaluation of the intensive care units _____ 391
Rui P. Moreno, Philipp G.H. Metnitz, Andrew Rhodes and Peter Bauer

Andreas Valentin

Patient safety –
An essential paradigm in intensive care medicine

The classic medical principle of "first, do no harm" refers primarily to the balance of risks and benefits of a specific treatment, but at the same time reflects a basic approach to patient safety. In a more advanced concept patient safety is considered as the assurance that a course of medical treatment will proceed correctly and provide the best possible chance to achieve a desired outcome. This definition is especially important in intensive care medicine. But the complexity of processes and medical conditions dealt with in intensive care units (ICUs) makes the system vulnerable and prone to error [1, 2]. In addition, the definition of intensive care medicine per se includes the care for patients with an inherent risk of an unfavourable outcome. Reducing this risk and enhancing safety for the most severely ill patients represents the very first mission of intensive care medicine [3].

How safe is intensive care?
The scope of the problem

Intensive care is characterised by a complex course of interaction among several medical specialties [4, 5], use of sophisticated healthcare technology [6], and significant time pressure. Considering the tight coupling between the complexity of the system and the high potential for harm

[7], most ICUs seem to function very well. But over the last decade, several articles have revealed a serious safety problem in intensive care medicine. In a landmark study, Donchin recorded an average of 178 activities per patient per day and an estimated number of 1.7 errors per patient per day [1]. A multinational study (Sentinel Events Evaluation) on patient safety in intensive care [8] confirmed that reports from single-centre studies reflect a widespread pattern of susceptibility to error in ICUs. In that study, 38.8 events per 100 patient days were detected in five categories:

- Medication
- Lines, catheters and drains
- Equipment
- Airway
- Alarms

A later study by the same research group from the European Society of Intensive Care Medicine focused on errors in the administration of parenteral drugs. In this multinational study, 74.5 events per 100 patient days were observed [9]. Table 1 displays the rate of events with respect to the five categories that were observed.

Both of these studies were based on a common definition of error as an occurrence that

Tab. 1 Observed rates of parenteral medication errors in the SEE 2 study (modified from [9]). Calculated per 100 patient days

	Events/ 100 pt days	lower 95 % CI	upper 95 % CI
All	74.5	69.5	79.4
Wrong time	33.4	30.1	36.7
Missed medication	22.4	19.7	25.1
Wrong dose	10.2	8.4	12.0
Wrong drug	5.3	4.0	6.6
Wrong route	3.2	2.2	4.2

harmed or could have harmed a patient. Research in patient safety is frequently based on this broad definition. Several reasons have gained this approach its current popularity. Probably the most important reason is the attempt to avoid an immediate search for blame and instead to look for the causes of error. An error does not necessarily lead to patient harm but highlights weak and unsafe steps in the process of care. From this perspective, every error carries the chance to reveal an unsafe practice or even to discover the reason why an error did not lead to an adverse event.

What do errors, critical incidents, and adverse events have in common?

In patient safety research, as well as in clinical practice, useful information is gained not only by studying actual incidents of harm, but by investigating risky situations or processes. If we aim to get the most comprehensive picture of patient safety in particular settings, we not only need to look at incidents that caused harm but must also retrieve useful information from errors that did not result in subsequent harm – so-called 'near misses'. Fortunately, not every error leads to a critical incident or an adverse event. A recent study in 70 french ICUs revealed that 15.4 % of medical errors lead to therapeutic or clinical consequences [10]. While incidents without subsequent harm happen more frequently than harmful events, they provide insight into the defence barriers that

prevent actual damage. Different types of events – with and without harm – can be summarised under the term 'critical incident'. A standardised terminology and classification scheme for collecting and organising patient safety data has been developed [11]. Because improvements in patient safety will only be achieved when causes, circumstances and contributing factors of error are known and subsequently altered, it is obviously necessary to look at the whole picture of critical incidents.

In many critical incidents, a common characteristic can be found. While healthcare providers act at the distal end of a process or structure, very often a system is the proximal cause of error [11]. Although the failure of a healthcare professional can be seen as an inevitable consequence of being human, the actual occurrence and outcome of an error are frequently due to the design of one or more systems. System failures range from simple organisational matters, like the maintenance of equipment, to complex issues such as ergonomics [12] or the culture of an institution.

For everyone who enters the medical profession, it very quickly becomes clear that adverse events can occur even when medical care is managed appropriately. An example is renal insufficiency after appropriate use and dosage of an antibiotic drug. It is therefore necessary to distinguish between nonpreventable and preventable adverse events. Any analysis of an adverse event should make this distinction. If a preventable adverse event is defined as the consequence of an unintercepted serious error in medical care, it will be necessary to prevent not only the future occurrence of the error but also its possible impact. For example, it has been shown that errors made during the administration of drugs occur with considerable frequency [9, 13]. But the impact of such an error might be mitigated by restrictions on the amount or concentration of a potentially dangerous drug in a previously prepared syringe.

Can we measure patient safety?

For patient safety, as well as for other areas of quality assurance and improvement, an important starting point is to assess the current status of development. With respect to patient safety, this is a difficult but not unachievable task. Several methods have been described, ranging from the use of observers [1] to self-reporting systems or retrospective chart review [14]. Determining which method is more appropriate depends mainly on the underlying intention. While a method using observers will likely be restricted to scientific purposes, the use of self-reporting systems has been shown to be practicable in clinical settings [15–17]. Of note is that different methods will retrieve different findings [18]. Although desirable, it is not always possible to retrieve information about the number of opportunities for error and the actual incidents. This is a frequent limitation of self-reporting systems. But one considerable advantage of self-reporting systems is that contextual information is provided by the medical staff directly involved. Another important advantage is the creation of a team culture that relies on an atmosphere of assurance instead of the conventional approach of 'blame and shame'. It is therefore of utmost importance that medical staff be assured that they can report errors without fear of reprisal. Although team culture is an essential prerequisite for improvements in patient safety, it is obviously not an easily observable dimension. For ICUs it would be desirable to see more tools for measuring healthcare climate, such as the recently published tool for measuring nursing climate [19].

To answer the question of how to reduce the number of adverse events and thus to measure advances in safety is a difficult undertaking. A simple measurement of event rates does not account for the unknown range of opportunities for harm. A valid measurement of advances in safety would require knowing the denominator (e.g. the population at risk) and the numerator (actual events). Actual harm is not always obvious and may only be detected by active screening (e.g. device-related infection, deep venous thrombosis).

A key step – Anticipation of hazards

Although recognising an error after the fact is an important prerequisite for making improvements, it is obviously preferable to catch safety concerns in advance. This is much more difficult than it sounds and requires continuous awareness and an essential change in perspective. The question is no longer 'What went wrong?' but 'What might go wrong?'. A simple example is the mix-up of medications that can be caused by "look-alike" or "sound-alike" drugs [20]. A system in which one drug can easily be confused with another is sure to bring harm to some patient at some point. An anticipatory approach would require staff to identify and review the look-alike and sound-alike drugs in a particular setting and to take action to prevent their being administered erroneously. In ICUs, standard situations such as patient transport, handover, information transfer, and intervention (e.g. intubation) are also important areas for anticipatory safety strategies. For instance, intra-hospital transport of patients through relatively insecure environments poses a high risk [21, 22] and requires an adequately trained staff and appropriate precautions [23]. This was highlighted by a report on intra-hospital transfer in which 39 % of 191 incidents were related to equipment failure (e.g. power supply) and 61 % were related to patient/staff management issues (e.g. inadequate monitoring) [24]. Obviously, adequate preparation would have avoided or mitigated most of the reported incidents.

Patient safety and risk reduction – An essential task in intensive care medicine

The actual risk of an unfavourable outcome in critically ill patients depends in considerable part on the quality of the process of care. Since such a process is potentially subject to change it will be possible to influence the extrinsic risk in ICU patients. Several interventions have been shown to reduce errors or even to decrease the rate of adverse events associated with particular ICU activities. A number of domains have been identified in which changes in infrastructure, process, and culture can result in a substantial risk reduction.

Human errors and ergonomic nightmares

With respect to human factors, the ICU has been described as a "hostile environment" [12]. Diffuse or flashy lighting, difficult access to the patient and/or equipment, a lack of space, and chaotic background noise are examples of environmental conditions most healthcare workers in ICUs are familiar with [25]. The negative impact of such an environment may become even greater when requirements for multitasking coupled with information overload are present [26]. In many instances, physicians and nurses need to act like an integrated clinical database, but often without the support of a properly structured information flow and without an environment designed with adherence to ergonomic principles [27, 28].

System factor – Workload

In a recent multinational study on errors in the administration stage of parenteral medication, the staff of participating ICUs reported workload, stress, and fatigue as contributing factors in 33 % of medication errors [9]. The same study showed that an increased patient-to-nurse ratio and an increased occupancy rate were associated with a higher risk for medication errors. It is well known that excessive workload, extended working hours, fatigue, and sleep deprivation affect the performance of physicians and nurses [29–33]. Another example of the impact of an inappropriate workload on patient safety relates to the risk of iatrogenic infection [34]. These risks are avoidable and have a negative impact not only on patient safety but also on the safety of healthcare providers [35–37]. Strategies to reduce such risks have been shown to be effective. In a study with interns in an ICU, an intervention to reduce the number of working hours per week and eliminate extended work shifts reduced serious errors by 26 % [38]. In a study on the effect of workload on infection risk, a higher staffing level was associated with a more than 30 % reduction in infection risk in critically ill patients [34].

Demanding tasks, time pressure and emotional stress add an additional burden for medical staff in ICUs [39]. Burnout and inadequate job strain can affect the quality of patient care [40, 41]. Although a clear association between burnout among ICU personnel and the causation of error has not been demonstrated, the reported numbers are of concern. In a national survey in French ICUs, 48 % of the physicians and 33 % of the nurses reported a high level of burnout [42, 43]. A similar survey in a Swiss ICU revealed that 49 % of the nursing team felt stressed and that 28 % of them showed a high level of burnout [44]. Knowing these facts, it is indisputably the duty of ICU managers and hospital administrators to optimise schedule design and ensure appropriate levels of staffing.

Cultural factor – Safety climate

While recognising that system design is the major source of error, the question then arises: What is the culture behind these systems? A major change is necessary to overcome a culture of blame and shame and to create a new attitude toward learning. The question 'Who is guilty?' should no longer be of interest; instead, the focus needs to be on the prevention and mitigation of future error. ICUs need to develop an increased alertness at all professional levels [45]. The steps in such a development will often evolve from a culture of denial ('We don't have that kind of incident'), to a reactive culture (reaction only after things have already gone wrong), to a general attitude of risk management as an integral part of the thinking of all professionals and managers (see Fig. 1). As a prerequisite, it is necessary to abandon the unrealistic goal of perfection, to accept the limitations of human nature, and to expect errors. Error detection and recovery are integral parts of such an approach. Of note, Patel and Cohen reported that experts made more errors than their less experienced colleagues during a 10-hour period of ICU practice but that they recovered from those errors faster and more often [46].

The transformation of traditional patterns of behaviour, including the assignment of blame, into a new culture focused on systemic improvements in patient safety relies on an atmosphere of trust and respect that allows open communication. Such an open communication is the prerequisite for a helpful error reporting system. As an encouraging signal it has been shown that an already existing critical incident reporting system was an independent predictor for a decreased risk of parenteral medication errors at the administration stage in ICUs [9].

In this context it is of utmost importance that responsible leaders foster teamwork, trust and individual commitment to patient care. The impact of such cultural changes is difficult to measure [47] but should not be underestimated. In a recent study, Zohar et al. [19] used a measure of

Generative culture
Risk management as integral part of the **thinking** of professionals and managers

Proactive culture
What might go wrong? Steps **before** something might go wrong

Bureaucratic culture
"As long as one keeps to **procedures** nothing can ever happen"

Reactive culture
Reaction only **after** things have already gone wrong

Denial
"We **don't** have that kind of incidents"

Fig. 1   Steps in the development of a safety culture

healthcare climate at the hospital and unit levels to investigate the influence of nurse managers and their professional peers on patient safety. Evaluation of climate was based on patient orientation, professional development, and teamwork. The authors found that patient safety was maximised when both hospital and unit climates were positive. Interestingly, a compensatory effect of a positive unit climate was seen when the hospital climate was poor. This observation emphasises the need for cultural change as a key to improved patient safety.

Education and training

Considering ICUs as complex systems for the management of complex situations, it becomes clear that the actions of operators in these systems require a high level of knowledge, skill, and competence. Guidelines [48] and core competencies [49] for training in intensive care medicine are available. Education and training need to be seen as an ongoing continuum throughout the practice of intensive care. The safety of patient care depends on it. For instance, in an analysis of "line-, tube-, and drain-related" incidents in critically ill patients, the knowledge and skills of the providers were significant preventive factors [50]. Other examples demonstrate that problem-focused education and training programmes in ICUs have a beneficial effect on patient safety. McMullin et al. reported that an educational intervention combined with implementation strategies increased sustained adherence to a guide-

line for heparin thromboprophylaxis [51]. A multi-centre study by Pronovost et al. showed an impressive and sustained reduction in catheter-related bloodstream infections after an intervention with strong educational elements [52, 53].

Key elements – Routine situations and continuity of care

Contrary to popular belief, errors occur most frequently in routine situations, not during unforeseeable events. As an example, the second multinational Sentinel Events Evaluation study revealed that 69 % of parenteral medication errors at the administration stage took place in routine situations [9]. But a simple organisational factor such as the routine check of perfusors and infusion pumps at nurses' shift changes was associated with a decreased risk for a medication error. Fortunately, every routine procedure in an ICU carries the potential to minimise the causes or at least the consequences of error. Several studies have demonstrated that a routine procedure such as the insertion and maintenance of a central venous line is amenable to considerable improvement. Central line-associated bloodstream infection rates were reduced by educational interventions as well as the implementation of protocols and bundles relating to the insertion, access, and maintenance of central venous lines [52–54]. Routine procedures are therefore a major starting point when looking systematically at opportunities to improve patient safety.

Another important area of concern is gaps in the continuity of care. Obviously, standard situations such as patient transport [22], information transfer, and shift changes are important targets for anticipatory safety strategies. A frequent routine procedure is the handover of patients between caregivers [55]. Since this process is characterised by the communication of complex information under time pressure, a structured approach might support this task [56]. Analogous situations in nonmedical professional areas can serve as a model. Catchpole et al. [57] used the expertise from a Formula i racing team and from aviation to develop a protocol for the handover between the operating theatre and the ICU. The authors showed that the number of technical errors, inadequate handover information, and duration of handover were reduced by using a protocol focused on leadership, task allocation, rhythm, standardised processes, checklists, awareness, anticipation, and communication.

Summary

Patient safety is an essential paradigm in the practice of intensive care medicine. Of note, patient safety consists not only of the absence of error, but even more, in the assurance that every patient will receive timely and appropriate, evidence-based medicine. Several reports have demonstrated an urgent need for ICUs to improve the safety of such key processes as the administration of drugs. A very first step in the effort to reduce the number of adverse events is to raise awareness and to recognise error. The use of critical incident reporting systems with self-reporting has been shown to be practicable and contribute to a considerable risk reduction. A more advanced approach includes the active search for hazards and system flaws and requires a sustained cultural change. Open communication and interprofessional exchange of information are essential in the development of such a safety culture. The intensive care community has already proved that patient safety is a top-priority issue. Several interventions have been shown to reduce errors or to decrease the number of adverse events. Important factors are working environment, workload and staffing, skills and competency, communication, and management of standard operations.

The author

Andreas Valentin, MD, MBA
General and Medical ICU
Second Medical Department
Rudolfstiftung Hospital
Juchgasse 25
1030 Vienna, Austria
E-mail: andreas.valentin@meduniwien.ac.at

References

1. Donchin Y, Gopher D, Olin M, Badihi Y, Biesky M, Sprung CL, et al. A look into the nature and causes of human errors in the intensive care unit. Crit Care Med. 1995 Feb;23(2):294–300.
2. Rothschild JM, Landrigan CP, Cronin JW, Kaushal R, Lockley SW, Burdick E, et al. The Critical Care Safety Study: The incidence and nature of adverse events and serious medical errors in intensive care. Crit Care Med. 2005 Aug;33(8):1694–700.
3. Moreno RP, Rhodes A, Donchin Y. Patient safety in intensive care medicine: the Declaration of Vienna. Intensive Care Med. 2009 Oct;35(10):1667–72.
4. Dodek PM, Raboud J. Explicit approach to rounds in an ICU improves communication and satisfaction of providers. Intensive Care Med. 2003 Sep;29(9):1584–8.
5. Reader TW, Flin R, Mearns K, Cuthbertson BH. Developing a team performance framework for the intensive care unit. Crit Care Med. 2009 May;37(5):1787–93.
6. Thomas AN, Galvin I. Patient safety incidents associated with equipment in critical care: a review of reports to the UK National Patient Safety Agency. Anaesthesia. 2008 Nov;63(11):1193–7.
7. Webster CS. The nuclear power industry as an alternative analogy for safety in anaesthesia and a novel approach for the conceptualisation of safety goals. Anaesthesia. 2005 Nov;60(11):1115–22.
8. Valentin A, Capuzzo M, Guidet B, Moreno RP, Dolanski L, Bauer P, et al. Patient safety in intensive care: results from the multinational Sentinel Events Evaluation (SEE) study. Intensive Care Med. 2006 Oct;32(10):1591–8.
9. Valentin A, Capuzzo M, Guidet B, Moreno R, Metnitz B, Bauer P, et al. Errors in administration of parenteral drugs in intensive care units: multinational prospective study. BMJ. 2009;338:b814.
10. Garrouste-Orgeas M, Timsit JF, Vesin A, Schwebel C, Arnodo P, Lefrant JY, et al. Selected medical errors in the intensive care unit: results of the IATROREF study: parts I and II. Am J Respir Crit Care Med. 2010 Jan 15;181(2):134–42.
11. Chang A, Schyve PM, Croteau RJ, O'Leary DS, Loeb JM. The JCAHO patient safety event taxonomy: a standard-

ized terminology and classification schema for near misses and adverse events. Int J Qual Health Care. 2005 Apr;17(2):95–105.

12. Donchin Y, Seagull FJ. The hostile environment of the intensive care unit. Curr Opin Crit Care. 2002 Aug;8(4):316–20.

13. Calabrese AD, Erstad BL, Brandl K, Barletta JF, Kane SL, Sherman DS. Medication administration errors in adult patients in the ICU. Intensive Care Med. 2001 Oct;27(10):1592–8.

14. Beckmann U, Bohringer C, Carless R, Gillies DM, Runciman WB, Wu AW, et al. Evaluation of two methods for quality improvement in intensive care: facilitated incident monitoring and retrospective medical chart review. Crit Care Med. 2003 Apr;31(4):1006–11.

15. Frey B, Kehrer B, Losa M, Braun H, Berweger L, Micallef J, et al. Comprehensive critical incident monitoring in a neonatal-pediatric intensive care unit: experience with the system approach. Intensive Care Med. 2000 Jan;26(1):69–74.

16. Ligi I, Arnaud F, Jouve E, Tardieu S, Sambuc R, Simeoni U. Iatrogenic events in admitted neonates: a prospective cohort study. Lancet. 2008 Feb 2;371(9610):404–10.

17. Harris CB, Krauss MJ, Coopersmith CM, Avidan M, Nast PA, Kollef MH, et al. Patient safety event reporting in critical care: a study of three intensive care units. Crit Care Med. 2007 Apr;35(4):1068–76.

18. Michel P, Quenon JL, de Sarasqueta AM, Scemama O. Comparison of three methods for estimating rates of adverse events and rates of preventable adverse events in acute care hospitals. BMJ. 2004 Jan 24;328(7433):199.

19. Zohar D, Livne Y, Tenne-Gazit O, Admi H, Donchin Y. Healthcare climate: a framework for measuring and improving patient safety. Crit Care Med. 2007 May;35(5):1312–7.

20. Medication safety issue brief. Look-alike, sound-alike drugs. Hosp Health Netw. 2005 Oct;79(10):57–8.

21. Gillman L, Leslie G, Williams T, Fawcett K, Bell R, McGibbon V. Adverse events experienced while transferring the critically ill patient from the emergency department to the intensive care unit. Emerg Med J. 2006 Nov;23(11):858–61.

22. Papson JP, Russell KL, Taylor DM. Unexpected events during the intrahospital transport of critically ill patients. Acad Emerg Med. 2007 Jun;14(6):574–7.

23. Warren J, Fromm RE, Jr., Orr RA, Rotello LC, Horst HM. Guidelines for the inter- and intrahospital transport of critically ill patients. Crit Care Med. 2004 Jan;32(1):256–62.

24. Beckmann U, Gillies DM, Berenholtz SM, Wu AW, Pronovost P. Incidents relating to the intra-hospital transfer of critically ill patients. An analysis of the reports submitted to the Australian Incident Monitoring Study in Intensive Care. Intensive Care Med. 2004 Aug;30(8):1579–85.

25. Elliott RM, McKinley SM, Eager D. A pilot study of sound levels in an Australian adult general intensive care unit. Noise Health. 2010 Jan-Mar;12(46):26–36.

26. Weigl M, Muller A, Zupanc A, Angerer P. Participant observation of time allocation, direct patient contact and simultaneous activities in hospital physicians. BMC Health Serv Res. 2009;9:110.

27. Sevdalis N, Brett SJ. Improving care by understanding the way we work: human factors and behavioural science in the context of intensive care. Crit Care. 2009;13(2):139.

28. Fackler JC, Watts C, Grome A, Miller T, Crandall B, Pronovost P. Critical care physician cognitive task analysis: an exploratory study. Crit Care. 2009;13(2):R33.

29. Barger LK, Ayas NT, Cade BE, Cronin JW, Rosner B, Speizer FE, et al. Impact of extended-duration shifts on medical errors, adverse events, and attentional failures. PLoS Med. 2006 Dec;3(12):e487.

30. Gander PH, Purnell HM, Garden A, Woodward A. Work Patterns and Fatigue-Related Risk Among Junior Doctors. Occup Environ Med. 2007 Mar 26;64(11):733–38.

31. Scott LD, Rogers AE, Hwang WT, Zhang Y. Effects of critical care nurses' work hours on vigilance and patients' safety. Am J Crit Care. 2006 Jan;15(1):30–7.

32. Rothschild JM, Keohane CA, Rogers S, Gardner R, Lipsitz SR, Salzberg CA, et al. Risks of complications by attending physicians after performing nighttime procedures. JAMA. 2009 Oct 14;302(14):1565–72.

33. West CP, Tan AD, Habermann TM, Sloan JA, Shanafelt TD. Association of resident fatigue and distress with perceived medical errors. JAMA. 2009 Sep 23;302(12):1294–300.

34. Hugonnet S, Chevrolet JC, Pittet D. The effect of workload on infection risk in critically ill patients. Crit Care Med. 2007 Jan;35(1):76–81.

35. Ayas NT, Barger LK, Cade BE, Hashimoto DM, Rosner B, Cronin JW, et al. Extended work duration and the risk of self-reported percutaneous injuries in interns. JAMA. 2006 Sep 6;296(9):1055–62.

36. Barger LK, Cade BE, Ayas NT, Cronin JW, Rosner B, Speizer FE, et al. Extended work shifts and the risk of motor vehicle crashes among interns. N Engl J Med. 2005 Jan 13;352(2):125–34.

37. Rauchenzauner M, Ernst F, Hintringer F, Ulmer H, Ebenbichler CF, Kasseroler MT, et al. Arrhythmias and increased neuro-endocrine stress response during physicians' night shifts: a randomized cross-over trial. Eur Heart J. 2009 Nov;30(21):2606–13.

38. Landrigan CP, Rothschild JM, Cronin JW, Kaushal R, Burdick E, Katz JT, et al. Effect of reducing interns' work hours on serious medical errors in intensive care units. N Engl J Med. 2004 Oct 28;351(18):1838–48.

39. Piquette D, Reeves S, LeBlanc VR. Stressful intensive care unit medical crises: How individual responses

impact on team performance. Crit Care Med. 2009 Apr;37(4):1251–5.

40. Reader TW, Cuthbertson BH, Decruyenaere J. Burnout in the ICU: Potential consequences for staff and patient well-being. Intensive Care Med. 2008 Jan;34(1):4–6.

41. Azoulay E, Timsit JF, Sprung CL, Soares M, Rusinova K, Lafabrie A, et al. Prevalence and factors of intensive care unit conflicts: the conflicus study. Am J Respir Crit Care Med. 2009 Nov 1;180(9):853–60.

42. Embriaco N, Azoulay E, Barrau K, Kentish N, Pochard F, Loundou A, et al. High level of burnout in intensivists: prevalence and associated factors. Am J Respir Crit Care Med. 2007 Apr 1;175(7):686–92.

43. Poncet MC, Toullic P, Papazian L, Kentish-Barnes N, Timsit JF, Pochard F, et al. Burnout syndrome in critical care nursing staff. Am J Respir Crit Care Med. 2007 Apr 1;175(7):698–704.

44. Verdon M, Merlani P, Perneger T, Ricou B. Burnout in a surgical ICU team. Intensive Care Med. 2008 Jan;34(1):152–6.

45. France DJ, Greevy RA, Jr., Liu X, Burgess H, Dittus RS, Weinger MB, et al. Measuring and comparing safety climate in intensive care units. Med Care. 2010 Mar;48(3):279–84.

46. Patel VL, Cohen T. New perspectives on error in critical care. Curr Opin Crit Care. 2008 Aug;14(4):456–9.

47. Huang DT, Clermont G, Sexton JB, Karlo CA, Miller RG, Weissfeld LA, et al. Perceptions of safety culture vary across the intensive care units of a single institution. Crit Care Med. 2007 Jan;35(1):165–76.

48. Dorman T, Angood PB, Angus DC, Clemmer TP, Cohen NH, Durbin CG, Jr., et al. Guidelines for critical care medicine training and continuing medical education. Crit Care Med. 2004 Jan;32(1):263–72.

49. Bion JF, Barrett H. Development of core competencies for an international training programme in intensive care medicine. Intensive Care Med. 2006 Sep;32(9):1371–83.

50. Needham DM, Sinopoli DJ, Thompson DA, Holzmueller CG, Dorman T, Lubomski LH, et al. A system factors analysis of "line, tube, and drain" incidents in the intensive care unit. Crit Care Med. 2005 Aug;33(8):1701–7.

51. McMullin J, Cook D, Griffith L, McDonald E, Clarke F, Guyatt G, et al. Minimizing errors of omission: behavioural reenforcement of heparin to avert venous emboli: the BEHAVE study. Crit Care Med. 2006 Mar;34(3):694–9.

52. Pronovost P, Needham D, Berenholtz S, Sinopoli D, Chu H, Cosgrove S, et al. An intervention to decrease catheter-related bloodstream infections in the ICU. N Engl J Med. 2006 Dec 28;355(26):2725–32.

53. Pronovost PJ, Goeschel CA, Colantuoni E, Watson S, Lubomski LH, Berenholtz SM, et al. Sustaining reductions in catheter related bloodstream infections in Michigan intensive care units: observational study. BMJ. 2010;340:c309.

54. Costello JM, Morrow DF, Graham DA, Potter-Bynoe G, Sandora TJ, Laussen PC. Systematic intervention to reduce central line-associated bloodstream infection rates in a pediatric cardiac intensive care unit. Pediatrics. 2008 May;121(5):915–23.

55. Perren A, Conte P, De Bitonti N, Limoni C, Merlani P. From the ICU to the ward: cross-checking of the physician's transfer report by intensive care nurses. Intensive Care Med. 2008 Nov;34(11):2054–61.

56. Berkenstadt H, Haviv Y, Tuval A, Shemesh Y, Megrill A, Perry A, et al. Improving handoff communications in critical care: utilizing simulation-based training toward process improvement in managing patient risk. Chest. 2008 Jul;134(1):158–62.

57. Catchpole KR, de Leval MR, McEwan A, Pigott N, Elliott MJ, McQuillan A, et al. Patient handover from surgery to intensive care: using Formula 1 pit-stop and aviation models to improve safety and quality. Paediatr Anaesth. 2007 May;17(5):470–8.

Stijn I. Blot, Sonia O. Labeau and Jordi Rello

Evaluating and reporting nosocomial infections

"Good surveillance does not necessarily ensure the making of the right decisions, but it reduces the chances of wrong ones."
                    Alexander D. Langmuir, 1963 [1]

Introduction – Why is surveillance and reporting of nosocomial infections important?

Nosocomial infection is the most common complication associated with hospitalisation and is responsible for a substantial clinical and economic burden [2, 3]. The attributable mortality varies according to the age of the patient, underlying condition, severity of illness, infection type, the causative pathogen, and adequacy of therapy [4]. As such, excess mortality rates may be rather low [5, 6], but can also rise up to 40 % [7, 8]. Surgical site infections are associated with an excess length of hospitalisation of 16 days [9] and an extra hospital cost of $ 4,091 [10]. The attributable cost associated with nosocomial bloodstream infection ranges from $ 6,000 to $ 56,000 while the extra length of hospitalisation varies from 5 to 24 days [11, 12]. In a meta-analysis, the average additional cost of ventilator-associated pneumonia was estimated at $ 10,019, while length of intensive care unit (ICU) stay was increased by an average of 6 days [7]. Additionally, infections caused by multi-drug-resistant pathogens cause an even higher toll in terms of clinical and economic outcomes [13–16]. As such, effective infection prevention can be converted into substantial savings of healthcare resources as well as patients' lives [17]. Therefore, infection prevention has become a priority in healthcare settings with several large-scale initiatives from policy makers, healthcare/medical societies, and academic institutions [18–21].

Setting up a solid system for the surveillance of nosocomial infection has been considered a first step in effective infection prevention and control. Surveillance can be defined as "the ongoing, systematic collection, analysis, interpretation, and dissemination of data regarding a health-related event for the use of public health action to reduce morbidity and mortality and to improve health" [22]. The two major goals of a surveillance programme in a healthcare setting are to improve the quality of healthcare, and to identify, implement, and evaluate strategies to prevent and control nosocomial infections [23]. As such, the four objectives of a surveillance programme are

1. to provide baseline, or endemic rates of infections,
2. to indentify increases in rates above the baseline, or expected rates of infection,
3. to indentify risk factors for infection, and
4. to evaluate the effectiveness of strategies to prevent and control nosocomial infections.

In daily practice, knowledge of baseline infection rates is necessary to detect problems in infection prevention and to define goals to better control these issues. As such, the data obtained by nosocomial infection surveillance are useful to steer quality improvement programmes. In the strive for increased patient safety, nosocomial infection rates are considered essential quality indicators. The existence of large (national or international) surveillance databases makes benchmarking possible. Through benchmarking clear goals in infection prevention can be defined and local surveillance data can be compared with the postulated standard on a regular basis. Such feedback mechanisms are useful to evaluate the process of infection prevention and to further motivate healthcare workers to continue the efforts made.

Surveillance programmes are not only valuable in terms of defining objectives in infection prevention and steering quality improvement initiatives through regular feedback. Developing a surveillance programme for nosocomial infection in itself appears to be beneficial for reducing infection rates. Surveillance systems combined with appropriate feedback have been shown to be an important strategy to reduce nosocomial infection rates [24–29]. This favourable side-effect of setting up a surveillance programme is (most probably) due to the increase in awareness regarding the problem of nosocomial infection. Furthermore, a surveillance programme focused on prompt reporting shortly after the diagnosis of infection allows for detailed route-cause analysis. In this approach, a thorough investigation of the origin of the problem is analysed with a strict evaluation of the processes that might have contributed to the infection or, in worse cases, outbreak.

Unfortunately, developing and organising surveillance programmes for nosocomial infection is not an easy task. The reliability of the programme depends on several issues that must be taken into account. These aspects include which infections to focus on, whether the surveillance will be organised at specific high-risk units or hospital-wide, which definitions to use, which denominator to choose, how to handle case mix, etcetera. Elementary aspects of surveillance reporting are outlined in this chapter.

Surveillance methods

No single surveillance system fits all organisations' needs. In order to maximise resources, surveillance systems must be tailored to the needs of the individual institution by targeting the in-

stitutional needs, priorities and patient populations' characteristics [30].

House-wide surveillance

House-wide surveillance, also called comprehensive or total surveillance, is described as a surveillance method in which all patients are continuously monitored for all healthcare-associated infections at all body sites [31]. Comprehensive surveillance was the most common type of surveillance conducted in hospitals throughout the United States in the 1970s, and the required surveillance method for all hospitals in the NNIS (National Nosocomial Infection Surveillance) system until the mid-1980s [23].

If adequately performed, house-wide surveillance could measure the occurrence and risk of healthcare-associated infection in an institution's entire patient population. This major advantage is nevertheless largely overruled by the serious drawbacks associated with this method of surveillance. Disadvantages comprise the fact that house-wide surveillance is extremely labour-intensive and requires the dedication of trained personnel. Moreover, it is hard to accomplish without additional resources such as computer-based applications and due technical support. Therefore the method's efficiency is called into question by several authorities. Additionally, house-wide surveillance does not take into account the fact that the risk of developing a healthcare-associated infection fluctuates depending on the patient population, the treatment supplied, the devices used, and the procedures provided. [23, 32–34]

Based on the reasons stated above, in 1986 the NNIS chose a new path towards promoting a targeted surveillance approach, and in the mid-1990s, the house-wide surveillance method was completely banned from the NNIS system [23].

Targeted surveillance

Targeted surveillance, also called focused, priority-directed, or surveillance by objective, is described as surveillance in which selected events or populations are monitored [23, 35, 36]. The focus of targeted programmes can be widely divergent and comprise specific units or wards, as well as selected procedures, device-associated infections, or epidemiologically important microorganisms [23, 36]. Overall, targeted surveillance programmes focus on healthcare-associated infections that are potentially avoidable and are considered high-risk, high-volume or high-cost [23]. Today, most organisations use a targeted surveillance methodology based on an annual risk assessment [37]. Following the demonstration of the effectiveness of surveillance in the prevention of nosocomial infection in the United States, several European countries started to set up national networks for the surveillance of nosocomial infections in the early 1990s. These networks were all target-oriented [38].

Periodic surveillance

The flexible nature of periodic or intermittent surveillance allows staff to increase opportunities for other activities, and the method permits the organisation to define long-term surveillance goals and activities. Serious disadvantages associated with this method include the fact that obtaining consistent baseline data is nevertheless extremely difficult, and that clusters of infection may be missed [33].

Prevalence surveillance

Prevalence surveillance is commonly used for risk factor identification, and the data acquired may be used to target future areas of surveillance. The method is quick, and the associated costs are relatively low. Prevalence surveillance does not, however, allow for comparison with incidence rates, nor for collecting information over a prolonged period of time. Finally, outbreaks or clusters of infection may be missed when surveillance is performed using this method [33].

Table 1 offers a schematic overview of the advantages and disadvantages of the different surveillance methods.

There is no single or 'right' method of surveillance design or implementation. Effective systems must be based on sound epidemiologic principles, and be well understood by key participants in the surveillance programme. Importantly, they should be supported by the senior man-

agement [30]. Frequently, combined surveillance methods are used in a single institution. Examples comprise institutions in which all patients are monitored for epidemiologically important organisms, while ventilator-associated pneumonia is solely monitored in ICU patients. Another example is the combination of site-specific and unit-specific surveillance to monitor healthcare-associated infection rates. The choice of strategies will be guided by the institution's particular needs or goals, which has been referred to as "surveillance by objectives" [36]. Time and personnel commitments to other activities of the infection control programme are the most frequently identified limiting factors [23].

Definitions in surveillance

The process of data collection must be based upon definable events. Examples of such definable events are catheter-related bloodstream infection and other definable device-related infections. Criteria, or case definitions, are a key element of any surveillance system. In Europe, case definitions were traditionally agreed upon within regional or national networks of hospitals. The HELICS (Hospitals in Europe Link for Infection Control through Surveillance) network, which is an international network aiming at the collection, analysis and dissemination of valid data on the risks of nosocomial infections in European hospitals, has made enormous efforts to harmonise the numerous differing definitions on a European level. In spite of the laborious job, some national networks today are still using definitions and surveillance methods that are not fully compatible with the European definitions [38, 39]. Meanwhile, the HELICS project has become part of the larger Improving Patient Safety in Europe (IPSE) project (http://ipse.univ-lyon1.fr).

To be acceptable to all users of the data, the criteria used in a surveillance programme should reflect generally accepted definitions of the specific infection. Whenever possible, previously published, standardised definitions should be used. Generally, criteria combine clinical findings with the results of laboratory and other diagnostic tests [23, 40].

Consistency in the use of these definitions is a crucial requirement to enable accurate analy-

Tab. 1 Advantages and disadvantages of surveillance strategies for surveillance of healthcare-associated infections [23, 33, 34]

Surveillance method	Advantages	Disadvantages
House-wide surveillance	Provides data from entire patient population	Labour-intensive
	Identifies patterns	Time-consuming
	Identifies outbreaks early	Expensive
	Provides baseline data	Impractical
		Risk factors are not taken into account
		Data obtained may be of little clinical significance
Targeted surveillance	High flexibility	Outbreaks or clusters of infection outside the surveillance area may be missed
	Ability to focus on important risk factors	Does not allow for defining hospital-wide baseline infection rates
	Allows for site-specificity	
	Allows for unit-specificity	
	Medium labour input	
Periodic surveillance	Allows for definition of long-term objectives	Outbreaks or clusters of infection may be missed
	Flexibility for staff	Provides little or no consistent baseline data
Prevalence surveillance	Inexpensive	Unable to compare prevalence rates with incidence rates/national benchmarks
	Time-efficient	Outbreaks or clusters of infection may be missed
	Can be performed periodically	Provides information for a restricted time interval
	Documents trends in healthcare-associated infections	Overestimates rates
	Identifies risk factors	

ses of surveillance data over time. All persons involved in the surveillance process, either by collecting, evaluating, analysing or using the data, must have a common understanding of the events being monitored. Moreover, all must use the same definitions, in the same way, all the time. In the absence of such consistency, accuracy and reproducibility of the results are not guaranteed. Consequently, a lack of uniformity will make it extremely hard, over even impossible, to assess the presence and the true incidence of a healthcare-associated infection, and to evaluate whether improvement efforts implemented are actually effective [23, 41]. Also, those using definitions must realise that incidence rates may change when a definition is changed, and this must be recognised when analysing surveillance data and noted when writing a surveillance report [23, 42]. Therefore, adequate education and

training of the infection control team should be given due attention with sufficient allocation of time and resources.

The difficulty of classifying some diseases when doing surveillance, especially pneumonia and bloodstream infection, has long been recognised. For classifying pneumonia, many different definitions have been proposed, but a consensus on a practical definition for this disease is still lacking [23, 42–44]. Sometimes, surveillance-based criteria are used which do not rely exclusively on the microbiological results obtained by invasive sampling techniques. Although this approach might be associated with misclassification bias, it is sometimes believed to be more suitable for surveillance purposes [42].

Differences between case definitions and surveillance methodologies lead to disparities in nosocomial infection rates. The ECDC (European Centers for Disease Control and Prevention) indicate that this issue is most obviously demonstrated by inter-country or intra-country comparisons. Examples of issues where crucial differences arise comprise whether the same patients are included in the denominator, whether only the first episode of an infection or all episodes are counted, and whether exposure is counted as up until the first infection or for the entire stay [38].

Since conventional surveillance definitions are prone to misclassification, algorithmic analysis of electronic health data is a promising alternative. Algorithms using combinations of diagnosis codes, microbiological analysis results, and/or administration of antimicrobial medications can identify healthcare-associated infections with sensitivities and positive predictive values that often match or are superior to those of conventional surveillance [37, 45].

Calculating and reporting infection frequency

Calculating an overall infection rate obtained by house-wide surveillance has been shown to be of little use, as such a rate is too insensitive to measure the influence of exposure to significant risk factors for developing healthcare-associated infection such as urinary catheterisation, mechanical ventilation, and surgical procedures. Instead of an overall rate, population-specific or event-related incidence rates, such as VAP rates in the ICU, should be calculated [23].

To guarantee the accuracy of calculated rates of infection frequency, the appropriate numerators and denominators must be used. The selection of an appropriate denominator is actually one of the most important aspects of measuring, and hence reporting, infection frequency. It is important to ensure that the number closely represents the true population at risk [23, 42].

It is obvious that infection rates will vary according to the denominator selected. This issue is clearly demonstrated by a remarkable study by Eggiman et al., who highlighted the effect of the use of different denominators on risk estimates for VAP [42]. During a two-year study period, 1,049 patients in a 2,300-bed tertiary care centre were surveyed for 1,068 distinct ICU stays. Subsequently, VAP rates were reported per 1,000 patient days, patient days at risk, ventilator days, and ventilator days at risk.

Within these 1,068 distinct ICU stays, VAP developed in 106 (23.5%) of mechanically ventilated patients. If all episodes of VAP (n = 127) were considered, infection rates were shown to be 27.3 episodes per 1,000 ICU patient days (95% confidence interval CI 22.6 to 32.1) and 42.8 episodes per 1,000 ventilator days (95% CI 35.3 to 50.2). When only the first episode of VAP was taken into account, the incidence was 22.8 per 1,000 patient days (95% CI 18.7 to 27.6), 29.6 per 1,000 patient days at risk (95% CI 24.2 to 35.8), 35.7 per 1,000 ventilator days (95% CI 29.2 to 43.2), and, finally, 44.0 per 1,000 ventilator days at risk (95% CI 36.0 to 53.2). Days at risk or ventilator days at risk were defined as the number of days or ventilator days before the onset of first infection. The results of this study clearly demonstrate that reported VAP rates are raised with increasing specificity of the denominator chosen.

VAP is most commonly reported as rates per patient days [46]. The use of this denominator, however, still does not take into account the main risk factor for infection, i.e. intubation and exposure to mechanical ventilation. Thus, it causes a significant underestimation of the true VAP incidence. Underestimation of the true VAP rates when using this method is additionally influenced by prolonged ICU stay. An analogous bias is noted when expressing rates per ventilator day: As the risk of developing VAP is highest at around day 5 post-intubation, VAP rates are lowered with increasing duration of mechanical ventilation. A more appropriate VAP risk estimate would be yielded by including only ventilator days at risk for calculating VAP rates [42].

Risk adjustment

Although expressing infection rates in terms of exposure time ("days at risk") is of the utmost importance to allow fair benchmarking, other population characteristics may confound comparison between units or hospitals. Optimal use of surveillance data requires the collection of specific patient characteristics which increase the risk of nosocomial infection. For example, ICUs with a greater number of trauma victims, including those with burn injuries, patients with solid organ transplantation, or patients with haematologic malignancies, will have a greater intrinsic risk of having high infection rates compared with units with predominantly elective surgery patients. In this regard, gathering data about admission category, severity of disease and acute illness is highly recommended. In this way adjustment for risk profile of infection is feasible, which makes a reasonable comparison between hospitals possible. Sax et al. investigated the influence of case-mix adjustment on comparisons of infection rates between small, intermediate, and large hospitals [47]. Compared to small hospitals, intermediate hospitals had significantly higher infection rates (odds ratio (OR) 1.69; 95% CI 1.33 to 2.90), and so did large hospitals (OR 1.97; 95% CI 1.33 to 2.90). However, after accurate case-mix adjustment the observed difference in infection risk was no longer statistically significant, with odds ratios of 1.54 for intermediate hospitals (95% CI 0.96 to 2.47) and 1.31 for large hospitals (95% CI 0.84 to 2.05). This study illustrates that benchmarking without considering differences in case mix may be highly questionable.

How to develop a surveillance programme?

In designing an effective surveillance programme, some elementary aspects should be taken into account [23]. Firstly, the outcomes that one wants to prevent should be targeted. In ICUs, if not all infections are considered, the infections most frequently targeted are device-related infections, such as ventilator-associated pneumonia and catheter-related bloodstream infection. In fact, particularly device-related infections are among the most preventable. Numerous programmes – even large-scale programmes – focused on reducing the number of these infections have proven successful, even in the long term [48, 49]. Secondly, one should assign priorities to the specific objectives. Since resources are limited, one has to rank the objectives according to their relative importance. Thirdly, time and resources should be allocated in relation to the assigned objectives. Allocating a great amount of resources to a rather small problem will result in an effective, but inefficient, surveillance programme. Fourthly, the surveillance, prevention and control strategies must be clearly designed with an accurate focus on the postulated objectives. Finally, after a defined period of time, the surveillance programme should be evaluated and, if necessary, revised. Table 2 shows – in more detail – the steps necessary to develop an effective surveillance programme [23].

Legal issues in surveillance

In Europe most surveillance systems for healthcare-associated infection today are still voluntary and confidential [50]. In the US, states are increas-

Tab. 2   Steps for developing an effective surveillance programme [data from 23]

Identify the preferred surveillance methodology.
Assess and define the population to be monitored, and select the events to be studied.
Determine the time period for observation and data collection.
Select surveillance criteria for each infection type.
Determine the data collection process.
Identify how to calculate infection rates and analyse data.
Determine the personnel and other resources needed to implement and sustain the programme.
Design an interpretive surveillance report.
Identify who will receive the report.
Develop a written surveillance plan.
Develop a mechanism for periodically evaluating the effectiveness of the surveillance programme.

ingly enacting laws mandating public reporting and disclosure of hospital-acquired infections [51]. As of 1 June 2009, some type of legislation or regulation regarding reporting has been instituted in all but 14 states [52]. Mandatory public reporting of healthcare-associated infection is a relatively new phenomenon that started in 2004. The first states to initiate some form of mandatory reporting were Pennsylvania, Illinois and Florida. Today, 20 states mandate that hospitals report their data through the CDC's NHSN (National Healthcare Safety Network). This network, which numbered less than 500 institutions in 2007, grew to comprise more than 2300 institutions in 2009. Nevertheless, it is important to note that state legislation and regulations across the nation are not uniform [52]. A systematic literature review was performed by the Healthcare Infection Control Practices Advisory Committee (HICPAC) to determine whether public reporting systems improve healthcare performance, and whether there was evidence of the effectiveness of confidential reporting systems in reducing healthcare-associated infection [53]. The investigators concluded that published studies do not provide strong support for the benefit of public reporting of healthcare-associated infection. Therefore, the HICPAC has not recommended for or against mandatory public reporting of healthcare-associated infection rates. It has, however, developed a guidance document based on established principles for public health and healthcare-associated infection reporting systems and intends to assist policymakers, programme planners, consumer advocacy organisations, and others tasked with designing and implementing public reporting systems for healthcare-associated infection [53].

Another important US federal policy change relates to payment reform. Specifically, as of 1 October 2008, the Centers for Medicare and Medicaid Services (CMS) changed its traditional viewpoint supporting its payment rules that the costs of hospital treatment-related complications should primarily be paid by patients and taxpayers, because hospitals were doing all they could to prevent such complications. Since, CMS no longer pays for a number of selected "preventable complications", some of which are healthcare-associated infections [54]. In particular, CMS no longer allows hospitals to receive additional payments for catheter-associated urinary tract infec-

tion, vascular catheter-associated infections and select surgical site infection. Moreover, it is considering adding ventilator-associated pneumonia, *Staphylococcus aureus* bloodstream infections, *Clostridium difficile*-associated disease and infections due to methicillin-resistant *Staphylococcus aureus* to this list of "never events" [23, 44, 52].

Meanwhile, it is still unclear whether the information provided by mandatory public reporting will empower consumers, or rather mislead or confuse them. It also remains to be seen whether these regulations will increase healthcare workers' and hospital administrators' motivation to strive for healthcare-associated infection reduction [50].

Conclusion

In each healthcare organisation, a well-implemented surveillance programme will play a pivotal part by providing systems for monitoring, measuring, and reporting important outcomes and processes, and by supporting initiatives that aim to improve quality of care. In order to achieve consistency, accuracy and reproducibility among all those collecting, evaluating, analysing and using the data, adequate education and training should be given. A European validation study based on a standardised validation methodology should be performed to further assess and improve the comparability and quality of the data collected in European healthcare-associated infections surveillance networks. Such a study would enable an exchange of experience between the European surveillance networks, as well as an assessment of their respective sensitivity.

The authors

Stijn I. Blot, RN, CCRN, MNSc, PhD[1, 2, 3]
Sonia O. Labeau, RN, MA, MNSc[2, 3]
Jordi Rello, MD, PhD[4]
  [1]Department of General
  Medicine & Infectious Diseases | Ghent
  University Hospital | Ghent, Belgium
  [2]Faculty of Medicine and Health Sciences |
  Ghent University | Ghent, Belgium
  [3]Faculty of Healthcare | University College
  Ghent | Ghent, Belgium
  [4]Critical Care Department | Hospital Vall
  d'Hebron | Barcelona, Spain

Address for correspondence
Jordi Rello
Critical Care Department
Vall d'Hebron University Hospital
P° de la Vall d'Hebron, 119–129
08035 Barcelona, Spain
E-mail: jrello.hj23.ics@gencat.cat

References

1. Langmuir AD. The surveillance of communicable diseases of national importance. N Engl J Med 1963;268:182–91.
2. Burke JP. Infection control – a problem for patient safety. N Engl J Med 2003;348:651–6.
3. Vandijck DM, Depaemelaere M, Labeau SO, Depuydt PO, Annemans L, Buyle FM, et al. Daily cost of antimicrobial therapy in patients with Intensive Care Unit-acquired, laboratory-confirmed bloodstream infection. Int J Antimicrob Agents 2008;31:161–5.
4. Blot S, Depuydt P, Vandewoude K, De Bacquer D. Measuring the impact of multidrug resistance in nosocomial infection. Curr Opin Infect Dis 2007;20:391–6.
5. Blot S, Vandewoude K, Hoste E, J DW, Kint K, Rosiers F, et al. Absence of excess mortality in critically ill patients with nosocomial Escherichia coli bacteremia. Infect Control Hosp Epidemiol 2003;24:912–5.
6. Rello J, Ochagavia A, Sabanes E, Roque M, Mariscal D, Reynaga E, et al. Evaluation of outcome of intravenous catheter-related infections in critically ill patients. Am J Respir Crit Care Med 2000;162:1027–30.
7. Safdar N, Dezfulian C, Collard HR, Saint S. Clinical and economic consequences of ventilator-associated pneumonia: a systematic review. Crit Care Med 2005;33:2184–93.
8. Vandewoude KH, Blot SI, Benoit D, Colardyn F, Vogelaers D. Invasive aspergillosis in critically ill patients: attributable mortality and excesses in length of ICU stay and ventilator dependence. J Hosp Infect 2004;56:269–76.
9. Weber WP, Zwahlen M, Reck S, Feder-Mengus C, Misteli H, Rosenthal R, et al. Economic Burden of Surgical Site Infections at a European University Hospital. Infect Control Hosp Epidemiol 2008.
10. Olsen MA, Chu-Ongsakul S, Brandt KE, Dietz JR, Mayfield J, Fraser VJ. Hospital-associated costs due to surgical site infection after breast surgery. Arch Surg 2008;143:53–60; discussion 1.
11. Blot SI, Depuydt P, Annemans L, Benoit D, Hoste E, De Waele JJ, et al. Clinical and economic outcomes in critically ill patients with nosocomial catheter-related bloodstream infections. Clin Infect Dis 2005;41:1591–8.
12. Digiovine B, Chenoweth C, Watts C, Higgins M. The attributable mortality and costs of primary nosocomial bloodstream infections in the intensive care unit. Am J Respir Critical Care Med 1999;160:976–81.
13. Blot SI, Vandewoude KH, Hoste EA, Colardyn FA. Outcome and attributable mortality in critically Ill patients with bacteremia involving methicillin-suscepti-ble and methicillin-resistant Staphylococcus aureus. Arch Intern Med 2002;162:2229–35.
14. Cosgrove SE, Carmeli Y. The impact of antimicrobial resistance on health and economic outcomes. Clin Infect Dis 2003;36:1433–7.
15. Schwaber MJ, Carmeli Y. Mortality and delay in effective therapy associated with extended-spectrum beta-lacta-mase production in Enterobacteriaceae bacteraemia: a systematic review and meta-analysis. J Antimicrob Chemother 2007;60:913–20.
16. Vandijck DM, Blot SI, Decruyenaere JM, Vanholder RC, De Waele JJ, Lameire NH, et al. Costs and length of stay associated with antimicrobial resistance in acute kidney injury patients with bloodstream infection. Acta Clin Belg 2008;63:31–8.
17. Blot S. Limiting the attributable mortality of nosocomial infection and multidrug resistance in intensive care units. Clin Microbiol Infect 2008;14:5–13.
18. Labeau S, Vandijck D, Rello J, Adam S, Rosa A, Wenisch C, et al. Evidence-based guidelines for the prevention of ventilator-associated pneumonia: results of a knowledge test among European intensive care nurses. J Hosp Infect 2008;70:180–5.
19. Labeau SO, Vandijck DM, Rello J, Adam S, Rosa A, Wenisch C, et al. Centers for Disease Control and Prevention guidelines for preventing central venous catheter-related infection: results of a knowledge test among 3405 European intensive care nurses. Crit Care Med 2009;37:320–3.
20. Berwick DM, Calkins DR, McCannon CJ, Hackbarth AD. The 100,000 lives campaign: setting a goal and a deadline for improving health care quality. Jama 2006;295:324–7.
21. Hawe CS, Ellis KS, Cairns CJ, Longmate A. Reduction of ventilator-associated pneumonia: active versus passive guideline implementation. Intensive Care Med 2009;35:1180–6.
22. Centers for Disease Control and Prevention. Updated guidelines for evaluating public health surveillance systems. MMWR 2001;50:1–35.
23. Arias KM. Outbreak investigation, prevention and control in health care settings: Critical issues for patient safety. Second ed. Sudbury, MA: Jones and Bartlett Publishers LLC 2010.
24. Condon RE, Schulte WJ, Malangoni MA, Anderson-Te-schendorf MJ. Effectiveness of a surgical wound surveillance program. Arch Surg 1983;118:303–7.
25. Gastmeier P, Geffers C. Prevention of catheter-related bloodstream infections: analysis of studies published between 2002 and 2005. J Hosp Infect 2006;64: 326–35.

26. Haley RW, Culver DH, White JW, Morgan WM, Emori TG, Munn VP, et al. The efficacy of infection surveillance and control programs in preventing nosocomial infections in US hospitals. Am J Epidemiol 1985;121:182–205.

27. Sykes PK, Brodribb RK, McLaws M-L, McGregor A. When continuous surgical site infection surveillance is interrupted: the Royal Hobart Hospital experience. Am J Infect Control 2005;33:422–7.

28. Cruse P. Wound infection surveillance. Rev Infect Dis 1981;4:734–7.

29. Cruse PJ, Foord R. The epidemiology of wound infection: a 10-year prospective study of 62,939 wounds. Surg Clin North Am 1980;60:27–40.

30. Lee T, Montgomery O, Marx J, Olmsted R, Scheckler W. Recommended practices for surveillance: Association for Professionals in Infection Control and Epidemiology (APIC), Inc. Am J Infect Control 2007;35:427–40.

31. Pottinger JM, Herwaldt LA, Peri TM. Basics of surveillance – an overview. Infect Control Hosp Epidemiol 1997;18:513–27.

32. Scheckler WE. Surveillance, foundation for the future: a historical overview and evolution of methodologies. Am J Infect Control 1997;25:106–11.

33. Edmiston CE, Jr., Wilson PJ, Grahn BF. Fundamentals of infection control and strategies for the Intensive Care Unit. In: Rello J, Kollef M, Diaz E, Rodriquez A, eds. Infectious diseases in critical care. Second ed. Berlin Heidelberg: Springer-Verlag 2007.

34. Emmerson M. Surveillance strategies for nosocomial infections. Curr Opin Infect Dis 1995;8:272–4.

35. Centers for Disease Control and Prevention. Outline For Healthcare-Associated Infections Surveillance, April 2006, Available at http://www.cdc.gov/nhsn/PDFS/OutlineForHAISurveillance.pdf, Accessed 27 February 2010. 2006.

36. Haley RW. Surveillance by objective: a new priority-directed approach to the control of nosocomial infections. The National Foundation for Infectious Diseases lecture. Am J Infect Control 1985;13:78–89.

37. Greene LR, Cain TA, Khoury R, Krystofiak SP, Patrick M, Streed S. APIC position paper: The importance of surveillance technologies in the prevention of health care-associated infections. Am J Infect Control 2009;37:510–3.

38. European Centre for Disease Prevention and Control. Annual epidemiological report on communicable diseases in Europe 2008: Report on the state of communicable diseases in the EU and EEA/EFTA countries. Stockholm; 2008.

39. Pittet D, Allegranzi B, Sax H, Bertinato L, Concia E, Cookson B, et al. Considerations for a WHO European strategy on health-care-associated infection, surveillance, and control. Lancet Infect Dis 2005;5:242–50.

40. Horan TC, Andrus M, Dudeck MA. CDC/NHSN surveillance definition of health care-associated infection and criteria for specific types of infections in the acute care setting. Am J Infect Control 2008;36:309–32.

41. Sherman ER, Heydon KH, St. John Keith H, Teszner E, Rettig Susan L, Alexander SK, et al. Administrative data fail to accurately identify cases of healthcare-associated infection. Infect Control Hosp Epidemiol 2006;27:332–7.

42. Eggimann P, Hugonnet S, Sax H, Touveneau S, Chevrolet J-C, Pittet D. Ventilator-associated pneumonia: caveats for benchmarking. Intensive Care Med 2003;29:2086–89.

43. Depuydt P, Myny D, Blot S. Nosocomial pneumonia: aetiology, diagnosis and treatment. Curr Opin Pulm Med 2006;12:192–7.

44. Klompas M, Platt R. Ventilator-Associated Pneumonia: The Wrong Quality Measure for Benchmarking. Ann Intern Med 2007;147:803–5.

45. Klompas M, Yokoe Deborah S. Healthcare epidemiology: Automated surveillance of health care-associated infections. Clin Infect Dis 2009;48:1268–75.

46. Eggimann P, Pittet D. Infection control in the ICU. Chest 2001;120:2059–93.

47. Sax H, Pittet D. Interhospital differences in nosocomial infection rates: importance of case-mix adjustment. Arch Intern Med 2002;162:2437–42.

48. Pronovost P, Needham D, Berenholtz S, Sinopoli D, Chu H, Cosgrove S, et al. An intervention to decrease catheter-related bloodstream infections in the ICU. N Engl J Med 2006;355:2725–32.

49. Pronovost PJ, Goeschel CA, Colantuoni E, Watson S, Lubomski LH, Berenholtz SM, et al. Sustaining reductions in catheter related bloodstream infections in Michigan intensive care units: observational study. BMJ (Clinical research ed;340:c309.

50. Gastmeier P. European perspective on surveillance. J Hosp Infect 2007;65:159–64.

51. Edmond MB, Bearman GML. Mandatory public reporting in the USA: an example to follow? J Hosp Infect 2007;65:182–8.

52. Stone P. Economic burden of healthcare-associated infections: an American perspective. Expert Rev Pharmacoecon Outcomes Res 2009;9:417–22.

53. McKibben L, Fowler G, Horan T, Brennan PJ. Ensuring rational public reporting systems for health care-associated infections: Systematic literature review and evaluation recommendations. Am J Infect Control 2006;34:142–9.

54. Milstein A. Ending extra payment for "never events" – stronger incentives for patients' safety. N Engl J Med 2009;360:2388–90.

Hans Flaatten

Self-reporting of errors and adverse events in the intensive care unit (ICU)

Errors and adverse events are thought to occur more frequently in the intensive care unit (ICU) than in other hospital wards, and the profiles, too, can be different [1]. The reasons are claimed to be partly due to the critical conditions of the patients, with small margins of error, loss of patient autonomy with reduced possibilities for "self-care", and partly the complex and potentially dangerous treatment and procedures often performed in the ICU.

Most researchers and clinicians will support the view that insight into the spectrum of errors and adverse events in a defined ICU is of importance. The reasons are mainly:

- Patient perspective: it is mandatory that patients and/or their families are provided with knowledge about errors and adverse events happening to them or their relatives.
- ICU unit perspective: errors and adverse events are an important source of input to the process of quality improvement
- Society perspective: it is important for regulatory and/or financial bodies to know about errors and events in their health care in general.

This chapter will shortly describe the epidemiology of errors and adverse events in the ICU, definitions, how to retrieve data and how to use such knowledge in a constructive way for the ICU.

The "epidemiology" of error and events in the ICU

There are several reports about adverse events and errors in the ICU. With support from the European Society of Intensive Care Medicine (ES-ICM), two studies have been conducted and published highlighting this problem. The so-called sentential events evaluation (SEE) have resulted in two studies: SEE1 and SEE2 [2, 3].

In the first study, performed in 255 ICUs, an overall frequency of incidents and errors was found to be approximately 40/100 patient days. The events were divided into drain and lines, artificial airway, equipment, alarms and medication errors. The last category was reported in approximately 10/100 patient days, and was chosen to be the main focus of the SEE2 study. In that investigation, all types of errors during the administration of parenteral medications in the ICU were studied. All such errors occurring during a 24-hour period in 113 ICUs in 27 countries were collected. This study documented 75 medication errors/100 patient days with most of the errors classified as errors of omission. Increased risk for at least one medication error to occur included:

- Increased number of vital organs in failure

- The number of parenteral medications ordered
- Increased number of ICU beds
- Increased number of patients per nurse
- Increased occupancy rate

The last study yielded several inputs on how an ICU should act in order to reduce the number of medication errors.

How can data be retrieved?

There is no ideal way to retrieve information and data about errors and events; several different methods can be used, and the kind of errors in focus may require different methods.

Retrospective searching of patient charts and records is a method which can be used intermittently in general and then later for specific problems. The method is resource-demanding, and being a retrospective method, it will not fulfil the patient perspective mentioned above. It may however be useful when studying the errors of omission, a part of error reporting not often found. Using these methods, researchers have found valuable information about hospital errors in general [4].

Direct observation of behaviour is probably the most sensitive method, able to pick up many more events than detected by the individual health worker and even more than by a search of records [5]. This method is of course very costly, since it will have to use a (trained) independent observer present at each patient bed, an effort unlikely to be sustained for more than a limited time period. This method was used in the well-known study of Donchin [6] where they could document one of the highest error and event rate in intensive care ever published. Use of this method was able to reveal more errors than any other method could, as it may indeed soon render a gold standard in regard to error and event reporting. The method, however, is not very sensitive towards detecting errors of omission.

The usual way to get insight into the occurrence of errors and events is the **self-reporting system**. They exist in many forms and shapes, but basically these are dependent on the reporting of all errors and events when it becomes apparent to the personnel. It is important that such a system is designed to function irrespective of who the personnel was, and where the

event started. Reporting may be very simple using manually filled-in schemes collected in a dedicated mailbox [7], or using online electronic systems [1, 8].

As an example, *if a nurse at the shift detects that the concentration of a dopamine infusion (syringe pump) is the double of that which is documented in the patient chart – with the consequence that twice the amount has been given over the last 8 hours – he or she should report it even if this error had not been initiated by themselves.*

The Institute for Healthcare Improvement (www.ihi.org) describes three factors for success when using self-reporting of errors and events:
- The staff must be able to recognize when errors occur
- The reporting system must be user-friendly, and neither difficult nor time-consuming
- The organisation must have a just culture, one that encourages and rewards any reporting, and one that does not focus on individual blame and punishment

Self-reporting error and event systems may be mandatory or voluntarily, they can be confidential (with full name of the reporter and the patient) or anonymous (at least the reporter is not revealed). They also differ with regard to their origin: being either a hospital or part of a regional system, covering several clinical units in different hospitals, or, they may be very unit-specific. The former system is often called a "top-down" reporting system, the other one "bottom up". The latter usually involves technically very simple systems, often created in the unit and relies on one or more very dedicated people to run it. The "top-down" is often regulated through the normal hospital hierarchy and seldom reflects a strong "ownership" at the individual unit level.

The existing literature of error and event reporting uses one or more of these three principals methods. The self-reporting system is more frequently in use, but is often reported to be the least sensitive method to reveal errors and events [5]. However, this is the only system which is capable of being integrated into part of the ICU structure, which means that it can be a system running routinely and not just intermittently. A great deal of evidence also comes from multicentre studies using self-reporting of errors.

Using information

No self-reporting systems have a value on their own. Registering the numbers and type of errors only in a passive manner will never lead to any improvement. It is extremely important that errors and events occurring in a unit are systemised and analysed locally; irrespective of its being a top-down or bottom up system. The "owner" of the event and error is the unit where it occurred. They are the only body that can place this into a meaningful context and clearly see what actions should be taken to prevent similar errors to happen in the future, or maybe even to reduce the consequences. Far too often errors are reported to external bodies with little or no insight into the organisation or working patterns in the unit where it happened. The value of such a passive recording of events can thus be questioned.

After analysing the events, the results must be brought back to the health care workers in the "micro-system" where the events and errors had happened. These workers are the "source" of errors and events, and must know what is going on since they are the only ones able to effectively do something about it. The so-called quality improvement circle is an excellent tool to use is this respect, and opens up the possibility for the problems to be discussed and solutions to be found at the local level (see Fig. 2 in chapter C "Evaluating and improving organizational outcome"). In many ways we can say that the errors and events are of little use for anyone outside the field where the occurred, but here they are a most valuable feedback in the continuous improvement process.

A positive "side effect" of having a running self-reporting system is the focus which this system sets on event and error reporting. Such happenings are frequent in the ICU and are not simply unusual events which affect only "bad apples". In fact, in a professional career as a physician or a nurse, one will be confronted with a number of small and large errors and events with a small or large contribution from oneself. This is an important aspect since the focus within the ICU should not be on poorly behaving individuals but rather on system failure and system improvement [9]. Luckily, in most hospitals the focus now is on the system rather than on the individual, and this is beneficial for the patients as well as for the working environment.

Experiences with a self-reported system for adverse events

At the Department of Anaesthesia and Intensive care, we have had since 1997 an integrated voluntary and anonymous system for reporting adverse events. The system has been used in three sections, the general ICU (10 beds), the postoperative unit (22 beds) and the postoperative cardiac surgery unit (6 beds). Our preliminary results have been published previously [7].

We used a very simple method with a paper-based registration form (see Fig. 1), and with a mailbox in each unit where the completed form could be delivered. A simple database made by the author (FileMaker Pro) was used for punching of the data and for analysis. A group of four people (two ICU nurses and two physicians) regularly screened incoming data and gave monthly feedback to unit leaders as well as to the staff. The unit leaders were responsible for all actions that were to be taken as a consequence of the reporting system.

In the 10-year period from 1997 to 2006, a total of 3192 events were reported through our self-reporting systems. Most events came from the ICU (see Fig. 2) and the number of events was fairly constant during these years. In Table 1, the events are broken down into the individual units and the number of events per patient. The

Tab. 1   The number of admission and events in the three reporting units 1997–2006

	General ICU	Cardiac surgery	Post-operative
Admissions	4,288	6,528	87,431
LOS (days)	21,203	6,994	25,406
Adverse events	1,747	603	842
Medications	29.7%	24.9%	22.1%
Infusions	10.7%	5.3%	6.8%
Procedures	31.9%	34%	43.3%
Technical equipment	16.4%	24%	5.5%
Other	12%	11.8%	22.3%
Events/patient	0.40	0.09	0.0096
Events/100 days	8.2	8.6	3.3

Form for report of Adverse Events -ICU

(deliver in the mail-box in the ICU)

Date   Time   Patient age   Reporter ☐ Physician ☐ Nurse ☐ Other

Patient O Postoperative   O ICU, stabile   Year   Month
         O Postopeative cardiac   O ICU, instabile

Place O ICU   O During transport
       O Postoperative cardiac O X-ray department
       O Postoperative general O Other

Medication error   O Yes O No   Type of error ☐ Wrong drug   ☐ Wrong administration
                                                      ☐ Wrong dose   ☐ Wrong ordination
                                                      ☐ Wrong concentration ☐ Other

IInfusion error   O Yes O No   Type of error ☐ Wrong solution   ☐ Wrong administration
                                                     ☐ Wrong concentration ☐ Other
                                                     ☐ Wrong voilume

Medications intended to give?

Medications actually given

Concentraion or d oseplanned

Concentration/dose given

Other adverse events   What? ☐ Incorrect use of medical device   ☐ Mismatch patient and test-result
   O Yes O No   ☐ Mal-function of medical device   ☐ Errors in the medical records
                                    ☐ Incorrectly performed procedure   ☐ Other

Consequences of the adverse events   ☐ None registered ☐ Hypoglycemia   ☐ Patient dead
                                     ☐ Circulatory   ☐ Hyperglycemia   ☐ Other
                                     ☐ respiratory   ☐ Physical injury to patient
                                     ☐ Skin/allergy   ☐ Bleeding

Degree of seriousness of the event   O 0= No observed change in condition
                                     O 1= Change (physiologic or biochemical), no intervention necessary
                                     O 2= Change (physiologic or biochemical), intervention necessary, no harm
                                     O 3= Change,Change (physiologic or biochemical), intervention, temporary harn
                                     O 4=Change (physiologic or biochemical), intervention, permanent harm
                                     O 5=Change (physiologic or biochemical), intervention, patient died

Your opinion of why this event happened
☐ Time pressure   ☐ No control   ☐ Impossible to read ordination
☐ No education in procedure   ☐ No double control (medications)   ☐ Poor communication
☐ Extra shift   ☐ Lack of equipment   ☐ Unconcentrated
☐ Double shift   ☐ Too many patients   ☐ Personal problems
☐ Not familiar in the unit   ☐ Lack of information about the patient ☐ Other (decribe)

A more detailed description of the event can be given here

What was done to correct the consequences?

©HAUKELAND UNIVERSITY HOSPITAL-ICU 2010

Fig. 1   The form for reporting adverse events in the ICU

number of events per 100 patient days is also given, illustrating that even if the number of events was infrequent in the two postoperative units, the events per 100 patient days were more similar; for example, these values were 8.2 in the ICU, 8.6 in the post cardiac surgery unit and 3.3 in the postoperative unit.

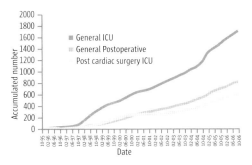

Fig. 2   The accumulated number of adverse events
reported over a 10-year period

Conclusion

In various types of industry it is often claimed that "A complaint is a gift", since this allows them to make use of customer feedback as a strategic tool for improvement [10]. In health care, such a type of feedback is not often available, and hence it is difficult to use complaints in the same way. As an alternative, one may be tempted to rephrase this into a medical context and declare "An event is gift" since it gives us an excellent opportunity to have a closer look at how health care – including intensive care – is actually delivered to individuals.

The author

Hans Flaatten, MD, PhD
    Haukeland University Hospital
    Department of Anaesthesia and Intensive Care
    Jonas Liesvei 65
    5021 Bergen, Norway
    E-mail: hans.flaatten@kir.uib.no

References

1. Kane-Gill SL, Kowiatek JG, Weber RJ. A comparison of voluntarily reported medication errors in intensive care and general care units. Qual Saf Health Care. 2010;19:55–9.
2. Valentin A, Capuzzo M, Guidet B, et al. Patient safety in intensive care: results from the multinational Sentinel Events Evaluation (SEE) study. Intensive Care Med. 2006;32:1591–8.
3. Valentin A, Capuzzo M, Guidet B, et al. Errors in administration of parenteral drugs in intensive care units: multinational prospective study. BMJ. 2009;338:b814.
4. Brennan TA, Leape LL, Laird NM, et al. Incidence of adverse events and negligence in hospitalized patients. Results of the Harvard Medical Practice Study I. N Engl J Med. 1991;324:370–6.
5. Haw C, Stubbs J, Dickens G. An observational study of medication administration errors in old-age psychiatric inpatients. Int J Qual Health Care. 2007;19:210–6.
6. Donchin Y, Gopher D, Olin M, et al. A look into the nature and causes of human errors in the intensive care unit. Crit Care Med. 1995;23:294–300.
7. Flaatten H, Hevroy O. Errors in the intensive care unit (ICU). Experiences with an anonymous registration. Acta Anaesthesiol Scand. 1999;43:614–7.
8. Milch CE, Salem DN, Pauker SG, et al. Voluntary electronic reporting of medical errors and adverse events. An analysis of 92,547 reports from 26 acute care hospitals. J Gen Intern Med. 2006;21:165–70.
9. Berwick DM, Leape LL. Reducing errors in medicine. BMJ. 1999;319:136–7.
10. Barlow J, Moller C. A complaint is a gift: Berrett-Koehler Publishers 1996.

Rui P. Moreno, Ana Cristina Diogo, Susana Afonso de Carvalho
and Andrew Rhodes

Benchmarking the intensive care unit

*"We will have to learn, before understanding
any task, to first ask the question, 'What information do I need, and in what form, and
when'. We should begin thinking about the
delivery system for the information only when
this is clear."*

Peter Drucker, 1990

Introduction

Intensive care medicine (ICM) is the science and art of
preventing, detecting and managing patients at risk of,
or already with, established critical illness in order to
achieve the best possible outcomes. Care is often a complex process that is carried out within a variety of healthcare systems and models on heterogeneous groups of
patient populations that are influenced by a number of
religious and cultural beliefs [1]. ICM is also a very expensive activity, consuming, at least in the more developed world, a significant portion of the healthcare budget and is considered to be one of the most expensive
hospital assets [2]. At a time of financial constraints, and
in the absence of clear and intuitive data about the quality and the adequacy of many ICM practices, it is vital
for us to be able to assess the performance of individual
units to ensure that our resources are wisely spent. This

requires a marker of quality (or performance) that can
be used both within and between hospitals in an objective and trustworthy fashion.

Probably the most robust and objective marker of
performance is patient mortality. Since the early 1980s,
investigators have concluded that for this to be used as
an assessment of quality, however, it must be adjusted
for the major determinants of prognosis, of which age,
comorbidities, acute reason for ICU admission and presence and degree of physiological derangement are the
most important. As a direct consequence of this need
for risk adjustment in the ICU, a series of models have
been proposed, trying to take into account this variability in the patient population characteristics. In other
words, there is a need to standardise different groups of
patients regarding outcome. These risk adjustment
methods then allow us to take into account all of the
patient characteristics known to affect their outcomes,
irrespective of the treatment received.

As it is impossible to set a priori mortality targets –
given the difficulty to forecast all the characteristics of
the patients that will be admitted in the future, the
evaluation of the performance of an ICU in the strictest
sense (the degree to which the pre-defined objectives
of each ICU are met) has been replaced in real life by
the relative evaluation of ICU performance, in which the
population of each ICU is compared (after the applica-

tion of some method for risk adjustment) to a reference database. This process, known as benchmarking, is based on the comparison of the risk-adjusted mortality of each ICU to – as defined in the New Oxford American Dictionary – a standard or point of reference against which things may be compared or assessed. Traditionally based on mortality, this process is now being applied to other outcomes, most, if not all, being related to costs. Perhaps the most popular of these is the risk-adjusted length of stay (LOS) (which is more or less a proxy for the cost of each patient).

The objective of this chapter is to analyse the principles of risk adjustment in the critically ill patient and their application to the benchmarking process.

Principles of risk adjustment in the ICU

Despite the increasing use of process-related performance measures [3], the evaluation of ICU throughput until recently has been based almost exclusively on severity-adjusted hospital mortality and on severity-adjusted length of stay (in the ICU or in the hospital). Other outputs have been proposed, such as the rates of admission for low-risk patients admitted just for monitoring [4, 5], or, on the other extreme, the rate of admissions for potentially futile care [6, 7]. Both, however, depend on a set of assumptions that can and have been challenged and thus have never gained widespread use. Unfortunately, given the probabilistic nature of the instruments used for risk adjustment and the fact that all of them are calibrated with the assumption that the patient will be admitted and cared for in an ICU, it is – by definition – impossible to apply these instruments to individual patients or to know what would be the outcome for any given patient if they were not admitted to the ICU. Consequently, we will focus this chapter on severity-adjusted hospital mortality and on severity-adjusted length of stay (in the ICU or in the hospital).

Severity-adjusted hospital mortality

The evaluation of severity of illness in a critically ill patient is made through the use of general severity scores and general outcome prognosis models. Severity scores are instruments that aim to stratify patients according to their severity, as-

signing to each patient an increasing number of points (or score) as their severity of illness increases; prognostic models, apart from their ability to stratify patients according to their severity of illness aim to predict a certain outcome – usually the vital status at hospital discharge – based on a given set of prognostic variables and a specific modelling equation. Other outcomes, both for the short and long term can eventually be considered, but most of them are more prone to bias and manipulation or are of little interest to patients, their families and the healthcare providers [1].

Today, all instruments used to predict mortality in patients admitted to an ICU are still based on the original concepts developed by William Knaus and co-workers in the acute physiology and chronic health evaluation (APACHE II) system [8] and by Jean-Roger Le Gall and co-workers on the new simplified acute physiological score (SAPS II) [9]. Both consist of a score, used to measure the severity of illness, and a modelling equation (using just the score or the score plus additional variables) that predicts the outcome at hospital discharge. Although the methods for selecting the predictive variables vary, all of them use standard logistic regression to develop the equation relating the predictive variables to the probability of the outcome of interest. They allow the user to adjust for the underlying characteristics of the admitted population (case mix) and to perform an indirect standardisation of the outcome of different groups of patients, irrespective of the treatment received in the intensive care unit (ICU). Although they are designed to be applied in heterogeneous groups of patients, they predict what should be the aggregate mortality at hospital discharge of a group of patients, with a certain degree of physiologic dysfunction, as if they had been treated in a virtual ICU such as was used to develop the model. Many other systems have been developed and proposed but have never gained the widespread use of these two original models. The most recent generations of these instruments have been extensively reviewed and discussed [10]: the APACHE models [11], the SAPS models [12], the Mortality Probability Models [13] and the Intensive Care National Audit & Research Centre (ICNARC) model [14].

An important debate exists about the ideal characteristics of the reference population. This pertains to whether the reference population should be local with the score adjusted to a certain region or group of ICUs or if it should include heterogeneity to improve the chances to learn with variation [15]. At the moment, the consensual view seems to be that for benchmarking purposes it is better to sacrifice the greater potential of large, heterogeneous databases to focus on the more homogeneous, permanent, high-quality systems. This allows us to maximise our capability to collect reliable data that is more likely to be adjusted for known, and unknown, confounders, many of them potentially context-dependent [16], and also enables the dataset to be constantly updated, preventing progress and changes with time from degrading the model [17].

No matter which system is chosen, it is vitally important that all the data needed for computation of the model can be collected in a standard and reliable fashion. This includes such issues as handling of the data before analysis that must be performed according to the original description of the model, the inclusion of the majority of admissions to the ICU, the model accounting for all the major variables with prognostic significance and finally that the dimension of the sample under analysis is large enough to yield the power for detecting significant differences [18, 19]. The frequency of data collection also impacts the reliability for the calibration of the model. For instance, most systems were designed in a time when data collection was performed in a manual fashion. Nowadays many units have patient data management systems (PDMS). These can more reliably collect the data but at a much-increased frequency compared to the older manual mechanism. This will decrease the calibration of the models due to the high sampling rates introducing important systematic deviations in the severity scores. Higher sampling rates are associated with higher probabilities of detecting deviations from normality and consequently give higher severity scores (and lower observed to adjusted mortality ratios) [20, 21]. This problem is significantly greater for models that use a long observation period, for example the first 24 hours after ICU admission, and should be small in systems based on admission data only [22, 23]. A complete understanding of the methodology (including the methodological problems and limitations) of the severity scores and outcome prediction models

is crucial to understand their use as the basis for risk-adjusted evaluation of mortality [17, 24].

Severity-adjusted length of stay (in the ICU or in the hospital)

Despite the fact that mortality (as well as residual disability and quality of life after ICU discharge) are among the most important outcomes for all those involved in the process of dealing with and managing critical illness, there are other important outcomes. Everything in life has a price, and in this society resources are limited. This potential imbalance, if badly managed, can lead to several possible scenarios, none of them desirable. These include inappropriate triaging, limitations of care based on economic rather than scientific or human constraints, or even the complete denial of care to some parts of the population. We, as intensivists, have the duty to help decrease this imbalance, and the best way to achieve this is to increase productivity. In other words, providing more and better care at a lower cost. As a consequence of this need, methods to compare the cost-effectiveness of different medical practices have made their way into the hospital [25, 26] and more specifically, into the ICU [27]. One of these measures is the comparative evaluation of costs inside a certain cohort of ICUs, or cost benchmarking. Given the many problems in cost evaluation and cost comparison between different ICUs, even within the same country [28, 29], many researchers until now have focused on the evaluation of proxies for costs of providing intensive care. In general, three methods have been used: the direct comparison of costs, the use of weighted LOS as a proxy for costs and, more recently, the use of risk-adjusted LOS as a proxy for costs of providing intensive care.

The use of weighted LOS as a proxy for costs used data from European and North American ICUs to compute what the authors described as Weighted Hospital Days (WHD) as a proxy for costs, a method that gives higher weight to ICU days than to days in the hospital after ICU discharge (and a different weight to different days while the patient is in the ICU) to compute resource use [30, 31]. The latest development of this approach was the publication in 2007 by Nathanson et al. [32], using a Weighted Hospital Days scale (based on the same concepts as the original WHD-94 scale) to assess resource utilisation. The main difference from the original model was the redefinition of the WHD and the development of a new model to predict ICU-specific log average WHD from 39 candidate variables available in Project ImpACT. The updated WHD now contains four independent variables: percentage of patients dying in the hospital, percentage of unscheduled surgical patients, percentage of patients on mechanical ventilation within 1 hr of ICU admission, and percentage discharged from the ICU to an external post-acute care facility. According to the authors the model now performs better.

The risk-adjusted LOS methodology was first used by Rapoport in the 1990s [33] and then by the Knaus group in 2000 [34], as a way to explain the large variability found between different ICUs [35, 36]. Similar analyses have subsequently been conducted using the same methodology in other settings, such as in a cohort of ICUs in Scotland [37]. The most recent developments are based on the APACHE IV model [38], and were published in 2006 [39]. Essentially, a model is developed to adjust LOS for a number of important case mix factors. The important point to recognise, however, is that it is not possible to develop a model that takes into account *every* relevant factor, only most of them. In the original database described above, only 21.5% of the variation in ICU stay across individual patients and 62% across ICUs was explained by the model, with a resulting difference between mean observed and predicted length of stay being reduced for patients with a short or long ICU stay and/or a low or high risk of death on ICU day 1. Thus, despite providing useful information about ICU length of stay predictions for critically ill patient groups (and consequently for benchmarking ICUs), the applicability of the model to individual patients was very limited. A similar approach was followed and published by Rothen et al. as a method to understand variations in costs between ICUs, using the SAPS 3 system to adjust for severity of illness [40].

The multidimensional nature of benchmarking

In a complex activity such as the provision of intensive care, benchmarking needs to be a multidimensional process, in which the assessment of resource use and outcomes must be viewed as being complementary to each other. Other indicators are certainly important, such as communication with the families [41] and respect for their spiritual needs and values [42, 43], or end-of-life practices [44–46], but these two are particularly important, because – when assessed together in a standardised way – they can help with the evaluation of the cost-effectiveness of the ICU, perhaps a more important issue to benchmark that just hospital mortality or cost alone. Furthermore, this measure can be used to study the link between ICU structures and the process of care, on the one hand, and resource use and outcome on the other [40].

This issue has recently been addressed using the SAPS 3 database [40]. This group was able to demonstrate a very large variation between different ICUs, encompassing a broad range of structures and processes, within and between geographical regions, based on standardised data collection. Unfortunately, despite these efforts, only a few factors of ICU structure and process were associated with efficient use of the ICU (e.g. multi-professional rounds, presence of an emergency department in the hospital), which suggests that many other confounding factors may play an important role in this variation. The proposed measures in this model were for outcome, the standardised mortality ratio based on the SAPS 3 model (SMR), and for resource use, the standardised resource use (SRU), based on the length of stay in the ICU, adjusted for severity of acute illness (as measured by the SAPS 3 model). The cross-tabulation of these two values allows the authors to split the ICUs into four groups, based on the median SMR and median SRU: "most efficient" included all units whose SMR and SRU were below the median SMR and SRU, respectively; "least efficient" included units in which SMR and SRU were both above the median; "overachieving" or relatively wasteful: low SMR but high SRU; and "underachieving", with a high SMR but low SRU.

This method has never been compared to the method proposed by Rapoport in 1994 [30] based on WHD and MPM SMR, the so-called Rapoport-Teres graph, in which standardised resource use was plotted against standardised clinical performance use. A new variation of the method was proposed by Nathanson [32], using a different way to compute the WHD and the SMR (this time based on the data from Project IMPACT (Cerner Corporation, KS City, MO) used to develop the MPM III model [23] that is used as the performance indicator). Apart from a Rapoport-Teres plot based on more actual data, the new method did not introduce any new concepts to the field. Certainly more research is needed in this area.

Doubts and prospects for the future

These methodologies have been criticised by some authors. They argue that ICUs should neither be assessed nor benchmarked by a system which at its core has a low signal (preventable deaths) to high noise (deaths from other causes) ratio that could lead to potentially inaccurate data [47, 48]. We all recognise that the quality of the data on which benchmarking systems are based must be optimised and controlled to avoid bias and manipulation, that the statistical methods used to generate the SMR are subject to methodological flaws, and that these methods are not intrinsically able to control for all variables that may affect prognosis (but certainly control for the major ones). However, to argue that risk-adjusted mortality should not be used as a performance indicator unless we can restrict the mortality analysis to preventable deaths is to argue that ICUs should only admit patients in which death is preventable. Unfortunately, currently used clinical criteria do not allow us to predict the patients that will benefit from ICU with the 100 % specificity and sensitivity required. At the moment it is not possible in many instances to predict which patients will certainly die irrespective of medical intervention (a non-preventable death), thus we are often faced with admitting patients for a trial of therapy knowing that sometimes we will do not more than delay an unavoidable outcome. Our role regarding this group is to ensure that when intervention becomes futile, care is optimised and delivered in such a way that death is as humane and dignified as possible.

Conclusions

As our case mix adjustment models become more sophisticated and we understand the competing influenc-

es on patient outcome, we are becoming better placed to comprehend both outcome prediction and resource utilisation. This enables us to benchmark our performance against other similar institutions. Whilst we would still advocate caution in extrapolating and over-concluding from these systems, in particular with regards resource allocation, we believe that they can give valuable insights into our practice that should enable us to review what we are doing with the purpose of higher quality care at less cost. But this is the ultimate call of our profession, as defined many years ago by Sir William Osler in his immortal words:

> "[The practice of medicine is] an art, not a trade; a calling, not a business; a calling in which your heart will be exercised equally with your head. Often the best part of your work will have nothing to do with potions and powders, but with the exercise of an influence of the strong upon the weak, of the righteous upon the wicked, of the wise upon the foolish."

The authors

Rui P. Moreno, MD, PhD[1]
Ana Cristina Diogo, MD[1]
Susana Afonso de Carvalho, MD[1]
Andrew Rhodes, FRCP FRCA[2]
  [1] Unidade de Cuidados Intensivos
  Polivalente | Hospital de Santo António
  dos Capuchos | Centro Hospitalar de Lisboa
  Central, E.P.E. | Lisbon, Portugal
  [2] General Intensive Care | St George's
  Hospital | London, UK

Address for correspondence
  Rui P. Moreno
  Unidade de Cuidados Intensivos Polivalente
  Hospital de Santo António dos Capuchos
  Centro Hospitalar de Lisboa Central, E.P.E.
  Alameda de Santo António dos Capuchos
  1169-050 Lisbon, Portugal
  E-mail: r.moreno@mail.telepac.pt

References

1. Moreno RP, Jardim AL, Godinho de Matos R, Metnitz PGH. Principles of risk-adjustment in the critically ill patient. In: Kuhlen R, Moreno R, Ranieri M,

Rhodes A, eds. 25 Years of Progress and Innovation in Intensive Care Medicine. Berlin: Medizinisch Wissenschaftliche Verlagsgesellschaft, 2007:409–17.

2. Halpern NA, Pastores SM. Critical care medicine in the United States 2000–2005: An analysis of bed numbers, occupancy rates, payer mix, and costs. Crit Care Med 2010;38:65–71.

3. Randall Curtis J, Cook DJ, Wall RJ, Angus DC, BionxJ, Kacmarek R, Kane-Gill SL, Kirchhoff KT, Levy M, Mitchell PH, Moreno R, Pronovost P, Puntillo K. Intensive care unit quality improvement: a "how-to" guide for the interdisciplinary team. Crit Care Med 2006;34:211–8.

4. Wagner DP, Knaus WA, Draper EA. Identification of low-risk monitor admissions to medical-surgical ICUs. Chest 1987;92:423–8.

5. Wagner DP, Knaus WA, Draper EA, et al. Identification of low-risk monitor patients within a medical-surgical ICU. Med Care 1983;21:425–33.

6. Esserman L, Belkora J, Lenert L. Potentially ineffective care. A new outcome to assess the limits of critical care. JAMA 1995;274:1544–51.

7. Zimmerman JE. Potentially ineffective care:A useful step forward. Crit Care Med 2002;30:1920–1.

8. Knaus WA, Draper EA, Wagner DP, Zimmerman JE. APACHE II: a severity of disease classification system. Crit Care Med 1985;13:818–29.

9. Le Gall JR, Lemeshow S, Saulnier F. A new simplified acute physiology score (SAPS II) based on a European/ North American multicenter study. JAMA 1993;270:2957–63.

10. Moreno RP. Outcome prediction in intensive care: why we need to reinvent the wheel. Curr Opin Crit Care 2008;14:483–4.

11. Zimmerman JE, Kramer AA. Outcome prediction in critical care: the Acute Physiology and Chronic Health Evaluation models. Curr Opin Crit Care 2008;14:491–7.

12. Capuzzo M, Moreno RP, Le Gall J-R. Outcome prediction in critical care: the Simplified Acute Physiology Score models. Curr Opin Crit Care 2008;14:485–90.

13. Higgins TL, Teres D, Nathanson B. Outcome prediction in critical care: the Mortality Probability Models. Curr Opin Crit Care 2008;14:498–505.

14. Harrison DA, Rowan KM. Outcome prediction in critical care: the ICNARC model. Curr Opin Crit Care 2008;14:506–12.

15. Moreno RP, Afonso S. Building and using outcome prediction models: Should we be lumpers or splitters? In: Kuhlen R, Moreno R, Ranieri M, Rhodes A, eds. Controversies in Intensive Care Medicine. Berlin: Medizinisch Wissenschaftiche Verlagsgesellschaft, 2008:415–9.

16. Poole D, Rossi C, Anghileri A, Giardino M, Latronico N, Radrizzani D, Langer M, Bertolini G. External validation of the Simplified Acute Physiology Score (SAPS) 3 in a cohort of 28,357 patients from 147 Italian intensive care units. Intensive Care Med 2009.

17. Poole D, Bertolini G. Outcome-based benchmarking in the ICU Part I: Statistical tools for the creation and validation of severity scores. In: Chice J-D, Moreno R, Putensen C, Rhodes A, eds. Patient Safety and Quality of Care In Intensive Care Medicine. Berlin: Medizinisch Wissenschaftiche Verlagsgesellschaft, 2009:vol 141–150).

18. Rowan K. The reliability of case mix measurements in intensive care. Curr Opin Crit Care 1996;2:209–13.

19. Black NA, Jenkinson C, Hayes JA, Young D, Vella K, Rowan KM, Daly K, Ridley S. Review of outcome measures used in adult critical care. Crit Care Med 2001;29:2119–24.

20. Bosman RJ, Oudemane van Straaten HM, Zandstra DF. The use of intensive care information systems alters outcome prediction. Intensive Care Med 1998;24:953–8.

21. Suistomaa M, Kari A, Ruokonen E, Takala J. Sampling rate causes bias in APACHE II and SAPS II scores. Intensive Care Med 2000;26:1773–8.

22. Moreno RP, Metnitz PG, Almeida E, Jordan B, Bauer P, Campos RA, Iapichino G, Edbrooke D, Capuzzo M, Le Gall JR, SAPS 3 Investigators. SAPS 3. From evaluation of the patient to evaluation of the intensive care unit. Part 2: Development of a prognostic model for hospital mortality at ICU admission. Intensive Care Med 2005;31:1345–55.

23. Higgins TL, Teres D, Copes WS, Nathanson BH, Stark M, Kramer AA. Assessing contemporary intensive care unit outcome: An updated Mortality Probability Admission Model (MPMo-III). Crit Care Med 2007;35:827–35.

24. Poole D, Bertolini G. Outcome-based benchmarking in the ICU Part I: Use and limitations of severity scores in critical care. In: Chiche J-D, Moreno R, Putensen C, Rhodes A, eds. Patient Safety and Quality of Care in Intensive Care Medicine. Berlin: Medizinisch Wissenschaftiche Verlagsgesellschaft, 2009:151–60.

25. Murray CJL, Evans DB, Acharya A, Baltussen RMPM. Development of WHO guidelines for generalized cost-effectiveness analysis. Health Econ 2000;9:235–51.

26. Russell LB, Gold MR, Siegel JE, Daniels N, Weinstein MC, for the Panel on Cost-Effectiveness in Health and Medicine. The Role of Cost-effectiveness Analysis in Health and Medicine. JAMA 1996;276:1172–7.

27. Zilberberg MD. Understanding Cost-Effectiveness in the ICU. Seminars in Respiratory and Critical Care Medicine 2010;31:13–8.

28. Edbrooke DL, Wilson AJ, Gerrish SP, Mann AJ. The Shefield costing system for intensive care. Care Criti Ill 1995;11:106–10.

29. Edbrooke DL, Hibbert CL, Corcoran M. Investigating the costs of intensive care. Intensive Care Monitor 1999;4:43–7.

30. Rapoport J, Teres D, Lemeshow S, Gehlbach S. A method for assessing the clinical performance and cost-effec-

tiveness of intensive care units: a multicenter inception cohort study. Crit Care Med 1994;22:1385–91.

31. Rapoport J, Teres D, Zhao Y, Lemeshow S. Length of stay data as a guide to hospital economic performance for ICU patients. Med Care 2003;41:386–97.

32. Nathanson BH, Higgins TL, Teres D, Copes WS, Kramer A, Stark M. A revised method to assess intensive care unit clinical performance and resource utilization. Crit Care Med 2007;35:1853–62.

33. Rapoport J, Teres D, Lemeshow S, Avrunin JS, Haber R. Explaining variability of cost using a severity of illness measure for ICU patients. Med Care 1990;28:338–48.

34. Rosenberg AL, Zimmerman JE, Alzola C, Draper EA, Knaus WA. Intensive care unit length of stay: recent changes and future challenges. Crit Care Med 2000;28:3465–73.

35. Knaus WA, Wagner DP, Zimmerman JE, Draper EA. Variations in mortality and length of stay in Intensive Care Units. Ann Intern Med 1993;118:753–61.

36. Zimmerman JE, Shortell SM, Knaus WA, Rousseau DM, Wagner DP, Gillies RR, Draper EA, Devers K. Value and cost of teaching hospitals: a prospective, multicenter, inception cohort study. Crit Care Med 1993;21:1432–42.

37. Woods AW, MacKirdy FN, Livingston BM, Norrie J, Howie JC. Evaluation of predicted and actual length of stay in 22 Scottish intensive care units using the APACHE III system. Acute Physiology and Chronic Health Evaluation. Anaesthesia 2000;55:1058–65.

38. Zimmerman JE, Kramer AA, McNair DS, Malila FM. Acute Physiology and Chronic Health Evaluation (APACHE) IV: Hospital mortality assessment for today's critically ill patients. Crit Care Med 2006;34:1297–310.

39. Zimmerman JE, Kramer AA, McNair DS, Malila FM, Shaffer VL. Intensive care unit length of stay: Benchmarking based on Acute Physiology and Chronic Health Evaluation (APACHE) IV. Crit Care Med 2006;34:2517–29.

40. Rothen HU, Stricker K, Einfalt J, Bauer P, Metnitz PGH, Moreno RP, Takala J. Variability in outcome and resource use in intensive care units. Intensive Care Med 2007;33:1329–36.

41. Levy M. Including families in quality measurement in critical care. Crit Care Med 2007;35:324–5.

42. Wall RJ, Engelberg RA, Gries CJ, Glavan B, Randall Curtis J. Spiritual care of families in the intensive care unit. Crit Care Med 2007;35:1084–90.

43. Sprung CL, Maia P, Bulow H-H, Ricou B, Armaganidis A, Baras M, Wennberg E, Reinhart K, Cohen SL, Fries DR, Nakos G, Thijs LG, the Ethicus Study Group. The importance of religious affiliation and culture on end-of-life decisions in European intensive care units. Intensive Care Med 2007;33:1732–9.

44. Bertolini G, Boffelli S, Malacarne S, Peta M, Marchesi M, Barbisan C, Tomelleri S, Spada S, Satolli R, Gridelli B, Lizzola I, Mazzon D. End-of-life decision-making and quality of ICU performance: an observational study in 84 Italian units. Intensive Care Med 2010.

45. Azoulay E, Metnitz B, Sprung C-L, Timsit J-F, Lemaire F, Bauer P, Schlemmer B, Moreno R, Metnitz P. End-of-life practices in 282 intensive care units: data from the SAPS 3 database. Intensive Care Med 2009;35:623–30.

46. Randall Curtis J. End-of-life care for patients in the Intensive Care Unit. In: Kuhlen R, Moreno R, Ranieri M, Rhodes A, eds. 25 Years of Progress and Innovation in Intensive Care Medicine. Berlin: Medizinisch Wissenschaftliche Verlagsgesellschaft, 2007:469–79.

47. Lilford R, Pronovost P. Using hospital mortality rates to judge hospital performance: a bad idea that just won't go away. Br Med J 2010;340:955–7.

48. Black N. Assessing the quality of hospitals. Hospital standardised mortality ratios should be abandoned. Br Med J 2010;340.

Mercedes Palomar Martínez

Nosocomial infection: outcome indicator?

Quality of care has been defined as "the degree to which health services for individuals and populations increase the likelihood of desired heath outcomes and are consistent with current professional knowledge" [1]. Scientific societies, hospital leaders, health authorities, politicians and also consumers are interested in improving the quality of care of health services, as much as in reducing health costs arising from complications. Although quality of care is on the agenda in most health care systems, in most countries there is no mandatory control of the care delivered to citizens.

Ensuring patients' safety during their hospital stay requires as a first step, mechanisms to determine the incidence of adverse effects. Today, healthcare-associated infection (HAIs) are considered preventable errors and surveillance systems have shown that HAIs are key errors because of their frequency and also the impact on patient outcome. Each year, in the EU approximately 4 million patients acquire a HAI and around 37,000 of them die as the direct result of the infection [2]. In the United States, the figure is approximately 2 million of HAI annually. These infections result in substantial morbidity, mortality, and cost. The excess duration of hospitalization secondary to nosocomial infections has been estimated to be 1 to 4 days for urinary tract infections, 7 to 8 days for surgical site infections, 7 to 21 days for bloodstream infections, and 6 to 30 days for pneumonia.

The estimated mortalities associated with nosocomial bloodstream infections and pneumonia are 23.8 % to 50 % and 14.8 % to 71 % (overall), or 16.3 % to 35 % and 6.8 % to 30 % (attributable), respectively [3]. Recent changes in some regulatory and financial reimbursement systems, reflect the new attitude of paying less and no more when these HAIs occur [4].

National surveillance of HAI was initiated in the United States in 1970. Since that time, the Centers for Disease Control and Prevention's (CDC) National Nosocomial Infections Surveillance (NNIS) system has provided standardized methods for collecting and comparing healthcare-associated infection rates, publishing the rates for major HAI [5]. Since 2000, the surveillance of surgical site infections and ICU-acquired infections has been coordinated at the European Union (EU) level by the DG Sanco funded HELICS project (Hospitals in Europe Link for Infection Control through Surveillance) and from 2005 to June 2008, as part of the IPSE (Improving Patient Safety in Europe) network [6]. In July 2008, the coordination of the IPSE network was transferred to ECDC [7]. To support clinicians in monitoring standards of practice, it is possible to obtain quality indicators through surveillance.

Quality indicators are defined as information that determines the degree of adherence to a standard goal by describing a situation in a simple, validated, reliable, and operational way with standard definitions that are reproducible, both in time and among observers [8]. National networks for the surveillance of HAI provide participating hospitals with a standardized methodology and reference data (quality indicators) to make risk-adjusted comparisons of HAI rates and follow-up the effect of infection control measures [9, 10]. HAI surveillance protocols target specific infection types, being the most frequent urinary tract infections, pneumonia, surgical site infections, bloodstream infections and gastrointestinal infections. ICUs account for 20–25 % of reported HAI. Basic process indicators in ICUs include VAP and CRBSI.

Clinical indicators

The clinical indicators can document the quality of care, although they are not a direct measure of quality. They help in making comparisons, not only between institutions (benchmarking) but over time in the same centre. Moreover, they facilitate the accreditation of hospitals [11], allow priorities to be set, support quality improvement, and in some health systems, patient choice of providers.

To be useful, clinical indicators should have some characteristics such as clear definitions, describing things exclusively and precisely. Apart from this, they have to be specific and quite sensitive. They also need to be valid and reliable, that is, reproducible and consistent as well as useful discriminators of good and bad quality. All these conditions permit us to make comparisons between ICUs, hospitals, regions, or health systems. Finally, clinical indicators must, above all, be relevant for clinical practice and based on the best evidence.

Clinical indicators can be classified in different ways [12, 13]. They can be rate-based versus sentinel; generic or disease-specific; related to the type of care: preventive, acute or chronic; according to function: screening, diagnosis, treatment or follow-up. One of the most useful classifications is to relate to structure, process and outcome of health care.

Indicators for structure are those which measure aspects related to organizational, technological or human resources. Structure indicators also need to reflect the system characteristics such as facilities, equipment and the number or qualification of the staff. No less important are aspects that affect organization including continuous training or the availability of updated protocols.

Process indicators monitor the availability, utilization and quality of care giving to the patients, that is, what the provider did and how well it was done. To be valid, process indicators must have been demonstrated to produce a better outcome. The same requirement is valid for the structure indicators.

Indicators for outcome measure the consequences of the healthcare process, expressed as complications, mortality or quality of life. We need to remember that the individual characteristics of each patient will exert influence on evolution.

It should be noted that in choosing the type of indicator, we obtain different information and therefore we do not properly interpret equivalent results [14, 15]. Table 1 shows some examples of indicators in HAI.

Tab. 1   Examples of indicators in HAI

Indicators for structure in HAI

Proportion of specialists (physicians and nurses)

Nurse staffing

Education/Certification

Updated clinical guidelines

Isolation capacity

Infection preventionist staffing

Indicators for performance in HAI

Proportion of patients receiving CVC bundle

Proportion of patients receiving ventilator bundle

Proportion of surgical patients receiving adequate antimicrobial prophylaxis

Proportion of surgical patients receiving surgical bundle

Indicators for outcome in HAI

Incidence of device-related infections (VAP, CR-BSI; UTI) and surgical infections

Multiresistant microorganism (MRSA, VRE)

Attributable excess length of stay

Attributable mortality

Attributable cost

One of the points that reinforce the use of outcome indicators is that they may reflect, at least in part, the quality of care delivered. On the other hand, process measures are only of value if they have a link to outcome. In many countries, nosocomial infection rates – an outcome indicator – have been incorporated into the quality programs and are required in the process of accreditation of hospitals (11). However, questions about the validity of the comparability of rates in different hospitals are more and more frequent and some authors have expressed their concern about the use of indicators as a "league table" [16].

Factors influencing differences in outcome indicators

The purpose of reporting indicators is to allow health systems to assess, compare, and improve the care delivered by hospital and health workers, but external observers are often unable to fully consider important factors in the interpretation of infection rates [17]. Several factors can be responsible for variations in outcome indicators, but the most important are:

- differences in case mix
- differences in measurements
- chance
- differences in quality of care

The patients' characteristics are relevant, and for example, patients admitted to the largest teaching hospitals, had a greater number of co-morbidities and their conditions are more frequently ultimately fatal, and could explain in part why rates of HAI are usually higher in bigger hospitals [18]. The admission category is one of the most important risk factor for HAI. ICUs are classified by diagnostic category in the USA, and mean rates of HAI vary widely depending on the type of patient. Burn and traumatic units show in general the highest rates for HAI, while cardiothoracic ICUs have the lowest [10]. However, in Europe, ICUs are often mixed, and a set of risk factors for risk adjustment of HAI rates is needed [19].

The surveillance methods may lead to important variations in outcome indicators. The way of expressing the indicators of infections related to device use can lead to confusion. Rates per 100 patients or incidence densities per 1000 days of stay or per 1000 days of device use are not equivalent. Nevertheless, incidence density per days of exposure to risk factors are the most helpful and allow intra-unit comparisons, but the risk of developing pneumonia of 100 patients ventilated for 1 day is not equivalent to the risk of 10 patients ventilated for 10 days (classically, patients in reanimation units versus ICU patients).

Probably, the lack of uniformity in the definitions is the most influential factor in the variability of HAI rates. This is especially complex for surgical infections, in some episodes of ventilator-associated pneumonia and in the calculation of the denominators used for calculating rates of catheter-associated bacteremia.

VAP is the ICU-AI with the higher variability in microbiological diagnostic tests, not only between countries or areas, but between units too [20–22]. In 2008, the CDC/NHSN launched the new definitions for surveillance of HCAI [9]. Pneumonia was categorized in 3 types:

1. clinically defined pneumonia (PNU1),
2. pneumonia with specific laboratory findings (PNU2) and
3. pneumonia in immunocompromised patients (PNU3).

Clinical diagnosis alone was not considered to be an acceptable criterium for health care-associated pneumonia, due to the multitude of processes that can mimic a VAP. However in PNU2, the accepted respiratory samples did not include quantitative or non-quantitative cultures from possible lower respiratory tract such as sputum or tracheal aspirate, which are the most commonly used diagnostic techniques in many ICUs. In the European surveillance, HELICS criteria for pneumonia definition is different and includes 5 categories based on the microbiology diagnostic technique used. In PN1, the bacteriologic diagnosis is performed by positive quantitative culture from minimally contaminated lower respiratory tract (LRT) such as broncho-alveolar lavage (BAL), protected brush (PB) or distal protected aspirate (DPA). In PN2, diagnosis is performed by positive quantitative cultures from possibly contaminated LRT specimen. PN3 include alternative microbiology methods as positive culture from blood, pleural fluid, pleural or pulmonary abscess, histological positive exam, seroconversion, detection of antigens in urine etc. PN4 is based on positive sputum culture or non-quantitative LRT specimen culture, and PN5, without positive microbiology, would be the equivalent to CDC-PNU1.

In addition to the differences in definitions, when we compare pneumonia diagnosis within European networks, we see the enormous variability of microbiological methods used in the 10 countries participating in the year 2007, which undoubtedly have an impact on VAP rates (see Fig. 1).

Although less relevant than for VAP, definition problems are also present in surveillance of Central Line Associated Bloodstream Infection (CLABSI), the second most frequent infection in ICUs. Using a questionnaire containing clinical cases, reproducibility of NNIS surveillance definition for CLABSI was assessed in an Australian cohort of infection control professionals participating in the Victorian Hospital Acquired Infection Surveillance System (VICNISS). The same questionnaire was then used to evaluate the reproducibility of the National Healthcare Safety Network (NHSN) surveillance definition for CLABSI. Target hospitals were defined as large

metropolitan or other large hospitals. Questionnaire responses of Centers for Disease Control and Prevention NHSN surveillance experts were used as the gold standard comparator. Eighteen centres participated in the survey. Overall concordance with the gold standard was 57.1%, and agreement was highest for large metropolitan hospitals (60.6%). The proportion of congruently classified cases varied according to NNIS criteria:

- criterion 1 (recognized pathogen), 52.8%;
- criterion 2a (skin contaminant in 2 or more blood cultures), 83.3%;
- criterion 2b (skin contaminant in 1 blood culture and appropriate antimicrobial therapy instituted), 58.3%;
- non-CLABSI cases, 51.4%.

When survey questions regarding identification of cases of CLABSI criterion 2b were removed (consistent with the current NHSN definition), overall percentage concordance increased to 62.5% (72.2% for large metropolitan centres). The conclusion of the authors was that further educational interventions are required to improve the discrimination of primary and secondary causes of bloodstream infection [23].

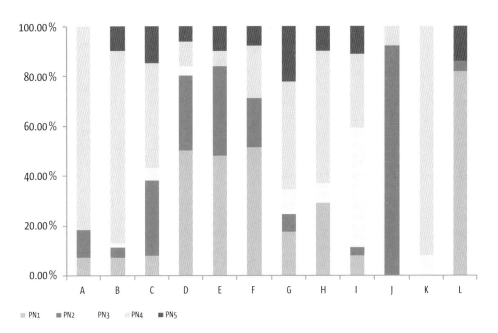

Fig. 1   HELICS 2007. Differences in diagnostic practices of ICU-acquired pneumonia in the participant countries

Moreover, if we compare NNISS surveillance with the European, monitoring of bacteraemia in the American system does not include bacteraemia clearly secondary to other sources different from CLABSI such as respiratory, abdominal etc, which are included in the rates of these infections. In contrast, the European program HELICS-ICU, included in the bacteraemia rates not only those secondary to CVC and those of unknown origin (primary), but also all bacteraemia episodes secondary to other sites. Clearly the incidence of bacteraemia is higher in the European program.

Random events can easily introduce variability in the results if the monitoring includes a small number of cases. Therefore, duration of surveillance could be relevant in small ICUs with limited number of admissions, especially if the number of patients collected is less than 100. It would be desirable to extend the period of surveillance in these cases. Likewise, seasonality or presence of outbreaks can also modify rates.

In the case of Surgical Site Infections (SSI), time of surveillance is crucial. As many patients are discharged home early after procedure, the follow-up of infections will vary the incidence if monitoring does not extend to home, the rates being lower, mainly for the superficial SSI.

The success of reporting systems requires several conditions including confidentiality and independence. Not only should the identity of the patient be protected, but the identity of the reporter and institution as well. The program should be independent with respect to authorities with power to punish, to avoid the fear of the reporters for the consequences and even the possibility of modifying the results, hiding episodes of HAI which may reflect in a negative way on the reputation of the institution involved.

But HAI rates depend on many other factors, including structural and functional conditions [25–27]. These represent the architecture of the units (single rooms versus open spaces) which provides the option of isolation and hence reduces any cross transmission. The availability of hand hygiene facilities, especially alcohol solutions, now accepted as crucial in preventing HAI. The number and training of nurses, the presence of educational programs, updated protocols, together with the use of some interventions such as continuous subglottic secretions aspiration, oral hygiene with clorhexidine, use of selective digestive decontamination, etc, will contribute to decrease the risk of developing HAI. In summary, these are conditions which could be considered as good practice, and which can be measured by the process indicators [28].

Which type of indicators should we use for nosocomial infections surveillance and control?

Indicators are measurement tools, useful as a guide to monitor, assess and improve quality of care, identifying opportunities for improvement and demonstrating effective performance [29]. After having basal data, it is necessary to flag areas requiring investigation or improvement, to focus on quality improvement activities and to monitor effects of implementing programs of change.

Outcome indicators are always relevant and attractive for patients and payers of care. Outcome measurement reflects all aspects of the processes of care, including some that are not measurable (such as technical skills). Outcome indicators provide a baseline data upon which to establish priorities and targets. On the other hand, outcome indicators may require fewer resources, and in some cases are available from routine administrative information in several institutions or countries. However, some studies have shown important discrepancies between "personal" and administrative surveillance in the case of some infections such as VAP, but are more acceptable for others like bacteraemia [30].

Another issue is whether outcome indicators are powerful enough to detect significant differences in quality. Statistical power depends upon how common the episode is.

The list of medicare's "never events", first implemented in 2008, includes overt mistakes such as wrong-site surgeries, objects left in the patient after surgery, and transfusing the wrong blood type. But it also includes a variety of infectious complications that may not be entirely preventable (see Tab. 2). Some authors think that calling these complications "never events" and refusing to pay for their treatment may advantage high-quality caregivers, but it also will penalize providers which care for the most vulnerable patients or which perform procedures with higher-than-average risk [31]. A recent analysis of some 890,000 surgeries (colon resection, coronary artery bypass grafting, total hip replacement, abdominal hysterectomy, and aortofemoral bypass) performed in 1,368 hospitals showed that patient age and pre-existing conditions greatly increased the risk of eight "never event" complications: MRSA, C. difficile, mediastinitis after coronary artery bypass graft (CABG), catheter-associated vascular and urinary tract infections, post-operative pneumonia, and decubitus ulcers [32]. Patient as well as hospital variables were significantly associated with rates of these events. Only mediastinitis after CABG surgery and catheter-associated urinary tract infections had C-statistics below the cut-off when hospital variables were removed. For each of the eight complications, certain patient factors were associated with substantial increased risks: older age, malnutrition, weight loss and chronic kidney failure. Odds ratios ranged from 1.8 for emergency admission as a risk factor for C. difficile enterocolitis to 16.4 for malnutrition and weight loss as a predictor of intravascular device infection. Aortofemoral bypass procedures increased the risk of five complications – C. difficile and MRSA infections, post-operative pneumonia, intravascular device infections, and decubitus ulcers – with odds ratios ranging from 2.3 to 11.9 compared with abdominal hysterectomy.

But yet, the inclusion of hospital variables as risk factors for the development of complications in the previous study, supports the contention that achievable improvements in quality of care can reduce the incidence of these complications. Process indicators can help in striving for this goal. They are more sensitive to detect differences in the quality of care than outcome indicators, because a lower number of cases are required. Another relevant advantage is that process indicators are easy to interpret and help in monitoring effects of implementing changes. Therefore, providers are quite interested in this type of clinical indicators.

In recent years, the use of "bundles" for prevention has been promoted by Institutions and Scientific Societies, ICUs [33–35]. But just having a bundle policy is not enough to reduce CLABSI, VAP or SSI rates; it is also necessary to monitor and maintain compliance. The single most important deficiency in health care today is that we frequently fail to adhere to evidence-based best practices. Improvement on a process level could favourably change the outcome. The last National Quality Forum (NQF) recommendations for Public Reporting included new performance measures in HAI. Besides the old incidence rates, the adherence to the bundles for prevention of CLABSI, VAP etc is now promoted [36]. Table 3 shows these performance indicators.

Tab. 3   National Quality Forum (NQF) recommendations for public reporting: new performance measures in HAI

Central line-associated bloodstream infection (CLABSI)

- Hand hygiene
- Maximal barrier precautions upon insertion
- Clorhexidine skin antisepsis
- Optimal catheter site selection (subclavian vein as preferred site for nontunneled catheters in patients aged 18 years and older)
- Daily review of line necessity with prompt removal of unnecessary lines

Previous reference: CLABSI rate

Ventilator-associated pneumonia (VAP)

- Head of the bed elevation > 30° (unless medically contraindicated)
- Daily "sedation interruption" and daily assessment of readiness to extubate
- Peptic ulcer disease prophylaxis
- Deep venous thrombosis prophylaxis

Previous reference: VAP rate

Respiratory illness

- Number of healthcare personnel who received influenza vaccination

Catheter-associated urinary tract infections (CAUTI)

Previous reference: CAUTI rate

Tab. 2   List of Medicare's infectious "never events"

MRSA

C. difficile

Surgical site infections

Catheter-associated urinary tract infections

Catheter-associated vascular infections

Mediastinitis after coronary artery bypass graft (CABG)

Post-operative pneumonia

Surgical site infections (SSI)

- Prophylactic antibiotics received within 1 hour before surgical incision
- Prophylactic antibiotics selection for surgical patients
- Prophylactic antibiotics discontinued within 24 hours after surgery
- Patients undergoing cardiac surgery who had controlled 6.00 AM postoperative serum glucose level
- Surgical patients who undergo appropriate hair removal

Previous reference: SSI rate

Conclusions

The existence of a surveillance program is a marker of quality of care recognized by different rating agencies. Outcome measures for nosocomial infections are indicators of health and may identify deviations from national rates as well as opportunities for improvement. Nevertheless, patient health outcomes are determined by many other factors besides the quality of care delivered, and risk adjustments are necessary to benchmark using outcome data. Standardising collection of data is essential to reduce variations in rates.

The arguments against the use of nosocomial infection rates as outcome indicators have been frequent in recent years. However, despite their limitations, we cannot completely rule out their use, which could be supplemented with process indicators. Process indicators for HAI will allow the quality of care to be monitored, but they have to be consistently linked to evidence-based practices

The author

Mercedes Palomar Martínez, MD, PhD
   Associated Professor Universitat Autonoma
   Barcelona and Intensive Care Medicine
   Hospital Vall Hebron
   P Vall Hebron 119–129
   08035 Barcelona, Spain
   E-mail: mpalomar@telefonica.net

References

1. Lohr KN. Medicare: A Strategy for Quality Assurance. Vol I and II. Washintong, DC: National Academy Press 1990.
2. Hospital in Europe Link for Infection Control through Surveillance. IPSE annual report 2006. http://ipse.univ-lyon1.fr/Documents/IPSE_Annual_Report_2006.pdf.
3. Rosenthal, MB, Landon BE, Normand SL, Frank RG, Epstein AM, Pay per performance in commercial HMOs NEJM 2006; 355:1895–1902.
4. Yokos DS, Classen D. Improving patient safety through infection control. A new healthcare imperative. Infect Control Hosp Epidemiol 2008;29:S3–S11.
5. Nosocomial infection rates for interhospital comparison: limitations and possible solutions. A Report from the National Nosocomial Infections Surveillance (NNIS) System. Infect Control Hosp Epidemiol 1991;12:609–621.
6. Suetens C, Savey A, Labeeuw J, Morales I and the working group HELICS-ICU. The ICU-HELICS programme: towards European surveillance of hospital-acquired infections in intensive care units. Euro Surveill 2002. 7:127–128.
7. The ECDC Annual Epidemiological Report on Communicable Diseases in the European Union http_//www.ecdc.europa.eu/en/publications/Pages/surveillance_reports.
8. Durocher A. Nosocomial infections as an indicator of the healthcare quality in intensive care units HygièneS 2004;7:561–9.
9. Horan TC, Andrus M, Dudeck MA. CDC/NHSN surveillance definition of health care-associated infection and criteria for specific types of infections in the acute care setting. Am J Infect Control 2008;36:309–32.
10. Edwards JR, Peterson KD, Andrus ML, Dudeck MA, Pollock DA, Horan TC; National Healthcare Safety Network Facilities.National Healthcare Safety Network (NHSN) Report, data summary for 2006 through 2007, Am J Infect Control 2008.36(9):609–26.
11. Joint Comisión on Accreditation of Healthcare Organizations: Infection Control. In: JCAHO, Accreditation Manual for Hospitals. Chicago: Joint Commision on Accreditation of Healthcare Organizations, 1990.
12. Mainz J: defining and classifying clinical indicators for quality improvement. Int J Quality Health Care 2003;15,6:523–530.
13. Donavedian A. The quality of care. How can it be assessed? J Am Med Asocc 1988;260:1743–1748.
14. Rubin HR, Pronovost P, Diette GB. The advantages and disadvantages of process-based measures of health quality. Int J Qual Health Care 2001;13:469–474.
15. Rubin HR, Pronovost P, Diette GB. From a process of care to a measure: the development and testing of a quality indicator. Int J Qual Health Care 2001;13:489–496.
16. Gibbert R, Hancock S, Howley P, Richards K. Using indicators to quantify the potential to improve the quality of health care. Int J Qual Health Care 2004;16:37–43.

17. Gastmeier P, Sohr D, Geffers C, Nassauer A, Daschner F, Ruden H. Are nosocomial infection rates in intensive care units useful benchmark parameters? Infection 2000;28:346–50.
18. Sax H, Pittet D, Swiss-NOSO Network. Interhospital differences in nosocomial infection rates: importance of case- mix adjustment. Arch Intern Med 2002;162:2437–42.
19. Suetens C, Lepape A, Palomar M, Hiesmayer M. Impact of risk adjustment on inter countries comparisons of ICU infections indicators. ESCAIDE. 2007, Stockholm, 18–20 October available at http://helics.univ-lyon1.fr.
20. Thiago Lisboa, Jordi Rello. Ventilator-associated pneumonia prevalence: To benchmark or not to benchmark. Critical Care Medicine 2009;37:9,2657–2659.
21. Uçkay I, Ahmed QA, Sax H, Pittet D.Ventilator-associated pneumonia as a quality indicator for patient safety?. Clin Infect Dis. 2008; 15;46(4):557–63.
22. Pittet D, Zingg W. Reducing ventilator-associated pneumonia: When process control allows outcome improvement and even benchmarking. Crit Care Medicine 2010;38:3,983–984.
23. McBryde ES, Brett J, Russo PL, Worth LJ, Bull AL, Richards MJ. Validation of central line associated bloodstream infection intensive care unit surveillance data from VICNISS. Infect Control Hosp Epidemiol 2009;30:1045–9.
24. Fridkin, SK, Pear, SM, Williamson, TH, Galgiani, JN, Jarvis, WR. The Role of Understaffing in Central Venous Catheter-Related Bloodstream Infections Infect Control Hosp Epidemiol 1996;17:150–158.
25. Clements A, Halton K, Graves N, Pettitt A, Morton A, Looke D, Whitby M. Overcrowding and understaffing in modern health-care systems: key determinants in Meticillin-Resistant Staphylococcus Aureus (MRSA) transmission Lancet Infect Dis 2008;8(7):427–34.
26. Gastmeier P, Schwab F, Geffers C, Rüden H. To isolate or not to isolate? Analysis of data from the German nosocomial infection surveillance system regarding the placement of patients with methicillin-resistant Staphylococcus aureus in private rooms in intensive care units. Infect Control Hosp Epidemiol 2004;25:109–113.
27. Bracco D, Dubois MJ, Bouali R, Eggimann P. Single rooms may help to prevent nosocomial bloodstream infection and cross-transmission of methicillin-resistant Staphylococcus aureus in intensive care-units. Intensive Care Med 2007;33:836–840.
28. Mant J. Process versus outcome indicators in the assessment of quality of health care. Int J Qual Health Care 2001;13:475–480.
29. Palomar M, Vaque J, Alvarez Lerma F, Pastor V, Olaechea P. Indicadores de infección nosocomial.Med Clin (Barcelona) 2008;131 Supl. 3 p. 48–55.
30. Claridge JA, Golob JF, Fadlalla AM, D'Amico B, Peerles JR, Yowler CJ, Malangoni MA. Who is monitoring your Infections: Shouldn't You Be?. Surgical Infections 2009;10:59–64.
31. Brown J, Doloresco Iii F, Mylotte JM. "Never events": not every hospital-acquired infection is presentable.Clin Infect Dis. 2009;49(5):743–6.
32. Fry DE, Pine M, Barbara MBA, Jones L, Roger MA, Meimban J, Patient Characteristics and the Occurrence of Never Events. Arch Surg. 2010;145(2):148–151.
33. Institute for Healthcare Improvement. Getting started kit: prevent ventilator-associated pneumonia. How-to guide. 2008. Available at: http://www.premierinc.com/safety/topics/bundling/downloads/03-vap-how-to-guide.pdf. Accessed January 3, 2009.
34. Pronovost P, Needham D, Berenholtz S, Sinopoli D, Chu H, Cosgrove S et al. An intervention to decrease catheter-related bloodstream infections in the ICU. N Engl J Med.2006;355 (26):2725–32.
35. Bonello RS, Fletcher CE, Becker WK, Clutter KL, Arjes SL, Cook JJ, Petzel RA. An intensive care unit quality improvement collaborative in nine Department of Veterans Affairs hospitals: reducing ventilator-associated pneumonia and catheter-related bloodstream infection rates. Jt Comm J Qual Patient Saf 2008;34(11):639–45.
36. National Quality Forum: Essentials of public reporting of healthcare – associated infections: a tool kit. January 2007. Available at: http//www.cdc.gov//ncidod//dhqp/pdf//ar/06.

Rui P. Moreno, Philipp G.H. Metnitz, Andrew Rhodes and Peter Bauer

The role of risk profile management
in the evaluation of the intensive care units

Introduction

General outcome prediction models (GOPM) have been developed for, and used by, adult intensive care units (ICU) since the 1980s [1]. Most models have been used to compute a proxy for ICU performance, the observed-to-predicted (O/E) mortality ratio or standardised mortality ratio (SMR). In order to develop this ratio, a number of similar approaches have been used, and these include:

- A general outcome prediction model (GOPM) that is developed from a specific database, and that is used to standardise mortality according to the elements of case-mix included in the model;
- The application of this model to almost all patients in the ICU during a certain period (excluding only some specific patient typologies such as burns, children, etc);
- The derivation of the quotient with respective confidence intervals between the observed and the expected mortality at hospital discharge (based on the risk-adjustment provided by the GOPM selected). This is known as the O/E ratio or SMR.
- This one-point estimate is then used to assess the (risk-adjusted) performance of the ICU. A value of lower than 1 implies that the ICU is performing better than the cohort in which the GOPM was derived, and

a value of higher than 1 when the performance of the ICU is judged to be worse. An ongoing discussion among experts is whether the GOPM should be externally derived, or derived from the analysed cohort.

This methodology has been in widespread use since 1985 with several different databases and GOPMs, for example APACHE II [1], APACHE III [2], APACHE IV [3], SAPS II [4] or the SAPS 3 [5]. The use of these databases for differing geographical or socio-economic regions has been proposed by some groups, but often with the conclusion that a new GOPM that is calibrated for the specific circumstances under assessment is required to better reflect the overall database used as comparator [6, 7].

Although this methodology is easy to understand and simplistically provides a straightforward number that can be used for comparison, it is perhaps overly simplistic. Metnitz and colleagues [8] described several limitations to this approach. The basic assumption behind this approach is that the risk-adjusted mortality (or performance) is independent on the severity of illness of the admitted patients. The severity of illness (and case-mix) obviously differs between different ICUs; however previous authors have always assumed that performance is constant over the whole spectrum of severity of illness. An ICU with a "good" performance (low SMR) is assumed to be uniformly good for both low-risk and high-risk patients; likewise, an ICU with a "bad" performance (high SMR) is assumed to be uniformly bad. This assumption is probably not entirely true, as performance can clearly differ over the spectrum from severely unwell to less sick patients. The major concern is that an overall SMR of 1.0 may mask the fact that an ICU has very major problems with the management of the very sick patients, as the overall number is masked by better performance at the less sick range. The loss of this data is therefore masking potential problems which could be remedied to the benefit of the unit and its patients. This will help the end-user to transform an instrument to measure performance into an instrument to change performance (by pointing at the weak points of the ICU). The reasons for these possible changes in performance at differing levels of severity are legion, but may include at least: staff patterns and workload [9, 10], availability and use of technology [11], volume-outcome relationships [12–15], overaggressive treatment of low-risk patients [16, 17], or under-treatment of very high-risk patients [18, 19].

The relationship between the performance of an ICU and the severity of illness of the admitted patients

In the past there have been attempts made to understand this relationship by looking at the risk ratio at discrete severity points. For instance, the EURICUS-I study [20] looked at three performance variables which they computed for each ICU:

- P20 (performance in low-risk patients, evaluated at the 20th percentile of the severity distribution),
- P50 (performance with medium-risk patients, evaluated at the median of the severity distribution) and
- P80 (performance with high-risk patients, evaluated at the 80th percentile of the severity distribution).

This method used a second-level customization of the SAPS II score in the EURICUS-I database using logistic regression with random effects. It allowed for the comparison of the performance of an ICU at three different points, although not for the continuum of severity of illness. Similar results were obtained during the development of the SAPS 3 model, when the relationship between severity of illness and observed mortality was found to differ greatly between different geographical areas, as published in 2005 [8].

Using the database of the Austrian Center of Documentation and Quality Assurance in Intensive Care Medicine (ASDI), an Austrian not for profit intensive care benchmarking organization [21], Moreno and colleagues have recently published a model for describing the relationship between performance and severity of illness. This prospectively collected, very high-quality database contains socio-demographic data; reason(s) for ICU admission; severity of illness, as measured by several GOPM (including SAPS II [4]); length of ICU and hospital stay; and outcome data from all patients consecutively admitted to 77 Austrian ICUs between January 1 1998, and December 31 2007 (for a total of 176,703 admissions). For this descriptive analysis, 102,561 patients were included, following the exclusion of all patients which had been at least readmitted to ICU, were under 18 years of age, had incomplete outcome data or were without a complete SAPS II score. In order to avoid a possible over or under estimation of the relative risks for patients in either extremely low or high risk zones, patients were also excluded if they had a predicted hospital mortality of < 5 % or > 95 %.

The reference GOPM used was the SAPS II model, as described originally by Le Gall et al in 1993 [4]. This model was then re-calibrated for each unit for the current relationship between severity of illness and outcome in order to develop an 'observed and adjusted' function of hospital mortality that could be then compared against the reference list published originally. The ratio of this observed to referenced function was then used to describe the 'risk' of dying across the continuum of severity from 5 to 95 % predicted risk for each ICU. This ICU-specific function, derived from logistic regression analysis, was then plotted as a smooth curve together with its 95 % confidence intervals, calculated using the customized models and assuming that the expected risk from the original model was occurring in a non-random fashion. This graphical plot essentially provides a risk profile for each individual ICU over the whole range of severity of illness, thus allowing for direct comparisons to be made and potentially allowing the management of that risk according to the observed pattern.

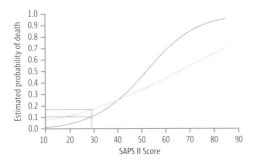

Fig. 1   Association between SAPS II score and predicted mortality in the reference cohort and a single ICU (n = 2202). The dark grey line represents the relationship between the SAPS II score and the predicted probability of death using the original SAPS II function. The light grey line represents the customized function for the specific ICU.

Figure 1 shows the association between the expected and observed probability of dying for an individual ICU. It can be clearly seen that the risk (ratio of observed to predicted probability) varies across the spectrum of severity. Overall, the risk of dying for a patient with a SAPS II score of approximately 29 was 10 % in the reference cohort, whereas it is actually observed to be 17 % in reality. This equates to a risk ratio of 1.7 (17/10) for a predicted risk of 0.1. With logistic regression modelling, these risk ratios can be plotted across the spectra of predicted risks and this gives us an assessment of the performance of an individual ICU for all degrees of severity of illness.

Figure 2 demonstrates three examples of how some units can have a performance which is independent of severity, whereas some can perform better at low severities and others better at the high end.

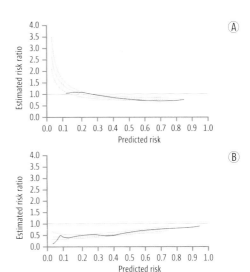

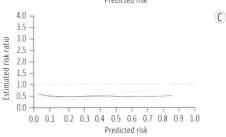

Fig. 2   Examples of three different relationships between the performance of the ICU and the severity of illness of the admitted patients. The thick grey lines represent the risk profile model. The thinner grey lines represent the confidence interval. The black lines represent the associated LOWESS curve [22]. Data were aggregated between 1998 and 2007.
A: ICU in which the clinical performance increased as the severity of illness increased.
B: ICU in which the clinical performance decreased as the severity of illness increased.
C: ICU in which the clinical performance was better than in the reference population and almost independent from the severity of illness.

Conclusion

These new modelling systems allow us to evaluate the performance of an ICU, not just as a single point across the entire population of patients studied, but as a graphical view allowing estimation across all the spectrum of severity. This gives us far greater insights into what is actually happening for a given unit and would allow us to better explore the avenues of increasing performance.

The authors

Rui P. Moreno, MD, PhD[1]
Philipp G.H. Metnitz, MD, PhD, EDIC, DEAA[2]
Andrew Rhodes, FRCA FRCP[3]
Peter Bauer, PhD, Prof.[4]
    [1]Unidade de Cuidados Intensivos Polivalente | Hospital de Santo António dos Capuchos | Centro Hospitalar de Lisboa Central | Lisbon, Portugal

[2]Dept. of Anaesthesiology and General Intensive Care | Medical University of Vienna | Vienna, Austria
[3]General Intensive Care | St George's Hospital | London, UK
[4]Chairman | Dept. of Medical Statistics | Medical University of Vienna | Vienna, Austria

Address for correspondence
Rui P. Moreno
Unidade de Cuidados Intensivos Polivalente
Hospital de Santo António dos Capuchos
Centro Hospitalar de Lisboa Central, E.P.E.
Alameda de Santo António dos Capuchos
1169-050 Lisbon, Portugal
E-mail: r.moreno@mail.telepac.pt

References

1. Knaus WA, Draper EA, Wagner DP, Zimmerman JE. APACHE II: a severity of disease classification system. Crit Care Med 1985;13:818–29.

2. Knaus WA, Wagner DP, Draper EA, Zimmerman JE, Bergner M, Bastos PG, Sirio CA, Murphy DJ, Lotring T, Damiano A, Harrell Jr. FE. The APACHE III prognostic system. Risk prediction of hospital mortality for critically ill hospitalized adults. Chest 1991;100:1619–36.

3. Zimmerman JE, Kramer AA, McNair DS, Malila FM. Acute Physiology and Chronic Health Evaluation (APACHE) IV: Hospital mortality assessment for today's critically ill patients. Crit Care Med 2006;34:1297–310.

4. Le Gall JR, Lemeshow S, Saulnier F. A new simplified acute physiology score (SAPS II) based on a European / North American multicenter study. JAMA 1993;270:2957–63.

5. Moreno RP, Metnitz PG, Almeida E, Jordan B, Bauer P, Campos RA, Iapichino G, Edbrooke D, Capuzzo M, Le Gall JR, SAPS 3 Investigators. SAPS 3. From evaluation of the patient to evaluation of the intensive care unit. Part 2: Development of a prognostic model for hospital mortality at ICU admission. Intensive Care Med 2005;31:1345–55.

6. Poole D, Bertolini G. Outcome-based benchmarking in the ICU Part I: Use and limitations of severity scores in critical care. In: Chiche J-D, Moreno R, Putensen C, Rhodes A, eds. Patient Safety and Quality of Care in Intensive Care Medicine. Berlin: Medizinisch Wissenschaftiche Verlagsgesellschaft, 2009:151–60.

7. Poole D, Bertolini G. Outcome-based benchmarking in the ICU Part I: Statistical tools for the creation and validation of severity scores. In: Chice J-D, Moreno R, Putensen C, Rhodes A, eds. Patient Safety and Quality of Care In Intensive Care Medicine. Berlin: Medizinisch Wissenschaftiche Verlagsgesellschaft, 2009:vol 141–150).

8. Metnitz PG, Moreno RP, Almeida E, Jordan B, Bauer P, Campos RA, Iapichino G, Edbrooke D, Capuzzo M, Le Gall JR, SAPS 3 Investigators. SAPS 3. From evaluation of the patient to evaluation of the intensive care unit. Part 1: Objectives, methods and cohort description. Intensive Care Med 2005;31:1336–44.

9. Moreno R, Reis Miranda D. Nursing staff in intensive care in Europe. The mismatch between planning and practice. Chest 1998;113:752–8.

10. The UK Neonatal Staffing Study Group. Patient volume, staffing, and workload in relation to risk adjusted outcomes in a random stratified sample of UK neonatal intensive care units: a prospective evaluation. Lancet 2002;359:99–107.

11. Bastos PG, Knaus WA, Zimmerman JE, Magalhães Jr A, Wagner DP, The Brazil APACHE III Study Group. The importance of technology for achieving superior outcomes from intensive care. Intensive Care Med 1996;22:664–9.

12. Jones J, Rowan K. Is there a relationship between the volume of work carried out in intensive care and its outcome? Int J Technol Assess Health Care 1995;11:762–9.

13. Kahn JM, Goss CH, Heagerty PJ, Kramer AA, O'Brien CR, Rubenfeld GD. Hospital volume and the outcomes of mechanical ventilation. N Engl J Med 2006;355:41–50.

14. Metnitz B, Metnitz PG, Bauer P, Valentin A, ASDI Study Group. Patient volume affects outcome in critically ill patients. Wien Klin Wochenschr 2009;121:34–40.

15. Kahn JM. Volume and outcome in intensive care. In: Chice J-D, Moreno R, Putensen C, Rhodes A, eds. Patient Safety and Quality of Care In Intensive Care Medicine. Berlin: Medizinisch Wissenschaftiche Verlagsgesellschaft, 2009:161–70.

16. Sakr Y, Vincent J-L, Groeneveld J, Michalopoulos A, Sprung C, Artigas A, Ranieri VM, on behalf of the SOAP investigators. High tidal volume and positive fluid balance are associated with worse outcome in Acute Lung Injuty. Chest 2003;128:3098–108.

17. Rosenberg AL, Dechert RE, Park PK, Bartlett RH, for the NIH NHLBI ARDS Network. Association of Cumulative Fluid Balance on Outcome in Acute Lung Injury: A Retrospective Review of the ARDSnet Tidal Volume Study Cohort. J Intensive Care Med 2009;24:35–46.

18. Metnitz PG, Reiter A, Jordan B, Lang T. More interventions do not necessarily improve outcome in critically ill patients. Intensive Care Med 2004;30:1586–93.

19. Connors AF, Speroff T, Dawson NV, Thomas C, Harrell Jr. FE, Wagner D, Desbiens N, Goldman L, Wu AW, Califf RM, Fulkerson WJ, Vidaillet H, Broste S, Bellamy P, Lynn J, Knaus WA, The SUPPORT investigators. The effectiveness of right heart catheterization in the initial care of critically ill patients. JAMA 1996;276:889–97.

20. Organization and management of Intensive Care: a prospective study in 12 European countries. Berlin Heidelberg: Springer-Verlag, 1997 (Reis Miranda D, Ryan DW, Schaufeli WB, Fidler V, eds. vol 29).

21. Moreno RP, Hochrieser H, Metnitz B, Bauer P, Metnitz PGH. Characterizing the risk profiles of intensive care units. Intensive Care Med 2010;0:1–6.

22. Cleveland WS. LOWESS: a program for smoothing scatterplots by robust locally weighted regression. Am Stat 1981;35:54.

E. Future approaches

The intensive care unit of the future _____ 399
Rui P. Moreno and Andrew Rhodes

Rui P. Moreno and Andrew Rhodes

The intensive care unit of the future

"We are what we repeatedly do. Excellence, then, is not an act, but a habit"

Aristotle

Intensive care medicine (ICU), the speciality that deals with the most critically ill patients, has been growing in recent years. In the early 2000s, it was estimated that intensive care beds represented 13.4% of all hospital beds in the United States of America (USA), costing upwards of $ 55.5 billions of USD, accounting for 13.3% of all hospital costs and 0.56% of the gross domestic product (GDP). In the last few years, the panorama has continued to change, as recently described by Halpern and Pastores [1], with the number of intensive care beds, days (as a percentage of the total hospital days) and occupancy rates continuing to increase. Also, the costs per day of intensive care medicine increased by 30.4% with a corresponding increase in the annual costs associated with this specialty of 44.2%, representing in 2005 13.4% of hospital costs, 4.1% of national health expenditures, and 0.66% of the gross domestic product, If we add to this number the other costs incurred by caring for the patients with a critical illness, the overall number accounts to 1% of the gross domestic product in the USA.

In Europe, despite the fact that the heterogeneity is much greater, either across countries [2] or even inside one and the same country [3] the mean costs per intensive care bed per year could be as low as 30,990 Euros or as high as between 225,000 and 471,330 Euros in the UK (depending on the level of care) [3], which represents values similar to those seen in Germany [4]. Despite the fact that these numbers are consistently lower than the numbers presented the USA, the pressure on the economy remains an issue.

These costs result partly from the high utilization (and costs) of monitoring and therapeutic devices, including medication, but are mainly explained by the labour-intensive, super-specialized nature of intensive care, which must be provided by a large multidisciplinary, highly specialised team of professionals, with a very high nurse-to-patient and physician-to patient-ratio. These facts, as well as the critical nature of the patients cared for inside of those four walls (plus those cared for by intensivists outside of those four walls) – along with a high percentage of deaths and a high percentage of patients with residual disabilities after ICU discharge – have transformed the evaluation of the performance of the ICU into a natural target for comparative evaluation. The hospital manager wants to know the results (in terms of prevented deaths or added health benefits) for all of the money spent, the population and society in general want to know if the best care is being provided in exchange for that huge capital investment, and the professionals of intensive care medicine want to know if their practices are effective.

This panorama is likely to change, due to the increasing age of the population, with the increasing prevalence of co-morbid diseases, together with significant advances (and costs) associated with medical science. These factors when combined result in the application of more complex and costly procedures to an increasing fragile population, where complications will have greater consequences due to the increasingly narrow cost-effective margin of a significant number of interventions. As a direct consequence of these changes, there has been a shift from the almost exclusive presentation in medical conferences and medical journals of new devices and drugs to an increasing discussion of topics that 15 years ago would not have been accepted in a large major conference, or would have been presented in a small room at the back. Examples are the increasing efforts put on patient safety [5–7], detection and prevention of adverse events [8–10], and cultural changes regarding patient safety and error management [11–15]. A major example of these changes in priorities and culture was the signature by more than 80 scientific societies, industry representatives and patient representatives of the declaration in Vienna, during the last annual congress of the European Society of Intensive Care Medicine, a public call for attention and action to these issues. This declaration was just a first step in an ongoing-process that includes the public presentation of a revised version of the structural norms for European ICUs [16]) or the revision of mandatory indicators for ICU evaluation. Benchmarking and other methods of comparative evaluation of the effectiveness and the cost-effectiveness of ICUs will have a growing impact in the decisions made by purchasers of intensive care [17, 18]

In the future, the maximization of the volume-outcome relationship will certainly lead to the fusion (or the closure) of small ICUs [19–23] and to the re-arrangement of existing ICUs and services in large networks, trained and evaluated for organizational performance and not just for clinical performance [24].

New drugs and devices will be subjected to an ever greater scrutiny before utilization, with the quality of the trials in which they proved their efficacy (and cost-efficacy) being more highly scrutinized for adverse events than done previously, and no longer neglected, restricted, distorted, nor silenced during the presentation of the results as pointed-out in a landmark paper by Michael Ioannidis [25] and clearly separating practice guidelines and clinical orientations from industry campaigns – something that has not always been done in recent years [26, 27]. Certainly we will have new tools and devices, new drugs and interventions [28], but we cannot just sit and wait for a magic bullet to appear, we must be proactive in applying existing (and new) interventions to decrease mortality [29], that generate evidence and translate evidence into practice [30].

This optimization in the use of resources will allow us to develop better and earlier triage criteria and a more extensive use of ICU trials, in which a patient is admitted to an ICU with clear limits on time for revaluation of the clinical condition and the response to therapy, with full therapy being applied during this period of time, usually varying between 3 and 5 days [31]. As the utilization of critical care expands, we will need to be increasingly conscientious that our efforts are being applied only to those patients most likely to benefit from them. End-of-life practices must therefore be incorporated into the assessment of quality [32, 33]. For this to be fair, clear, honest and transparent, these issues have to be better and more openly discussed with the patients and their families [34–36]. This debate must start before admission to intensive care with a discussion and re-education that resets the expectations, desires and perceptions of the general public to allow for more rational decision making and an assurance that these therapies are directed only to those most likely to benefit.

The education and training of the next generation of intensivists, that has been neglected for many years in Europe despite the many alarming signs coming from the USA [37–39], needs to be re-evaluated. In the USA, it is probable that the pendulum has already swung beyond the point where the equilibrium between the need for these specialists and the ability to provide them can be restored just by training alone. This will inevitably result in increased outsourcing of several medical interventions to other professional groups, for instance the increase in the use of physicians-assistants and nursing practitioners. New technologies such as tele-ICU [40] can help to solve this problem but their effectiveness has not yet been demonstrated in a convincing fashion, as shown recently [41, 42].

Europe, the home country of the closed ICU model and of the fully trained, fully dedicated intensivist, will make an effort to meet the increasing demand with more intensivists, shifting education and training programmes from time-based to competency-based programmes [43, 44] such as those by the CoBaTrICE collaboration [45] and by an increased use of simulation for critical situations [46, 47]. This will not be an easy process. It will need to change our perception of teaching and the skills of our teachers [48, 49], but it can and should be done. The social and egalitarian tradition of Europe and the respect for our patients' needs will help us to keep this view and win this challenge. As once said by Joel A. Barker (in the training video "The Power of Vision"):

"Vision without action is a dream. Action without vision is simply passing the time. Action with Vision is making a positive difference."

The authors

Rui P. Moreno, MD, PhD[1]
Andrew Rhodes, FRCP FRCA[2]
[1]Unidade de Cuidados Intensivos Polivalente | Hospital de Santo António dos Capuchos | Centro Hospitalar de Lisboa Central, E.P.E. | Lisbon, Portugal
[2]General Intensive Care | St George's Hospital | London, UK

Address for correspondence
Rui P. Moreno
Unidade de Cuidados Intensivos Polivalente
Hospital de Santo António dos Capuchos
Centro Hospitalar de Lisboa Central, E.P.E.
Alameda de Santo António dos Capuchos
1169-050 Lisbon, Portugal
E-mail: r.moreno@mail.telepac.pt

References

1. Halpern NA, Pastores SM. Critical care medicine in the United States 2000–2005: An analysis of bed numbers, occupancy rates, payer mix, and costs. Crit Care Med 2010;38:65–71.
2. Csomós A, Janecsko M, Edbrooke D. Comparative costing analysis of intensive care services between Hungary and United Kingdom. Intensive Care Med 2005;31:1280–3.
3. Edbrooke DL, Ridley S, Hibbert CL, Corcoran M. Variations in expenditure between adult general intensive care units in the UK. Anaesthesia 2001;56:208–16.
4. Prien T, Groll O, Geldner G, Martin J, Weiler T, Dahmen KG, Sorgatz H, Bach A. Ist-Kosten Intensivmedizin deutscher Anasthesieabteilungen-Bezugsjahr 1999. Anasthesiol Intensivmed 2002;43:244–54.
5. Haller G, Stoelwinder J, Myles PS, McNeil J. Quality and Safety Indicators in Anesthesia. A Systematic Review. Anesthesiology 2009;110:1158–75.
6. Moreno RP, Rhodes A, Donchin Y. Patient safety in intensive care medicine: the Declaration of Vienna. Intensive Care Med 2009;35:1667–72.
7. Chakravarthy M. Errors in cardiac anesthesia – A deterrent to patient safety. Annals of Cardiac Anaesthesia 2010;13:87–8.
8. Donchin Y, Gopher D, Olin M, Badihi Y, Biesky M, Sprung CL, Pizov R, Cotev S. A look into the nature and causes of human errors in the intensive care unit. Crit Care Med 1995;23:294–300.
9. Valentin A, Capuzzo M, Guidet B, Moreno RP, Dolanski L, Bauer P, Metnitz PG. Patient safety in intensive care: results from the multinational Sentinel Events Evaluation (SEE) study. Intensive Care Med 2006;32:1591–8.
10. Beydon L, Ledenmat PY, Soltner C, Lebreton F, Hardin V, Benhamou D, Clergue F, Laguenie G. Adverse Events with Medical Devices in Anesthesia and Intensive Care Unit Patients Recorded in the French Safety Database in 2005–2006. Anesthesiology 2010;112:364–72.
11. Zohar D, Livne Y, Tenne-Gazit O, Admi H, Donchin Y. Healthcare climate: A framework for measuring and improving patient safety. Crit Care Med 2007;35:1312–7.
12. Wiegmann DA, Dunn WF. Changing Culture. A New View of Human Error and Patient Safety. Chest 2010;137:250–2.
13. Livne Y, Donchin Y. Building a safety culture within the ICU. In: Chiche J-D, Moreno R, Putensen C, Rhodes A, eds. Patient Safety and Quality of Care in Intensive Care Medicine. Berlin: Medizinisch Wissenschaftiche Verlagsgesellschaft, 2009:39–46.
14. O'Connor MF. Safety culture: Easy to advocate, difficult to create. Crit Care Med 2007;35:1429.

15. Sexton JB, Helmreich RL, Neilands TB, Rowan K, Vella K, Boyden J, Roberts PR, Thomas EJ. The Safety Attitudes Questionnaire: psychometric properties, benchmarking data, and emerging research. BMC Health Services Research 2006;6:44.

16. Ferdinande P, Members of the Task Force of the European Society of Intensive Care Medicine. Recommendations on minimal requirements for Intensive Care Departments. Intensive Care Med 1997;23:226–32.

17. Poole D, Rossi C, Anghileri A, Giardino M, Latronico N, Radrizzani D, Langer M, Bertolini G. External validation of the Simplified Acute Physiology Score (SAPS) 3 in a cohort of 28,357 patients from 147 Italian intensive care units. Intensive Care Med 2009.

18. Poole D, Bertolini G. Outcome-based benchmarking in the ICU Part I: Use and limitations of severity scores in critical care. In: Chiche J-D, Moreno R, Putensen C, Rhodes A, eds. Patient Safety and Quality of Care in Intensive Care Medicine. Berlin: Medizinisch Wissenschaftiche Verlagsgesellschaft, 2009:151–60.

19. Aujesky D, Mor MK, Geng M, Fine MJ, Renaud B, Ibrahim SA. Hospital volume and patient outcomes in pulmonary embolism. Can Med Assoc J 2008;178:27–33.

20. Lindenauer PK, Behal R, Murray CK, Nsa W, Houck PM, Bratzler DW. Volume, Quality of Care, and Outcome in Pneumonia. Ann Intern Med 2006;144:262–9.

21. Glance LG, Dick AW, Osler TM, Mukamel DB. The relation between surgeon volume and outcome following off-pump vs on-pump coronary artery bypass graft surgery. Chest 2005;128:829–37.

22. Kahn JM. Volume and outcome in intensive care. In: Chice J-D, Moreno R, Putensen C, Rhodes A, eds. Patient Safety and Quality of Care In Intensive Care Medicine. Berlin: Medizinisch Wissenschaftiche Verlagsgesell-schaft, 2009:161–70.

23. Matti R, Sari K, Tero V, Ilkka P, Esko R, Marjut V, Tero A K, Ville P. Are small hospitals with small intensive care units able to treat patients with severe sepsis? Intensive Care Med 2009;36:673–9.

24. Minvielle E, Aegerter P, Dervaux B, Boumendil A, Retbif A, Jars-Guincestre MC, Guidet B, for the CUB-REA network. Assessing organizational performance in intensive care units: A French experience. J Crit Care 2008;23:236–44.

25. Ioannidis JPA. Adverse Events in Randomized Trials. Neglected, Restricted, Distorted, and Silenced. Arch Intern Med 2009;169:1737–9.

26. Eichacker PQ, Natanson C, Danner RL. Separating practice guidelines from pharmaceutical marketing [Letter]. Crit Care Med 2007;35:2877–8.

27. Eichacker PQ, Natanson C, Danner RL. Surviving Sepsis – Practice Guidelines, Marketing Campaigns, and Eli Lilly. N Engl J Med 2006;355:1640–2.

28. Vincent J-L, Singer M, Marini JJ, Moreno M, Levy M, Matthay MA, Pinsky M, Rhodes A, Ferguson ND, Evans T, Annane D, Hall JB. Thirty years of critical care medicine. Crit Care 2010;14.

29. Pronovost pj, Berenholtz sm, Goeschel c, Thom i, Watson sr, Holzmueller cg, Lyon js, Lubomski lh, Thompson DA, Needham D, Hyzy R, Welsh R, Roth G, Bander J, Morlock L, Bryan Sexton J. Improving patient safety in intensive care units in Michigan. J Crit Care 2008;23:207–21.

30. Winters BD, Gurses AP, Lehmann H, Sexton JB, Rampersad CJ, Pronovost PJ. Clinical review: Checklists – translating evidence into practice. Crit Care 2009;13.

31. Lecuyer L, Chevret S, Thiery G, Darmon M, Schlemmer B, Azoulay E. The ICU Trial: A new admission policy for cancer patients requiring mechanical ventilation. Crit Care Med 2007;35:808–14.

32. Azoulay E, Metnitz B, Sprung C-L, Timsit J-F, Lemaire F, Bauer P, Schlemmer B, Moreno R, Metnitz P. End-of-life practices in 282 intensive care units: data from the SAPS 3 database. Intensive Care Med 2009;35:623–30.

33. Bertolini G, Boffelli, Malacarne S, Peta M, Marchesi M, Barbisan C, Tomelleri S, Spada S, Satolli R, Gridelli B, Lizzola I, Mazzon D. End-of-life decision-making and quality of ICU performance: an observational study in 84 Italian units. Intensive Care Med 2010.

34. Fassier T, Darmon M, Laplace C, Chevret S, Schlemmer B, Pochard F, Azoulay B, the FAMIREA Study Group. One-day quantitative cross-sectional study of family information time in 90 intensive care units in France. Crit Care Med 2007;35:177–83.

35. Siegel MD. Lost in translation: Family conferences for families that do not speak English. Crit Care Med 2009;37:340–1.

36. Azoulay E, Pochard F, Chevret S, Lemaire F, Mokhtari M, Le Gall J-R, Dhainaut JF, Schlemmer B, for the French FAMIREA Group. Meeting the Needs of Intensive Care Unit Patient Families. A Multicenter Study. Am J Respir Crit Care Med 2001;163:135–9.

37. Goodman DC, Fisher ES. Physician Workforce Crisis? Wrong Diagnosis, Wrong Prescription. N Engl J Med 2008;358:1658–61.

38. Samb B, Celletti F, Holloway J, Van Damme W, De Cock KM, Dybul M. Rapid Expansion of the Health Workforce in Response to the HIV Epidemic. N Engl J Med 2007;357:2510–4.

39. Angus DC, Kelley MA, Schmitz RJ, White A, Popovich J, for the Committee in Manpower for Pulmonary and Critical Care Societies (COMPACCS). Caring for the critically ill patient. Current and projected workforce requirements for care of the critically ill and patients with pulmonary disease: can we meet the requirements of an aging population? 284 2000;21.

40. Sapirstein A, Lone N, Latif A, Fackler J, Pronovost PJ. Tele ICU: paradox or panacea? Best Practice & Research Clinical Anaesthesiology 2009;23:115–26.

41. Yoo EJ, Dedley RA. Evaluating Telemedicine in the ICU. JAMA 2009;302:2705–6.

42. Thomas EJ, Lucke JF, Wueste L, Weavind L, Patel B. Association of Telemedicine for Remote Monitoring of Intensive Care Patients With Mortality, Complications, and Length of Stay. JAMA 2009;302:2671–8.

43. Bion J, Reay H, Bullock A. Training in intensive care medicine. In: Kuhlen R, Moreno R, Ranieri M, Rhodes A, eds. 25 Years of Progress and Innovation in Intensive Care Medicine. Berlin: Medizinisch Wissenschaftliche Verlagsgesellschaft, 2007:351–8.

44. Perkins GD, Barrett H, Bullock I, Gabbott DA, Nolan JP, Mitchell S, Short A, Smith CM, Smith GB, Todd S, Bion JF. The Acute Care Undergraduate TEaching (ACUTE) Initiative: consensus development of core competencies in acute care for undergraduates in the United Kingdom. Intensive Care Med 2005;31:1627–33.

45. The CoBaTrICE Collaboration. The educational environment for training in intensive care medicine: structures, processes, outcomes and challenges in the European region. Intensive Care Med 2009;35:1575–83.

46. Park CS, Rochlen LR, Yaghmour E, Higgins N, Bauchat JR, Wojciechowski KG, Sullivan JT, McCarthy RJ. Acquisition of Critical Intraoperative Event Management Skills in Novice Anesthesiology Residents by Using High-fidelity Simulation-based Training. Anesthesiology 2010;112:202–11.

47. Cooper JB, Murray D. Simulation Training and Assessment. A More Efficient Method to Develop Expertise than Apprenticeship. Anesthesiology 2010;112:8–9.

48. Pardo Jr M. Anesthesia: How to Organize and Train Our Teachers. Anesthesiology 2010;112:773–4.

49. McMahon GT, Katz JT, Thorndike ME, Levy BD, Loscalzo J. Evaluation of a Redesign Initiative in an Internal-Medicine Residency. N Engl J Med 2010;362:1304–11.